SICKNESS AND HEALTH IN AMERICA

Readings in the History of Medicine and Public Health

Edited by
JUDITH WALZER LEAVITT
and
RONALD L. NUMBERS

The University of Wisconsin Press

Published 1978

The University of Wisconsin Press
Box 1379, Madison, Wisconsin 53701

The University of Wisconsin Press, Ltd.
70 Great Russell Street, London

First printing
Printed in the United States of America

For LC CIP information see the colophon

ISBN 0-299-07620-2 cloth; 0-299-07624-5 paper

To Our Students
Past, Present, and Future

Contents

Sickness and Health in America: *An Overview* 3

Part I: Medical Practice and Institutions

THEORY 13

1. The Disease of Masturbation: *Values and the Concept of Disease* 15
H. Tristram Engelhardt, Jr.

2. The Uses of a Diagnosis: *Doctors, Patients, and Neurasthenia* 25
Barbara Sicherman

PRACTICE 39

3. A Portrait of the Colonial Physician 41
Whitfield J. Bell, Jr.

4. The Practice of Medicine in New York a Century Ago 55
Charles E. Rosenberg

THERAPEUTICS 75

5. The Heroic Approach in 19th-Century Therapeutics 77
Alex Berman

6. Do-It-Yourself the Sectarian Way 87
Ronald L. Numbers

7. Device Quackery in America 97
James Harvey Young

EDUCATION 103

8. Abraham Flexner in Perspective: *American Medical Education, 1865–1910* 105
Robert P. Hudson

9. The "Connecting Link": *The Case for the Woman Doctor in 19th-Century America* 117
Regina Markell Morantz

IMAGE AND INCOME 129

10. The Changing Image of the American Physician 131
John Duffy

11. The Third Party: *Health Insurance in America* 139
Ronald L. Numbers

INSTITUTIONS 155

12. SOCIAL CLASS AND MEDICAL CARE IN 19TH-CENTURY AMERICA: *The Rise and Fall of the Dispensary* 157
Charles E. Rosenberg

13. PATRONS, PRACTITIONERS, AND PATIENTS: *The Voluntary Hospital in Mid-Victorian Boston* 173
Morris J. Vogel

14. THE FIRST NEIGHBORHOOD HEALTH CENTER MOVEMENT — *Its Rise and Fall* 185
George Rosen

ALLIED PROFESSIONS 201

15. NURSING EMERGES AS A PROFESSION: *The American Experience* 203
Richard Harrison Shryock

16. THE AMERICAN MIDWIFE CONTROVERSY: *A Crisis of Professionalization* 217
Frances E. Kobrin

Part II: Public Health and Personal Hygiene

EPIDEMICS 229

17. THE INOCULATION CONTROVERSY IN BOSTON: 1721–1722 231
John B. Blake

18. POLITICS, PARTIES, AND PESTILENCE: *Epidemic Yellow Fever in Philadelphia and the Rise of the First Party System* 241
Martin S. Pernick

19. THE CAUSE OF CHOLERA: *Aspects of Etiological Thought in 19th-Century America* 257
Charles E. Rosenberg

SANITATION 273

20. A HISTORY OF THE PURIFICATION OF MILK IN NEW YORK, *or, "How Now, Brown Cow"* 275
Norman Shaftel

21. RAISING AND WATERING A CITY: *Ellis Sylvester Chesbrough and Chicago's First Sanitation System* 293
Louis P. Cain

22. THE FLAMBOYANT COLONEL WARING: *An Anticontagionist Holds the American Stage in the Age of Pasteur and Koch* 305
James H. Cassedy

HYGIENE 313

23. "TEMPEST IN A FLESH-POT": *The Formulation of a Physiological Rationale for Vegetarianism* 315
James C. Whorton

24. WHEN SOCIETY FIRST TOOK A BATH 331
Harold Donaldson Eberlein

REFORM 343

25. PIETISM AND THE ORIGINS OF THE AMERICAN PUBLIC HEALTH MOVEMENT: *A Note on John H. Griscom and Robert M. Hartley* 345
Charles E. Rosenberg and Carroll Smith-Rosenberg

26. SANITARY REFORM IN NEW YORK CITY: *Stephen Smith and the Passage of the Metropolitan Health Bill* 359
Gert H. Brieger

27. THE MOVEMENT TOWARD A SAFE MATERNITY: *Physician Accountability in New York City, 1915–1940* 375
Joyce Antler and Daniel M. Fox

POLITICS 393

28. SOCIAL IMPACT OF DISEASE IN THE LATE 19TH CENTURY 395
John Duffy

29. POLITICS AND PUBLIC HEALTH: *Smallpox in Milwaukee, 1894–1895* 403
Judith Walzer Leavitt

30. SOCIAL POLICY AND CITY POLITICS: *Tuberculosis Reporting in New York, 1889–1900* 415
Daniel M. Fox

A GUIDE TO FURTHER READING 433

ABBREVIATIONS OF JOURNAL TITLES 443

INDEX 447

A pictorial essay
on sickness and health in America
follows page 225

Sickness and Health in America

Sickness and Health in America: An Overview

The history of health care in America is much more than the accomplishments of a few prominent physicians. It encompasses all efforts to cure and prevent illness — lay as well as professional, the failures as well as the successes. In recognition of this diversity, we have included in this collection essays ranging from the colonial physician to the 20th-century quack, from masturbation to smallpox, from bathing to bacteriology. Food and filth often play as important roles as doctors and hospitals. Although, for example, we recognize the skill of surgeons who extended a few lives by dramatically transplanting human hearts, their historical significance pales in comparison with their contemporaries who organized comprehensive health centers in the rural South, markedly reducing infant mortality through unglamorous improvements in diet, sanitation, and preventive medicine.

When we look at the broad picture of sickness and health in America, two trends immediately capture our attention: the conspicuous decline in mortality and the corresponding increase in life expectancy for all ages. Although health records before 1900 are fragmentary and precision is illusory, there is little doubt that average Americans today live more than twice as long as their colonial forebears, whose life expectancy at birth was under 30 years and half of whose children died before their tenth birthdays (see Fig. 1). Unfortunately, not all Americans have benefitted equally from these changes. Women live increasingly longer than men, while whites continue to outlive nonwhites (see Figs. 1 and 2).

The changing disease pattern in America presents several problems for the historian. Health statistics before 1933, when the United States adopted uniform registration procedures for reporting diseases, must be used with caution. They are seldom complete and often inconsistent in classifying diseases. Many of today's clinical distinctions did not exist in the past, and those that did were frequently blurred by practitioners with little diagnostic sophistication. To compound our difficulties, disease patterns varied widely from city to city and state to state, so that what is typical of one region may have been rare in another. Nevertheless, we should not let these problems deter us from attempting qualified generalizations.

Early settlers in America often suffered from malnutrition, which increased their vulnerability to infectious diseases. These maladies, transmitted from one person to another, can be either *endemic*, that is, always present, or *epidemic*, appearing from time to time with great intensity. The gravest threats to life and health were malaria and dysentery in summer and respiratory ailments, like influenza and pneumonia, in winter. Sporadic outbreaks of smallpox, yellow fever, and diphtheria created widespread panic, but over the long run they took far fewer lives than the more familiar scourges.

As living conditions improved during the 18th and early 19th centuries, so apparently did the health of Americans. But with increasing urbanization and industrialization the situation in the cities soon deteriorated. In Boston, New York, Philadelphia, and New Orleans, for example, the death rate per 1,000 rose from 28.1 for the quarter century 1815–1839 to 30.2 for the following 25 years.[1] By mid-century some American cities were scarcely better off than the notorious industrial centers of Europe. Lemuel Shattuck of Massachusetts sadly reported in 1850 that "London, with its imperfect supply of water, — its narrow, crowded streets, — its foul cesspools, — its hopeless pauperism — its crowded grave-yards, — and its other monstrous sanitary evils, is as healthy a city as Boston, and in some respects more so."[2]

The mid-century increases in urban mortality

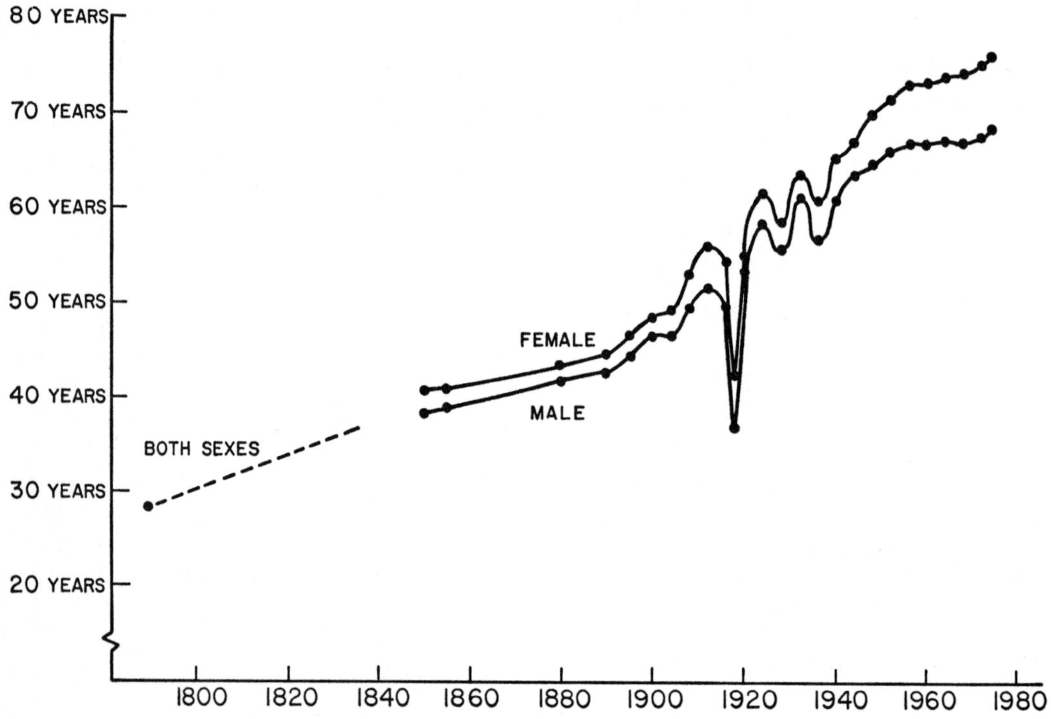

Fig. 1: Life expectancy at birth, 1789–1974, United States. Sources: Frederick L. Hoffman, "American mortality progress during the last half century," in *A Half Century of Public Health*, ed. Mazyck P. Ravenel (New York: American Public Health Association, 1921), p. 98; U.S. Bureau of the Census, *Historical Statistics of the United States: Colonial Times to 1970* (Washington, D.C.: Government Printing Office, 1975), Part 1, pp. 55–56; U.S. Bureau of the Census, *Statistical Abstract of the United States, 1976* (Washington, D.C.: Government Printing Office, 1976), p. 60. Note: The figure for 1789 is for Massachusetts and New Hampshire only, and the data between 1850 and 1900 are for Massachusetts only. The decrease in life expectancy in 1918–1919 is largely attributable to a severe influenza epidemic.

resulted primarily from the numerous infectious diseases that attacked the nation's increasingly dense population centers. Besides intermittent epidemics of yellow fever, cholera, and smallpox, which caused more fear than mortality, there were the ever-present influenza and pneumonia, typhus, typhoid fever, diphtheria, scarlet fever, measles, whooping cough, dysentery, and — above all — tuberculosis. Tuberculosis, sometimes called consumption or phthisis, was the greatest killer of 19th-century Americans. Although present in America since the settling of Jamestown, it did not acquire its deadly reputation until it attacked heavily crowded cities. As early as the 1810s Boston, for example, experienced a tuberculosis mortality rate of 472 per 100,000 inhabitants. By the close of the century this rate had fallen by more than half, and in the mid-1970s tuberculosis killed fewer than two Americans out of every 100,000 (see Fig. 3).

The American health picture began to improve by the late 19th century, as evidenced by the declining urban death rate. The cities of Boston, New York, Philadelphia, and New Orleans, which had suffered under a death rate of 30.2 per 100,000 between 1840 and 1864, saw this figure drop to 25.7 between 1865 and 1889 and down to 18.9 between 1890 and 1914.[3] Even more dramatic was the precipitous fall of infant mortality rates. During the first three decades of the 20th century infant mortality decreased by more than 50 percent, and fell at an even greater rate during the next 20 years (see Fig. 4). But despite these improvements, the United States continued to lag behind many other industrialized nations in reducing infant

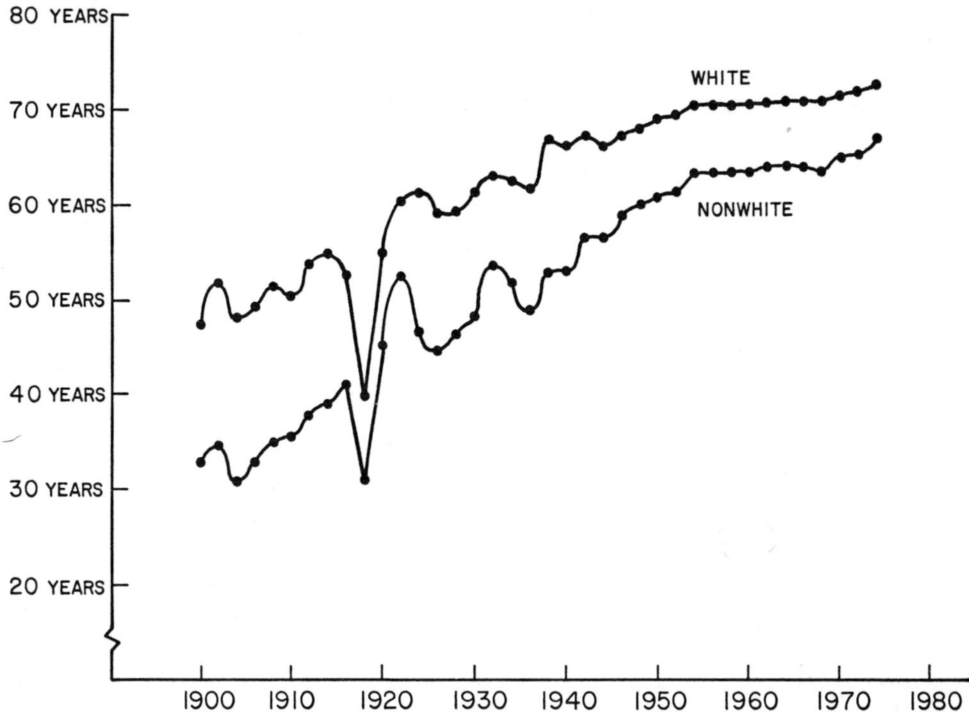

Fig. 2: Racial differences in life expectancy, 1900–1974, United States. Sources: U.S. Bureau of the Census, *Historical Statistics of the United States: Colonial Times to 1970* (Washington, D.C.: Government Printing Office, 1975), Part 1, p. 55; U.S. Bureau of the Census, *Statistical Abstract of the United States, 1976* (Washington, D.C.: Government Printing Office, 1976), p. 60.

deaths, a symbolic indicator of national health standards.

As the familiar infectious diseases of the 19th century diminished in virulence, a host of chronic, degenerative diseases appeared to take their place (see Figs. 5 and 6). By the mid-1970s tuberculosis, gastritis, and diphtheria no longer ranked among the nation's top ten killers, but heart problems, cancer, and cerebrovascular disorders (e.g., strokes), all typical of an older population, headed the list.

Given the available evidence, it is not easy to find an explanation for the decline of infectious diseases and the increase in life expectancy. But the three most likely candidates are medical practice, public health measures, and improvements in diet, housing, and personal hygiene.

Popularizers of medical history like to glorify the intrepid "doctors on horseback" and the marvelous "magic bullets" of white-coated medical scientists in explaining the miracles of the past hundred years. The historical record, however, suggests a different interpretation. Clearly, the brief improvement of health conditions in the 18th century owed little to the efforts of physicians, who probably did their patients more harm than good. Dr. William Douglass, a prominent Boston physician, observed at mid-century that "more die of the practitioner than of the natural course of the disease."[4] If this was true of the 18th century, it was probably even more so in the early 19th century during the heyday of "heroic" medicine, when regular physicians intemperately bled, purged, and puked their patients. Until the latter part of the century doctors possessed few specific remedies besides quinine for malaria, digitalis for dropsy, and lime juice for scurvy.

America's experience with three diseases — tuberculosis, diphtheria, and smallpox — further illustrates the limitations of 19th-century

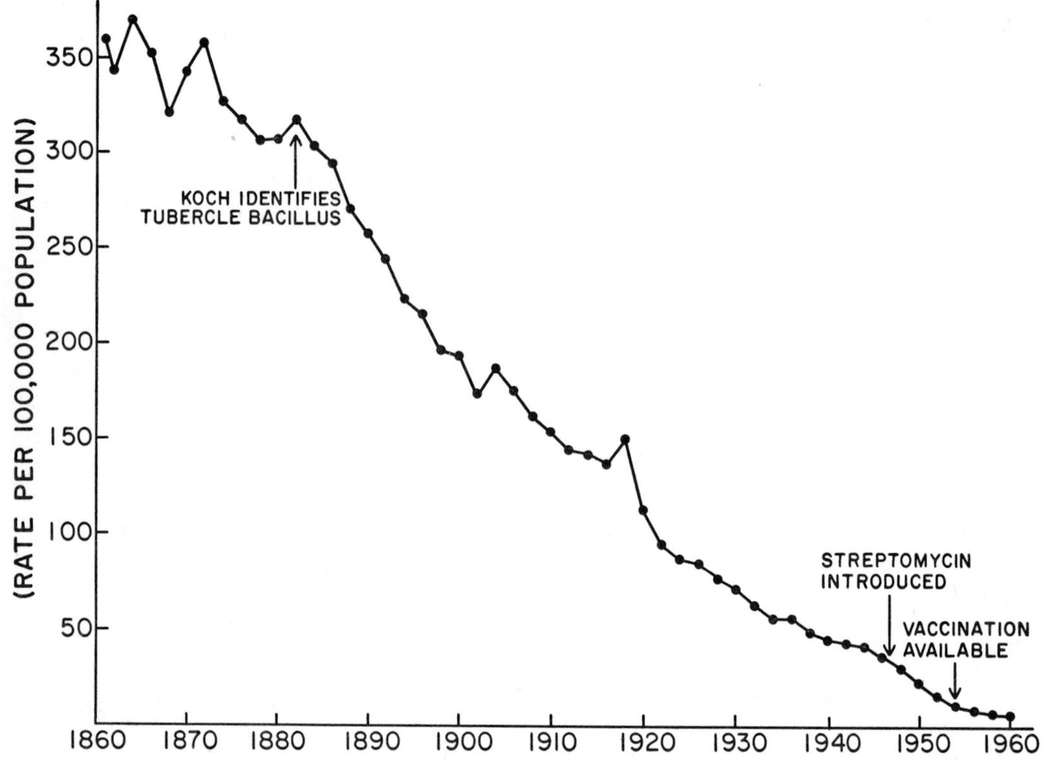

Fig. 3: Death rate for tuberculosis, 1860–1960, United States. Source: U.S. Bureau of the Census, *Historical Statistics of the United States: Colonial Times to 1970* (Washington, D.C.: Government Printing Office, 1975), Part 1, pp. 58, 63. Note: Data between 1860 and 1900 for Massachusetts only.

medicine. Tuberculosis, the most deadly of the three in Victorian America, declined for almost a century before physicians discovered an effective way to treat or prevent it (see Fig. 3). By the time streptomycin was introduced in 1947, the death rate from tuberculosis had already dropped to 33.5 per 100,000. The use of chemotherapy markedly accelerated the rate of decline, from 44.9 percent during the 1940s to 69.7 percent in the 1950s, but even without this therapy, it seems likely that the death rate would have continued its decline.

For diphtheria, the story is somewhat different. Although the death rate from this disease dropped dramatically after antitoxin became available in 1894 (see Fig. 7), it is debatable how much of the decline is attributable to this measure. First, the national death rate for diphtheria had been fluctuating downward for almost two decades prior to the introduction of antitoxin; second, antitoxin was neither systematically nor consistently used throughout the country. Thus it is probable that other nonmedical factors also contributed to the downfall of diphtheria in the 1890s.

In the case of smallpox, medicine *did* offer a means of protection, as early as the 1720s, when Cotton Mather introduced inoculation (variolation). This method gave treated persons a mild case of smallpox, which provided lifetime immunity. Although inoculation often spread the disease, it also appears to have lessened mortality in the 18th century. At the turn of the 19th century vaccination with cowpox virus, an even safer method, became available. But despite these measures, smallpox continued to plague Americans until the 20th century (see Fig. 8), primarily because many chose to ignore the protection medicine offered them.

If we can generalize from these three examples, it seems that medicine contributed little to the ini-

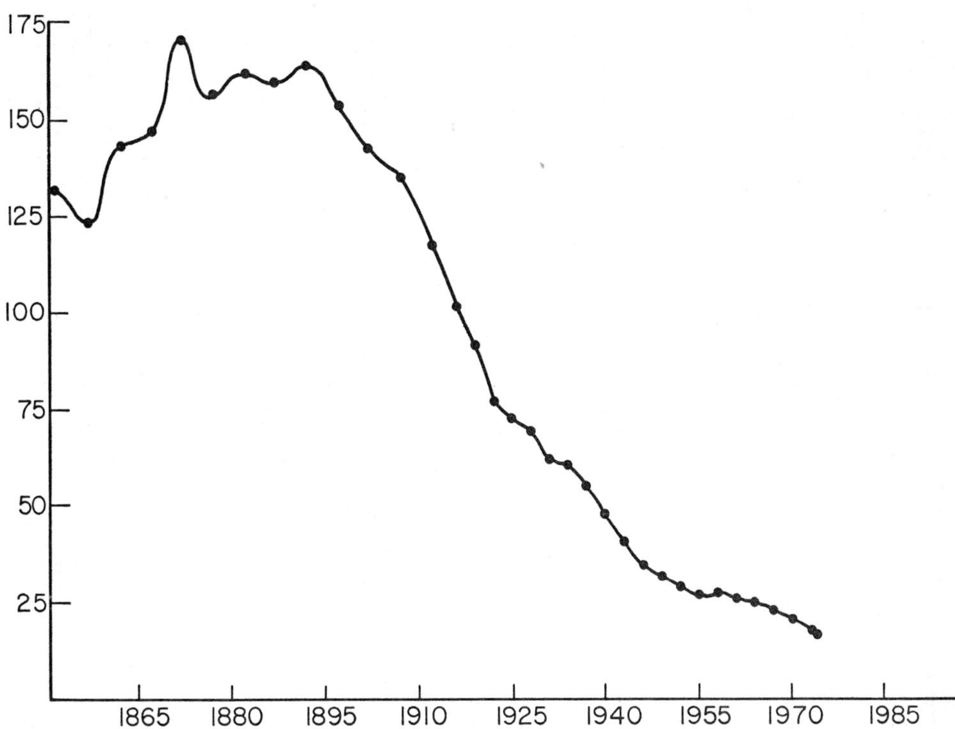

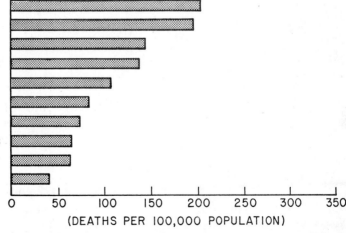

Fig. 4: Infant mortality rate per 1,000 live births, 1851–1974, United States. Sources: U.S. Bureau of the Census, *Historical Statistics of the United States: Colonial Times to 1970* (Washington, D.C.: Government Printing Office, 1975), Part 1, p. 57; U.S. Bureau of the Census, *Statistical Abstract of the United States, 1976* (Washington, D.C.: Government Printing Office, 1976), p. 64. Note: Data between 1851 and 1913 are for Massachusetts only.

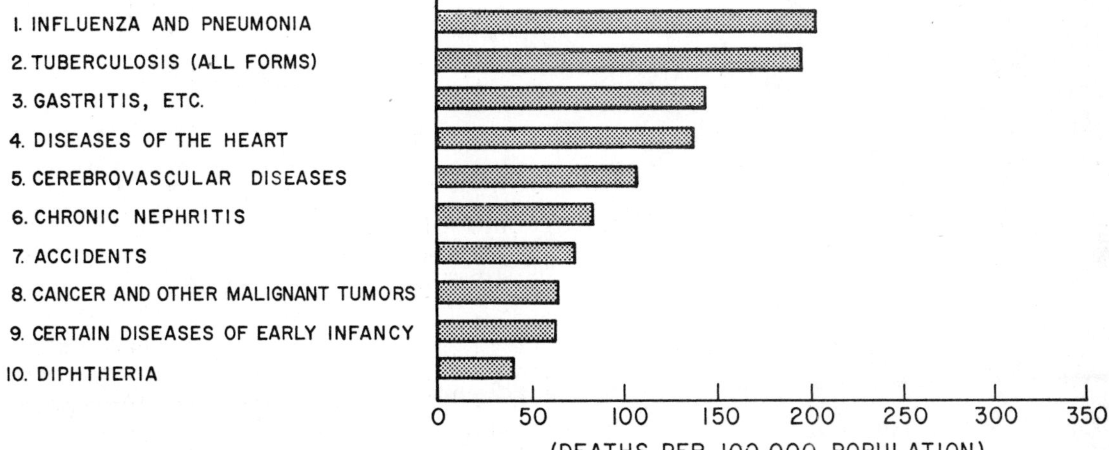

Fig. 5: Leading causes of death in the United States, 1900. Source: Monroe Lerner and Odin W. Anderson, *Health Progress in the United States: 1900–1960* (Chicago: Univ. of Chicago Press, 1963), p. 16.

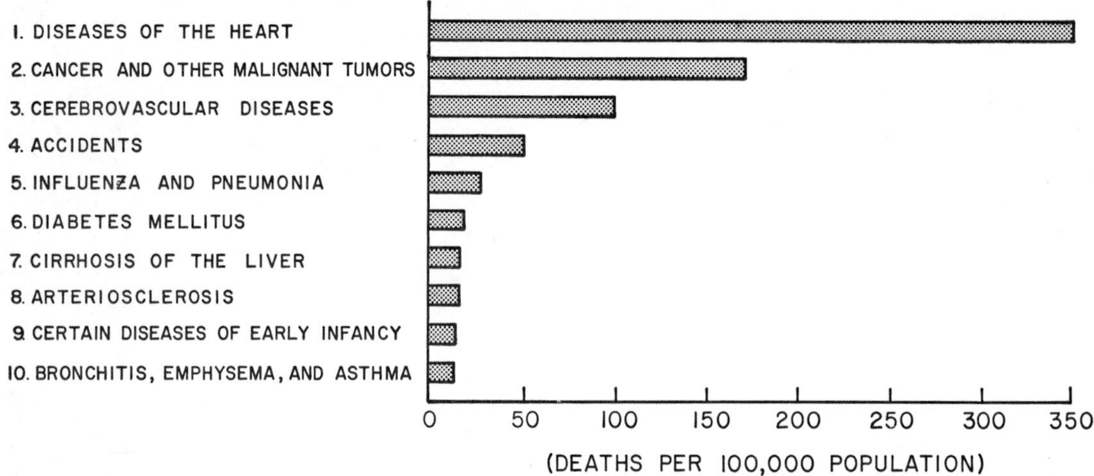

Fig. 6: Leading causes of death in the United States, 1974. Source: U.S. Bureau of the Census, *Statistical Abstract of the United States, 1976* (Washington, D.C.: Government Printing Office, 1976), p. 66.

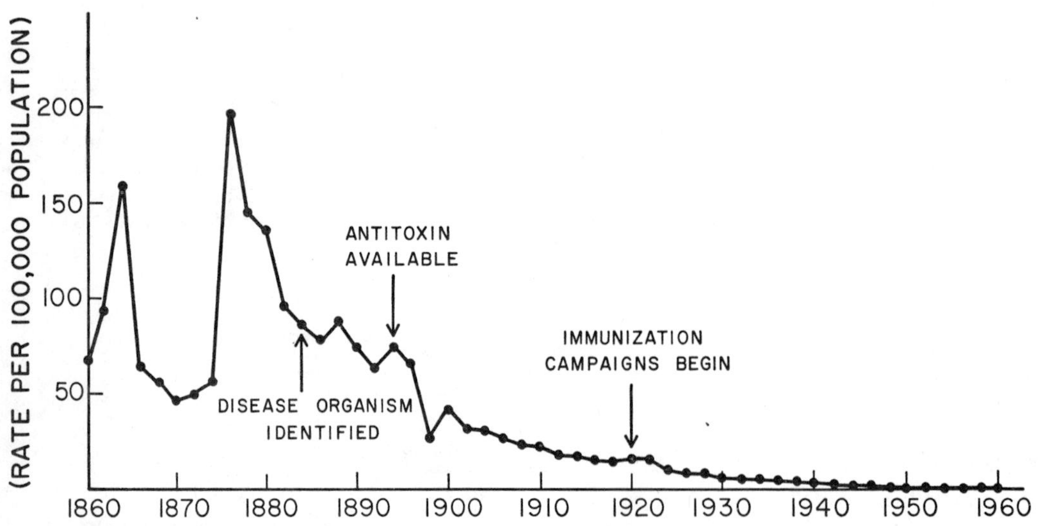

Fig. 7: Death rate for diphtheria, 1860–1960, United States. Source: U.S. Bureau of the Census, *Historical Statistics of the United States: Colonial Times to 1970* (Washington, D.C.: Government Printing Office, 1975), Part 1, pp. 58, 63. Note: Data between 1860 and 1900 are for Massachusetts only.

tial decline of infectious diseases in the United States, but sometimes played a crucial role in the 20th century. The discovery in the 1930s and 1940s of powerful new drugs, like the sulphonamides and antibiotics, finally gave physicians effective weapons with which to fight infection.

The public health movement proved more effective than medicine in combatting communicable diseases during the 19th century. It reduced exposure to infectious diseases by cleaning up the physical environment and improving living conditions, and it helped to lower the incidence of waterborne infections like cholera and dysentery by regulating urban water sources and sewerage.

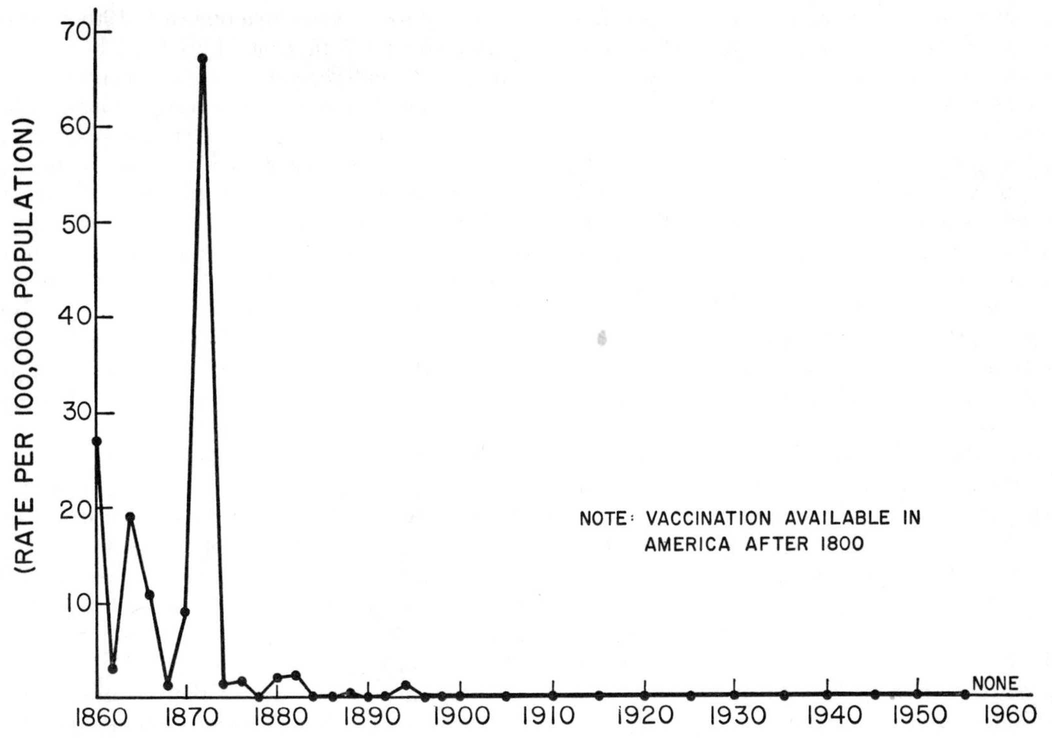

Fig. 8: Death rate for smallpox, 1860–1960, Massachusetts. Source: U.S. Bureau of the Census, *Historical Statistics of the United States: Colonial Times to 1970* (Washington, D.C.: Government Printing Office, 1975), Part 1, p. 63.

Filth was the premier public health problem in the 19th century. Most physicians thought that dirt caused disease and that cleaning up the cities was the best preventative to high mortality. But as traditional methods of keeping cities clean broke down in the wake of massive population increases, those responsible for public health faced unprecedented problems. Festering piles of garbage littered urban streets, dead animals lay where they fell, privies and cesspools overran into drainless, unpaved streets. Horses defecated indiscriminately. Municipal employees spent countless hours trying to staunch the seemingly endless flow of waste products, and, to varying degrees, they were successful. They removed garbage, emptied privies, drained stagnant pools, improved and extended water and sewer systems, and slowly created an environment in which it was possible to walk down the street without dragging one's skirt in the filth or having to hold a handkerchief over one's nose. Health departments also regulated food and housing, at least minimally. Undoubtedly these efforts, to the extent they were successful, significantly reduced the spread of infectious diseases that thrived in unhygienic, congested environments. Their precise impact cannot be measured, because conditions at the local level varied so greatly. But it hardly seems coincidental that mortality from communicable diseases declined at the very time American cities were waging vigorous sanitation campaigns.

Improved water supplies and sewerage provided additional protection against infectious diseases. As more and more American cities installed municipal water systems, urbanites no longer had to consume water from contaminated wells and polluted rivers. The construction of sewers, which carried off tons of septic waste products each day, eliminated another source of infection. All of these public health measures, plus the isolation of the sick during times of epidemics and the regulation of foodstuffs, helped to turn mortality rates downward.

It also seems likely that living conditions — diet, housing, and personal hygiene — contributed to reducing mortality. Recent studies, for example, have demonstrated a high correlation between malnutrition and susceptibility to infectious diseases. Unfortunately, historical data regarding the way people lived are so scarce, we must rely more on inference than hard evidence.

Seventeenth-century colonists frequently suffered from severe food shortages and consequent malnutrition. As one pioneer observed in 1628, "for want of wholesome Diet and convenient Lodgings, many die of Scurvys and other Distempers."[5] These shortages largely disappeared as agricultural production stabilized in the 18th century, but the staple American diet of corn and pork, though ample in quantity, hardly provided a balanced diet.

It was not until the coming of railroads in the 1840s and 1850s and the development of the canning industry after 1860 that products like milk, fruit, and vegetables became readily available year-round, especially to urban dwellers. It is impossible to tell exactly how much the availability of these products increased the consumption of them, but we do know that one early 19th-century family spent 9.7 percent of its food budget on milk, fruit, and vegetables, while a century later another family spent 40.8 percent.[6] This revolution in American eating habits, suggests one historian, "may have contributed as fully to the development of a healthful, vigorous manhood as major measures of sanitary reform and preventive medicine."[7] Certainly it was an important factor.

In the 20th century diet continued to influence the nation's health, though its effect was often negative. As affluent Americans ate more fats and sugar and less fruit, vegetables, and grain products, they fell victim to a form of malnutrition that some authorities predicted might be "as profoundly damaging to the Nation's health as the widespread contagious diseases of the early part of the century." By the mid-1970s six of the ten leading causes of death — heart disease, cancer, cerebrovascular disease, diabetes, arteriosclerosis, and cirrhosis of the liver — could be tied to dietary habits like the over-consumption of saturated fats, cholesterol, sugar, salt, and alcohol.[8] Such evidence clearly demonstrates that to understand sickness and health in America we must study not only medicine, but public health and life-style as well.[9]

NOTES

1 Frederick L. Hoffman, "American mortality progress during the last half century," in *A Half Century of Public Health*, ed. Mazyck P. Ravenel (New York: American Public Health Association, 1921), p. 101.

2 *Report of the Sanitary Commission of Massachusetts* (Boston: Dutton and Wentworth, 1850), p. 281.

3 Hoffman, "American mortality progress," p. 101.

4 Quoted in John Duffy, *Epidemics in Colonial America* (Baton Rouge: Louisiana State Univ. Press, 1971), p. 4.

5 Quoted *ibid.*, p. 11.

6 Chase Going Woodhouse, "The standard of living at the professional level, 1816–17 and 1926–27," *J. Polit. Econ.*, 1929, *37*: 565–567.

7 Richard Osborn Cummings, *The American and His Food: A History of Food Habits in the United States* (Chicago: Univ. of Chicago Press, 1941), p. 52.

8 U.S. Senate Select Committee on Nutrition and Human Needs, *Dietary Goals for the United States* (Washington, D.C.: Government Printing Office, 1977), p. 9.

9 Thomas McKeown's provocative *The Modern Rise of Population* (New York: Academic Press, 1976) inspired this essay.

PART I

Medical Practice and Institutions

Theory

Ideas, like individuals and institutions, have their own histories, and concepts of sickness and health are no exception. What one generation of Americans may have considered an illness, another regarded as perfectly normal. As both Tristram Engelhardt and Barbara Sicherman show, the existence of disease entities may relate as much to the needs of doctors and patients as to objective phenomena.

The history of masturbation, described by Engelhardt, illustrates a common progression from sin to sickness to normal, healthy behavior. Prior to the 19th century Americans widely regarded "self-abuse" as a bad habit, condemned by Scripture and society. During the Victorian age, however, this practice partially escaped its immoral past and metamorphosed into a disease, with distinctive etiology and therapy. Still later, it dropped its pathological connotation and emerged as an acceptable, if not quite respectable, activity. Other practices once attributed to character defects have undergone similar transformations. Today alcoholism, drug addiction, and obesity all seem to be winning recognition as legitimate illnesses, freeing their sufferers from moral blame. At times the change of label from sin to sickness appears arbitrary, as when the Supreme Court in 1962 declared drug addiction to be a disease rather than a crime, and when psychiatrists in 1973 decided that homosexuality was not a form of mental illness.

Sicherman's study provides still another example of changing disease concepts. Neurasthenia, once "the national disease," quietly disappeared in the 20th century, when it no longer served the purpose for which it had been invented a half-century earlier. Americans continued to suffer and die from nervous exhaustion, but physicians, aided by new diagnostic techniques, now interpreted exhaustion as a mere symptom of other diseases. Benjamin Rush's theory of the unity of disease experienced a similar fate. Rush, the foremost physician and medical educator of the early Republic, assured his students in 1796 that "there is but one disease in the world," the essence of which was vascular tension. Within a short time, however, diagnostic sophistication and a new philosophy of medicine had reduced vascular tension to the status of a symptom.

Because illness is a departure from the normal, the more familiar a condition, the less likely it is to be labeled a disease. Malaria, for example, was so common in the Midwest during the mid-19th century, one medical historian, Erwin Ackerknecht, has argued that it briefly lost its identity as a disease. Views of childbirth likewise changed over time. During most of the 18th and 19th centuries, women, who bore many children at home without the aid of a physician, regarded delivery as a normal — if risky — part of life. But when women began having fewer children, and having them in hospitals attended by physicians, the event took on the characteristics of an illness.

1

The Disease of Masturbation: Values and the Concept of Disease

H. TRISTRAM ENGELHARDT, JR.

Masturbation in the 18th and especially in the 19th century was widely believed to produce a spectrum of serious signs and symptoms, and was held to be a dangerous disease entity. Explanation of this phenomenon entails a basic reexamination of the concept of disease. It presupposes that one think of disease neither as an objective entity in the world nor as a concept that admits of a single universal definition: there is not, nor need there be, one concept of disease.[1] Rather, one chooses concepts for certain purposes, depending on values and hopes concerning the world.[2] The disease of masturbation is an eloquent example of the value-laden nature of science in general and of medicine in particular. In explaining the world, one judges what is to be significant or insignificant. For example, mathematical formulae are chosen in terms of elegance and simplicity, though elegance and simplicity are not attributes to be found in the world as such. The problem is even more involved in the case of medicine which judges what the human organism should be (i.e., what counts as "health") and is thus involved in the entire range of human values. This paper will sketch the nature of the model of the disease of masturbation in the 19th century, particularly in America, and indicate the scope of this "disease entity" and the therapies it evoked. The goal will be to outline some of the interrelations between evaluation and explanation.

The moral offense of masturbation was transformed into a disease with somatic not just psychological dimensions. Though sexual overindulgence generally was considered debilitating since at least the time of Hippocrates,[3] masturbation was not widely accepted as a disease until a book by the title *Onania* appeared anonymously in Holland in 1700 and met with great success.[4] This success was reinforced by the appearance of S. A. Tissot's book on onanism.[5] Tissot held that all sexual activity was potentially debilitating and that the debilitation was merely more exaggerated in the case of masturbation. The primary basis for the debilitation was, according to Tissot, loss of seminal fluid, 1 ounce being equivalent to the loss of 40 ounces of blood.[6] When this loss of fluid took place in an other than recumbent position (which Tissot held often to be the case with masturbation), this exaggerated the ill effects.[7] In attempting to document his contention, Tissot provided a comprehensive monograph on masturbation, synthesizing and appropriating the views of classical authors who had been suspicious of the effects of sexual overindulgence. He focused these suspicions clearly on masturbation. In this he was very successful, for Tissot's book appears to have widely established the medical opinion that masturbation was associated with serious physical and mental maladies.[8]

There appears to have been some disagreement whether the effect of frequent intercourse was in any respect different from that of masturbation. The presupposition that masturbation was not in accordance with the dictates of nature suggested that it would tend to be more subversive of the constitution than excessive sexual intercourse. Accounts of this difference in terms of the differential effect of the excitation involved are for the most part obscure. It was, though, advanced that "during sexual intercourse the expenditure of nerve force is compensated by the magnetism of the

H. Tristram Engelhardt is Rosemary Kennedy Professor of the Philosophy of Medicine at the Kennedy Institute, Center for Bioethics, Georgetown University, Washington, D.C.

Reprinted with permission from the *Bulletin of the History of Medicine*, 1974, *48*: 234–248.

partner."[9] Tissot suggested that a beautiful sexual partner was of particular benefit or was at least less exhausting.[10] In any event, masturbation was held to be potentially more deleterious since it was unnatural, and, therefore, less satisfying and more likely to lead to a disturbance or disordering of nerve tone.

At first, the wide range of illnesses attributed to masturbation is striking. Masturbation was held to be the cause of dyspepsia,[11] constrictions of the urethra,[12] epilepsy,[13] blindness,[14] vertigo, loss of hearing,[15] headache, impotency, loss of memory, "irregular action of the heart," general loss of health and strength,[16] rickets,[17] leucorrhea in women,[18] and chronic catarrhal conjunctivitis.[19] Nymphomania was found to arise from masturbation, occurring more commonly in blonds than in brunettes.[20] Further, changes in the external genitalia were attributed to masturbation: elongation of the clitoris, reddening and congestion of the labia majora, elongation of the labia minora,[21] and a thinning and decrease in size of the penis.[22] Chronic masturbation was held to lead to the development of a particular type, including enlargement of the superficial veins of the hands and feet, moist and clammy hands, stooped shoulders, pale sallow face with heavy dark circles around the eyes, a "draggy" gait, and acne.[23] Careful case studies were published establishing masturbation as a cause of insanity,[24] and evidence indicated that it was a cause of hereditary insanity as well.[25] Masturbation was held also to cause an hereditary predisposition to consumption.[26] Finally, masturbation was believed to lead to general debility. "From health and vigor, and intelligence and loveliness of character, they became thin and pale and cadaverous; their amiability and loveliness departed, and in their stead irritability, moroseness and anger were prominent characteristics. . . . The child loses its flesh and becomes pale and weak."[27] The natural history was one of progressive loss of vigor, both physical and mental.

In short, a broad and heterogeneous class of signs and symptoms were recognized in the 19th century as a part of what was tantamount to a syndrome, if not a disease: masturbation. If one thinks of a syndrome as the concurrence or running together of signs and symptoms into a recognizable pattern, surely masturbation was such a pattern. It was more, though, in that a cause was attributed to the syndrome providing an etiological framework for a disease entity. That is, if one views the development of disease concepts as the progression from the mere collection of signs and symptoms to their interrelation in terms of a recognized causal mechanism, the disease of masturbation was fairly well evolved. A strikingly heterogeneous set of signs and symptoms was unified and comprehended under one causal mechanism. One could thus move from mere observation and description to explanation.

Since the signs and symptoms brought within the concept of masturbation were of a serious order associated with marked debility, it is not unexpected that there would be occasional deaths. The annual reports of the Charity Hospital of Louisiana in New Orleans which show hospitalizations for masturbation over an 86-year period indicate that, indeed, two masturbators were recorded as having died in the hospital. In 1872, the reports show that there were two masturbators hospitalized, one of whom was discharged, the other one having died.[28] The records of 1887 show that of the five masturbators hospitalized that year two improved, two were unimproved, and one died.[29] The records of the hospital give no evidence concerning the patient who died in 1872. The records for 1887, however, name the patient, showing him to have been hospitalized on Tuesday, January 6, 1887, for masturbation. A 45-year-old native of Indiana, a resident of New Orleans for the previous 35 years, single, and a laborer, he died in the hospital on April 8, 1887.[30] There is no indication of the course of the illness. It is interesting to note, though, that in 1888 there was a death from anemia associated with masturbation, the cause of death being recorded under anemia. The records indicate that the patient was hospitalized on August 17, 1887, and died on February 11, 1888, was a lifelong resident of New Orleans, and was likewise a laborer and single.[31] His case suggests something concerning the two deaths recorded under masturbation: that they, too, suffered from a debilitating disease whose signs and symptoms were referred to masturbation as the underlying cause. In short, the concept of masturbation as a disease probably acted as a schema for organizing various signs and symptoms which we would now gather under different nosological categories.

As with all diseases, there was a struggle to develop a workable nosology. This is reflected in the reports of the Charity Hospital of Louisiana (in New Orleans) where over the years the disease was placed under various categories and numerous nomenclatures were employed. In 1848, for example, the first entry was given as "masturbation," in 1853 "onanism" was substituted, and in 1857 this was changed to "onanysmus."[32] Later, as the records began to classify the diseases under general headings, a place had to be found for masturbation. Initially in 1874, the disease "masturbation" was placed under the heading "Male Diseases of Generative Organs." In 1877 this was changed to "Diseases of the Nervous System," and finally in 1884 the disease of "onanism" was classified as a "Cerebral-Spinal Disease." In 1890 it was reclassified under the heading "Diseases of the Nervous System," and remained classified as such until 1906 when it was placed as "masturbation" under the title of "Genito-Urinary System, Diseases of (Functional Disturbances of Male Sexual Organs.)" It remained classified as a functional disturbance until the last entry in 1933. The vacillation in the use of headings probably indicates hesitation on the part of the recorders as to the nature of the disease. On the one hand, it is understandable why a disease, which was held to have such grossly physical components, would itself be considered to have some variety of physical basis. On the other hand, the recorders appear to have been drawn by the obviously psychological aspects of the phenomenon of masturbation to classify it in the end as a functional disturbance.

As mentioned, the concept of the disease of masturbation developed on the basis of a general suspicion that sexual activity was debilitating.[33] This development is not really unexpected: if one examines the world with a tacit presupposition of a parallelism between what is good for one's soul and what is good for one's health, then one would expect to find disease correlates for immoral sexual behavior.[34] Also, this was influenced by a concurrent inclination to translate a moral issue into medical terms and relieve it of the associated moral opprobrium in a fashion similar to the translation of alcoholism from a moral into a medical problem.[35] Further, disease as a departure from a state of stability due to excess or under-excitation offered the skeleton of a psychosomatic theory of the somatic alterations attributed to the excitation associated with masturbation.[36] The categories of over- and under-excitation suggest cogent, basic categories of medical explanation: over- and under-excitation, each examples of excess, imply deleterious influences on the stability of the organism. Jonathan Hutchinson succinctly described the etiological mechanism in this fashion, holding that "the habit in question is very injurious to the nerve-tone, and that it frequently originates and keeps up maladies which but for it might have been avoided or cured."[37] This schema of causality presents the signs and symptoms attendant to masturbation as due to "the nerveshock attending the substitute for the venereal act, or the act itself, which, either in onanism or copulation frequently indulged, breaks men down."[38] "The excitement incident to the habitual and frequent indulgence of the unnatural practice of masturbation leads to the most serious constitutional effects. . . ."[39] The effects were held to be magnified during youth when such "shocks" undermined normal development.[40]

Similarly, Freud remarks in a draft of a paper to Wilhelm Fliess dated February 8, 1893, that "Sexual exhaustion can by itself alone provoke neurasthenia. If it fails to achieve this by itself, it has such an effect on the disposition of the nervous system that physical illness, depressive affects and overwork (toxic influences) can no longer be tolerated without [leading to] neurasthenia. . . . *neurasthenia in males* is acquired at puberty and becomes manifest in the patient's twenties. Its source is masturbation, the frequency of which runs completely parallel with the frequency of male neurasthenia."[41] And Freud later stated, "It is the prolonged and intense action of this pernicious sexual satisfaction which is enough on its own account to provoke a neurasthenic neurosis. . . ."[42] Again, it is a model of excessive stimulation of a certain quality leading to specific disabilities. This position of the theoreticians of masturbation in the 19th century is not dissimilar to positions currently held concerning other diseases. For example, the first Diagnostic and Statistical Manual of the American Psychiatric Association says with regard to "psychophysiologic autonomic and visceral disorders" that "The symptoms are due to a chronic and exaggerated state of the normal physiological expression of emotion, with the feeling, or subjective part, repressed. Such long continued visceral states may eventually lead to structural changes."[43] This theoretical formulation is one that would have been compatible with theories concerning masturbation in the 19th century.

Other models of etiology were employed besides those based upon excess stimulation. They, for the most part, accounted for the signs and symptoms on the basis of the guilt associated with the act of masturbation. These more liberal positions developed during a time of reaction against the more drastic therapies such as Baker Brown's use of clitoridectomy.[44] These alternative models can be distinguished according to whether the guilt was held to be essential or adventitious. Those who held that masturbation was an unnatural act were likely to hold that the associated guilt feelings and anxiety were natural, unavoidable consequences of performing an unnatural act. Though not phrased in the more ethically neutral terms of excess stimulation, still the explanation was in terms of a pathophysiological state involving a departure from biological norms. "The masturbator feels that his act degrades his manhood, while the man who indulges in legitimate intercourse is satisfied that he has fulfilled one of his principal natural functions. There is a healthy instinctive expression of passion in one case, an illegitimate perversion of function in the other."[45] The operative assumption was that when sexual activity failed to produce an "exhilaration of spirits and clearness of intellect" and when associated with anxiety or guilt it would lead to deleterious effects.[46] This analysis suggested that it was guilt, not excitation, which led to the phenomena associated with masturbation. "Now it happens in a large number of cases, that these young masturbators sooner or later become alarmed at their practices, in consequence of some information they receive. Often this latter is of a most mischievous character. Occasionally too, the religious element is predominant, and the mental condition of these young men becomes truly pitiable. . . . The facts are nearly these: Masturbation is not a crime nor a sin, but a vice."[47] Others appreciated the evil and guilt primarily in terms of the solitary and egoistic nature of the act.[48]

Such positions concerning etiology graded over into models in which masturbation's untoward signs and symptoms were viewed as merely the result of guilt and anxiety felt because of particular cultural norms, which norms had no essential basis in biology. "Whatever may be abnormal, there is nothing unnatural."[49] In short, there was also a model of interpretation which saw the phenomena associated with masturbation as mere adventitious, as due to a particular culture's condemnation of the act. This last interpretation implied that no more was required than to realize that there was nothing essentially wrong with masturbation. "Our wisest course is to recognize the inevitableness of the vice of masturbation under the perpetual restraints of civilized life, and, while avoiding any attitude of indifference, to avoid also an attitude of excessive horror, for that would only lead to the facts being effectually veiled from our sight, and serve to manufacture artificially a greater evil than that which we seek to combat."[50] This last point of view appears to have gained prominence in the development of thought concerning masturbation as reflected in the shift from the employment of mechanical and surgical therapy in the late 19th century to the use of more progressive means (i.e., including education that guilt and anxiety were merely relative to certain cultural norms) by the end of the century and the first half of the 20th century.[51]

To recapitulate, 19th-century reflection on the etiology of masturbation led to the development of an authentic disease of masturbation: excessive sexual stimulation was seen to produce particular and discrete pathophysiological changes.[52] First, there were strict approaches in terms of disordered nerve-tone due to excess and/or unnatural sexual excitation. Over-excitation was seen to lead to significant and serious physical alterations in the patient, and in this vein a somewhat refined causal model of the disease was developed. Second, there were those who saw the signs and symptoms as arising from the unavoidable guilt and anxiety associated with the performance of an unnatural act. Third, there were a few who appreciated masturbation's sequelae as merely the response of a person in a culture which condemned the activity.

Those who held the disease of masturbation to be more than a culturally dependent phenomenon often employed somewhat drastic therapies. Restraining devices were devised,[53] infibulation of placing a ring in the prepuce was used to make masturbation painful,[54] and no one less than Jonathan Hutchinson held that circumcision acted as a preventive.[55] Acid burns or thermoelectrocautery[56] were utilized to make masturbation painful and, therefore, to discourage it. The alleged seriousness of this disease in females led, as Professor John Duffy has shown, to the employment of the rather radical treatment of clitoridectomy.[57] The classic monograph recommending clitoridectomy, written by the British surgeon Baker Brown, advocated the procedure to terminate the "long continued peripheral excitement, causing frequent and increasing losses of nerve force, . . ."[58] Brown recommended that "the patient having been placed completely under the influence of chloroform, the clitoris [be] freely excised either by scissors or knive — I always prefer the scissors."[59] The supposed sequelae of female masturbation, such as sterility, paresis, hysteria, dysmenorrhea, idiocy, and insanity, were also held to be remedied by the operation.

Male masturbation was likewise treated by means of surgical procedures. Some recommended vasectomy[60] while others found this procedure ineffective and employed castration.[61] One illustrative case involved the castration of a physician who had been confined as insane for seven years and who subsequently was able to return to practice.[62] Another case involved the castration of a 22-year-old epileptic "at the request of the county judge, and with the consent of his father . . . the father saying he would be perfectly satisfied if the masturbation could be stopped, so that he could take him home, without having his family continually humiliated and disgusted by his loathsome habit."[63] The patient was described as facing the operation morosely, "like a coon in a hollow."[64] Following the operation, masturbation ceased and the frequency of fits decreased. An editor of the *Texas Medical Practitioner*, J. B. Shelmire, added a remark to the article: "Were this procedure oftener adopted for the cure of these desperate cases, many, who are sent to insane asylums, soon to succumb to the effects of this habit, would live to become useful citizens."[65] Though such approaches met with ridicule from some quarters,[66] still various novel treatments were devised in order to remedy the alleged sequelae of chronic masturbation such as spermatorrhea and impotency. These included acupuncture of the prostate in which "needles from two to three inches in length are passed through the perineum into the prostate gland and the neck of the bladder. . . . Some surgeons recommend the introduction of needles into the testicles and spermatic cord for the same purpose."[67] Insertion of electrodes into the bladder and rectum and cauterization of the prostatic urethra were also utilized.[68] Thus, a wide range of rather heroic methods were devised to treat masturbation and a near fascination developed on the part of some for the employment of mechanical and electrical means of restoring "health."

There were, though, more tolerant approaches, ranging from hard work and simple diet[69] to suggestions that "If the masturbator is totally continent, sexual intercourse is advisable."[70] This latter approach to therapy led some physicians to recommend that masturbators cure their disease by frequenting houses of prostitution,[71] or acquiring a mistress.[72] Though these treatments would appear ad hoc, more theoretically sound proposals were made by many physicians in terms of the model of excitability. They suggested that the disease and its sequelae could be adequately controlled by treating the excitation and debility consequent upon masturbation. Towards this end, "active tonics" and the use of cold baths at night just before bedtime were suggested.[73] Much more in a "Brownian" mode was the proposal that treatment with opium would be effective. An initial treatment with 1/12 of a grain of morphine sulfate daily by injection was followed after ten days by a dose of 1/16 of a grain. This dose was continued for three weeks and gradually diminished to 1/30 of a grain a day. At the end of a month the patient was dismissed from treatment "the picture of health, having fattened very much, and lost every trace of anaemia and mental imbecility."[74] The author, after his researches with opium and masturbation, concluded, "*We may find in opium a new and important aid in the treatment of the victims of the habit of masturbation by means of which their moral and physical forces may be so increased that they may be enabled to enter the true physiological path.*"[75] This last example eloquently collects the elements of the concept of the disease of masturbation as a pathophysiological entity: excitation leads to physical debilitation requiring a physical remedy. Masturbation as a pathophysiological entity was thus incorporated within an acceptable medical model of diagnosis and therapy.

In summary, in the 19th century, biomedical scientists attempted to correlate a vast number of signs and symptoms with a disapproved activity found in many patients afflicted with various maladies. Given an inviting theoretical framework, it was very conducive to think of this range of signs and symptoms as having one cause. The theoretical framework, though, as has been indicated, was not value free but structured by the values and expectations of the times. In the 19th century, one was pleased to think that not "one bride in a hundred, of delicate, educated, sensitive women, accepts matrimony from any desire of sexual gratification: when she thinks of this at all, it is with shrinking, or even with horror, rather than with desire."[76] In contrast, in the 20th century, articles are published for the instruction of women in the use of masturbation to overcome the disease of frigidity or orgasmic dysfunction.[77] In both cases, expectations concerning what should be significant structure the appreciation of reality by medicine. The variations are not due to mere fallacies of scientific method,[78] but involve a basic dependence of the logic of scientific discovery and explanation upon prior evaluations of reality.[79] A sought-for coincidence of morality and nature gives goals to explanation and therapy.[80] Values influence the purpose and direction of investigations and treatment. Moreover, the disease of masturbation has other analogues. In the 19th century, there were such diseases in the South as "Drapetomania, the disease causing slaves to run away," and the disease "Dysaesthesia Aethiopis or hebetude of mind and obtuse sensibility of body — a disease peculiar to negroes — called by overseers 'rascality'."[81] In Europe, there was the disease of *morbus democritus*.[82] Some would hold that current analogues exist in diseases such as alcoholism and drug abuse.[83] In short, the disease of masturbation indicates that evaluations play a role in the development of explanatory models and that this may not be an isolated phenomenon.

This analysis, then, suggests the following conclusion: although vice and virtue are not equivalent to disease and health, they bear a direct relation to these concepts. Insofar as a vice is taken to be a deviation from an ideal of human perfection, or "well-being," it can be translated into disease language. In shifting to disease language, one no longer speaks in moralistic terms (e.g., "You are evil"), but one speaks in terms of a deviation from a norm which implies a degree of imperfection (e.g., "You are a deviant"). The shift is from an explicitly ethical language to a language of natural teleology. To be ill is to fail to realize the perfection of an ideal type; to be sick is to be defective rather than to be evil. The concern is no longer with what is naturally, morally good, but what is naturally beautiful. Medicine turns to what has been judged to be naturally ugly or deviant, and then develops etiological accounts in order to explain and treat in a coherent fashion a manifold of displeasing signs and symptoms. The notion of the "deviant" structures the concept of disease providing a purpose and direction for explanation and for action, that is, for diagnosis and prognosis, and for therapy. A "disease entity" operates as a conceptual form organizing phenomena in a fashion deemed useful for certain goals. The goals, though, involve choice by man and are not objective facts, data "given" by nature. They are ideals imputed to nature. The disease of masturbation is an eloquent example of the role of evaluation in explanation and the structure values give to our picture of reality.

NOTES

Read at the 46th annual meeting of the American Association for the History of Medicine, Cincinnati, Ohio, May 5, 1973. I am grateful for the suggestions of Professor John Duffy, and the kind assistance of Louanna K. Bennett and Robert S. Baxter, Jr.

1 Alvan R. Feinstein, "Taxonomy and logic in clinical data," *Ann. N.Y. Acad. Sci.*, 1969, *161*: 450–459.

2 Horacio Fabrega, Jr., "Concepts of disease: logical features and social implications," *Perspect. Biol. & Med.*, 1972, *15*: 583–616.

3 For example, Hippocrates correlated gout with sexual intercourse, *Aphorisms*, VI, 30. Numerous passages in the *Corpus* recommend the avoidance of overindulgence especially during certain illnesses.

4 René A. Spitz, "Authority and masturbation. Some remarks on a bibliographical investigation," *Yearbook of Psychoanalysis*, 1953, *9*: 116. Also, Robert H. MacDonald, "The frightful consequences of onanism: notes on the history of a delusion," *J. Hist. Ideas*, 1967, *28*: 423–431.

5 Simon-André Tissot, *Tentamen de Morbis ex Manustrupatione* (Lausanne: M. M. Bousquet, 1758). An anonymous American translation appeared in the early 19th century: *Onanism* (New York: Collins & Hannay, 1832). Interestingly, the copy of Tissot's book held by the New York Academy of Medicine was given by Austin Flint. Austin Flint in turn was quoted as an authority on the effects of masturbation: see Joseph W. Howe's *Excessive Venery, Masturbation and Continence* (New York: Bermingham, 1884), p. 97. Also the American edition of Tissot's book, to show its concurrence with an American authority, added in a footnote a reference to Benjamin Rush's opinion concerning the pernicious consequences of masturbation. See Tissot, *Onanism*, p. 19, and Benjamin Rush's *Medical Inquiries and Observations Upon the Diseases of the Mind* (Philadelphia: Kimber and Richardson, 1812), pp. 348–349; also Tissot, *Onanism*, p. 21.

6 Simon-André Tissot, *Onanism* (New York: Collins & Hannay, 1832), p. 5.

7 *Ibid.*, p. 50.

8 E. H. Hare, "Masturbatory insanity: the history of an idea," *J. Mental Sci.*, 1962, *108*: 2–3. It is worth noting that Tissot, as others, at times appears to have grouped together female masturbation and female homosexuality. See Vern L. Bullough and Martha Voght, "Homosexuality and its confusion with the 'secret sin' in pre-Freudian America," *J. Hist. Med.*, 1973, *28*: 143–155.

9 Howe, *Excessive Venery*, pp. 76–77.

10 Tissot, *Onanism*, p. 51.

11 J. A. Mayes, "Spermatorrhoea, treated by the lately invented rings," *Charleston Med. J. & Rev.*, 1854, *9*: 352.

12 Allen W. Hagenbach, "Masturbation as a cause of insanity," *J. Nerv. & Ment. Dis.*, 1879, *6*: 609.

13 Baker Brown, *On the Curability of Certain Forms of Insanity, Epilepsy, Catalepsy, and Hysteria in Females* (London: Hardwicke, 1866). Brown phrased the cause discreetly in terms of "peripheral irritation, arising originally in some branches of the pudic nerve, more particularly the incident nerve supplying the clitoris. . . ." (p. 7)

14 F. A. Burdem, "Self pollution in children," *Mass. Med. J.*, 1896, *16*:340.

15 Weber Liel, "The influence of sexual irritation upon the diseases of the ear," *New Orleans Med. & Surg. J.*, 1884, *11*: 786–788.

16 Joseph Jones, "Diseases of the nervous system," *Tr. La. St. Med. Soc.* (New Orleans: L. Graham & Son, 1889), p. 170.

17 Howe, *Excessive Venery*, p. 93.

18 J. Castellanos, "Influence of sewing machines upon the health and morality of the females using them," *Southern J. Med. Sci.*, 1866–1867, *1*: 495–496.

19 Comment, "Masturbation and ophthalmia," *New Orleans Med. & Surg. J.*, 1881–1882, *9*: 67.

20 Howe, *Excessive Venery*, pp. 108–111.

21 *Ibid.*, pp. 41, 72.

22 *Ibid.*, p. 68.

23 *Ibid.*, p. 73.

24 Hagenbach, "Masturbation as a cause of insanity," pp. 603–612.

25 Jones, "Diseases of the nervous system," p. 170.

26 Howe, *Excessive Venery*, p. 95.

27 Burdem, "Self pollution," pp. 339, 341.

28 *Report of the Board of Administrators of the Charity Hospital to the General Assembly of Louisiana* (for 1872) (New Orleans: The Republican Office, 1873), p. 30.

29 *Report of the Board of Administrators of the Charity Hospital to the General Assembly of Louisiana* (for 1887) (New Orleans: A. W. Hyatt, 1888), p. 53.

30 Record Archives of the Charity Hospital of Louisiana [in New Orleans] MS, "Admission Book #41 from December 1, 1885 to March 31, 1888 Charity Hospital," p. 198. I am indebted to Mrs. Eddie Cooksy for access to the record archives.

31 *Ibid.*, p. 287.

32 This and the following information concerning entries is taken from a review of the *Report of the Board of Administrators of the Charity Hospital*, New Orleans, Louisiana, from 1848 to 1933. The reports were not available for the years 1850–1851, 1854–1855, 1862–1863, and 1865.

33 Even Boerhaave remarked that "an excessive discharge of semen causes fatigue, weakness, decrease in activity, convulsions, emaciation, dehydration, heat and pains in the membranes of the brain, a loss in the acuity of the senses, particularly of vision, *tabes dorsalis*, simplemindedness, and various similar disorders." My translation of Hermanno Boerhaave's *Institutiones Medicae* (Vienna: J. T. Trattner, 1775), p. 315, paragraph 776.

34 "We have seen that masturbation is more pernicious than excessive intercourse with females. Those who believe in a special providence, account for it by a special ordinance of the Deity to punish this crime." Tissot, *Onanism*, p. 45.

35 ". . . the best remedy was not to tell the poor children that they were damning their souls, but to tell them that they might seriously hurt their bodies, and to explain to them the nature and purport of the functions they were abusing." Lawson Tait, "Masturba-

tion. A clinical lecture," *Med. News, N.Y.*, 1888, *53*: 2.

36 Though it has not been possible to trace a direct influence by John Brown's system of medicine upon the development of accounts of the disease of masturbation, yet a connection is suggestive. Brown had left a mark on the minds of many in the 18th and 19th centuries, and given greater currency to the use of concepts of over and under excitation in the explanation of the etiology of disease. Guenter B. Risse, "The quest for certainty in medicine: John Brown's system of medicine in France," *Bull. Hist. Med.*, 1971, *45*: 1–12.

37 Jonathan Hutchinson, "On circumcision as preventive of masturbation," *Arch. Surg.*, 1890–1891, *2*: 268.

38 Theophilus Parvin, "The hygiene of the sexual functions," *New Orleans Med. & Surg. J.*, 1884, *11*: 606.

39 Jones, "Diseases of the nervous system," p. 170. It is interesting to note that documentation for the constitutional effects of masturbation was sought even from post-mortem examination. A report from Birmingham, England, concerning an autopsy on a dead masturbator, concluded that masturbation "... seems to have acted upon the cord in the same manner as repeated small haemorrhages affect the brain, slowly sapping its energies, until it succumbed soon after the last application of the exhausting influence, probably through the instrumentality of an atrophic process previously induced, as evidenced by the diseased state of the minute vessels" ([James] Russell, "Cases illustrating the influence of exhaustion of the spinal cord in inducing paraplegia," *Med. Times & Gaz., Lond.*, 1863, *2*: 456). The examination included microscopic inspection of material to demonstrate pathological changes. Again, the explanation of the phenomena turned on the supposed intense excitement attendant to masturbation. "In this fatal vice the venereal passion is carried at each indulgence to the state of highest tension by the aid of the mind, and on each occasion the cord is subjected to the strongest excitement which sensation and imagination in combination can produce, for we cannot regard the mere secretion of the seminal fluid as constituting the chief drain upon the energies of the cord, but rather as being the exponent of the nervous stimulation by which it has been ejaculated" (*ibid.*, p. 456). The model was one of mental tension and excitement "exhausting" the nervous system by "excessive functional activity" leading to consequent "weakening" of the nervous system. Baker Brown listed eight stages in the progress of the disease in females: hysteria, spinal irritation, hysterical epilepsy, cataleptic fits, epileptic fits, idiocy, mania and finally death; Brown, *Curability*, p. 7.

40 "Any shock to this growth and development, and especially that of masturbation, must for a time suspend the process of nutrition; and a succession of such shocks will blast both body and mind, and terminate in perpetual vacuity." Burdem, "Self pollution," p. 339. In this regard, not only adolescent but childhood masturbation was the concern of 19th-century practitioners; e.g., Russell, "Influence of exhaustion," p. 456.

41 Sigmund Freud, *The Standard Edition of the Complete Psychological Works of Sigmund Freud*, I (London: The Hogarth Press, 1971), 180.

42 *Ibid.*, III, "Heredity and the Aetiology of the Neuroses," p. 150.

43 *Diagnostic and Statistical Manual: Mental Disorders* (Washington, D.C.: American Psychiatric Association, 1952), p. 29.

44 "Mr. Baker Brown was not a very accurate observer, nor a logical reasoner. He found that a number of semi-demented epileptics were habitual masturbators, and that the masturbation was, in women, chiefly effected by excitement of the mucous membrane on and around the clitoris. Jumping over two grave omissions in the syllogism, and putting the cart altogether before the horse, he arrived at the conclusion that removal of the clitoris would stop the pernicious habit, and therefore cure the epilepsy." Tait, "Masturbation," p. 2.

45 Howe, *Excessive Venery*, p. 77.

46 *Ibid.*, p. 77.

47 James Nevins Hyde, "On the masturbation, spermatorrhoea and impotence of adolescence," *Chicago Med. J. & Exam.*, 1879, *38*: 451–452.

48 "There can be no doubt that the habit is, temporarily at least, morally degrading; but if we bear in mind the selfish, solitary nature of the act, the entire absence in it of aught akin to love or sympathy, the innate repulsiveness of intense selfishness or egoism of any kind, we may see how it may be morally degrading, while its effect on the physical and mental organism is practically nil." A. C. McClanahan, "An investigation into the effects of masturbation," *N.Y. Med. J.*, 1897, *66*: 502.

49 *Ibid.*, p. 500.

50 Augustin J. Himel, "Some minor studies in psychology, with special reference to masturbation," *New Orleans Med. & Surg. J.*, 1907, *60*: 452.

51 Spitz, "Authority and masturbation," esp. p. 119.

52 That is, masturbation as a disease was more than a mere collection of signs and symptoms usually "running together" in a syndrome. It became a legitimate disease entity, a causally related set of signs and symptoms.

53 C. D. W. Colby, "Mechanical restraint of masturbation in a young girl," *Med. Rec. in N.Y.*, 1897, *52*: 206.

54 Louis Bauer, "Infibulation as a remedy for epilepsy and seminal losses," *St. Louis Clin. Rec.*, 1879, *6*: 163–165. See also Gerhart S. Schwarz, "Infibulation, population control, and the medical profession," *Bull. N.Y. Acad. Med.*, 1970, *46*: 979, 990.

55 Hutchinson, "Circumcision," pp. 267–269.

56 William J. Robinson, "Masturbation and its treatment," *Am. J. Clin. Med.*, 1907, *14*: 349.

57 John Duffy, "Masturbation and clitoridectomy. A nineteenth-century view," *J.A.M.A.*, 1963, *186*: 246–248.

58 Brown, "Curability," p. 11.

59 *Ibid.*, p. 17.

60 Timothy Haynes, "Surgical treatment of hopeless cases of masturbation and nocturnal emissions," *Boston Med. & Surg. J.*, 1883, *109*: 130.

61 J. H. Marshall, "Insanity cured by castration," *Med. & Surg. Reptr.*, 1865, *13*: 363–364.

62 "The patient soon evinced marked evidences of being a changed man, becoming quiet, kind, and docile." *Ibid.*, p. 363.

63 R. D. Potts, "Castration for masturbation, with report of a case," *Texas Med. Practitioner*, 1898, *11*: 8.

64 *Ibid.*, p. 8.

65 *Ibid.*, p. 9.

66 Editorial, "Castration for the relief of epilepsy," *Boston Med. & Surg. J.*, 1859, *60*: 163.

67 Howe, *Excessive Venery*, p. 260.

68 *Ibid.*, pp. 254–255, 258–260.

69 Editorial, "Review of European legislation for the control of prostitution," *New Orleans Med. & Surg. J.*, 1854–1855, *11*: 704.

70 Robinson, "Masturbation and its treatment," p. 350.

71 Parvin, "Hygiene," p. 606.

72 Mayes, "Spermatorrhoea," p. 352.

73 Haynes, "Surgical treatment," p. 130.

74 B. A. Pope, "Opium as a tonic and alternative; with remarks upon the hypodermic use of the sulfate of morphia, and its use in the debility and amorosis consequent upon onanism," *New Orleans Med. & Surg. J.*, 1879, *6*: 725.

75 *Ibid.*, p. 727.

76 Parvin, "Hygiene," p. 607.

77 Joseph LoPiccolo and W. Charles Lobitz, "The role of masturbation in the treatment of orgasmic dysfunction," *Arch. Sexual Behavior*, 1972, *2*: 163–171.

78 E. Hare, "Masturbatory insanity," pp. 15–19.

79 Norwood Hanson, *Patterns of Discovery* (London: Cambridge Univ. Press, 1965).

80 Tissot, *Onanism*, p. 45. As Immanuel Kant, a contemporary of S.-A. Tissot remarked, "Also, in all probability, it was through this moral interest [in the moral law governing the world] that attentiveness to beauty and the ends of nature was first aroused." (*Kants Werke*, Vol. 5, *Kritik der Urtheilskraft* [Berlin: Walter de Gruyter & Co., 1968], p. 459, A 439. My translation.) That is, moral values influence the search for goals in nature, and direct attention to what will be considered natural, normal, and nondeviant. This would also imply a relationship between the aesthetic, especially what was judged to be naturally beautiful, and what was held to be the goals of nature.

81 Samuel A. Cartwright, "Report on the diseases and physical peculiarities of the negro race," *New Orleans Med. & Surg. J.*, 1850–1851, 7: 707–709. An interesting examination of these diseases is given by Thomas S. Szasz, "The sane slave," *Am. J. Psychoth.*, 1971, *25*: 228–239.

82 Heinz Hartmann, "Towards a concept of mental health," *Brit J. Med. Psychol.*, 1960, *33*: 248.

83 Thomas S. Szasz, "Bad habits are not diseases: a refutation of the claim that alcoholism is a disease," *Lancet*, 1972, *2*: 83–84; and Szasz, "The ethics of addiction," *Am. J. Psychiatry*, 1971, *128*: 541–546.

2

The Uses of a Diagnosis: Doctors, Patients, and Neurasthenia

BARBARA SICHERMAN

In 1869 George M. Beard suggested a common origin and the designation "neurasthenia" for a staggering variety of symptoms that had long taxed the ingenuity and the patience of physicians. A pioneer specialist in neurology, Beard made his reputation in New York City by treating the functional nervous disorders, that is, those for which no gross pathology could be found.[1] Neurasthenia was one of these, a disease characterized by profound physical and mental exhaustion. It was also a protean condition that might attack any organ or function. Its characteristic symptoms included sick headache, noises in the ear, atonic voice, deficient mental control, bad dreams, insomnia, nervous dyspepsia, heaviness of the loin and limb, flushing and fidgetiness, palpitations, vague pains and flying neuralgia, spinal irritation, uterine irritability, impotence, hopelessness, and such morbid fears as claustrophobia and dread of contamination.[2]

To a modern observer, as to a contemporary critic, Beard appears to have "greatly overloaded his subject."[3] But by suggesting a common pathology, prognosis, history, and treatment for such varied behavioral attributes, Beard was attempting to bring order to the chaotic field of the functional nervous disorders. In the absence of clear anatomical changes, or hard and fast tests, such conditions not only tested the physician's diagnostic skills, but invited the disbelief of friends and relatives. Beard acknowledged that neurasthenia was subjective, its symptoms "slippery, fleeting, and vague." But he insisted that it was as real a disease, with as genuinely somatic a course, as smallpox or cholera. "In strictness," he wrote, "nothing in disease can be imaginary. If I bring on a pain by worrying, by dwelling on myself, that pain is as real as though it were brought on by an objective influence."[4]

Beard had not discovered a new disease, as even he acknowledged. But until his premature death in 1883, he labored to secure for neurasthenia an honored place in the medical lexicon. Motivated in part by personal need — he had wrestled with the symptoms of the disease in his youth — Beard was able to transform his own struggles into a disease syndrome that struck a responsive chord among his contemporaries. By interpreting diverse physical and mental symptoms as the common consequence of an excessive expenditure of nervous energy, he brilliantly blended scientific theories about the nature of the nervous impulse, the conservation of energy, and biological evolution into a plausible disease entity.

Beard defined neurasthenia as an "impoverishment of nervous force. . . . 'Nervousness' is really nervelessness." Physicians in the late 19th century believed that each individual possessed a fixed amount of nervous energy, determined mainly by heredity, which acted as a messenger between various parts of the body. Neurasthenia resulted when demand exceeded supply; even a tiny excess could cause the entire system to break down. Immoderate toil or worry, lack of food or rest, could induce an acute attack or even a chronic condition. The exhaustion of any one bodily system — the brain, for instance — could by the principle of reflex irritation spread to the reproductive and digestive systems, causing a total breakdown. Two popular metaphors — the overloaded electrical circuit and the overdrawn bank account — graphi-

---

BARBARA SICHERMAN is editor of the Supplement to *Notable American Women*, Radcliffe College, Cambridge, Massachusetts.

Reprinted with permission from the *Journal of the History of Medicine and Allied Sciences*, 1977, *32*: 33–54.

cally illustrated the process for layman and physician alike.[5]

Just as physicians considered nervous energy limited, they believed that contemporary society placed inordinate demands on that supply. The dynamism of the Gilded Age, so welcome in other respects, thus became a source of social and psychological as well as physical stress. Beard drew on evolutionary theory to support his belief that nervousness was peculiarly an American phenomenon. In his long list of causes, he gave special attention to the periodical press, steampower, the telegraph, the sciences, and the increased mental activity of women. By encouraging men and women to experience life more fully, these five characteristic features of 19th-century civilization — most advanced in America — placed too many demands on their limited supplies of nervous energy. Civilized society also demanded repression of the emotions, a refinement from which savages were exempt, and thus additionally drained human energies.[6]

Beard thought his work had initially been ignored, but by 1880 he contended that the subject "after long standing and waiting at the doors of science, has, at last, gained admission." A large popular and technical literature supported his claim. A tract by S. Weir Mitchell, the Philadelphia neurologist who developed the rest cure for neurasthenia, choicely titled *Wear and Tear*, sold out in ten days and went through five editions between 1871 and 1881; his *Fat and Blood* did even better. In the late 1880s a *Journal of Nervous Exhaustion* appeared briefly. And in the 1890s, two Shattuck lecturers, charged with enlightening members of the Massachusetts Medical Society on diseases prevalent in the Commonwealth, chose neurasthenia as their subject. When Beard's one-time partner, A. D. Rockwell, brought out a new edition of Beard's treatise for physicians in 1901, he noted that "neurasthenia is now almost a household word." Whether accurate or not, he continued, the diagnosis proved "often as satisfactory to the patient as it is easy to the physician."[7]

Even as Rockwell wrote, Beard's classic formulation of neurasthenia as a syndrome characterized by a deficiency of energy had begun to break down. The diagnosis had become so widespread, its use so imprecise, that many physicians believed it had outlived its usefulness. One called it the newest garbage can of medicine.[8] No longer able to provide a coherent explanation for the symptoms it had once readily encompassed, neurasthenia lost ground in the first two decades of the 20th century both to demonstrably organic ills and to conditions increasingly assumed to be of psychological origin. New diagnostic tests made it possible to distinguish a number of conditions characterized by exhaustion, among them anemia, pulmonary tuberculosis, incipient paresis, lead poisoning, and Addison's disease together with other endocrine disorders.[9] Just as the diagnosis fever had earlier given way to more precise formulations, so exhaustion came to be viewed less as an essence than as a symptom.

A preference for psychological interpretations of the psychoneuroses was also apparent by 1900, a consequence mainly of the discovery of unconscious mental states. Pioneer psychopathologists like Pierre Janet and Sigmund Freud proposed psychodynamic interpretations of many physical and psychological symptoms formerly assumed to be of somatic origin. Thus Janet substituted the term *psychasthenia* for neuroses in which obsessions and phobias predominated. He attributed these to reduced psychic energy and discarded neurasthenia because he found no evidence of any physiological etiology. Freud retained the term, but wished to limit it to the relatively infrequent cases of physical exhaustion brought on by masturbation or nocturnal emissions. He considered it an actual neurosis as distinct from the more common psychoneuroses that psychoanalysis did so much to elucidate.[10] American physicians debated these concepts and, although some still accorded neurasthenia a limited place, Beard's earlier synthesis was effectively demolished by 1920.[11]

In retrospect it is clear that what was called neurasthenia actually comprehended a range of conditions that included depressive, obsessive, and phobic states later classified as psychoneuroses; mildly psychotic and borderline states; palpable physical ills that could not then be adequately diagnosed; and a host of symptoms that are today considered psychophysiological. Leonard Woolf was quite correct when he called neurasthenia "a name, a label, like neuralgia or rheumatism, which covered a multitude of sins, symptoms, and miseries."[12]

This modern diagnostic nemesis has recently attracted the attention of historians precisely because it so neatly illustrates the interplay of scientific theory and cultural values in the fashioning of a disease entity. Concentrating on physicians' generalizations about the disease, scholars for the most part have considered neurasthenia within the framework of intellectual history. The best of these studies securely anchors Beard's work in the medical and social structures of the Gilded Age, taking seriously his now dated explanatory model as a measure of the intellectual temper of the time.[13] Others, unable to see past the colorful etiology of the disease, have claimed that the term *neurasthenia* "stood for conflicting . . . ideologies," and, on the patient's part, was "a reservoir of class prejudices, status desires, urban arrogance, repressed sexuality, and indulgent self-centeredness."[14]

However imprecise the label *neurasthenia* now appears, it is surely unfair to doctors and especially to patients to view illness purely as an intellectual construct. To ignore the clinical context in which disease is identified is to miss the distinguishing feature of medical practice. For it is in the consulting room, the hospital clinic, and at the bedside that the daily drama of diagnosis and treatment takes place. There the patient offers up the symptoms that have already caused sufficient distress to prompt the encounter. As a psychoanalyst reminds us: "For the patient illness is always an uncanny experience. He feels something has gone wrong with him, something that might, or certainly will, do him harm unless dealt with properly and swiftly. What 'it' is, is difficult to know."[15]

In what is frequently a highly charged atmosphere, the physician's primary task is to identify "it," to transform the diffuse symptoms of his patient into a condition that can be rationally understood and treated. To such an encounter each party brings his own preconceptions about illness, expectations of the other, and more or less enduring personality traits, shaped by class and social position as well as individual need. If the physician fails to make sense of the patient's troubles — or to relieve them — neither he nor his patient will retain much confidence in his skill. If the interpretation is unacceptable, the patient may take his business elsewhere.

In the late 19th century, neurasthenia proved a satisfactory label to doctors and patients alike. By incorporating into a disease picture a host of behavioral symptoms, many of which would otherwise have been deemed self-willed and thus deviant, the diagnosis legitimized new roles for physicians and their patients. For patients, it provided the most respectable label for distressing, but not life-threatening, complaints, one that conferred many of the benefits — and fewest of the liabilities — associated with illness. Certainly it was preferable to its nearest alternatives — hypochondria, hysteria and insanity, not to mention malingering.

At a time when psychiatry was limited to the institutional care of psychotic patients, those who specialized in the functional nervous disorders were actually providing psychiatric services for many patients. Thoughtful clinicians understood that deep-rooted personality needs often influenced the onset of an illness, and that the relationship between doctor and patient affected the patient's capacity to recover. Although their suspicion of psychology kept them from exploring this relationship fully, physicians sometimes acknowledged that they ministered to the soul as well as the body. As confessors, they concerned themselves with all aspects of the patient's behavior. Neurasthenia was thus an important chapter in the expansion of the medical sphere that has characterized modern American society.

As a diagnosis on the borderland of medicine and psychiatry, neurasthenia augmented therapeutic approaches in both fields. Medicine had reached an ambiguous stage when the disparity between actual achievement and future promise was especially great. Scientists, by correlating clinical and pathological data, had identified the basic diseases in modern form by mid-century. As typhus and malaria replaced the symptomatic designation fever, it became possible to search for pathogenic microorganisms. The first such organism was identified in 1876, but two decades elapsed before the great medical discoveries yielded practical results. In the meantime, death rates remained high and the art of therapeutics perilously low. Recognizing that there were few specific remedies, medical leaders repudiated many traditional therapies as unavailing or positively harmful. This therapeutic nihilism, although an advance over the heavy drugging of the past, left the practitioner in a peculiarly vulnerable position. For, as the authors of guides for aspiring physicians noted, patients expected medicines and even specific courses of treatment. If they did not receive them from members of the regular profession, they might patronize adherents of medical sects who still offered a holistic view of disease, or one of the numerous vendors of patent medicines.[16]

The laboratory cast of mind of professional leaders at the end of the century further highlighted the practitioner's impotence. In this era of extreme somaticism, a respectable disease required a specific and identifiable etiology, pathology, and therapy. The discovery that microorganisms caused specific diseases contributed to this outlook. So did insistence on a localized pathology exemplified in Rudolf Virchow's famous dictum: "There are no general diseases . . . only diseases of organs and cells." In their efforts to make medicine an exact science the most prominent physicians often overlooked — and certainly underrated — the importance of clinical medicine. Their emphasis on basic research in chemistry, bacteriology, and anatomy, so productive in other respects, did little to help either the ambitious practitioner or the anxious patient in their mutual quest.[17]

Neurasthenia offered the practitioner a way out of this therapeutic dilemma. The new label, with its implied precision, emphasized what physicians could do for their patients rather than their impotence. At a time when physicians felt comfortable only with clearly organic disorders, a diagnosis of neurasthenia permitted some to address themselves to less tangible clinical issues and to provide an essentially psychological therapy under a somatic label. The diagnosis and its treatment helped physicians to justify a traditional role, threatened by the one-sided emphasis on science, of providing advice and comfort to patients and their families. In view of the impoverished state of medical therapeutics in the late 19th century, this was by no means an insignificant achievement.[18]

Conditions of weakness had long been known to physicians by a variety of names, among them debility. But the emphasis on weakness of the nerves coincided with the rise of neurology as a medical specialty in the years after the Civil War. Knowledge of the brain and nervous system advanced rapidly in Europe after 1860 as experimental physiologists demonstrated that fixed parts of the brain controlled specific motor activities. Important clinical advances, especially J. Hughlings Jackson's work on epilepsy and Jean-Martin Charcot's delineations of several classic neurological disorders, followed. By the late 1860s, important teaching and hospital positions in neurology had been established in England, France, and the German-speaking world, a sign that the specialty had come of age.[19]

Beard and Mitchell belonged to the pioneer generation of physicians who established neurology on a firm professional footing in the United States. Concentrated in large cities on the eastern seaboard and Chicago, they began in the 1870s to found the journals and societies that constitute the core of a professional identity. In their bid for recognition, the neurologists encountered resistance from general practitioners opposed to specialization of any kind, and outright hostility from the medical superintendents of asylums for the insane who since the 1840s had claimed exclusive authority over the care of the mentally ill. At a time when all experts considered insanity a disease of the brain, neurologists legitimately claimed competence in the field of mental as well as neurological disorders. But because the two fields had developed separately in the United States, ambitious young specialists like Beard found it necessary to challenge what amounted to the superintendents' monopoly in caring for the mentally ill. Rivalry between competing specialists was particularly intense during the 1870s and 1880s. In the struggle for professional status and monetary rewards, neurasthenia helped the neurologists build up their clienteles. Since the organic nervous disorders were relatively rare, specialists welcomed patients with less tangible ills who crowded their waiting rooms. Some earned sizable fees for this work; Weir Mitchell reputedly made $70,000 in a good year, much of it in consulting fees.[20]

Professional needs help to explain the advantage of a new diagnosis. But to discern how and why neurasthenia was used, one must turn from the institutional to the clinical setting. The typical neurasthenic patient presented the physician with a rich variety of symptoms. A diagnosis by exclusion, neurasthenia could be established only after a thorough physical examination and appraisal of the patient's actual, as distinct from stated, discomfort had ruled out any other condition. (Beard once listed 48 ailments with which it might be confounded.[21]) Once satisfied that the patient had no organic disease, the physician must decide what label to attach to the condition.

Neurasthenia had most often to be distinguished from hysteria and hypochondria, the other major functional nervous disorders. Hysteria, long the most frequent nervous disease of women, had become in Weir Mitchell's view "the nosological limbo of all unnamed female maladies. It were as well called mysteria." The typical hysteric manifested bizarre symptoms — convulsive fits, trances, choking, tearing the hair, and rapid fluctuations of mood. Where languor characterized the neurasthenic, Beard considered "acuteness, violence, activity, and severity" the essence of hysteria. Moral considerations as well as the physician's empathy for particular patients undoubtedly influenced diagnostic decisions in ambiguous cases. Where neurasthenics seemed deeply concerned about their condition and eager to cooperate, hysterics were accused of evasiveness — *la belle indifférence* — and even intentional deception. Physicians sometimes contrasted the hysteric's lack of moral sense with the neurasthenic's refined and unselfish nature. "The sense of moral obligation [in the hysteric] is so generally defective as to render it difficult to determine whether the patient is mad or simply bad." By contrast, patients suffering from "impaired vitality" were "of good position in society . . . just the kind of women one likes to meet with — sensible, not over sensitive or emotional, exhibiting a proper amount of illness . . . and a willingness to perform their share of work quietly and to the best of their ability."[22]

Hypochondria had been the most common diagnosis for men with ill-defined complaints. Once a medically respectable disease, by the 1870s hypochondriasis had acquired the connotation of an imaginary illness. Neurasthenics and hypochondriacs both displayed inordinate interest in the vagaries of their bodies, but physicians considered the former more often the victims of circumstances, or lack of prudence, while the difficulties of the latter, if not dismissed entirely, appeared to be distinctly self-induced.[23]

Although 19th-century physicians and historians alike have written at length about women's ill health, the subject of illness in men has been neglected.[24] Yet neurasthenia seems to have been a particularly useful label for men. If women were sometimes expected, and perhaps even encouraged, to be weak and sickly, an ethos of fortitude made it difficult for men to exhibit weakness of any kind. Illness, in all its presumed objectivity, was one of the permissible exceptions. It is significant, therefore, that several physicians — mistakenly — considered neurasthenia a male disease, a striking assertion at a time when the profession rarely lost an opportunity to decry the ill-health of American women.[25] While acknowledging that neurasthenia afflicted women more often than men, Beard was especially eager to legitimize it as a diagnosis for men. He insisted that hypochondria, which he defined as "groundless fear of disease," was extremely rare; the label too often covered the diagnostician's failure to detect the real trouble.[26]

Neurasthenia then was the diagnosis of choice for men and women whose diffuse symptoms might otherwise have been dismissed as hypochondria or hysteria. As a new diagnosis, neurasthenia escaped the pejorative connotations associated with its nearest alternatives. Doctors had often suffered from neurasthenia themselves — Beard estimated that physicians constituted one-tenth of his clientele — and empathized with similarly distressed patients.[27] Certainly many of its putative causes — overwork or the too solicitous care of sick relatives — resulted from an excess of essentially admirable traits.

Neurasthenia was also preferable to a diagnosis of insanity, then considered an incurable disease. Despite their rivalry, American neurologists and superintendents agreed with Beard that neurasthenia was "the door that opens into so many phases of mental disease." It was a warning signal, which, if unheeded, might lead from a temporary physical breakdown to a permanent state of melancholia. Edward Cowles, the influential superintendent of McLean Asylum, went so far as to suggest in his Shattuck lecture of 1891 that "all people of previously sound health and constitutions, who become insane with ordinary functional mental disorders, have their psychoses dependent upon neurasthenic conditions of the organism."[28]

Neurasthenics suffered from many of the symptoms of those hospitalized for insanity, including loss of mental control, depression, morbid fears, and obsessions. Presumably the persistence and severity of these symptoms helped to separate the insane from the neurasthenic, but diagnostic criteria were by no means clear. Class considerations, the tolerance of physicians for particular symptoms, and the ability of family members to care for patients undoubtedly influenced diagnostic decisions, then as now. Like Virginia Woolf, an upper-class patient suffering from hallucinations and severe feeding disorders might frequently be diagnosed as neurasthenic.[29] An individual with similar problems, but fewer financial resources and less loyal family and friends, might have been declared insane and placed in an asylum. Given the importance of the therapist's expectations on the patient's chances of recovery, the more optimistic diagnosis may have kept some individuals who would today be considered schizophrenic or borderline from long hospital stays and possible deterioration.[30]

Class prejudice undoubtedly influenced the attitudes of upper- and middle-class patients and their physicians toward the asylums, as the rhetorical query of one neurologist suggests: "Should the psychical symptoms of instability, distrust, and confusion of mind be used as an excuse for, and can such a condition be most effectively combated by, sending such a delicate, sensitive, nervous invalid to an insane asylum? We think not." But at a time when public hospitals suffered from overcrowding, understaffing, and low recovery rates, treatment at home or in one of the new nerve retreats was the rational choice for those who could afford it. Such individuals could also escape the stigmatizing label of insanity. For even after recovery, formerly hospitalized patients often continued to be reminded that they had been "crazy a number of years ago."[31]

Many late 19th-century physicians accepted Beard's generalization that neurasthenia was principally a disease of the "comfortable classes." Like Beard, their patients were probably drawn largely from the business and professional classes in large cities. Those with diverse clienteles reached other conclusions. In 1869, the year Beard published his first article on the subject, a superintendent in Michigan independently discovered neurasthenia — and so labeled it — in the hardworking farm women near his hospital. To his surprise, Weir Mitchell diagnosed it in such unlikely victims as working-class male clinic patients. By the early years of the 20th century, neurasthenia had become the most frequent diagnosis of the working-class patients who attended the neurological outpatient clinics at Boston City and Massachusetts General Hospitals. The deficient energy syndrome could be applied to the most varied individuals, and was not just a euphemism for serious mental illness in middle-class patients.[32]

It would appear that age and marital status had more to do with the disease, or at least with the diagnosis, than either class or sex. Many neurasthenic patients were young and single. In one study of 333 neurasthenics, two-thirds were between the ages of 20 and 40, with the incidence highest among those 20 to 30 and the average age 33.3. Almost one-third of the women and over two-fifths of the men were single, a figure no doubt partly related to their age.[33] Observing the relationship between neurasthenia and young adulthood, Beard noted that the "dark valley of nervous depression" often disappeared between the ages of 25 and 35. Once cured, the former sufferer went on to a "healthy and happy maturity."[34]

Beard spoke from personal experience. Between the ages of 17, when he completed his preparatory course at Phillips Andover Academy, and 23, when he graduated from Yale, Beard suffered from ringing in the ears, pains in the side, acute dyspepsia, nervousness, morbid fears, and "lack of vitality." His journal reveals a young man beset by religious and vocational indecision. Reared in an austere and religious family that rejected drinking and smoking and warned its children of the snares of worldly success, Beard chastized himself for his coldness and "hanging back" in religious matters. Health and joy finally came with his decision to become a physician (which was equally a rejection of the ministry, the occupation of his father and two brothers). Beard entered medicine with a passionate commitment to medical and hygienic reform. By this time, too, he had begun to enjoy the worldly pleasures of champagne and Turkish tobacco, and soon after became engaged. His recovery seems to have been permanent. A minister who knew Beard in later life described him as a man who "put courage, hope, strength into one's heart, and his atmosphere was always healthy. He did not gush with over-warmth, or freeze with over-cold."[35]

In conjunction with other case materials, Beard's experience suggests that for many middle-class men and women neurasthenia incorporated elements of today's fashionable identity crisis. Clearly individuals reaching maturity in the second half of the 19th century had no monopoly on the trials of establishing a satisfactory adult identity. But cultural imperatives may have made the task particularly problematic. Intellectuals who struggled to emancipate themselves from the introspective and gloomy religious teachings of their childhood often suffered acutely from the loss of faith that accompanied Darwinism, higher criticism of the Bible, and the growing authority of Science. In a society of changing and often conflicting values, the decline of spiritual certitude intensified feelings of isolation. Educated women struggled to reconcile their desire for independence with still potent family expectations that they would live out traditional female roles. For men, longer professional training and the desire to achieve a higher standard of living necessitated later marriages; prescriptions for "masculinity" often meant disavowing "feminine" emotional impulses. Both men and women encountered a sexual code that demanded purity in thought as well as in deed, restraint within marriage as well as abstinence outside it. But men were sometimes also expected to be rough and ready.[36]

William James is a good example of a Victorian incapacitated by psychosomatic ills, mental anguish, indecision, and an inability to believe. As a young man he developed digestive and eye troubles, weakness of the back, and a "feeling of loneliness and intellectual and moral deadness." He feared being alone in the dark, had morbid obsessions, and for a time felt continually on the verge of committing suicide. His family considered his condition hypochondriacal, but James claimed he was "a victim of neurasthenia, and of the sense of hollowness and unreality that goes with it." Relief first came with his decision to believe in free will. Of the same generation as Beard, James tried to reconcile science and religion, resisted determinism in both, and struggled to find a genuine vocation. He successively tried art, natural history, medicine, and psychology and did not commit himself to philosophy, his first love, until the age of 57. It has recently been suggested that James's intense relationship with his domineering Swedenborgian father complicated this struggle, and that his illness gave him a psychic moratorium and a legitimate reason for disobeying parental wishes. His symptoms subsided following his first professional position (at 30) and marriage (at 36).[37]

If men sometimes found it difficult to choose the right profession, educated women faced a dilemma merely by wanting to have a vocation. Those who chose to defy convention as well as those who gave up their aspirations might find life equally intolerable. Jane Addams has described the years of backaches, depression, and purposelessness that followed her graduation from college. She even consulted Weir Mitchell, with little benefit. She diagnosed her problem as an inability to find a practical way to fulfill the ideals she had acquired in college and a disinclination to follow the course favored by her stepmother, including marriage and the dilettantish pursuit of culture. For Jane Addams and, she believed, for others like her, the decision to found a social settlement and create a new kind of community proved immensely liberating.[38] Charlotte Perkins Gilman experienced a more severe breakdown following her marriage and birth of a daughter. Her vague but exalted hopes of helping mankind seemed threatened by these events, so inescapable a part of most women's lives. In her case, Mitchell's advice compounded her difficulties and reduced her to playing with a rag doll on the floor. Her symptoms finally abated when she separated from her husband and began to pursue an independent course as a writer and lecturer.[39]

Because evidence about sexual behavior is harder to come by than information about vocational and religious conflict, it is difficult to assess its role in neurasthenia. Beard for one was acutely sensitive to the difficulties that contemporary sexual mores posed for his patients. It is possible that he had personally experienced such stress, for shortly after his engagement he asked God's blessing for his spiritual interests. He went on to declare: "The most solemn and weighty of any experience with the exception of religious experience is the love life of a man."[40]

In his posthumously published *Sexual Neurasthenia*, Beard insisted that sexual complaints had been vastly underestimated as a cause of nervousness, in men especially. He believed that sexual desire, like neurasthenia itself, plagued the sensitive men and women of the middle classes more than those of phlegmatic temperament who lived and worked outdoors. Masturbation he viewed as a nearly universal practice, for women as well as men, and did not think it invariably harmful if not begun too early in life or indulged in too often. As for other sexual difficulties, such as impotence and nocturnal emissions, Beard advised his patients not to worry about them: "Live generously. Work hard. . . . As soon as convenient, get married, but at all events keep diligently at work." Most important, he offered reassurance: "*I have known personally of very many young men who have passed through difficulties of the kind and are now well and the fathers of healthy families.*" Perhaps it was advice of this sort that prompted the comment, by a minister-friend at the memorial service for Beard, that: "Many joy children were born of his kindly words and kindly deeds, while of sad ones there were none to moan."[41]

The self-study of a neurasthenic patient, herself a specialist in mental and nervous disorders, suggests some of the conflicts that must have been central to many neurasthenic individuals, particularly those who resigned themselves to lives of partial nervous invalidism. Written in 1910 with pre-Freudian innocence, *The Autobiography of a Neurasthene* by Margaret Cleaves is a classic study of unresolved dependency needs that were at least partly met by her long-term relationship with her physician.[42]

Dr. Cleaves describes herself as hardworking to a fault, so completely devoted to her patients that "they are my family and my friends. I have none other, and science is my mistress." Overwork led first to a "sprained" brain and later to a "complete crash," accompanied by the sensation of hot blood pouring into her ears, an inability to concentrate or to "bear a touch heavier than the brush of a butterfly's wing," depression, copious weeping, fears of going insane, and other typical neurasthenic symptoms. Learning to live within the margin of her slender nervous endowment proved difficult, but essential, for she suffered "utter lassitude of body," "weariness of mind," and a "sense of physiologic sin" from the slightest indiscretion, even an excess in diet. Social events proved particularly tiring, for she could not control them. Always she fought against her illness, which she took pains to distinguish from hysteria.

Between acute attacks she carried on her work. But even as she took pride in her ability to care for her patients, it is clear that she resented her responsibilities, particularly because there "was no one to look after [her] needs." She attributed her illness (which she considered constitutional) to feeding insufficiencies in infancy, aggravated by the death of her father when she was 14. Thus she notes that the too early arrival of a younger sister interfered with her babyhood by depriving her of milk. Upbraided throughout her life for her failure to eat, she attributed her later preference for milk products to this early deprivation. When she was acutely ill, milk was often her only source of nourishment. She thought of her father, a physician after whom she seems to have modeled herself, as her best friend and, following the death of the family's only son, tried to become her "father's boy." She must bitterly have resented his death, even as it devastated her, for she insisted that he would have protected her against the stresses and strains she encountered in later life. For years she had a recurrent dream of being a child cradled in her father's arms. The dream disappeared after her most severe breakdown, and she missed the comfort it had afforded her.

The patient was fortunate enough to find a sympathetic physician who cared for her for many years, often visiting her daily during her acute attacks. If he did not completely understand her condition — at least until he had himself suffered a neurasthenic breakdown — he was compassionate: "I told him all this tale of woe, of my past life . . . [and] laid bare my soul to my professional confessor." She depended on her physician greatly, and in times of special need on a trained nurse as well. When others responded to her needs, she reported: "It seemed worthwhile to have suffered for the sake of all this comfort." Her course of treatment — rest, limitation of activities, tonics, massage — was designed to replenish her meager supply of "neuronic energy." But given this patient's personality and her isolated life in New York City, the close relationship with her physician-confessor, by providing a substitute for other forms of intimacy, was obviously the crucial element.

The patient's struggles with her propensity toward invalidism were familiar enough to therapists, who insisted that each case required individualized treatment. Prescribing rest for one patient might be restorative, while for another with similar symptoms, it could be completely wrong. Clinicians thus recognized that the relationship between doctor and patient was often the most potent agency in effecting a cure. Given contemporary insistence that disease was an entirely objective phenomenon, they could not pursue such insights very far. Beard, for example, outraged fellow members of the American Neurological Association when he reported a series of experiments with "definite expectation" — what a later generation called suggestion — in which he cured patients of rheumatism and neuralgic sleeplessness by prescribing placebos. One colleague denied the existence of mental therapeutics entirely, a second considered it more dangerous than handling the most powerful drugs, while still another claimed that doctors had known about royal touch cures for centuries, but before practicing such deceits should "give up our medicines and enter a convent."[43]

The therapeutic guidelines of S. Weir Mitchell, member of Philadelphia's upper class and a popular novelist, proved less controversial. Mitchell first tried out the rest cure on Civil War soldiers suffering from acute exhaustion brought on by marching. He did not repeat it until 1874 when, despairing of any other treatment, he ordered an exhausted invalid to bed. He carried the principle of rest to what he later admitted was "an almost absurd extreme." The patient — a 95-pound invalid who had tried every available cure — was fed and washed by others, forbidden to read, use her hands, or talk. At first a maid even turned her when she wished to move. Mitchell subsequently systematized the treatment to include total isolation of the patient from the family, a trained nurse, a carefully regulated diet (often limited initially to milk), tonics for the nerves, rest, and massage. The treatment's success could be explained in the somatic terms so appealing to this generation, and Mitchell emphasized the benefits of building up the patient's fat and blood by this method.[44]

But Mitchell also appreciated the moral aspects of the rest cure. The separation of patients from the moral poison of their accustomed environments, especially the attentions of too solicitous relatives, was often an essential condition for recovery. Isolation also enhanced the physician's influence over the patient, which Mitchell considered of supreme importance: "The man who can insure belief in his opinions and obedience to his decrees secures very often most brilliant and sometimes easy success." Confidence in the physician produced "that calmness of trustful belief which alone will secure the rest of mind we want." At first he found it surprising "that we ever get from any human being such childlike obedience. Yet we do get it, even from men."[45]

The similarity between the rest cure — with its bland diet, lack of external stimuli, and complete dependence on the physician — and infancy is apparent. Indeed, the enforced regression may well account for its success. The rest cure permitted individuals who ordinarily survived only by desperate effort to remove themselves from daily life and to submit for a time to the attentions of a charismatic physician like Mitchell. The physician in turn imposed reciprocal obligations. During convalescence, Mitchell lectured patients on the value of self-control and used his by then considerable influence to exact a "promise to fight every desire to cry, or twitch, or grow excited."[46] The paternalism of this therapy may help to explain why Charlotte Perkins Gilman and Jane Addams — women who temperamentally rejected the subordinate role assigned to their sex — were among Mitchell's most conspicuous failures.

Clearly there was often a therapeutic fit between physicians like Beard and Mitchell who had mastered their own nervous crises and their neurasthenic patients, many of whom — like the doctors themselves — were from the middle and upper classes. But class was not the sole determinant of a physician's response to patients. A. A. Brill, one of Freud's earliest American disciples, described the rapt attention with which as a medical student he attended the clinic on neurasthenia: "In contrast to the psychotics, the neurasthenics inspired one with a sympathetic interest; they spoke feelingly about their symptoms and apparently wanted to be helped."[47] What more could a young physician, eager to be of service, ask of a patient?

The perception of pain, the significance attached to symptoms, even the symptoms themselves vary greatly, depending not only on individual personality needs but on class and ethnic patterns. Today middle-class individuals are more willing to consult psychiatrists and to discuss emotional problems. And, despite the somatic orientation of medicine in the late 19th century, articulate individuals like William James often considered their illness in the context of their search for a meaningful personal identity.[48]

Although working-class men and women may lack a vocabulary of psychological distress, they are by no means immune from the effects of emotional stress; indeed, today they tend to be more subject to psychophysiological illnesses than members of other social groups. Recent clinical and sociological studies also indicate that visits to physicians for minor symptoms are often prompted by such needs as a desire for reassurance, for a close relationship with someone, for sanction to escape onerous duties or conflicts — needs which are often intensified during periods of severe psychological stress.[49]

It is likely that also in the late 19th century many of the conflicts of less articulate individuals manifested themselves in the myriad of physical symptoms that constitute the central clinical picture of neurasthenia. Not only were working-class patients treated for neurasthenia in outpatient clinics, but they sometimes entered Massachusetts General Hospital (then primarily an institution for charity patients) for extended periods. Nor were physicians unsympathetic to such patients. Hospital case records were not devoid of moral judgments, but the individuals described as "stupid," "lacking gumption," or "intent on deception" were more often diagnosed as hysterical than as neurasthenic. Doctors carefully recorded the complaints of individuals who were run down or "unable to keep about" after overworking or an imperfect recovery from an illness. Patients might complain of sinking feelings about the heart, an inability to bear the weight of their own hands, seeing stars, sensations of smothering, and "bearing down" pains. Their physical symptoms included palpitations and shortness of breath and a rich variety of gastric complaints (anorexia, vomiting, belching, constipation). The interpretation of these symptoms was entirely somatic. An occasional entry reported a recent death in the family, but attributed the breakdown to excessive exposure to cold or rain at the funeral rather than to the psychological effects of the loss.[50]

What is most surprising is that cigarmakers, millworkers, seamstresses, and housewives received modified versions of the rest cure for weeks and even months. Like the middle-class patients seen in private practice, they received a variety of physical therapies — including tonics, bromides, cannabis, massage, and blisters over tender spots. Special diets ranged from milk, cream toast, and eggnogs to oysters, whiskey, sherry, and beer. The entry for a particularly frail woman read, "keep her quiet and stuff with food." The treatment seemed to work, for within three weeks the patient left the hospital much relieved, with the notation that "rest was apparently all that she needed." Many patients seemed to enjoy their hospital stays — one entry recorded a patient who "seemed disposed to remain indefinitely" — and a few kept their physicians informed of their latest symptoms after discharge. Since so many of these patients were single, it is likely that their illness and hospital sojourns provided some with psychological as well as physical care that they could obtain in no other way.[51]

During its brief reign as the national disease, neurasthenia gave physicians a rationale for diagnosing and treating many types of stress. Whatever the limitations of their construct, physicians like Beard and Mitchell pioneered in developing respectable therapies for patients with problems otherwise excluded by medicine and psychiatry. Although asylum superintendents maintained that neurasthenia might lead to insanity if not treated early enough, their isolation from general medicine and restricted conception of their role gave them no way of reaching men and women before serious trouble occurred. The rest cure and related therapies provided individuals with alternatives to inaction or incarceration.

During the first two decades of the 20th century the scope of psychiatry expanded almost beyond recognition. Physicians openly practiced psychotherapy in offices and in outpatient clinics in general and psychiatric hospitals. Some participated in prophylactic programs in schools, prisons, and industry. Most practitioners still worked in mental hospitals, but professional spokesmen insisted that psychiatry must concern itself not only with the psychoses but with "the smallest diseases and the minutest defects of the mind" and even with the efficiency of normal individuals. The new practitioner was "educator, preacher, sociologist" as well as asylum superintendent and dispenser of drugs.[52]

Specialists in the functional nervous disorders

had pioneered in the expansion of the physician's social role. Even by diagnosing neurasthenia, they were interpreting behavioral symptoms that some found morally reprehensible (an inability to work for no apparent cause, compulsive or phobic behavior, bizarre thoughts) as signs of illness rather than wilfulness. They thus legitimized the right of individuals with such difficulties to be considered, and to consider themselves, victims of disease, and their own right as healers, to treat them.

Beard went further than most in asserting the physician's obligation to become a power in society. He not only insisted that neurasthenia be taken seriously, but urged that the categories kleptomania, inebriety, and pyromania — all safely medical — replace the traditional moralistic designations of stealing, drunkenness, and arson. A rebel against the evangelical faith of his childhood, Beard relished the substitution of physician for priest as arbiter of social and personal mores. Mitchell, noting the similarity between the physician's role and that of the priest, also thought members of his profession more fitted to probe human character: "The priest hears the crime or folly of the hour, but to the physician are oftener told the long, sad tales of a whole life."[53]

So much attention to a disease that could easily have been dismissed as minor also reveals a changed attitude toward health and disease. Long before the popularization of psychoanalysis, physicians interested in mental and nervous disorders proclaimed the relativity of health and illness. One superintendent declared that "perfect health of mind is probably . . . exceptional." And an influential lay philanthropist went so far as to claim: "The question to be considered is, not whether such and such a person is insane, — that is, indisposed mentally: of course he is, more or less, like the rest of us, — but, *How much* out of health is he?" Many no doubt reached such conclusions on the basis of personal experience. A fictional physician drawn by Weir Mitchell — a self-portrait — noted that even "to the most healthy nature, at times [come] inexplicable desires, moments of unreason, impulses which defy analytic research, even brief insanities." To the extent that individuals considered such conditions mental aberrations rather than sinful thoughts, they would consult physicians rather than ministers.[54]

The relationships between symptoms and diagnosis, disease and culture, doctors and patients are inevitably complex. Any attempt to understand them historically must take account of the clinical context in which doctors and patients interact; certainly this must be the case for a disease as subjective as neurasthenia. The available clinical materials suggest that neurasthenia was a complex reality for the doctors and patients charged with interpreting puzzling mental and physical difficulties they did not fully understand. If the particular insights of late 19th-century physicians into the psychological and psychophysiological aspects of illness disappoint us, it is not altogether certain that we have, even today, found satisfactory solutions to conditions of this sort.

NOTES

Work on this article was greatly assisted by fellowships from the Radcliffe Institute and the Peter B. Livingston Fund. I am indebted to Phyllis Ackman, Martin Duberman, Nathan G. Hale, Jr., Dolores Kreisman, Charles E. Rosenberg, Barbara G. Rosenkrantz, Bennett Simon, and Martha Vicinus for their comments on earlier drafts and to Catherine Lord for research assistance. I also want to thank Dr. G. Octo Barnett and James Vaccarino for permission to use the medical records of the Massachusetts General Hospital, 1875–1900.

1 The best analysis of Beard's career is Charles E. Rosenberg, "The place of George M. Beard in nineteenth-century psychiatry," *Bull. Hist. Med.*, 1962, *36*: 245–259. See also Henry Alden Bunker, Jr., "From Beard to Freud: a brief history of the concept of neurasthenia," *Med. Rev. Rev.*, 1930, *36*: 108–114.

2 George M. Beard, *A Practical Treatise on Nervous Exhaustion (Neurasthenia): Its Symptoms, Nature, Sequences, Treatment*, 2nd ed., rev. (New York, 1880), pp. 11–85. See also George M. Beard, *American Nervousness: Its Causes and Consequences* (New York, 1881), pp. 7–8.

3 "The question of the existence of neurasthenia," *Med Rec.*, 1886, *29*: 185–186.

4 Beard, *Nervous Exhaustion*, pp. 85, 80.

5 George M. Beard, *Sexual Neurasthenia (Nervous*

Exhaustion): Its Hygiene, Causes, Symptoms, and Treatment, with a Chapter on Diet for the Nervous, ed. A. D. Rockwell (New York, 1884), p. 36; cf. pp. 61–62 and Beard, *American Nervousness*, p. 9.

6 Beard, *American Nervousness*, pp. 96–192.

7 Beard, *Nervous Exhaustion*, p. xix; Edward Cowles, "Neurasthenia and its mental symptoms," *Boston Med. & Surg. J.*, 1891, *125*: 49–52, 73–76, 97–100, 125–128, 153–157, 181–186, 209–214; Robert T. Edes, "The New England invalid," *Boston Med. & Surg. J.*, 1895, *133*: 53–57, 77–81; 101–107; Beard, *Nervous Exhaustion*, 4th ed., rev. and enl. A. D. Rockwell (New York, 1901), p. 3. Numerous references to neurasthenia may be found in the several series of the *Index-Catalogue of the Library of the Surgeon General's Office*.

8 Quoted in A. A. Brill, "Diagnostic errors in neurasthenia," *Med. Rev. Rev.*, 1930, *36*: 123.

9 I. S. Wechsler, "Is neurasthenia an organic disease?" *Med. Rev. Rev.*, 1930, *36*: 115–121; I. S. Wechsler, "The psychoneuroses and the internal secretions," *Neurol. Bull.*, 1919, *2*: 199–208; Edes, "The New England invalid," pp. 78–80.

10 On the shift in diagnostic styles, see Henri F. Ellenberger, *The Discovery of the Unconscious: The History and Evolution of Dynamic Psychiatry* (New York, 1970); and Nathan G. Hale, Jr., *Freud and the Americans: The Beginnings of Psychoanalysis in the United States, 1876–1917* (New York, 1971), esp. pp. 71–173.

11 See, for example, Charles L. Dana, "The partial passing of neurasthenia," *Boston Med. & Surg. J.*, 1904, *150*: 339–344, and G. Alder Blumer, "The coming of psychasthenia," *J. Nerv. & Ment. Dis.* 1906, *33*: 336–353. Widely used in World War I, the term *neurasthenia* largely disappeared in the United States by the 1930s and reappeared in the 1968 diagnostic manual of the American Psychiatric Association. See John C. Chatel and Roger Peele, "A centennial review of neurasthenia," *Am. J. Psychiatry*, 1970, *126*: 1404–1413.

12 Leonard Woolf, *Beginning Again: An Autobiography of the Years 1911 to 1918* (New York, 1964), pp. 75–76.

13 Rosenberg, "The place of George M. Beard." Cf. Chatel and Peele, "A centennial review," Bunker, "From Beard to Freud," and S. P. Fullinwider, Neurasthenia: the genteel caste's journey inward," *Rocky Mount. Social Sci. J.*, 1974, *2*, 1–9.

14 John S. Haller, Jr., and Robin M. Haller, *The Physician and Sexuality in Victorian America* (Urbana and Chicago, 1974), pp. 5–43.

15 Michael Balint, *The Doctor, His Patient and the Illness*, 2nd ed. rev. (London, 1964), p. 41. This work is an excellent introduction to the psychological aspects of general medicine.

16 Richard Harrison Shryock, "The interplay of social and internal factors in modern medicine: an historical analysis," in *Medicine in America: Historical Essays* (Baltimore, 1966), pp. 307–332; Richard Harrison Shryock, *The Development of Modern Medicine: An Interpretation of the Social and Scientific Factors Involved* (New York, 1947), pp. 248–303.

17 Cf. Erwin H. Ackerknecht, *Rudolf Virchow: Doctor, Statesman, Anthropologist* (Madison, 1953). For a critical view of the laboratory approach to medicine, see Knud Faber, *Nosography: The Evolution of Clinical Medicine in Modern Times*, 2nd ed. rev. (New York, 1930), esp. pp. 68–71, 76, 87.

18 On the ambiguities of medical practice in the late 19th century, see Charles Rosenberg, "The practice of medicine in New York a century ago," *Bull. Hist. Med.*, 1967, *41*: 223–253. [See pp. 55–74 in this book.]

19 There is no adequate history of neurology in English. But see Erwin Ackerknecht, *A Short History of Psychiatry*, trans. Sulammith Wolff (London and New York, 1959).

20 On early American neurology, see Charles L. Dana, "Early neurology in the United States," *J.A.M.A.* 1928, *90*: 1421–1424; Louis Casamajor, "Notes for an intimate history of neurology and psychiatry in America," *J. Nerv. & Ment. Dis.*, 1943, *98*: 600–608; and Barbara Sicherman, "The quest for mental health in America, 1880–1917," (Ph.D. dissertation, Columbia Univ., 1967), pp. 35–45, 231–239.

21 Beard, *Sexual Neurasthenia*, pp. 32–33; and Beard, *Nervous Exhaustion*, pp. 86–117. For contemporary views on this type of illness, see Gerald Chrzanowski, "Neurasthenia and hypochondriasis," in Alfred M. Freedman and Harold I. Kaplan, *Comprehensive Textbook of Psychiatry* (Baltimore, 1967), pp. 1163–1168, and David Mechanic, "Social psychological factors affecting the presentation of bodily complaints," *New Eng. J. Med.*, 1972, *286*: 1132–1139.

22 S. Weir Mitchell, *Rest in Nervous Disease: Its Use and Abuse*, in *A Series of American Clinical Lectures*, ed. E. C. Sequin, I (New York, 1875), 94; Beard, *Nervous Exhaustion*, p. 103; A. S. Myrtle, "On a common form of impaired vitality," *Med. Press Circular*, 1874, *17*: 375–376. Cf. Carroll Smith-Rosenberg, "The hysterical woman: sex roles and role conflict in 19th-century America," *Social Research*, 1972, *39*: 652–678; and Ilza Veith, *Hysteria: The History of a Disease* (Chicago, 1965).

23 Esther Fischer-Homberger, "Hypochondriasis of the eighteenth century — neurosis of the present century," *Bull. Hist. Med.*, 1972, *46*: 391–401.

24 Cf. Ann Douglas Wood, "'The fashionable diseases':

women's complaints and their treatment in nineteenth-century America," *J. Interdisc. Hist.*, 1973, *4*: 25–52; Carroll Smith-Rosenberg and Charles Rosenberg, "The female animal: medical and biological views of woman and her role in nineteenth-century America," *J. Am. Hist.*, 1973, *60*: 332–356; and Regina Morantz, "The lady and her physician," in *Clio's Consciousness Raised: New Perspectives on the History of Women*, ed. Mary S. Hartman and Lois Banner (New York, 1974), pp. 38–53.

25 See Joseph Collins and Carlin Phillips, "The etiology and treatment of neurasthenia. An analysis of three hundred and thirty-three cases," *Med. Rec.*, 1899, *55*: 413–422; and Paul Schilder, "Neurasthenia and hypochondria: introduction to the study of the neurasthenic-hypochondriac character," *Med. Rev. Rev.*, 1930, *36*: 165.

26 Beard, *Nervous Exhaustion*, pp. 96–98.

27 *Ibid.*, p. 80. Mitchell too suffered from neurasthenia. See Margaret C.-L. Gildea and Edwin F. Gildea, "Personalities of American psychotherapists," *Am. J. Psychiatry*, 1945, *101*: 464–466; and Anna Robeson Burr, *Weir Mitchell: His Life and Letters* (New York, 1929).

28 George M. Beard, "The problems of insanity," *Physn. & Bull. Medico-Legal Soc.*, 1880, *13*: 244; Cowles, "Neurasthenia," p. 50.

29 *The Letters of Virginia Woolf. Volume I: 1888–1912*, ed. Nigel Nicolson and Joanne Trautmann (New York and London, 1975), pp. 141–142.

30 The classic work on the relationship between social class and the diagnosis and treatment of psychiatric illness is August B. Hollingshead and Frederick C. Redlich, *Social Class and Mental Illness: A Community Study* (New York, 1958). Gerald N. Grob discusses the ways class, race, and ethnicity influenced treatment in mental hospitals. See *Mental Institutions in America: Social Policy to 1875* (New York, 1973), esp. pp. 221–256.

31 Edward C. Mann, "A plea for lunacy reform," *Medico-Legal J.*, 1884, *1*: 159; discussion of William A. Hammond, "The non-asylum treatment of the insane," *Tr. Med. Soc. St. N.Y.* (1879), p. 297.

32 E. H. van Deusen, "Observations on a form of nervous prostration (neurasthenia), culminating in insanity," *Am. J. Insanity*, 1869, *25*: 445–461; S. Weir Mitchell, "Clinical lecture on nervousness in the male," *Med. News Libr.*, 1877, *35*: 177–184. See also Cecil MacCoy, "Some observations on the treatment of neurasthenia at the dispensary clinic," *Brooklyn Med. J.*, 1903, *17*: 399–401; and annual reports of Boston City and Massachusetts General Hospitals.

33 Collins and Phillips, "Treatment of neurasthenia," pp. 413–422. My own research in Massachusetts General Hospital records reveals a similarly high proportion of neurasthenic patients between the ages of 20 and 40 and an even higher proportion of single patients.

34 Beard, *American Nervousness*, pp. 282–284.

35 Beard's case is discussed in Barbara Sicherman, "The paradox of prudence: mental health in the gilded age," *J. Am. Hist.*, 1976, *62*: 890–912. The quotation from the minister appears in *Sermon by the Rev. J. L. Willard, of Westville, Connecticut at the Funeral Services of Elizabeth A. Beard. Together with Comments upon the Life and Career of the Late Dr. George M. Beard* (Grand Hotel, New York [1883]), p. 4, in George M. Beard Papers, Yale University Library, New Haven, Conn.

36 In addition to works discussed in n. 22 and n. 24, see Hale, *Freud and the Americans*, pp. 24–46; and Charles E. Rosenberg, "Sexuality, class and role in 19th-century America," *Am. Quart.*, 1973, *25*: 131–153.

37 Cushing Strout, "William James and the twice-born sick soul," in *Philosophers and Kings: Studies in Leadership*, ed. Dankwart A. Rustow (New York, 1970), pp. 491–511; Erik H. Erikson, *Identity: Youth and Crisis* (New York, 1968), pp. 19–22, 150–155. Compare the similar case of G. Stanley Hall, the psychologist who later formulated the modern concept of adolescence, in Dorothy Ross, *G. Stanley Hall: The Psychologist as Prophet* (Chicago, 1972), pp. 309–340.

38 Jane Addams, *Twenty Years at Hull-House. With Autobiographical Notes* (New York, 1911), pp. 64–88, 113–127. Cf. Allen F. Davis, *American Heroine: The Life and Legend of Jane Addams* (New York, 1973), pp. 24–37.

39 Charlotte Perkins Gilman, *The Living of Charlotte Perkins Gilman: An Autobiography* (New York, 1975; originally published in 1935), pp. 78–106. See also her short story about the same events, "The yellow wall-paper," reprinted in *The Oven Birds: American Women on Womanhood, 1820–1920*, ed. Gail Parker (Garden City, 1972), pp. 317–334.

40 George M. Beard, "Private Journal," p. 217, Beard Papers.

41 Beard, *Sexual Neurasthenia*, pp. 102–103, 122, 119–120; Willard, Beard Papers, p. 4.

42 Margaret A. Cleaves, *An Autobiography of a Neurasthene. As Told by One of Them and Recorded by Margaret A. Cleaves* (Boston, 1910). Although presented as an as-told-to autobiography, this work is probably the story of Margaret Cleaves herself. Insofar as they are known, the facts of Margaret Cleaves's family background, early life, and professional career closely resemble those of the subject of the autobiography.

43 "American Neurological Association," *J. Nerv. & Ment. Dis.*, 1876, *3*: 429–437.

44 S. Weir Mitchell, "The evolution of the rest treatment," *J. Nerv. & Ment. Dis.*, 1904, *31*: 368–372; Mitchell, *Rest in Nervous Disease*, esp. pp. 94–96; S. Weir Mitchell, *Fat and Blood: An Essay on the Treatment of Certain Forms of Neurasthenia and Hysteria*, 5th ed. (Philadelphia, 1888); and S. Weir Mitchell, *Lectures on Diseases of the Nervous System, Especially in Women*, 2nd ed. rev. (Philadelphia, 1885), esp. pp. 265–283.

45 Mitchell, *Fat and Blood*, pp. 40–42, 47–49, 55–62; Mitchell, *Rest in Nervous Disease*, p. 84.

46 Mitchell, *Rest in Nervous Disease*, p. 94; Mitchell, *Diseases of the Nervous System*, p. 38. For a discussion of regression as a psychoanalytic technique, see Karl Menninger, *Theory of Psychoanalytic Technique* (New York, 1958), esp. pp. 43–76.

47 Brill, "Diagnostic errors in neurasthenia," p. 122.

48 Cf. Dewitt L. Crandell and Bruce P. Dohrenwend, "Some relations among psychiatric symptoms, organic illness, and social class," *Am. J. Psychiatry*, 1967, *123*: 1527–1538; and Mechanic, "Bodily complaints," pp. 1132–1139. See also William James's letters to James Jackson Putnam in the James Jackson Putnam Papers, at The Francis A. Countway Library of Medicine, Boston.

49 Cf. John D. Stoeckle, Irving K. Zola, and Gerald E. Davidson, "The quantity and significance of psychological distress in medical patients: some preliminary observations about the decision to seek medical aid," *J. Chron. Dis.*, 1964, *17*: 959–970.

50 The material in the next two paragraphs is drawn from Massachusetts General Hospital, Medical Records (East and West Wings), 1880–1900. See, for example, Vol. 381 (1885), p. 82, and Vol. 455 (1893), p. 124. For judgmental comments, see Vol. 349 (1880), p. 198; Vol. 381 (1885), p. 250. Charles Rosenberg informs me that he found similar material on working-class patients at Pennsylvania General Hospital.

51 *Ibid.*, Vol. 487 (1897), p. 42. One of these letters appears in Vol. 451 (1893), p. 56. The comment about wanting to stay refers to the same patient during a second hospitalization. Cf. Vol. 457 (1894), p. 306.

52 E. E. Southard, "Cross sections of mental hygiene, 1844, 1869, 1894," *Am. J. Insanity*, 1919, *76*: 109; Charles L. Dana, "The future of neurology," *J. Nerv. & Ment. Dis.*, 1913, *40*: 753–757.

53 George M. Beard, *Our Home Physician: A New and Popular Guide to the Arts of Preserving Health and Treating Disease* (New York, 1870), pp. xxi, 672; Mitchell, *Doctor and Patient*, 3rd ed. (Philadelphia, 1889), p. 10; cf. p. 6.

54 Peter Bryce, "The mind and how to preserve it," *Tr. Med. Assn. St. Ala.*, 1880, p. 260; Philip Garrett, "President's address," *Proc. Nat. Conf. Charities & Correction*, 1885, *12*, 20; S. Weir Mitchell, *Dr. North and His Friends* (New York, 1900), p. 389.

Practice

The colonial American physician, portrayed by Whitfield J. Bell, Jr., practiced medicine, performed surgery, and prescribed drugs. Some historians have argued that this type of general practice resulted from the democratizing effect of the New World environment on Old World distinctions that rigidly separated the duties of physician, surgeon, and apothecary. Other historians have pointed out that even in England such strict divisions of labor seldom held outside London; in the provinces medical practitioners performed all the healing arts. Besides, few members of the upper classes, to which university-educated physicians belonged, immigrated to the colonies. Thus medicine in America from the beginning fell largely into the hands of surgeon-apothecaries and others already accustomed to a mixed practice.

Most American doctors of the 18th and early 19th centuries lived in small towns or villages where they ministered to perhaps three or four hundred families. Although they frequently kept medicines, instruments, and a few books in an office at home, they conducted most of their practice in the homes of patients, visiting them on horseback with their supplies in saddlebags. Many physicians combined the practice of medicine with some other trade, like farming, since their professional fees seldom sufficed to support a family.

By the 1860s the practice of medicine was becoming more complex, especially in cities like New York. According to Charles Rosenberg, some urban physicians were beginning to focus their practice on one specialty, such as surgery or ophthalmology, and the best often saw patients in dispensaries or hospitals as well as in their homes.

The next half-century saw a revolution in the practice of medicine. First the telephone and then the automobile drastically reduced the hours spent on the road and allowed physicians to remain in constant contact with their patients. Most doctors closed their offices at home and opened ones "downtown," often in proximity to the local hospital, where much of their practice now centered. Some physicians gathered in groups, in imitation of the Mayo Clinic in Rochester, Minnesota, where equipment could be shared and responsibilities divided. By the 1930s almost one-half of all practitioners in the United States were at least partial specialists, and in large cities those in general practice were already a minority.

Within a few more decades solo practice virtually disappeared. Even general practitioners surround themselves with receptionists, nurses, bookkeepers, and technicians, to say nothing of colleagues. House calls became a nostalgic symbol of times past. Physicians no longer visited the sick; the sick visited physicians, who efficiently examined them in assembly-line fashion. As assistants multiplied and forms proliferated, many physicians began to feel more like managers than healers. In three hundred years the practice of medicine had evolved from a cottage industry into big business.

3

A Portrait of the Colonial Physician

WHITFIELD J. BELL, JR.

Unlike some of my predecessors in this series I cannot claim to have known Fielding H. Garrison; but I can — and do, most warmly — express my sense of grateful obligation to the Association for appointing me to this lectureship in his memory. In common with many others who have studied the history of medicine at any level, I cheerfully acknowledge my indebtedness to Colonel Garrison's published writings. Among the various subjects presented by Garrison lecturers in former years, there is probably none for which his *History of Medicine* or his essays do not contain useful information or helpful insights. About medicine in early America, to which, almost as an afterthought, he allotted a few pages at the end of his chapter on the Eighteenth Century, Garrison pronounced a chilling judgment: "There was no American medical literature to speak of until long after the American Revolution."[1] The dictum may well daunt anyone who proposes to speak on that subject and time; but it should also have the salutary effect of keeping him from uttering superlatives and making unwarranted claims. In confession and avoidance I can only plead my topic is not American medical *literature*, but an aspect of the American medical profession: I shall sketch a few strokes in A Portrait of the Colonial Physician.

Biographies of only a small percentage of the physicians of colonial America have been written in modern times, critically, extensively, using all surviving data. Of an estimated 3,500 practitioners in 1775,[2] all but a few hundred are only names; of that small number fewer than 50 are usually cited in any description of the profession in the 18th century. Textbooks are content to mention Zabdiel Boylston and Benjamin Rush; general social and cultural historians add half a dozen more — Mark Catesby, John Mitchell, Lionel Chalmers, Joseph Warren; men who were often distinguished as much for careers in science or politics as in medicine. Practically all the names in any discussion of medicine in 18th century America are those of men who obtained European degrees, practiced in larger towns, founded medical institutions, or played prominent roles in public life, and, generally, can be cited as evidences of the maturation of American society and culture.

To sketch the profession in terms of its leaders and of institutions like Edinburgh University, the Pennsylvania Hospital, and the New Jersey Medical Society, however, is to draw a partial and distorted picture. The historian-biographer should take into account the hundreds of practitioners in towns and villages and in the countryside on scattered farms, not graduates of Edinburgh or founders of some medical society, who, for better or worse, formed the great bulk of the profession, provided the greatest amount of medical care, and gave the profession its prevailing tone. The names of Redman, Shippen, Rush, Physick, Coxe, and Wistar shine brightly in any catalogue of Philadelphia physicians at the close of the 18th century; but two-thirds of the 85 physicians and surgeons listed in the city directory of 1800 were not members of the College of Physicians or graduates of any medical school, and they are today mostly unknown. Who were George Alberti, David Bertron, Arthur Blaney, Bernard Frexo, Nathan Norgrave, Isaac Sermon, Albertus Shilack, John Weaver, and, above all, Martha Brand of North Six Street, whose name appears not among the nurses, midwives, or surgeons, but as one of the physicians?[3]

WHITFIELD J. BELL, JR., is Executive Officer and Librarian of the American Philosophical Society, Philadelphia, Pennsylvania.

Reprinted with permission from the *Bulletin of the History of Medicine*, 1970, *44*: 497–517.

If it is misleading to describe the profession in colonial America in terms of only its most visible and articulate leaders, it is also deceptive to liken or contrast those leaders with the famous physicians in Europe. It flattered Philadelphians and Charlestonians to think their cities at the close of the colonial period were smaller Londons; but I submit there is no sound basis for comparing an American town of 30,000 inhabitants with the British capital with 500,000. The difference in size is a difference in kind. Philadelphia was not a lesser London, but a provincial center like Bristol, Manchester, Norwich, and Edinburgh, and bore somewhat the same relation to the capital that they did. The historian of medicine in the American colonial period, in short, should not only consider the careers of the nearly anonymous and almost forgotten physicians of the time, but also compare the profession in competence, organization, and reputation with the doctors of Essex, Norfolk, and West Country towns and villages.

Addressing a local medical society at Sharon, Connecticut, which had named itself grandly "The First Medical Society in the Thirteen United States of America," James Potter in 1780 presented a highly colored picture of medicine in America in the preceding century and a half. He recalled to his audience all the familiar scenes and characters — the "howling and uncultivated wilderness," the "inhuman barbarians" who patrolled the woods "seeking to imbrue their hands in English blood," the "terrisonous accents of stern Bellona" drowning out "the agreeable voice of medical learning." In these circumstances the sick must resort to "some ignorant person who had only a superficial knowledge of the medicinal virtues of a few barbarous plants." When, in time, the harsh tasks of settlement and survival were completed and the colonists got more doctors and European drugs, they found they were no better off. A more terrible scene now opened — doctors, thoughtlessly following some manual or system, dosed and bled without reason or restraint, until the unhappy patient was "sent as it were dreaming out of the world."[4]

Though Dr. Potter's rhetoric owed something to patriotic emotion and a need to measure the advances of his day by a past thought to be primitive and debased, his views were by no means unique. Dr. John Morgan, at the opening of the first medical college in the colonies in 1765, had said similar things in hardly less impassioned prose. Uneducated physicians, Morgan asserted, spread havoc "on every side," robbing husbands of their wives, making wives helpless widows, increasing the number of orphans, laying whole families desolate. "Remorseless foe to mankind! actuated by more than savage cruelty! hold, hold thy exterminating hand."[5] And the strictures of Dr. William Douglass of Boston still earlier in the century are well known: "In general, the physical Practice in our Colonies, is so perniciously bad, that excepting in Surgery, and some very acute Cases, it is better to let Nature under a proper regimen take her Course . . . than to trust to the Honesty and Sagacity of the Practitioner. . . . Frequently there is *more Danger* from the Physician, than from the Distemper. . . ." The mode of practice, a native New England physician told Douglass, was uniformly "bleeding, vomiting, blistering, purging, Anodyne, &c. If the Illness continued, there was *repetendi* and finally *murderandi*."[6]

Though many physicians were ill-trained, even untrained, there were a good many of them; the colonies were not quite so destitute of doctors as Potter described them.[7] In planned settlements a reasonably competent medical practitioner usually accompanied each first shipload of emigrants. At Jamestown Lawrence Bohune (d. 1621) was described by Captain John Smith as "a worthy Valiant Gentleman, a long time brought up amongst the most learned Surgeons and Physitions in Netherlands"; and he was succeeded by John Pott (d. *c.* 1642), "well practised in Chirurgerie and Physique, and expert allso in distilling of waters" (an art which helped undo him). Samuel Fuller (d. 1633) of Plymouth, "the first regularly educated physician that visited New England," and a deacon of the church, was called on to care for bodies and souls in Salem and Charleston as well as in Plymouth. At New Amsterdam was George Hack (fl. 1623–c. 1665), a native of Cologne who was said to have studied at the university of that city. Griffith Owen (1647–1717), who had practiced some time in Lancashire, came over with William Penn. These men, all among the first settlers, practiced medicine while they discharged a variety of civic functions and pursued private business interests, giving their neighbors as good medical care as was available in most of the villages of Britain and

Germany. Perhaps the standard of medical care was relatively higher during the first period of settlement, when strong religious and political forces might act on a well-trained physician, than a generation or two later, when pressures and inducements to come to America were weaker.

By the second third of the 18th century the colonies were all, if hardly thickly settled, at least firmly established. "The first Drudgery of Settling new Colonies," Franklin had pointed out in 1743, was "now pretty well over."[8] The arts and sciences and the professions and trades that promoted them were emerging into steady growth; and the beginnings of specialization were at least noticeable. Such qualities of maturity also characterized the medical profession, which now displayed what Potter called "the first physical aurora in this American empire."[9] Far from being simple and accommodated to what some have supposed was the uncomplicated state of colonial society, medical practice was almost as complex and its practitioners nearly as varied as in the oldest nations of Europe.

First in prestige, though not in numbers or always in influence (since the opinions of the large number of mediocre physicians in a sense outweighed the judgments of a smaller number of well-trained doctors), were the "regular" physicians. The term cannot be defined precisely — it connotes a combination of formal preparation, ethical conduct, and demonstrated success in practice. Certainly graduates and students of a medical college — Leyden, Edinburgh, or Philadelphia, for example — were considered as having been "regularly" trained. There was never a doubt in Boston that James Lloyd (1728–1810) was a regular physician, for he had served a good apprenticeship and followed that with attendance on the lectures of Cheselden and Hunter in London; while in Philadelphia Thomas Parke (1749–1835), who had only a bachelor of medicine degree from the College of Philadelphia but had studied at Edinburgh, was always "Doctor" Parke, a member of the hospital staff, and ultimately president of the College of Physicians of Philadelphia. American college graduates, like Robert Harris (1731?–1815), an alumnus of the College of New Jersey, who served an apprenticeship of three or four years, might also be ranked among the regulars, for, like graduate M.D.'s, they had some theoretical base for practice. Finally, in the ranks of regular physicians were admitted some who, without formal professional or undergraduate education, had nonetheless served a good apprenticeship and practiced some time to general approbation. The case of the elder William Shippen (1712–1801) of Philadelphia is illustrative: he was an apothecary in the 1730s, but, as he acquired knowledge and experience, he gave up his shop and limited himself to the practice of medicine, with the result that in 1753, now reckoned one of "the faculty," he was elected a physician to the newly founded Pennsylvania Hospital — the only one without a medical degree.[10] Needless to say, had Shippen still been the proprietor of the Sign of Paracelsus' Head, he would not have been chosen a hospital physician.

On the whole the regular physicians were fairly well organized. They recognized one another, called one another into consultation, and in general strove to raise the standards of the profession, which they were agreed were shockingly low. In the 1740s Boston physicians met regularly in a "Physical Club." At Edinburgh in 1760 Virginia medical students, looking forward to practice, formed a club for mutual improvement in anatomy which obligated its members to work for the reform of medicine at home. All the members of the Philadelphia Medical Society of 1766 were regular physicians (though not all the regulars were members of the society; but that is another story); and so were the New Jersey physicians who in the same year organized to raise the level of professional education and practice in that province.[11] Port and quarantine physicians were generally drawn from the ranks of regular physicians; and it was usually the regulars, like William Aspinwall (1743–1823) of Brookline, Massachusetts, who organized inoculation hospitals and took the lead in most measures for the public health.

Had there been doctors who limited their practice to surgery or midwifery, they would probably not have been accepted as regular physicians. In fact, of course, there were few such practitioners. Medicine and surgery were practiced by the same person, and he was acknowledged or rejected by the regular profession for reasons of education and conduct, not because of an arbitrary distinction. The distinction was, of course, jealously maintained in London; some British-born physicians sought to perpetuate it; and Dr. John Morgan wanted to establish it in America. But the proposal received little support. Even in Britain the separation of physicians and medicine from surgeons and surgery was not universally approved: Dr. John Gregory of Edinburgh denounced it as the source of much bad practice; and the book in which this sentiment was expressed was reprinted several times in the American colonies.[12]

For all that, some practitioners emphasized medicine or surgery without limiting themselves to it. A few, like Samuel Danforth (1740–1827) of Boston and James McClurg (1746–1823) of Williamsburg, simply had no taste for surgery — McClurg's biographer alludes to "the great delicacy of his nerves" — but others discovered they had a knack for the art, proved to be successful operators, and thereafter attracted more surgical cases than their brethren. They remained physicians nonetheless, unreservedly members of the regular profession. James Hutchinson (1752–1793) of Philadelphia was such a one. After graduating bachelor of medicine from the College of Philadelphia, on the advice of Dr. Fothergill who thought the city had enough physicians but needed a surgeon, Hutchinson studied anatomy and surgery in London; but on his return he practiced medicine as well as surgery and died prematurely, not of an infected surgical wound but of yellow fever caught from a patient. It was the same with midwifery. William Shippen, Jr. (1736–1808) of Philadelphia, James Lloyd (1728–1810) and his successor Isaac Rand (1743–1822) of Boston, and Hall Jackson (1739–1797) of Portsmouth, New Hampshire, made obstetrics something of a specialty but were never considered anything but regularly bred physicians and ornaments of "the faculty."

Below the regular physicians was the vastly larger number of practitioners who had studied medicine for a winter or two with a more or less reputable country physician or, motivated in various ways, had taught themselves medicine and set up as doctors. Thomas Green (1699–1773) of Leicester, Massachusetts, progenitor of a line of doctors, is said to have "received his first medical impressions and impulse" from a book given him by a British naval surgeon who was billeted at his father's and "took an interest in his [the lad's] vigorous and opening intellect." Young Green began practice in western Massachusetts with a gun, an axe, a sack, a cow, and a medical book; and, with the aid of that book and a knowledge of simples gained from the Indians, was soon able to treat the common maladies of his neighbors. However successful men like Green might prove to be, they seem to have had little professional esprit; indeed, living on the edges of the profession, sensitive to the limitations of their knowledge, they were a little inclined to scoff at the regular profession — though they usually saw to it that their sons who followed them into medicine got sounder training.[13]

For better or worse these men provided medical care of most kinds over vast areas. The best of them were conscientious, observant, devoted to their patients. They were not quacks; their common practice was hardly to be distinguished from that of the regularly trained; and in the end a few achieved more than local reputation. Dr. Alexander Hamilton of Annapolis, rarely disposed to think well of the medical practitioners he met on his gentleman's progress to and from Boston in 1744, was astonished to discover that Peter Bouchelle, "the famous yaw doctor" of Bohemia Manor, Maryland, was intelligent, knowledgeable, modest, and "not insensible of his depth in physical literature."[14]

Often practicing in the same communities with such doctors as these, sometimes offering the only medical care available in remote settlements, were the clerical physicians. A clergyman was usually drawn into medicine out of local necessity. He might be the only educated person within miles, the only one with a handbook of domestic medicine, and therefore the only one able to diagnose and prescribe with confidence. There were always some in his flock who could not afford the charges of regular physicians or might fall into the hands of unscrupulous quacks; and again the clergyman, moved by Christian compassion, offered his help. "Since doctors are few and far between," explained the Lutheran patriarch Reverend Heinrich Melchior Muhlenberg (1711–1787), who cared for the bodies as well as the souls of the rural Pennsylvania Germans, "I necessarily had to take a hand myself." Called to comfort the sick and dying, the minister sometimes found that a drug would help as much as faith. "I asked my dear colleagues to unite in prayer to God for his life and true welfare," Muhlenberg wrote of a visit to a sick man; "and in the meantime I prepared a few poultices. . . ."[15]

As practitioners of medicine, the clerical physicians should be considered along with other doctors. Some, with good training and wide experience, were in fact accepted as professional equals. The first president of the New Jersey Medical Society in 1766, for example, was the Reverend Robert McKean (1732–1767), rector of St. Peter's Church, Perth Amboy, a missionary of the Anglican Society for the Propagation of the Gospel; while the Reverend Jonathan Odell (1737–1818), of Burlington, New Jersey, was admitted to membership without examination, "being well known by many of the Society." Pastor Muhlenberg had acquired some medical knowledge during his student years at Halle; he regularly imported medicines from Germany and dispensed them freely among the sick poor of his extended parish. "Because . . . genuine *doctores medicinae* are rare in this country," he wrote, "I had to muddle through as best I could."[16] He respected the trained physicians in his neighborhood, generally calling them into any difficult case; and he had nothing but angry contempt for the empiricks, water-casters, and "quacksalvers" who gulled his people. He complained of the want of supervision of ministers and physicians alike. "We have only a very few properly educated and experienced doctors. Most of them are *empirici*, or at least *chirurgi*. The real *doctores* are not respected as they deserve to be, and are not used. The *empirici* are very busy and do a great deal of harm, for they are without supervision or order."[17] In the sickroom Muhlenberg performed with a resolute, no-nonsense attitude, even with a kind of grim humor, as when, summoned to offer spiritual counsel to a German physician or surgeon about to be hanged for receiving stolen goods, he called on the poor man to bear up and remember his anatomy — "death by strangulation was not much different from that by apoplexy."[18]

The combination of medical and spiritual advisor in one person held special risks. For one, the clerical physician found himself the recipient of all sorts of complaints and confidences — Muhlenberg once likened himself to a "privy to which all those with loose bowels come running from all directions to relieve themselves."[19] Another objection was that patient-parishioners were sometimes reluctant to pay the doctor's fees. Christ, they pointed out, had healed the sick and sent no bills; why should not His ministers follow that holy example?[20]

It is not easy to distinguish empirics of little or no training from failed physicians from Europe, runaway surgeons of ships, quacks, and near-quacks. John Hall, who hobbled into Philadelphia on crutches in 1758, claimed to have studied under a famous lithotomist of Bristol, served some years in British vessels on the African coast and in the West Indies, and practiced a while at St. Kitts.[21] Who were William Henderson, "Practitioner in Physick and Surgery," Hendrick van Bebber, and Hugh Graham, who practiced in Philadelphia in 1732? What, one wonders, were the real qualifications of the Dr. Ludwig who came to Philadelphia in 1775 announcing that he had studied physic and surgery "at the most renowned Universities in Germany" and practiced "in the best Hospitals and Infirmaries" and in the army?[22] Some of these men were probably itinerants, who provided a good deal of the medical care available in the colonies. Many of this tribe "specialized" in particular diseases, as did James Graham (1745–1794), who offered his services "in all the Disorders of the Eye and its Appendages; and in every Species of Deafness, Hardness of Hearing, Noise, Ulcerations of the Ear, &c."[23] We may judge the quality of the care they dispensed by the same "Doctor" Graham, for he soon returned to London, where, opening a temple of health and Hymen, he offered the services of a "celestial bed" to barren and other couples.

"Quacks," wrote William Smith in his *History of the Province of New York* in 1757, "abound like Locusts in Egypt, and too many have recommended themselves to a full Practice and Profitable Subsistence."[24] With no medical societies, no licensing laws, and limited confidence that the regular profession could effect cures, the colonies were a hotbed of autodidacts. Dr. Hamilton encountered such a self-starter on Long Island: he had been a shoemaker until, "happening . . . to cure an old woman of a pestilent mortal disease," he began to be "applied to from all quarters," and gave up cobbling for physic — which he had "practiced" several years with sufficient success.[25] Another self-starting medic was Philip George Sibble, the Anspach orderly to an officer billeted on Henry Drinker during the British occupation of Philadelphia in 1777–78: enticed by the prospect of a better life in America and the charms of the Drinkers' maid, he deserted, married the girl, and fled to Easton, Pennsylvania, where he set up among the Germans there as a physician and, in Mrs. Drinker's phrase, "sells medicine, and makes money fast, German like."[26]

Though they may not have made money fast, most regular practitioners in towns and larger villages appear to have had decent incomes; a few, by good economy and judicious investments, died rich. Country physicians usually lived on working farms — something Rush recommended for both personal and professional reasons: the produce would augment the physician's small cash income, while in his local character as farmer, he would more readily win the approval of prospective patients.[27] But country practice, Pastor Muhlenberg warned, was nothing for anyone unaccustomed to rural life — a townsman in such a situation would need some independent income to make ends meet.[28] On the other hand, ill-educated physicians, doctors in remote, poor, and sparsely settled areas, quacks, and itinerants resorted to a variety of expedients to eke out a living. Young Benjamin Franklin's friend, John Browne (1667–1737) of Burlington, New Jersey, kept a tavern;[29] some marketed a panacea or other "cure"; a few stooped to crime. The poor remuneration of most physicians may have been a reason why so many eagerly accepted public offices and military commissions with their cash fees and regular salaries.

Economics was not the only reason, however. Prestige was another. The practice of medicine in colonial America did not rank with the law or the ministry in the intellectual endowments it required or, therefore, in the social rank it conferred. The parents of Charles Jarvis (1748–1807) of Boston would have preferred that he study law, but they thought him too shy and diffident, and so sent him into medicine, where, in fact, he had a distinguished career. Similarly, Samuel Holten (1738–1816) of Danvers, Massachusetts, because of an early illness, could not attend college; but he could study medicine. The private knowledge of some doctors, that medicine had not been their first choice for a calling, understandably debased the profession in their own eyes. Not a few took up medicine after quitting the ministry, often for reasons of health, as did Joshua Brackett (1733–1802) of Portsmouth, New Hampshire, and Aeneas Monson (1734–1826) of New Haven, Connecticut, who had been a chaplain in the French and Indian War. The explanation is that whereas the ministry required long hours of study and writing bent over a desk, the practicing physician might look forward to healthful days making his rounds on horseback. It is therefore not entirely surprising that a good many physicians left the profession, temporarily or permanently, as soon as better opportunity offered. Holten quit medicine completely after 16 years of practice; William Bradford (1729–1808) of Bristol, Rhode Island, and Nathaniel Freeman (1741–1827) of Sandwich, Massachusetts, both took up law; and a good many, during and after the Revolution, abandoned the profession for public service.

How did these physicians conduct themselves in their professions and as citizens? What did they do? What did the leaders and spokesmen of the profession say they did, or should do? Which qualities and achievements were particularly mentioned by contemporaries, both colleagues and patients, as worthy of praise or censure? What kind of man, in short, was the colonial doctor? Some answers to these questions may be found in contemporary biographical notices and eulogies and in admonitory lectures to medical students and addresses to physicians.

Here several warnings should be uttered. In the first place, the surviving data are neither representative nor impartial. One would like to have biographies, or significant materials for biographies, for all, or at least a substantial number of, practicing physicians of the period; but they do not exist. In general, we know anything about only the successful, locally prominent, or otherwise outstanding physicians. In the second place, many of the available data even about these outstanding figures provide no answers to the more penetrating questions we have about the profession, such as why a man went into medicine, or what his professional income came to. Finally, many judgments and opinions about the profession which we can find do not apply uniquely to colonial America. Complaints about punctuality of attendance, for example, are made at every time and place; they may be found in the Roman satirists and are not unknown in the 20th century. All that one can do is point to those qualities which seem to have been uppermost in the minds of those who commented on the physicians of 18th-century America.

Medical students about to receive their diplomas were sure to be reminded, as young graduates always are, that they were only beginning, not concluding, their studies; that there was no substitute for the regular reading of medical literature, and that they must expect to spend laborious hours over books and journals if they would achieve success in practice and promote the dignity of the profession. Yet even as they addressed their hopeful juniors, the professors realized that few of the lads would ever own more than a shelf of books; that most of them would acquire skill in the profession, if at all, by experience and observation. Only here and there did a country practitioner manage to acquire a few professional works as they appeared. The fact that Joseph Orne (1749–1786) of Salem, Massachusetts, read European journals was so unusual that biographers commented on it with approval and astonishment.

Foreign physicians in America were sometimes noticeable because they pursued a scholarly interest, often to the neglect of practice. Thomas Moffatt (d. 1787), a graduate of Edinburgh, and John Brett (fl. 1740), who had studied at Leyden and had a degree from Rheims, liked to peer through their microscopes, make little experiments, and discourse with strangers on the order, elegance, and uniformity of nature as displayed in the texture of animate and inanimate bodies.[30] More often than not, however, too notorious an interest in reading and experimental science excited popular suspicions that the doctor was a "notional" man, not quite sound or reliable in practice; at best, the interest was cited in disapproving tones as a sample of exotic eccentricity.

Far scarcer than books were opportunities for post-mortem examinations. Whenever you lose a patient, Samuel Bard counselled in 1769, "let it be your constant Aim to convert, particular Misfortunes into general Blessings, by carefully inspecting the Bodies of the Dead, inquiring into the Causes of their Diseases, and thence improving your own Knowledge, and making further and useful Discoveries in the healing Art."[31] The advice was unexceptionable, but almost irrelevant, for opportunities almost never arose. Physicians in larger towns might occasionally examine the body of a criminal or suicide, but every project for more regular provision invariably evoked strong objections and even violent resistance. In the event, a physician who had ever examined a dead body at length, as John Bard (1716–1799) and Peter Middleton (d. 1781) did in New York in 1752,[32] was likely to cite the achievement to his credit thereafter and to gain reputation from it. But such post-mortems, though undeniably useful, were not so valuable as examining a deceased patient, as Bard had recommended.

Though reading medical texts and recording medical data were enjoined on the younger physicians and were usually mentioned approvingly by eulogists and biographers, too obvious a reliance upon texts in practice was something else. Far more praiseworthy was demonstrated capacity for accurate observations and sound thinking based on experience. Abner Hersey (1721–1787) of Hingham, Massachusetts, "never wearied his mind with theoretical investigation, but contented himself with simple practical observations." Of Benjamin Shattuck (1742–1794) of Worcester County, Massachusetts, his biographer wrote, "His knowledge was considerable, but his wisdom was superior to his knowledge. He knew much of the thought of other men, but was governed by a system formed from his own." Seth Bird (1733–1805) of Litchfield, Connecticut, was more distinguished for "acute sagacity, correct judgment, and talent at discrimination, than for learning or science"; his prescriptions were "simple, often inelegant, but always well adapted to the circumstances of his cases." William Douglass (*c.* 1691–1752), who had a Leyden degree, achieved an easy ascendancy over some young physicians of Boston by loudly rejecting formal systems and reminding his hearers that he had once called the great Boerhaave a mere compiler of books.[33] Empiricism, though a term of reproach among the learned, was, if successful, usually approved by the public, which liked its doctors to practice medicine with the same forthrightness they might bring to carpentry or farming.

Though medical care would probably have been better had physicians read and pondered more, it is also probably true that in some instances their professional skepticism and rejection of professional nonsense — at its worst, their ignorance of notions — was a salutary check on uncritical acceptance of untested theories and extreme systems of practice. Marshall Spring (1742–1818) of

Watertown, Massachusetts, who "was no book man,"

> appeared to learn more from the nature of the diseases of his patients by the eye than by the ear. He asked few questions. . . . He often effected cures by directing changes of habits, of diet and regimen. He used little medicine, always giving nature fair play. . . . He was . . . no friend to the profuse use of medicines, abhorred the tricks and mummery of the profession, used no learned terms, to make the vulgar either in or out of the profession stare.[34]

And Samuel Danforth (1740–1827) of Boston rejected bleeding when that procedure was everywhere strongly recommended: he believed it weakened the body's powers of resistance and had no effect on the disease.

Colonial American physicians do not appear to have treated the poor with much consideration or charity. At least medical students were so often adjured to treat rich and poor alike, deceased physicians were so often praised because they had done just that, that one must conclude that doctors gave scant thought to the plight of the sick poor. Ezekiel Hersey (1708–1772) of Hingham, Massachusetts, was praised, as were some others, because he had never sued but one person, and that for £ 8 for two journeys of more than 60 miles each and a serious operation. It was long remembered to his credit that on a cold, snowy night he had responded to a call to a Negro woman eight miles away, saying to those who would have dissuaded him, "Whether black or white, she is of the human family and shall have my assistance." In Philadelphia someone whom Benjamin Rush described as "a trader in medicine" constantly refused to attend the poor and, if called on to visit them, would drive the messenger from his door with angry curses.[35]

This attitude should not be too surprising, for 18th-century men were great respecters of persons, and gentlemen had little knowledge of, and less sympathy for, the poor. Boerhaave, Fothergill, and Cullen, Rush would remind his students, were often seen coming out of the hovels of the poor — an edifying sight that vastly increased the esteem in which they were held by the wealthy.[36] But the argument apparently convinced few. To many physicians medicine was a trade, and, like other tradesmen, they preferred the custom of those who paid well and promptly.

Physicians were notoriously skeptics in religion; some were irreligious, a few even atheists. Educated in the sciences, trained to look for causes rather than to contemplate a First Cause, less certain than the clergy that God was always wise and merciful, having a clear notion of what their own intervention had achieved, physicians did not readily accept all the orthodox teachings of the church. At their worst, they had an offensive confidence in their own powers: to a patient who replied to the question how he was, "Much better, thank God!" a doctor retorted, "'Thank God!' Thank me; it is I who cured you."[37]

Skepticism was tolerated in the latter 18th century, but in the orthodox reaction following the French Revolution, physicians with rationalistic, deistical views were apt to be regarded as "singular," "wavering," "loose and unsettled." Too active skepticism might even injure a man's reputation. Nathaniel Peabody (1741–1823) of Plaistow, New Hampshire, despite a distinguished career as a soldier, legislator, delegate to the Constitutional Congress, and speaker of the New Hampshire House, because he was a staunch republican and a "favorer of infidelity," died regarded by many of his virtuous neighbors as a "degraded character" — but in extenuation of this stern judgment it should be added that Peabody was also a great admirer and good judge of horse flesh and was once imprisoned for debt. Lemuel Hopkins (1750–1801) of Hartford, Connecticut, who admired Voltaire, Rousseau, d'Alembert, Volney, and other "infidel" writers, escaped condemnation because his character was otherwise irreproachable; he took up the Bible late in life and made a satisfying death. John Browne of Burlington, New Jersey, on the other hand, not only held, but propagated, unorthodox views — he parodied the Bible in doggerel verse — so that no matter what his professional competence might have been, he could hardly have expected to win much practice or personal reputation.

Many physicians were sensitive to the charge of irreligion, which they vigorously rejected in public, while in private accepting the criticism and offering in addresses to their fellow physicians and medical students elaborate reasons why a physician should be a believer. Rush, as usual, had a simple remedy: if physicians only attended church regularly, their religious faith would be sufficient. Even physicians who welcomed Sunday calls as an honorable excuse, could appreciate the economic and social benefits from regular church attendance. Rush went further still, taking the positive view that religious faith was an advantage in practice. It often supplied the want of professional skill, he advised; pious words from the physician were sometimes effectual where medicine failed. William Aspinwall (1743–1823) of Brookline, Massachusetts, gave religious counsel at the sickbed, as all clerical physicians did. "There is no substitute for this cordial in the materia medica," Rush declared firmly.[38]

A physician arriving at a patient's house after a long country ride in cold or wet weather was likely to be met at the door with a warming glass. John Green, Jr. (1763–1808) of Leicester, Massachusetts, "was never known to yield to the well-intended proffer of that kind of momentary refreshment"; but others were. William McKissack (1754–1831) of Bound Brook, New Jersey, became a heavy drinker in consequence of this country custom;[39] while James Hurlbut (1717–1794) of Wethersfield, Connecticut, was addicted not only to ardent spirits but to opium as well.

> He would not prescribe or even look at a patient in the last years of his life, till the full bottle was placed in his entire control, and daily replenished; it was his practice to take very frequently small potations, and at the same time swallow enormous quantities of opium. For many of his last years all the avails of his medical practice were expended in the purchase of this one drug; his spirits he obtained from his employers, which was a heavy tax, and he probably took as much opium as the most devoted Turk. He was rarely intoxicated, and when so much under the influence of alcohol as not to be able to stand, his mind would appear to be clear, and his judgment unimpaired.[40]

Though Dr. Hurlbut's excess was not typical of the profession, intemperance was. At least, older physicians constantly warned the younger against it. As late as 1826 David Hosack spoke out strongly on the subject, assuring his readers that the intemperate physician "under the influence of his daily inebriating potion" was "not a fancied picture." On one surviving copy of Hosack's address a proper Philadelphian penned a refutation. "I have never known a drunken physician in Pennsylvania," wrote Peter S. DuPonceau and then added significantly: "The possibility of the existence of a *drunken* Physician, should never have been admitted. It will injure this Country abroad and make foreigners believe that drunkenness is a common vice among our Medical Men."[41]

Except in times of epidemic, most physicians, especially those in small towns and the country, were probably not very busy; and their attendance on patients was marked by the same casual and leisurely pace that characterized rural life generally. Promptness and punctuality were unusual; at least they were constantly enjoined on young graduates by their professors and mentioned to the credit of every physician who observed them. Equally appreciated, wherever present, was a quiet manner, kindliness, and sensitive feeling for the patient and his family. Not a few practitioners, since they had not had the advantage of genteel rearing or of a college education, seem to have been rough, coarse, and abrupt; some even cultivated such a manner. Rush cited one physician who, being called to attend a very sick man, was urged to hurry because the patient was dying. "Then I can do him no service," the doctor replied. "Let him die, and be damned."[42] Vulgar, offensive, unmannerly were adjectives often applied to practitioners by those who had been better bred; we can only guess what their patients must have thought of them.

Professions have their badges and regalia; and physicians were no different from others. London practitioners affected large wigs and gold-headed canes, often bore themselves in a ridiculously stately manner, and spoke with absurd solemnity. Though there was less of this sort of thing in America, the tendencies were there, and Rush and others warned their students against them. Singularity in dress, manners, and speech, Rush declared, was "incompatible with the simplicity of science, and the real dignity of physic. There is more than one way of playing the quack."[43] There was indeed. Benjamin Waterhouse carried a gold-headed cane, but that was at the end of his life. A physician whom Dr. Hamilton met at Wrentham, Massachusetts, dressed outlandishly in a weatherbeaten black wig, an old striped collimancoe banian, an antique brass spur on his right ankle, and a pair of thick-soled shoes tied with points[44] — but this was probably New England eccentricity rather than a claim to professional notice; as was the behavior of Samuel Savage (1748–1831) of Barnstable on Cape Cod, who on the approach of the stage used to clamber atop a large boulder at the entrance to the village and cry out that he was a physician and surgeon.

The most important event in the life of every physician alive in 1755 was the American Revolution. Colonel Garrison declared that it was "the making of medicine in this country."[45] Like the French and Indian War before it, the Revolution afforded apprentices and young doctors an exceptional school of experience; it brought them into association with better trained men, inspired some to undertake further study — surgeon's mates were released from duty during the winter to attend medical lectures at Philadelphia — and provided observant physicians with materials for the medical communications that would at last make American medical literature, in Garrison's phrase, worth speaking about. The war and the efforts thereafter to establish and maintain effective governments also offered opportunities for profit, promotion, and new careers. It was perhaps to be expected that the great majority of physicians should support independence sooner or later. Those who did not, unless they made themselves singularly obnoxious, were generally unmolested or, if proscribed, were allowed, like John Jeffries (1744–1819) of Boston and Adam Kuhn (1741–1817) of Philadelphia, to return afterwards and resume practice. But it is a little surprising to mark how many neglected or abandoned their practices to answer to civil or military calls. In that republican era, of course, service to the state was the most urgent obligation of all; but the excitements of war and politics probably seemed more alluring in human terms than the humdrum of medical practice.

The doctors responded even before the first shots. Samuel Prescott (1751–1777) of Concord, Massachusetts, son and grandson of physicians, completed Paul Revere's ride. Next morning several doctors appeared on the battlefield between Concord and Boston, not as surgeons, but as minutemen carrying rifles. Many wished to continue to serve in the field, though most were persuaded to accept appointments in the military hospitals by none other than Joseph Warren (1741–1775) of Boston, who did not take his own advice and was killed with the fighting troops at Bunker Hill. Other physicians, like Edward Hand (1744–1802) of Lancaster, Pennsylvania, William Irvine (1741–1804) of Carlisle, Pennsylvania, John Brooks (1752–1825) of Reading, Massachusetts, Hugh Mercer (c. 1725–1777) of Fredericksburg, Virginia, and John Beatty (1749–1826) of Princeton, New Jersey, received commissions in the army and led troops in battle with success and distinction. Others, like the elder Josiah Bartlett (1729–1795) of Kingston, New Hampshire, who had been colonel of a regiment in the French and Indian War, served principally in civil offices: he was in succession a member of the provincial legislature, a justice of the peace, a delegate to the Continental Congress, chief justice of New Hampshire, United States senator, and governor of New Hampshire. Nathaniel Freeman of Sandwich on Cape Cod seems to have laid aside all practice for the duration of the war. Jonathan Elmer (1745–1817) of Bridgeton, New Jersey, known in medical-historical annals as a member of the first medical graduating class at the College of Philadelphia, preferred politics to practice and from 1772 onwards was almost constantly in public office. So was Thomas Henderson (1743–1824) of Freehold, New Jersey, who began as a member of the Monmouth County Committee of Observation on the eve of the Revolution, served in the war as an officer and thereafter in the state assembly, on the bench, and finally as a member of Congress.

The Revolution, Benjamin Rush wrote soon after the close of the war, "rescued physic from its former slavish rank in society." Certainly many doctors had demonstrated what they could do as patriotic men of affairs. Some were revealed as the natural leaders of the community, freer than the clergy to accept most kinds of public service. The popular esteem thus gained for the profession Rush was determined to preserve. He used to exhort his students thereafter to have "a regard to all the interests of your country," informing the nation about useful arts and seizing opportunities to diffuse useful knowledge and sound opinions of every kind. Doctors no less than others should speak out on public questions.[46] Rush himself exemplified his lesson. In time, however, as the profession became better organized and more respected for professional achievements, and as more persons of other professions came forward, the physicians dropped out of public life. Rush himself in his latter years confided to Hosack that he thought he had spent too much time in concerns outside his profession. And Hosack declared that the legislatures of the nation would be better off if physicians were barred from election to them.[47]

It would be reasonable to expect that the infusion of physicians into the legislatures and the courts of the new states would have benefited the profession. Ought not these doctors-turned-legislators have taken an informed interest in measures for the public health? Might they not have been expected to take a lead in, or at least give support to, enacting licensing laws and establishing standards of admission to practice? Ought it not have mattered in the councils of the state that they were or had been physicians? It does not appear to have done so. The explanation may simply be that most of the doctors in public service were not outstanding physicians (they were physicians who were otherwise outstanding); many had withdrawn from medicine into politics early in life; and, by the time they had power to do something for the profession, they hardly thought of themselves as physicians at all. The title "Doctor" signified a profession and for some a modest social position; it did not mean influence in the state medical society; and most of the medical statesmen preferred to be addressed, as soon as they earned the right, as "General," "Judge," or "Governor."

Despite its palpable effects and influence on American life and thought, the American Revolution hardly marks a clear breaking point in the conditions of medical practice and of the profession in America. Many physicians who had read medicine and begun practice before 1775 did not retire until the 1820s. Able and ambitious young men continued to go to London and Edinburgh and did so in greater numbers than before the war. Ill-educated physicians were as common after 1790 as before; ministers accepted responsibility for the sick; quacks flourished everywhere — and sometimes organized schools and issued diplomas. The same advice and warnings that Samuel Bard and Benjamin Rush gave their students were being given 40 years later by Hosack, John Godman, and others.[48]

Yet if the war itself had made little difference, time had. There had been no medical school in the British American colonies before 1765; at the end of the century there were several, and it was not unreasonable that the citizens of a long-established village should expect to be treated by a doctor with formal medical training. Medical journals were appearing and, thanks to improving postal service, physicians in even remote places could receive them. Medical literature in the 18th century may have been, as Colonel Garrison asserted, hardly worth talking about; but in the early years of the 19th century there would be the work and writings of Elisha Bartlett, William Beaumont, Daniel Drake, William E. Horner, Philip Syng Physick, Wright Post, Samuel G. Morton, Nathan Smith, John Warren, and Caspar Wistar — as well, of course, as of hundreds, thousands, of undistinguished, forgotten, but typical practitioners, the counterparts in 1820 of the Aspinwalls, Birds, Greens, Herseys, Ornes, Springs, and even Martha Brands of an earlier generation.

NOTES

Delivered as the Fielding H. Garrison Lecture at the 42nd annual meeting of the American Association for the History of Medicine, Baltimore, Maryland, May 9, 1969.

1 Fielding H. Garrison, *An Introduction to the History of Medicine* (Philadelphia: Saunders, 1914), p. 306.

2 Joseph M. Toner, *Contributions to the Annals of Medical Progress and Medical Education in the United States before and during the War of Independence* (Washington, D.C.: 1874), pp. 105–106.

3 *The New Trade Directory for Philadelphia*, Anno *1800* (Philadelphia, 1799), pp. 130–132, 172.

4 James Potter, *On the Rise and Progress of Physic in America: Pronounced before the First Medical Society in the Thirteen United States of America* (Hartford, 1781), pp. 4–7.

5 John Morgan, *A Discourse upon the Institution of Medical Schools in America* (Philadelphia, 1765), p. 24.

6 William Douglass, *A Summary, Historical and Political, . . . of the British Settlements in North-America* (Boston, 1749–53), II, 350–352.

7 Biographical data in this lecture have been taken principally from the *Dictionary of American Biography*; James Thacher, *American Medical Biography* (Boston,

1828); and *Sibley's Harvard Graduates*. A facsimile edition of Thacher, with biographical introduction and bibliographical notes, was published by Da Capo Press, New York, 1967.

8 *The Papers of Benjamin Franklin*, ed. Leonard W. Labaree et al. (New Haven: Yale Univ. Press, 1959–), II, 378.

9 Potter, *Rise and Progress*, p. 7.

10 Whitfield J. Bell, Jr., "Medical practice in Colonial America," *Bull. Hist. Med.*, 1957, *31*: 445.

11 Carl Bridenbaugh, ed., *Gentleman's Progress: The Itinerarium of Dr. Alexander Hamilton, 1744* (Chapel Hill: Univ. of North Carolina Press, 1948), p. 116; Wyndham B. Blanton, *Medicine in Virginia in the Eighteenth Century* (Richmond: Garrett and Massie, 1931), p. 401; Stephen Wickes, *History of Medicine in New Jersey, and of its Medical Men* (Newark, 1879), pp. 43–49; Whitfield J. Bell, Jr., *John Morgan, Continental Doctor* (Philadelphia: Univ. of Pennsylvania Press, 1965), pp. 137–138.

12 [John Gregory], *Observations on the Duties and Offices of a Physician; and on the Method of Prosecuting Enquiries in Philosophy* (London, 1770), pp. 40–46.

13 Needless to say, the bleeders who worked on prescription and under direction of regular physicians, like Jacob Smith, whom Dr. Adam Kuhn sent to the Drinker family during the yellow fever epidemic of 1798, were the menials of the profession, ranking near the bottom of the professional hierarchy. Henry D. Biddle, ed., *Extracts from the Journal of Elizabeth Drinker, from 1759 to 1807* (Philadelphia, 1889), p. 331.

14 Hamilton, *Gentleman's Progress*, pp. 195–196.

15 *The Journals of Henry Melchior Muhlenberg*, tr. Theodore G. Tappert and John W. Doberstein (Philadelphia: Muhlenberg Press, 1942–58), I, 189–190.

16 *Ibid.*, p. 168.

17 *Ibid.*, pp. 381–382.

18 *Ibid.*, II, 68–69.

19 *Ibid.*, p. 268.

20 Wickes, *History of Medicine*, pp. 167–168.

21 *Pennsylvania Archives*, 6th series, XIV, 285–287.

22 *Pennsylvania Gazette*, March 15, 1775.

23 *Ibid.*, June 30, Dec. 22, 1773.

24 William Smith, *The History of the Province of New-York . . . to the Year M.DCC.XXXII* (London, 1757), p. 212.

25 Hamilton, *Gentleman's Progress*, p. 91. On a trip from Annapolis to Boston in 1744 Dr. Hamilton encountered a sorry assortment of doctors — in Cecil County, Maryland, a "greasy thumb'd fellow" who "professed physick and particularly surgery" and who extracted teeth "with a great clumsy pair of blacksmith's forceps"; at New York a drunken military surgeon of little education who damned Boerhaave for a fool and a blockhead; and at Albany physicians who chiefly prescribed local herbs and eked a living as barbers. One layman, fed up with doctors, told Hamilton that he had learned by experience to shun them as impostors and cheats and that "now no doctor for me but the great Doctor above." *Ibid.*, pp. 7, 53–54, 65–66, 179–180.

26 Drinker, *Journal*, p. 279. I do not include as a category physicians found guilty of crimes, as Dr. Benjamin Budd of Morris County, New Jersey, was of counterfeiting in 1773. He received a pardon but was expelled from the New Jersey Medical Socety, *New Jersey Archives*, 1st series, XXVIII, 611, XXIX, 17–18, 28, 48, 62, 128, 335; New Jersey Medical Society, *Minutes and Proceedings* (Newark, 1875), p. 35.

27 Benjamin Rush, "Observations on the duties of a physician, and the method of improving medicine," *Medical Inquiries and Observations*, 2nd ed. (Philadelphia, 1805), I, 305–408.

28 Muhlenberg, *Journals*, III, 559.

29 Fred B. Rogers, "Dr. John Browne: friend of Franklin," *Bull. Hist. Med.*, 1956, *30*: 1–6.

30 R. W. Innes Smith, *English-Speaking Students of Medicine at the University of Leyden* (Edinburgh: Oliver and Boyd, 1932), p. 30; Hamilton, *Gentleman's Progress*, p. 156.

31 Samuel Bard, *A Discourse upon the Duties of a Physician* (New York, 1769), pp. 13–14.

32 W. B. McDaniel, 2d, "The beginnings of American medical historiography," *Bull. Hist. Med.*, 1952, *26*: 45–53.

33 Hamilton, *Gentleman's Progress*, pp. 116–117, 131–132, 137–138.

34 Thacher, *American Medical Biography*, II, 98–99.

35 Rush, "On the vices and virtues of physicians," Nov. 2, 1801, *Sixteen Introductory Lectures* (Philadelphia, 1811), pp. 125–126.

36 Rush, "On the means of acquiring business and the causes which prevent the acquisition, and occasion the loss of it, in the profession of medicine," Nov. 4, 1807, *ibid.*, pp. 232–255.

37 Rush, "On the vices and virtues of physicians," p. 122.

38 *Ibid.* See also John P. Batchelder, *On the Causes Which Degrade the Practice of Physick* (Bellows Falls, Vt., 1818), p. 4. The "undevout" physician in Batchelder's view simply was "mad," and if he was guilty of infidelity, it was because he indulged in some vice imcompatible with religion.

39 Andrew D. Mellick, Jr., *Lesser Crossroads*, ed. Hubert G. Schmidt (New Brunswick: Rutgers Univ. Press, 1948), pp. 343–344.

40 Thacher, *American Medical Biography*, I, 309. Thomas P. Jones, *Charge to the Graduates in Medicine at the . . . Columbian College, D.C.* (Washington, 1830),

p. 7, urged physicians to cultivate intellectual traits; one result would be that they would not succumb to "the temptations to which the Physician, and particularly the country practitioner, is exposed . . . that of drinking stimulating liquids" — the greatest and most baneful of his temptations.

41 David Hosack, *Observations on the Medical Character* (New York, 1826), pp. 23–24. DuPonceau's commentary is in the American Philosophical Society copy.

42 Rush, *Sixteen Introductory Lectures*, p. 125.

43 Rush, "Duties of a physician," p. 391.

44 Hamilton, *Gentleman's Progress*, p. 148. A calamanco banian was a loose woolen gown. The gown (or shirt or jacket) was of Indian origin; but calamanco is a fabric of European manufacture.

45 Garrison, *History of Medicine*, p. 307.

46 Rush, "Duties of a physician," p. 393.

47 Hosack, *Medical Character*, pp. 6, 18.

48 See, for example, John Godman, *Professional Reputation. An Oration delivered before the Philadelphia Medical Society* (Philadelphia, 1826), as well as the essays of Hosack and Batchelder cited above.

4

The Practice of Medicine in New York a Century Ago

CHARLES E. ROSENBERG

The following pages represent an attempt to sketch the outlines of medical practice and assumption in one American city a century ago. The undertaking began with the author's casual acceptance of an invitation to speak on medical practice a century ago and his difficulty in finding materials pertinent to his subject or concepts with which to order it. Though hardly exhaustive, this study may, I hope, suggest the multiplicity of relationships visible in so clearly defined a context and perhaps the desirability of other such analyses.

I

According to the census of 1865, New York City and County had a population of 723,587. Well over 90 percent lived on Manhattan Island's southern half. The northern half of Manhattan Island, in a day before really convenient public transportation, was for all practical purposes empty and served indeed as a summer resort into the 1880s. South of these hills and meadows, New Yorkers lived in conditions more cramped than those of any other American city. New York, a contemporary estimated, was ten times as crowded as Philadelphia. A housing census taken late in 1865 reported 15,357 tenements containing 501,327 persons — over two-thirds of the city's population.[1] New York was as crowded as any city in the western world.

A congested jerry-built city, New York was notoriously unhealthy. It had the highest death rate (1 in 35) of any major American city, a rate higher than that of either Paris or London. Whereas one child in six born in London died before its first birthday, one in five New York infants died before reaching this milestone. Indeed, in the half-century since 1810 when the first more or less accurate statistics were published, New York's death rate had increased steadily. Sewage and sanitation arrangements were primitive. Fewer than half the city's inhabitants lived in houses or apartments containing bathing facilities; summer and the rivers provided the poor with their only opportunity to wash thoroughly.[2] Accidents were common, and the large amount of outdoor work in the city's streets and on its piers meant exposure to cold in winter, heat and sun in summer. Food supplies reached the city's markets in poor condition, a trial even to prosperous New Yorkers, while a good portion of New York's tenement population suffered from chronic if marginal malnutrition as well. "These decaying animal and vegetable remains," one physician wrote of the food purchased by the poor, "are daily entombed in the protuberant stomachs of thousands of children, whose pallid, expressionless faces and shrunken limbs are the familiar attributes of childhood in these localities."[3] Far more than in the 20th century, New York's physicians were faced with acute infectious diseases, with cases demanding frequent visits, anxiety, and intimate personal contact.

It is hardly surprising then that medical men placed so great an emphasis upon the peculiarity of city practice. Not only the poor, but New Yorkers generally were exposed to dirt and overcrowding. Though the poor were particularly debilitated by inadequate food and poor ventilation, the city, contemporary physicians believed, held dangers almost as great for the well-to-do. The idle wealthy and especially women of this class suffered, doctors assumed, from lack of exercise

---

CHARLES E. ROSENBERG is Professor of History at the University of Pennsylvania, Philadelphia, Pennsylvania.

Reprinted with permission from the *Bulletin of the History of Medicine*, 1967, *41*: 223–253.

coupled with improper diet and clothing. "Among the American ladies brought up in our dark parlours and rooms," one health enthusiast wrote, "crooked spines, decaying teeth, a pale sickly color of the skin, flabby muscles, weak digestion, tender spines and irritable nerves, are the rule."[4] Business men too suffered from improper diet and lack of exercise — both exacerbated by the anxieties of trade. Logically enough, textbooks of medicine and materia medica warned that city-dwellers could not tolerate dosages in strengths necessary for the hardy country-dweller. Milder, less heroic measures, were appropriate for city-folk.

If there were doubts in 1866 as to the healthfulness of city life, there could be none as to the vigor of the city's growth. New York's medical community was equally vigorous — or at least numerous. With practically no control of licensing, with even the best medical schools enforcing relatively lenient requirements, the number of physicians in proportion to the population was high and their competition for the available, paying clientele correspondingly intense. The *Medical Register for the City of New York for 1866* listed 806 regular practitioners, while the Homoeopathic Medical Society counted some 70 active members.[5] One must, moreover, include a good number of irregulars in order to arrive at the total number of practitioners. It would probably be a safe guess that about 1,500 New Yorkers treated the sick in some manner, a ratio of one physician to roughly 500 inhabitants.

Much of the treatment of sickness was not overseen by men calling themselves physicians. Midwives and "old ladies" (the latter a term favored by medical contemporaries in describing all laymen who routinely provided advice and simple remedies to family and neighbors) provided a good deal of informal practice. It is apparent as well from the number and generous claims of patent medicine manufacturers that these remedies with, as many physicians complained, the advice of a none-too-scrupulous breed of pharmacist, provided the first line of medical attention for many New Yorkers regardless of social class. Patients too casually refilled prescriptions if they thought them appropriate for what seemed to be a recurrence of the illness for which they had originally been prescribed.[6] Such casual self-prescribing was estimated by contemporaries to be the source of a majority of all prescriptions compounded.

Even assuming that we limit our discussion to medicine as practiced by persons calling and thinking of themselves as physicians and earning their livelihood exclusively by treating the sick, we will see that the situation was by no means a simple one. Ideological and ethical differences, in the absence of any governmental control, created a number of sub-communities within the medical world. Most confusing was the duplication of professional organization and function between homoeopathic and regular physicians, groups in some ways more similar than either would have admitted. But similarities in attitude toward education and ethics could not modify the peculiar therapeutic doctrines which kept homoeopaths apart from the main camp of regular practitioners.[7] In addition to these groups, there were many other healers in the city, some practicing without benefit of diploma or medical education of even the most perfunctory sort. A flourishing group of "pox doctors," for example, specialized in venereal disease, sterility, and sexual problems generally.[8] There were herb doctors and "electricians," specialists in cancer and lung complaints. Such practitioners, though certainly active, are difficult to trace and were in a real sense outside the medical profession — united perhaps in performing the same function but alien in values. One can, I think, without danger of distortion, simply acknowledge these irregulars' existence and devote the rest of these remarks to the better-educated, "regular" practitioners of medicine.

Though not as intricately organized as in mid-20th century, New York's physicians a century ago had already begun to show signs of differentiation. Both knowledge and status were distributed unevenly among New York's medical men. Institutional power especially was concentrated in comparatively few hands.

This can be easily demonstrated. The Medical and Surgical Society of New York, limited in membership to 34, was the most exclusive of the city's informal medical associations.[9] Seventeen of the society's members in 1866 held teaching positions in the city's three regular medical schools. Even more significant was the dominance of Society men in hospital appointments. They held collectively 97 consulting and attending appointments at the city's hospitals and dispensaries, roughly half of the total number available. Members of the society were also active in the councils of the New York Academy of Medicine — though conspicuously inactive in the County Medical Society. Gurdon Buck, for example, held eight hospital appointments, served as vice-president of the New York Medical Journal Association and the Alumni Association of the College of Physicians and Surgeons, as trustee of the College of Physicians, and as a member of the Academy of Medicine's Committee on Medical Education. Willard Parker enjoyed ten hospital appointments as well as being active in the Metropolitan Board of Health and serving as Professor of Practice at the College of Physicians. Only six members held no hospital appointments. One of these, however, Robert Watt, was Professor of Anatomy at the College of Physicians, and two, C. R. Agnew and Fessenden Otis, offered specialty clinics at the same medical school; two others, W. M. Blakeman and John G. Adams, were influential in the affairs of the Academy of Medicine. These were in the idiom of the time "the hospital men," the social and institutional leaders of the profession. And the dominance of these professors and attending physicians was clearly understood and resented, especially the favoritism which seemed to rule hospital appointments.[10]

The Medical and Surgical Society was, of course, only one among a number of medical societies, all representing status and knowledge in some proportion. The New York Academy of Medicine, for example, with its membership of 273 probably included almost all of the city's well-trained and financially secure physicians. Those with scientific pretensions belonged to the New York Pathological Society and, very likely, the Medical Journal Society as well. There were, of course, other roads to status and success outside the exclusive confines of the Medical and Surgical Society's membership. No immigrants, for example, were members of this establishment organization, yet a number of the city's leading medical scholars were Europeans, men like Abraham Jacobi and Ernst Krackowizer. These émigré physicians were highly respected for their specialized skills, active in the Society of German Physicians, and prominent in the affairs of New York's sizable German community. Within New York's specialty societies as well knowledge and ability provided avenues to leadership and recognition.

I do not mean to imply that social and intellectual status were unrelated. For the opposite, of course, is true. Twenty-two of the Medical and Surgical Society's 34 members — to return to our example — could be classified as specialists. Among them were some of the country's leading teachers of medicine, men like Austin Flint and Alonzo Clark. Clearly, however, intellectual and institutional leadership, while overlapping, were hardly coincidental — a fact which J. Marion Sims discovered abruptly some years earlier when he received a cold reception from the leaders of New York's medical establishment.[11] Among physicians in ordinary practice, of course, the drop in knowledge was immense. Much of ordinary practice was undoubtedly bad, even when judged by the flexible standards of the day. Knowledge trickled slowly down to the majority of practitioners. A Boston physician, for example, quoted approvingly a pathologist friend's cynical opinion that "if what is really *known* of the laws of disease were told to the members of the profession, more than half of them would indignantly discredit it."[12]

With so many doctors, competition was correspondingly intense, and although the rewards of success could be great, an established physician's income was probably somewhere in the vicinity of $1500 to $2000 a year. Valentine Mott, New York's most eminent surgeon of the previous generation, dying late in 1865, left an estate of almost a million dollars. But physicians beginning practice in the 1860s probably averaged close to $400 a year, a bit less than the $416 paid resident physicians at Bellevue and Charity Hospitals. The salary of the sanitary superintendent of the Metropolitan Board of Health was set at $4000 a year, police surgeons at $2250. These were adequate but not munificent salaries in an economy still affected by the inflation of the Civil War.[13]

II

There were, essentially, two kinds of medical practice in New York a century ago, charity and pay. The ideal practice, however, was one performed by a regular practitioner in the middle-class home, in contemporary terms, a "family practice." An office clientele was, at least in theory, considered something quite distinct and indeed a vaguely marginal kind of endeavor, one in which a hardworking physician might make useful contacts and acquire much-needed cash. (An office practice, as opposed to a family practice, was usually conducted on a cash basis.) It was not, however, considered to be the basis of a completely sound "business."[14]

A family practice was that in a very real sense. The physician attended father and mother, children, even servants. (It must be remembered the presence of servants in a respectable household was considered a century ago as much a necessity as a refrigerator today; when a servant lived in it was assumed that medical care would be her employer's responsibility.) Bills were commonly sent on an annual basis, perhaps semi-annually by the more efficient. As we have noted, this family practice was middle-class; a casual glance at any textbook of children's diseases in this period makes this clear, its discussion, for example, of the proper means of choosing a wet-nurse, its assumption that nursery maids were in many, if not most, cases the proper repository for directions in infant care.

A comparative superfluity of physicians in the still compact city helped maintain the visit as the basic unit of the physician's work day; the doctor's slate was still standard office-equipment. One visited nice persons in their homes; they did not ordinarily come to one's office. It was considered, indeed, a matter of good planning to visit frequently enough to oversee the progress of a case, but not so frequently as to give the impression that one was padding the bill. Respectable persons did not ordinarily enter hospitals for treatment; nor did the truly upright allow their servants to be sent to one. Thus, what is today the physician's hospital practice was, a hundred years ago, the heart of his daily round of visits — and this in a generation during which acute and protracted infectious diseases were still common. Physicians charged a special fee for overnight visits and expected to be awakened from their sleep to make calls. At the same time it was considered quite normal for a physician to visit homes for relatively minor complaints, to vaccinate for example, in theory even to advise on matters such as the location of a new house, proper plumbing, an appropriate diet.

Theory explained and justified this pattern of practice. Etiological thought still emphasized the role of constitutional and environmental factors in the causation of disease. It followed logically that the best physician was the one most familiar with individual circumstances and constitutional patterns of reaction to illness. If a model practice was that in middle-class homes, an ideal practitioner was the experienced physician who had come to know a family through several generations, becoming familiar with its characteristic strengths and weaknesses, its peculiarities in regard to the action of medicines or to changes in regime. As Oliver Wendell Holmes put it,

> The young man knows his patient, but the old man also knows his patient's family, dead and alive, up and down for generations. He can tell beforehand what diseases their unborn children will be subject to, what they will die of if they live long enough, and whether they had better live at all, or remain unrealized possibilities. . . .[15]

Both the regular and homoeopathic codes of ethics reflected the acceptance of a paradigmatic family practice, one in which it was assumed a personal as well as professional relationship would subsist between patient and physician. Both codes, for example, urged patients not to dismiss a physician without some formal explanation. It was hoped that there would be no bitter feelings. Somewhat similar considerations underlay the code's elaborate emphasis upon the formal etiquette of consultation. This was a situation which the unethical consultant might turn to his advantage, through casual slights and innuendoes discrediting the family physician and perhaps seducing away his patients. The emphasis of medical theory, however, upon the regular attendant's unique knowledge sanctioned the prominent role he was to play in the elaborately formalized ritual of consultation.[16]

This emphasis upon the ethics of consultation and the frequency of such occasions emphasizes another quality of the profession a century ago. I refer to its still essentially "horizontal," undifferentiated structure. Despite what has been said concerning the distribution of status within the profession, the organization of American medicine a century ago was still largely geographical and social, corresponding to the location and class of patients attended, only partially dependent upon education and institutional ties. Since almost all physicians did the same sort of things, consultants were ordinarily potential competitors. The general practitioner today sees, of course, little danger in referring cases demanding specialized knowledge to another physician; the functional differentiation of the profession within the past century has defined and thus limited the specialist's activities.[17] (And referral, of course, is infrequently an occcasion for the formal consultation so common a century ago.) Medical theory too has changed and these intellectual developments have in some ways paralleled the structural changes within the organization of the profession. Decreasing emphasis — at least until the relatively recent past — on familial, diathetical, and environmental factors in etiological and therapeutic thought has removed much of the theoretical justification for personal interaction between the general practitioner and specialist.

Without benefit of any generally convincing or specific etiology, medical attitudes toward disease causation a century ago were broadly inclusive. Practicing physicians cannot well afford the habitual luxury of confessing ignorance; models of disease causation were shifting schemes, equations in which the factors of heredity, habit, and environment could be judiciously balanced to explain either health or disease. Although heredity was emphasized, as we have seen in the words of Dr. Holmes, it provided only one given in the disease equation. And perhaps given is too strong a word, for heredity itself was a variable and constantly shifting attribute. "Hereditary tendency to disease," as one contemporary put it, "is one of the most certainly established facts in pathology; yet its operations and manifestations are most singular and uncertain." Heredity was not fixed, but could be altered by external influences at any point between conception and weaning. It was, for example, part of the physician's task to warn against emotional excitement during pregnancy, stress which might mark the child. Even during lactation, it was believed, maternal impressions might be transmitted to children. It was the physician's task, similarly, to warn against sexual intercourse while under the influence of alcohol or drugs; even a momentary indiscretion of this kind might balefully affect the constitution of a child conceived under such unfavorable circumstances.[18] The open-ended quality of etiological thought provided abundant opportunity for medical men to articulate and justify the moral convictions of their contemporaries.

Though heredity was a potent cause of illness, such ills might never manifest themselves if the individual were protected from the "cooperating" causes in the environment; for disease was considered the product ordinarily of an interaction between such environmental causes and hereditary attributes. "Herein," Austin Flint, probably New York's leading teacher of clinical medicine, wrote in 1866, "lies a truth of great practical importance." Diseases, he explained, "thus are preventable, notwithstanding a predisposition to them, insofar as they depend on the union of cooperating causes."[19] It was the task, then, of the family physician to avert through wise counsel the dangers posed by hereditary predisposition. Within the shifting etiological world, the physician's theoretical responsibility was far broader than mere diagnosis, prognosis, and treatment.

The practicing physician had to understand not only variations in individual constitution; the physical environment too was fluid, climate and temperature constantly changing, constantly interacting with human strengths and weaknesses. The idea of "epidemic constitution" was still generally unquestioned. Fatal epidemic diseases were, for example, still assumed to be preceded by the prevalence of similar but less serious ills. (A cholera epidemic might thus be expected to follow the prevalence of non-specific diarrhoeal complaints.) General patterns of disease incidence were as well affected by changes in climate; in certain seasons or localities bowel complaints, in others neurological disorders, might be peculiarly prevalent. The action of remedies was also modified by climatic changes. The Committee on Diseases of the Medical Society of the County of New York pointed out, for example, in the spring of 1866 that mercurials seemed to be losing their effectiveness, that it was increasingly difficult to salivate patients.[20] Thus, in prescribing, transitory climatic conditions as well as more permanent environmental factors had to be considered in conjunction with known constitutional differences, including those of sex, profession, temperament, and age. An educated and experienced regular physician, the argument inevitably followed, was the only one capable of understanding and evaluating this multiplicity of protean factors.

With such a kaleidoscope of etiological and therapeutic variables, it was only to be expected that general pathological designs were most popular with New York practitioners. Only in the most egregiously local lesions — those, for example, resulting from trauma — was there any general feeling that an exclusively local process might be involved.[21] From hysteria to carbuncles, all man's ills were made to fit a similarly open-ended pattern. Local affections exerted a general effect either through the blood or "reflex-action," while general influences might through the same agencies create local inflammations. In this scheme, of course, emotional and psychological influences played a significant role. Fear or anxiety, for example, might have so debilitating an effect on the nervous system or the blood's nutritional qualities as to cause physical or mental ills of the most varied sort.[22] Particularly striking was the manner in which the uterus in women and dentition in infants were presumed capable of inducing through these speculative mechanisms almost every conceivable pathological condition. (The more critical had indeed already come to the defense of the uterus, making light of the blanket charges habitually levelled against this hapless organ.[23]) The point, of course, is that physicians cannot well fulfill their social function without offering some explanation of the ills they treat; in the absence of knowledge they necessarily adopted the most flexible of etiological and pathological designs — ones in which explanations of health and disease could readily be cast.

Thus far we have been sketching a rather schematic description of private practice and the medical theory which paralleled and in some ways justified it. To illustrate this pattern in concrete, individual terms is a difficult matter. Numberless memoirs and autobiographies describe medical careers in this period; almost all lack the immediacy and often the accuracy of the contemporary diary or letter. I have been able to locate only one detailed diary kept by a New York practitioner in 1866. The diarist was John Burke, a prosperous and responsible physician, a member of the Academy of Medicine, a founder of the East River Medical Association, but by no means a member of the city's medical elite.

Dr. Burke worked very hard. This was especially true during the summer of 1866, when he lost 16 pounds.[24] On the evening of July 30, for example, he recorded having already made "28 outdoor visits besides prescribing for innumerable office patients, and I have some calls to make to night yet for it is now only 7 OC PM." His normal day, Dr. Burke noted on December 15, began when he rose soon after seven, saw his office patients, and then read his paper.

> If I have time, [he continued] have breakfast so that I may leave the house by 8½ OC I visit the lower part of town and get back to the house by 10½ — I then visit patient [*sic*] between this and [illeg but presumably a dispensary] by 12 or 12½ noon. It takes me nearly an hour there — I then visit the calls left at [illeg.] I try to get home from 3 to 4 P.M. I attend patients in the office. I have my dinner at 4½ or 5. I then try and have a snoose [*sic*] for an hour or so — I come down to the office by 7 OC — I attend there until 8½. After that hour I go out and visit more patients — I generally have from 3 to 5 to visit — I reach home for the night from 10 to 12. I lie down then after reading for an hour or so.

Dr. Burke's cases were enormously varied. In the summer, for example, there were large numbers of sun-stroke and intestinal complaints; winter brought an entirely different pattern of cases. On December 2, he noted visiting in their homes 2 cases of scarlatina, 7 bronchitis, 4 typhoid fever, 1 pneumonia, 2 tuberculosis, 1 vomiting and diarrhoea, 1 sore throat, 1 scald from porridge, 1 retention of urine, 1 injury to hip joint from fall on ice, 1 dysentery, 1 threatened miscarriage, 1 remittent fever, 1 "pains in abdomen — local peritonitis." This, he observed, "for one day and not a very busy one." Despite these wearing rounds, Dr. Burke did try to keep alert to professional developments. It was no easy task however. When he prepared a paper, for example on pneumonia, for his friends in the newly founded East River Medical Society, Burke had to find the time in the few hours he normally devoted to sleep.[25]

Dr. Burke may indeed have been somewhat atypical, and perhaps our delineation of a general pattern of medical practice has been excessively schematized. There were many different kinds of practice in New York a century ago. New York did have its specialists, its practitioners for the rich, for the simply well-to-do, and, as well, for those families only marginally established in the middle class — artisans, small shopkeepers, and the like.

The poor were treated on a different plan entirely. They were the beneficiaries of what today might be called public medicine, what a hundred years ago was called medical charity.

The basic unit in this system was the dispensary. These were independent, private charities, scattered by 1866 liberally throughout the city. Somewhat over 184,000 new cases were treated in eleven of these dispensaries during 1866, and, of these, more than 30,000, or roughly a sixth, visited in their homes.[26] New York's first dispensary was founded in the 1790s and, by 1866, their administration had become standardized. All had a salaried resident physician, available at the dispensary from roughly nine to five (though hours varied from institution to institution) and for several hours on Sunday. An apothecary was on duty during the same hours to make up prescriptions and in most cases to pull teeth as well. Treatment was administered by a staff of volunteer physicians, each available at stated hours during the week in clinics corresponding to the developing specialties of the day, diseases of the chest, of women and children, of the eye and ear, the skin, genito-urinary system, surgery, and the head and abdomen. These consultants were not salaried. The resident and visiting physicians however, normally somewhat younger men, did have regular if modest salaries. It was the task of the resident physician to treat simple emergencies, to vaccinate and — most importantly — to screen incoming patients, sending them to the appropriate clinic and entering the names of patients unable to leave their rooms on the visiting physician's ledger.

The visiting physician's task was particularly difficult. These young practitioners had to make their way through the dark and reeking halls of crowded tenements, at times unable even to find would-be patients; tenement dwellers, they explained, often did not know their neighbors' names. They had as well to deal with a poorly educated clientele which, they found, shunned fresh air as a major cause of disease and which took little interest in cleanliness — even when facilities for washing were available. It was also difficult, the visiting physicians complained, to see patients on a regular basis, to follow them even through the course of an acute disease. If a patient should die, there was, of course, almost no chance of obtaining permission for an autopsy. And the conditions they encountered were truly appalling. William Thoms, active in medical work for several dispensaries and a city mission, described, for example, one alley harboring an inordinate number of typhus cases. In a slanting attic room, its measurements 14 × 7½ × 7, Thoms reported finding 12 human beings; there were five typhus cases among them. There was no real furniture; the "inmates" slept on pallets arranged on the floor. During one of his visits, Thoms recalled, he found all the children in the group stripped and lying naked under the same bedclothes and on the same mattress, though several were suffering with active cases of typhus. The children's only clothes were, it seemed, being washed. The room itself was so crowded that on several calls, Dr. Thoms found it almost impossible to force a way to the corner where his patients lay.[27]

Not surprisingly, it was dispensary physicians such as Dr. Thoms who provided concerned New Yorkers with much of their knowledge of such intolerable conditions. Many of the physicians participating in the careful sanitary survey sponsored by New York's Citizen's Association in 1865 were, or had been, dispensary physicians. And despite the comparatively low social status generally afforded physicians who engaged in the public health work,[28] the task of the dispensary physician had its compensations: the few hundred dollars a year paid visiting physicians was a welcome addition to a beginning physician's slender income. Perhaps more important, it was an excellent way in which to sharpen clinical skills.

The larger dispensaries undertook a staggering amount of work. One of the largest, for example, was the Demilt at Twenty-third Street and Second Avenue. Its "district" was the East Side of Manhattan Island, from Fourteenth Street on the south to Fortieth on the north, from Sixth Avenue on the west to the East River. One-hundred-and-ten-thousand New Yorkers lived in this area, 75,000 in tenement houses. The dispensary treated 29,070 new cases in 1866, 4,625 in their homes, while the apothecary prepared 58,520 prescriptions. The dispensary treated thus an average of some 80 new cases a day and filled daily about 160 prescriptions.[29] Though the Demilt published no statistics on this point, the great majority of their patients must have been immigrants or their children. This was clearly the case with other dispensaries publishing such records and established in similar areas. Of 20,301 patients treated by the Northern Dispensary during 1866, 11,184 had been born in Ireland. At the North-western Dispensary, one district physician reported that of 684 patients he had visited, 311 were Irish by birth; less than half were born in the United States and of these, two-thirds were of foreign parentage.[30]

When such disadvantaged New Yorkers became gravely ill they entered a hospital. Without exception, these were purely eleemosynary institutions. Bellevue and Charity Hospital, the city's two great hospitals, dwarfed all others. Bellevue, with a thousand beds, treated 7,725 patients during the year, while another 7,574 were administered to at Charity Hospital on Blackwell's Island. No other hospital approached these figures, although the New York Ophthalmic Hospital and the New York Eye and Ear Infirmary treated impressive numbers of cases for special hospitals.[31]

A stay in one of New York's hospitals in 1866 could not have been too pleasant. Patients were regarded with condescension and still expected to work in the wards as soon as they had recovered sufficiently. Convalescent women helped everywhere to care for others still sicker; in Bellevue and Charity Hospitals women were set to work sewing, the men at carpentry and cleaning. A few formed the crew of the rowboat which plied twice-daily between Bellevue and Blackwell's Island. A pervasive moralism and — in the best hospitals — a species of heavy-handed paternalism, faced the patients as well. The Infant's Hospital, for example, charged seven dollars a month for children able to walk, but ten dollars for the illegitimate. Even St. Luke's, probably the most liberally administered of New York's hospitals, which allowed visitors on weekdays, forbade them on the Sabbath. Patients might, in addition, be expelled for blasphemy, indeed for any insubordination.[32] Many of the desperately ill, moreover, could not be admitted to the city's hospitals. Patients with ailments judged incurable, cancer for example, were forbidden admittance by all of New York's hospitals; they could turn only to the Alms-House or to their own families' resources.[33]

Nursing was casual, hygiene inadvertent. Some years earlier, for example, a young New York physician had in advocating hospital reform hopefully urged the installation of a spittoon in each ward, and the thorough airing of beds and bedding. Nurses, he suggested, should have some badge of their station, and be "compelled to dress in clean garments, and not be allowed to wander over the building looking like the off-scouring of the city."[34] Though many of the city's leading physicians held attending and consulting posts, the lack of thorough clinical training in contemporary medical schools must inevitably have meant a house-staff inadequate in many instances — even by the standards of the day. And the young men of the house-staff, of course, provided the bulk of medical care. Death rates for the several hospitals averaged in the vicinity of 10 percent, almost none lower and a few a bit higher. The highest death rate, one not included in this average, was among the foundlings brought to the Alms-House. Six-hundred and forty-four of the 771 admitted during the year died.[35] Hospitals were, finally, administered by lay boards, a fact which most physicians regarded with consistent hostility, and to which they attributed many of the hospital's inadequacies.[36]

Though perhaps not immediately apparent to the patients, these hospitals had already come to play a significant role in New York's medical growth. The elite among medical school graduates could compete for positions on the house staff and, increasingly, the medical schools themselves offered instruction utilizing the city's abundant clinical material. By 1866, some physicians at least were able to state that the principal function of the city's hospitals lay not in the alleviation of individual suffering, but in the teaching of medicine.[37] A few attending physicians had even begun to use their hospital facilities for the conduction of clinical investigations.

III

Diagnosis and therapy had in 1866 changed in some ways very little since the 18th century. Despite brave talk of reliance on hygiene, despite an invigorating scepticism in some circles toward the bulky materia medica, medicine was still in practical terms just that — the administration of medicine. "Prescribing for" a patient was still a synonym for seeing him. Diagnostic procedures too shifted slowly and with them the physician's prognostic ability. Inadequacies in therapeutics helped, of course, maintain the traditional importance of prognostic skills in determining a physician's success. "People in general," as Austin Flint put it, "are apt to estimate [the physician's] knowledge and ability by the correctness of his judgment in this regard."[38] In the hands of most practitioners, diagnosis was in all probability still based on the asking of questions, observing the patient's appearance, taking his pulse, examining — and sometimes tasting — his urine.[39] Physical diagnosis was not employed routinely by the ordinary practitioner, only by the better-trained and then, apparently, only when the case seemed a severe one.

It is extremely difficult, of course, to discover precisely how many physicians practiced physical diagnosis in New York a century ago and how expert they were. Some useful hints can be found, however, in the manuals prepared by the various insurance companies to guide their medical examiners. Insurance examiners were well-established physicians, certainly more skillful than the average practitioner; clearly, as well, their examination would be as thorough as the company's advisors could design. One learns from these manuals, for example, that auscultation and percussion were normally performed through underclothing.[40] The very detailed and explicit quality of the instructions indicates, moreover, that too much could not be assumed as to the physician's consistency in diagnosis. In 1866, physical diagnosis was not taught on an individual basis in medical schools; it was something which one had to learn either in practice, in the apprentice relationship (though this ancient mode of clinical instruction was falling increasingly into disuse), or more commonly in one of the small, semi-formal tutoring classes attached to the city's medical school. It would be safe, I think, to conclude that physical diagnosis was not an ordinary procedure in routine house-visits; it had still the aura of high-level practice. The lag between the general academic acceptance of auscultation and percussion and their introduction in routine practice demonstrates quite well the gap which existed in this period between the "best" practice and the day-to-day round of the average practitioner.

At the same time, of course, other newer modes of diagnosis were being introduced. Thermometry was known from the literature but was hardly considered by the general practitioner an appropriate part of his normal routine. In the fall of 1865, and then in 1866, clinical thermometry was introduced to New York City on an experimental basis, first at New York, then at Bellevue Hospitals; it is clear, however, even in enthusiastic pleas for their use that thermometers were considered unnecessary, indeed wildly impractical by the average practitioner.[41] The use of other aids to diagnosis, the ophthalmoscope and laryngoscope especially, were well known but, of course, used routinely only by those who specialized in ailments of the eye and ear and nose and throat.[42] The vaginal speculum was certainly used by many non-specialists; it is doubtful, however, that its employment could have been routine if only because of contemporary moral standards. The analysis of blood, despite the influence in theoretical matters of hematological pathologies, was still an experimental procedure — and most often a post-morten one at that.

Therapy, as we have noted, was still heavily dependent upon the administration of drugs, less heroic than in an earlier generation perhaps, but still strenuous enough. It is, of course, difficult to quantify, but a pattern of multiple prescriptions was seemingly universal. Dispensary apothecaries compounded an average of almost exactly two prescriptions per case.[43] Certainly the average would have been higher in private practice.

It cannot be denied that a certain critical scepticism in matters therapeutic had been present, even increasing in the quarter-century before 1866. Beginning most clearly with Jacob Bigelow, a respectable number of American medical leaders had warned against the routine and uncritical use of severe drugs and bleeding. The logic of Bigelow's position and that assumed by like-thinking physicians was based on the assumption that most diseases were self-limited, their natural tendency even if untreated being to recovery not death. The physician should therefore, the argument followed, be cautious in his therapy, attempting simply to strengthen the body's vital powers in their struggle with disease. For ills that were not self-limited, on the other hand, there was usually little that could be done. Reliance should, therefore, be placed upon good food, favorable hygienic conditions, upon stimulants such as alcohol and relaxing anodynes such as opium — as opposed to so-called depleting remedies, the traditional arsenal of cathartics and bleeding. By the 1860s, the position of Austin Flint was probably representative of the best therapeutic thinking in American medicine.[44] Flint called his therapeutic stance "conservative medicine." The term had in reality two separate but complementary meanings, conservative in the sense of conserving the body's natural powers and conservative in the sense of abjuring harsh and unproven modes of therapy. Flint, for example, was famous in this generation for his emphasis in the treatment of tuberculosis upon fresh air — and enormous quantities of whiskey.[45] The emphasis of fashionable clinicians in the late 1860s upon the administration of alcohol and other stimulants was not altogether popular. Temperance writers were bitterly hostile and more than a few older practitioners considered this new practice a rather naively self-confident Neo-Brunonianism.[46] It is apparent, however, from a survey of medicine and materia medica textbooks (including Austin Flint's *Practice*) that a rather elaborate drug therapy was assumed and suggested in the great majority of conditions.

Certainly, of course, the casual employment of severe bloodletting and the almost automatic prescribing of harsh emetics and cathartics had decreased, though again the gap between the more sophisticated academic or quasi-academic practitioners and their less pretentious colleagues is difficult to evaluate.[47] Nor should the problem of generations be ignored: older men must have found it difficult to change accustomed practices, to abandon faith in the calomel and phlebotomy which had, apparently, served them so well. Cupping and leeches were still used routinely, and while venesection was in intellectual disfavor, texts still pointed out that in children under three, blood might be drawn from the jugular if other veins were difficult to locate.[48] Blisters and setons were still a part of the therapeutic armory. Most important, however, the therapeutic implications of a logically severe emphasis on the self-limited quality of most ills were still heresy to most physicians. Both characteristic and revealing is the frequency with which physicians could write on one page of the evils of traditional therapeutics and the self-limited quality of most ailments and on the next emphasize their contempt for expectant therapy. Certainly there was virtue in drugs, as T. Gaillard Thomas, a vigorous advocate of the self-limited quality of most ills, put it: "There was a vantage ground between the two extremes, neither verging toward meddlesome interference on the one hand, nor imbecile neglect on the other."[49]

And the patients themselves were a sturdy bulwark against any nihilism in therapeutics. People seemed to want medicines, wished when the physician left to be in the comforting possession of a prescription. (One need, I think, to support this view simply mention the routine use of placebos by practitioners in this period — and their general conviction that such placebos played a significant, possibly even genuinely therapeutic, role in comforting patients and their families.) Devotees of homeopathy too quaffed countless doses — even if they had little physiological effect. Most of the drugs imbibed, moreover, were not prescribed by physicians. In addition to the omnipresent patent mixtures, drugs such as calomel, laudanum, even strychnine, were everywhere available at pharmacy counters.[50] Parents routinely administered cathartics to helpless children when they appeared a bit peaked; many others followed the dictates of traditional wisdom and administered purges every spring. Popular wisdom still held that infections in the blood would have to be driven out through the skin — resulting in the administration of countless doses of medicine, mustard plasters, and the like. And many Americans, of course, still felt comfortable with the calomel that had played so prominent a role in their own childhood.

With drug-taking so important in therapeutics, a central aspect of medical practice a century ago was the relationship between physician and pharmacist. A "course of treatment" was, as we have noted, essentially a series of prescriptions. It was the pharmacist's duty to fill these as carefully and accurately as possible; this was as far as his authority extended. At least in theory. In practice, apothecaries felt no hesitation in acting as medical advisors, suggesting particularly patent medicines and, more importantly, casually refilling prescriptions at the patient's request. (In 1867, New York City's East River Medical Association voted to boycott local pharmacies which did not agree to forego this practice.) There was, not surprisingly, a good deal of chronic ill-feeling between physicians and druggists. Apothecaries criticized physicians for occasionally extortionate demands for percentages of each prescription;[51] physicians, on the other hand, criticized pharmacists for carelessness and for selling everything but drugs in their stores.[52] Essentially, of course, the problem rested in the embryonic state of professionalism within the guild of pharmacists, exacerbated by the state's failure to exert any control over the druggist's training, licensing, or operations. With a similar *laissez-faire* prevailing in regard to physicians, this unsatisfactory state of things was inevitable.

IV

We have tended, thus far, in discussing medicine in New York a century ago, to emphasize factors which made for continuity. I should like, finally, to suggest a number of "unstable" areas within the profession itself and emphasize in these sectors the possibility, if not as yet the realization, of change. These aspects of medicine are education, specialization, and values.

In each of these areas, moreover, the city itself played a significant role; effects of scale and organization helped make New York medicine a century ago foreshadow in a number of ways the shape of American medicine generally in generations to come.[53] Some of the influences exerted by the city are obvious, some more subtle. Most apparent are the simple effects of scale, the availability of abundant clinical material, for example, or the presence of large numbers of wealthy prospective patients; both attracted ambitious physicians and intensified specialization. And all such effects are, of course, cumulative, each building upon and magnifying the next. The metropolis served as well as a node for the gathering and distribution of knowledge. New York, the nation's largest city, was also its leading port of entry. Inevitably, New York and other great cities provided a peculiarly stimulating context for the profession's institutional and intellectual growth.

Specialism was still a term of derision in the vocabulary of many physicians. General practitioners feared the specialist's competition and attacked any professed limitation of practice to specific classes of ailments as a symptom of quackery — which in the not-too-distant past it had usually been. (And which, it should be recalled, it still was in the case of numberless pox-doctors, cancer specialists, and the like proliferating at this time in American cities.) In 1866, coincidentally, the American Medical Association's Committee on Medical Ethics took a sceptical view of what the committee's majority termed exclusive specialism. Indeed, many forward-looking physicians of good-will were critical of exclusive and seemingly premature specialism, feeling that it should develop only out of the broad opportunities for observation enjoyed by the general practitioner.[54] Despite this not entirely friendly climate, on the other hand, specialism was by 1866 clearly well-established in New York.[55] Busy and intelligent practitioners gradually concentrated upon certain classes of ailments, seeking them out in hospitals and dispensary work, finally having colleagues refer such cases when they appeared in private practice. In a city, with its great numbers of people and its complex social structure, there was obviously room for specialists; in rural areas there could be little opportunity for them either to earn a living or to perfect clinical skills.

In the intense competition, moreover, specialism was clearly a road to reputation and status. How else, indeed, was distinction to be won in a day of rapidly accumulating knowledge and before a purely academic career provided a realistic aspiration for American physicians? The majority, as we have noted, of the Medical and Surgical Society's members were specialists.[56] Even outside the society's socially impeccable membership, specialism was intricately related to the acquisition of status. Men like Louis Elsberg, Abraham Jacobi, Emil Noeggerath, Ernst Krackowizer, and a few years later Hermann Knapp — to mention only a few distinguished German physicians active in New York a century ago — made reputations as specialists, eventually overlapping and merging with the establishment of "hospital men" seen in so concentrated a form in the membership of the Medical and Surgical Society. Not surprisingly, New York physicians played an extraordinarily prominent role in the founding of the first national specialty societies in this period.[57]

The new specialties were recognized not only in such informal terms, moreover, but institutionally as well in the creation of chairs in the city's medical schools and special clinics and services in the city's hospitals and dispensaries. Such institutional provisions are particularly significant, for they provide an opportunity for the ordered transmission of knowledge — while the availability of a sufficient number of cases made such institutional provisions feasible. And, once created, it is the tendency of all such arrangements to grow and consolidate themselves. With the increasing accumulation of knowledge and technique generally in medicine, with the trend within European clinical medicine quite clearly toward specialization, it was inevitable that similar and parallel developments should take place in this country. Certainly this was the case after the wedding — already achieved in New York by 1866 — of such intellectual influences with institutional contexts appropriate for their transmission and elaboration.

By 1866, in any case, the elite among New York's medical men were in large degree specialists — or surgeons, and even surgeons were beginning to show signs of specialization, with men like Lewis A. Sayre limiting themselves largely to orthopedic cases or Thomas Addis Emmett to gynecological surgery.[58] But this emphasis upon the emergence of specialism is easily exaggerated. Specialists in this period almost always acted to some extent also as general practitioners. Exclusive specialism, despite the anxieties of its critics, was still essentially in the future.

Medical education mirrored and at once fostered this growing differentiation within an as yet comparatively homogeneous group. For most would-be physicians, medical education had probably not changed for generations. Though somewhat longer, the regular session from October to March was filled with didactic, factual, and routinely pedantic lectures. The great majority of students graduating after such a two-year course must have been indeed ill-prepared to begin practice.[59]

For the better student, on the other hand, more highly motivated, more intelligent, wealthier perhaps, the possibilities of medical education within New York a century ago could be surprisingly broad. In an age of vigorous competition among medical schools, the availability of great clinical resources was an obvious inducement to be held out by the New York City schools to prospective students.[60] The city's three regular medical schools offered clinical instruction, both in hospital wards (open to students of all medical schools) and dispensary clinics. All three schools had as well by 1866 instituted special fall preliminary courses, optional but free of charge. Some offered summer courses as well. Both these innovations in the curriculum promised an emphasis upon clinical teaching greater than that possible in the constricted winter course. Many of the city's eminent teachers offered private instruction in diagnosis, or, more traditionally, quizzes in test-passing. Senior students were beginning to be entrusted with obstetric cases in the city's tenements. After graduation, there were desirable house-staff positions to be competed for; these posts, unlike senior consulting appointments, were awarded on the basis of a competitive examination, not simply through influence. Then, of course, there were the dispensaries and the possibility of perfecting one's skills, perhaps even developing a specialty in their clinics.[61]

Most students, of course, never took advantage of these opportunities. Many failed even to attend regularly scheduled clinics, for they were never specifically tested on such practical knowledge.[62] The better students, however, and especially those with adequate funds, were exposed to the possibility at least of a far more elaborate, if informal, medical education than one might have thought, at first glance possible. Ordinary practitioners, perhaps, did not take advantage of these opportunities, but the leaders-to-be of New York medicine certainly did. The New York medical education of William Welch, for example, clearly illustrates this pattern. Welch competed and studied throughout the city, seeking out the best teachers and the most desirable positions in which to develop his skills.[63] Just as we have seen in the beginning of specialization a gradual elaboration of structure within the medical profession, so we have in medical education the simultaneous creation of institutional mechanisms through which an elite, still small in numbers perhaps, might be trained in the values and techniques of the new clinical medicine.

It might be argued, of course, that Welch and many others like him completed their studies in Europe. Such foreign study, however, is not an act of arbitrary impulse. Although clinical and laboratory teaching may have been far more advanced in the Old World, the values which accepted this superiority and chafed against American inadequacies were already being formed in the New World. A spirit of urgent, and in some cases aggressive, positivism was widely disseminated among younger intellectuals in the profession.[64] Book reviews in both of New York's medical journals, the *Medical Record* and the *New York Medical Journal*, tended in the mid-1860s to exhibit a fine scorn for the subtleties of mere speculation; closet philosophy was no substitute for solid laboratory or clinical investigation. Certainly such a rationalistic spirit influenced the contemporary debate over therapeutics. American physicians were as well beginning to acknowledge their awareness of German knowledge and acumen, of the emergence of a new leader in world medicine. The New York Medical Journal Club, for example, which, like the New York Pathological Society, included in its membership the great majority of New York's scientifically oriented physicians, subscribed in 1866 to more German journals than it did to French, English — or even American.[65]

A significant role in the transfer of knowledge and values was played, moreover, by European physician emigrees, by the Seguins, for example, or Abraham Jacobi. All sought to spread the gospel of scholarship and investigation in a nation which must have seemed to them lamentably shoddy in the standards it demanded of its medical practitioners.[66] Such men would naturally choose to practice in New York or some similar eastern city; in addition to the other advantages of metropolitan life, its large immigrant population offered the possibility of conviviality and financial security. American physicians too flocked to New York City; in medicine as in business it promised boundless opportunity. The great majority of New York medicine's intellectual leaders in the latter part of the 19th century were born outside the city.[67]

The values of world science were, of course, still a minor, if somewhat disturbing, current in the total life of New York medicine. The acquisition of "business" was still the physician's primary concern. It was still possible for medical men to more or less casually abet malpractice suits, to squabble in private and public. Puffing, the planting of one's name in news columns, and the signing of endorsements for anything from patent medicines to galoshes were still favorite means of acquiring publicity. Most importantly, of course, it did not seem to most New York physicians that one could be a success in any full sense of the word without the attainment of financial independence.[68]

It is my hope in these pages to have suggested something of the texture of American medical practice a hundred years ago. Conclusions of any dogmatic sort are certainly premature, but this cross-sectional survey does, I think, indicate a number of general points. One is the interdependence of ideas and the institutional contexts in which they are elaborated. Another is the interrelation of status and learning, the existence of an already well-articulated pattern in which knowledge, practical success, and status were distributed within the profession.

American medicine was, a century ago, disturbed by a number of labile elements. The practitioner's status was uncertain, protected neither by state sanctions nor by the universal trust and admiration of laymen, certainly not by the transcendent faith accorded medical science today. Many aspects of the physician's practice and ideas have thus to be seen in terms of a need to secure his financial and social status. At the same time, a number of the more ambitious, academically successful practitioners, men atypically secure by contemporary standards, were disturbed by the challenge and availability of new ideas, new techniques, and — most important — new aspirations. From the hind-sight of a century, it seems clear enough that these contrasting and coexisting instabilities of status and values were ultimately to cancel each other. The progress of the scientific disciplines within medicine was eventually to raise the level of objective — and to the laymen increasingly visible — achievement, thus insuring the ultimate willingness of society to control both medical education and access to the profession. This limitation of access coupled with better and more specialized medical training in a society increasingly prosperous was in the 20th century to largely banish these anxieties of status.

NOTES

This investigation was supported by U.S. Public Health Service Research Grant LM-00013-02.

1 For tenement house statistics, see: New York *Evening Post*, Jan. 6, 1866, which reprints the annual report of the Board of Police Surgeons. For other statistics, see: New York State, *Annual Report of the Metropolitan Board of Health, 1866* (New York, 1867), Appendix C, pp. 61, 97, 102. The best general survey of tenement house conditions is to be found in the *Report of the Council of Hygiene and Public Health of the Citizens' Association of New York upon the Sanitary Condition of the City* (New York, 1865). The manuscript copy-books kept by the Council of Hygiene's District physicians, upon which this published report is based, are deposited in the manuscript division of the New York Historical Society; they contain somewhat more detail than is available in the published version. Until the end of the 19th century the northern reaches of Manhattan Island were regarded as dangerously malarious. Simon Baruch, "Malaria as an etiological factor in New York City," *Med. Rec.*, 1883, *24*: 505–509.

2 L. Emmett Holt, "Infant mortality and its reduction, especially in New York City," *J.A.M.A.*, 1910, *54*: 682–690; W. F. Thoms, "Health in country and cities. Illustrated by tables of the death-rates, sickness-rates, etc. . . . ," *Tr. A.M.A.*, 1866, *17*: 431–434, esp. p. 422. New York State, *Annual Report 1866*, p. 65. On inadequate bathing facilities in the city, see *ibid.*, p. 157, and Robert Ernst, *Immigrant Life in New York City, 1825–1863* (New York: King's Crown Press, 1949), p. 51.

3 Ezra R. Pullen, *Citizens' Association Report*, 1865, p. 59. Much descriptive material on the markets is to be found in the work of Thomas F. DeVoe, *The Market Assistant* (New York, 1867) and *The Market Book, Containing a Historical Account of the Public Markets in the Cities of New York, Boston*, . . . (New York, 1862).

4 John Ellis, *Suggestions to Young Men, on the Subject of Marriage and Hints to Young Ladies, and to Husbands and Wives* (New York, 1866), p. 9.

5 *The Medical Register of the City of New York for the Year Commencing June 1, 1866*, ed. Guido Furman (New York, 1866), pp. 217–243; *Tr. Homoeopathic Med. Soc. St. N.Y.*, 1866, pp. 268–270.

6 See, e.g., John H. Griscom's casual reprinting of a letter in which a patient reported giving several friends similarly afflicted "the apothecaries No. of your prescription." "Essay on the therapeutic value of certain articles in the materia medica," *Tr. Med. Soc. St. N.Y.*, 1868, p. 10.

7 Attitudes assumed by the leaders of the homeopathic medical community towards matters such as ethics, educational reform, and specialization were remarkably similar to those of regular medical men. This accounts, I think, partially for the longevity of homeopathy and the eventual assimilation of its remnants by regular medicine in this century. A modern study of homeopathy in America is much needed.

8 Prostitution, the prevalence of venereal disease, and social condemnation of the sexual license such ailments implied conspired to make these specialists in "secret diseases" both popular and successful. Modesty and fear made many patients suffering with other sexual problems also unwilling to turn to their family physician. The ads of these specialists in matters sexual were everywhere in New York newspapers a century ago. The more popular hired assistants and published books advertising their services and providing information and advice on sexual problems. A few of these treatises — all going through a number of editions — were: Edward B. Foote, *Medical Common Sense; Applied to the Causes, Prevention and Cure of Chronic Diseases and Unhappiness in Marriage. Rev. . . . ed.* (New York, 1864); Frederick Hollick, *A Popular Treatise on Venereal Disease* . . . (New York, [c. 1852]); L. J. Kahn, *Nervous Exhaustion: Its Cause and Cure . . . with Practical Information on Marriage, its Obligations and Impediments . . .* (New York, [c. 1870]). Such books ordinarily offered advice by mail, Dr. Kahn even urging patients to send samples of their urine by express for "microscopic examination." Regular physicians always charged extraordinarily high fees in cases of venereal disease and, contrary to their usual practice, demanded advance payment. George Rosen, *Fees and Fee Bills* (Baltimore: Johns Hopkins Press, 1946), pp. 21, 44, 59; D. W. Cathell, *The Physician Himself* (Baltimore, 1882), pp. 71, 186. Cathell's remarkably revealing and popular book provides, to my knowledge, the most vivid single picture available of American medical practice in the late 19th century. I have relied more upon it than any other single work in my general description of medical practice.

9 *The Medical Register*, 1866, pp. 54–56, provides a list of the members of the Medical and Surgical Society. Data on appointments and positions were gathered either from the rosters published in the *Medical Reg-*

ister or from the annual report of the appropriate institution. For a history of the society, see Philip Van Ingen's *A Brief Account of the First One Hundred Years of the New York Medical and Surgical Society* (n. p., 1946).

10 [George F. Shrady], "Medical appointments," *Med. Rec.*, 1866, *1*: 477–478; E. P., "Hospital appointments," *ibid.*, p. 459; Stephen Smith, *Doctor in Medicine: And Other Papers on Professional Subjects* (New York, 1872), pp. 247–250.

11 J. Marion Sims, *The Story of My Life*, ed. H. Marion-Simons (New York, 1894), pp. 269, 295; Thomas Addis Emmett, "Reminiscences of the founders of Woman's Hospital Association," *N.Y. J. Gynec. & Obst.*, 1893, *3*: 366. Of the seven prominent physicians mentioned specifically by Emmett as having opposed Sims, four (Willard Parker, Gurdon Buck, William Van Buren, and Alfred Post) were leading members of the Medical and Surgical Society. And the influence of the Society was, of course, a continuing one. When Edward Trudeau competed in the early 1870s for a position on the house-staff of the newly opened Stranger's Hospital, he was quizzed by the entire visiting staff, all four of whom (H. B. Sands, W. H. Draper, T. Gaillard Thomas, and Fessenden Otis) were members of the society. Trudeau, *An Autobiography* (Garden City: Doubleday, Doran, 1930), pp. 59–62.

12 Quoted, apparently, as having been made in 1865. Benjamin Cotting, *Medical Addresses* (Boston, 1875), p. 109 n. Dr. A. K. Gardner, a well-known New York obstetrician, described, for example, in the summer of 1866 the tribulations of a female patient, delivered of two successive children by two different but equally "stupid" physicians whose ignorance verged on malpractice. New York Academy of Medicine, Section on Diseases of Women and Children, "Minutes," Entry for June 18, 1866, p. 307. Rare Book Room, New York Academy of Medicine.

13 S. D. Gross, *Memoir of Valentine Mott., M.D., LL.D.* (Philadelphia, 1868), pp. 87–88. The salary of Bellevue house-staff members is noted in New York City, Commissioners of Charity and Correction, *7th Annual Report*, 1866, p. 19. *Med. Rec.*, 1866, *1*: 120 reported the Police Surgeon's salary and the *Annual Report, Metropolitan Board of Health, 1866*, p. 62, the Sanitary Superintendent's salary. The estimate of a beginning practitioner's income was made by A. D. Rockwell, who began practice in New York City in 1866. *Rambling Recollections* (New York, 1920), p. 181.

14 There are a number of indications that this "ideal" practice was, even in 1866, more accurate as a description of practice in small towns and rural areas than it was for a large city. Office practice, for example, in a city like New York with its shifting population and its many consultants, must have been more important than in rural areas. Even the most successful practitioners held generous daily office hours, usually in the morning or late afternoon, many three times, morning, afternoon, and evening. Most had office hours on Sunday as well. *The Medical Register, 1866*, pp. 217–243, provides the addresses and office hours of New York's regular practitioners. There was, of course, no such thing as a physician without a private practice or established office hours. Some of the more successful physicians seem, however, to have had younger graduate physicians associated with them in their office practice whose task it was to screen incoming patients.

15 Oliver Wendell Holmes, "The Young Practitioner," *Medical Essays* (Boston: Houghton, Mifflin, 1911), p. 377. This passage is excerpted from an address originally given March 1871 to the graduates of Bellevue Hospital Medical College. Some years later, S. Weir Mitchell pointed acidly to the clichéd faith which rested upon the hallowed but often undeserving figure of the "family physician." *Doctor and Patient* (Philadelphia, 1889), pp. 28–29. In keeping with this emphasis was the insistence of insurance companies upon certificates from family physicians in addition to the reports of their own medical examiners in evaluating risks. A clear-headed medical man would, it was believed, even when treating acute symptoms, acquire an understanding "of the tendencies toward a particular form of death." J. Adams Allen, *Medical Examinations for Life Insurance*, 2nd ed. rev. (Chicago, 1867), p. 50.

16 The A.M.A.'s 1847 Code of Ethics (Ch. I, Art. II, Par. 3) in discussing the duties of patients urged that one particular physician be chosen, for a medical man acquainted with the "peculiarities of constitution, habits, and predispositions, of those he attends, is more likely to be more successful in his treatment, than one who does not possess that knowledge." Cf. Ch. I, Art. II, Par. 8, and American Institute of Homeopathy, *Code of Medical Ethics, Constitution, By-Laws, and List of Members . . .* (Boston, 1869), pp. 8, 10, 13.

17 Those processes, moreover, which have brought about this specialization have at the same time raised standards and limited access to the profession — thus tending to remove a basic component of economic competition in medicine.

18 The quotation is from John J. Elwell, *A Medico-Legal Treatise on Malpractice and Medical Evidence . . .*, new ed. (New York, 1866), p. 40. As late as 1870, a critical physician noted acidly the prevalence of belief in the medical profession in the ability of maternal impressions to cause any degree of malformation. G. J.

Fisher, "Does maternal mental influence have any constructive or destructive power in the production of malformations or monstrosities . . . ?," *Am. J. Insanity*, 1870, *26*: 241–295. Cf. Edward Seguin's *Idiocy: and its Treatment by the Physiological Method* (New York, 1866), pp. 41–42. New York specialist Augustus K. Gardner warned in a popular treatise on sex not only against sexual intercourse when intoxicated, but also with old men, and when grief-stricken, despondent, or irate. *Conjugal Sins against the Laws of Life and Health and their Effects upon the Father, Mother and Child*, rev. ed. (New York, 1874), pp. 174–175, 194.

19 Austin Flint, *A Treatise on the Principles and Practice of Medicine* (Philadelphia, 1866), p. 95. Insurance companies at the time, however, unanimously urged medical examiners to be wary of applicants with a clouded hereditary background; tuberculosis was especially feared and its occurrence in near relatives was an automatic cause of refusal to insure. Cf. *Instructions to the Medical Examiners of the Mutual Insurance Company of New York* (New York, 1866), p. 19 and *passim.*

20 Medical Society, County of New York, Committee on Diseases, "Minutes," Entry for meeting of June 4, 1866, Rare Book Room, New York Academy of Medicine. On the epidemic constitution, see *ibid.*, "Report of Committee on Diseases for Month ending April 2, 1866," p. 13, which describes the month as being marked by a tendency to neurological complaints, "Persons suffering with very different forms of sickness seem often to be afflicted alike in this respect."

21 John J. Elwell in a popular text on medical jurisprudence explained in such terms the difficulties encountered even by the surgeon in producing consistent results. "Where a surgeon undertakes to treat a fractured limb, he has not only to apply the known facts and theoretical knowledge of his science, but he must contend with very many powerful and hidden influences; such as want of vital force, habit of life, hereditary diathesis, climate, the mental state, local circumstances, and a thousand other agencies. . . ." *A Medico-Legal Treatise*, p. 23.

22 In 1866, blood disorders were particularly popular as pathological mechanisms with which to explain disease; well-nigh all infectious diseases, for example, were presumed by progressive physicians to be blood conditions, spread from person to person by a substance or agency capable of bringing about some alteration in the patient's blood. J. Lewis Smith could, for example, define diphtheria as a "blood disease, which, like measles or scarlet fever, has a local inflammatory manifestation." *A Treatise on the Diseases of Infancy and Childhood* (Philadelphia, 1869), pp. 439, 450.

23 Smith, "The age of uterine disease," *Doctor in Medicine*, pp. 104–108; S. D. Gross, *Then and Now: A Discourse* . . . (Philadelphia, 1867). On dentition, see Abraham Jacobi, *Dentition and its Derangements* (New York, 1862).

24 The following passages, located by date, are from Burke's diary, in the possession of the Rare Book Room of the New York Academy of Medicine. The New York Academy also contains the "Diary and Case-Book" of Henry G. Cox for the period 1851–1866. Dr. Cox, who died early in 1866, kept only brief accounts of financial matters. They do, however, indicate a number of aspects of his practice: the infrequent settling of accounts by his patients, the inclusion of servants in the accounts of their employers, his staying overnight with difficult cases.

25 Entry for Jan. 14, 1866.

26 The eleven dispensaries mentioned were those dedicated to general medicine; there were others, of course, founded for the treatment of specific classes of disease. Where the annual reports of these dispensaries have not been available, statistics have been taken from *The Medical Register of the City of New York and Vicinity . . . for the Year Commencing June 1, 1867*, ed. John Shrady (New York, 1867). Homeopathic statistics were drawn from the annual reports of the New York Homoeopathic Dispensary and the Bond Street Homoeopathic Dispensary, both published in the *Tr. Homoeopathic Med. Soc. St. N.Y.*, 1866.

27 William Thoms, "Sanitary condition of Fish Alley and surroundings," *Tr. Med. Soc. St. N.Y.*, 1866, p. 151. For other descriptions of the difficulties faced by these visiting physicians, see *14th Annual Report Board of Managers of the North-Western Dispensary* . . . (New York, 1867), pp. 14–15; Henry M. Field, "The continued fever of New York City," *Tr. Med. Soc. St. N.Y.*, 1867, p. 322.

28 Smith, *Doctor in Medicine*, p. 152; Cathell, *The Physician Himself*, p. 20; B. Howard Rand, *Valedictory Address to the Graduates of the Jefferson Medical College* . . . (Philadelphia, 1868), p. 11.

29 These statistics are drawn from, The Demilt Dispensary in the City of New York, *16th Annual Report . . . for . . . 1866* (New York, 1867).

30 *North-Western Dispensary . . . 14th Annual Report*, p. 7; Northern Dispensary, *40th Annual Report* (New York, 1867), p. 17.

31 New York, Commissioners of Charities and Correction, *Annual Report, 1866*, "Annual Report of the Warden of Bellevue Hospital," p. 4. The New York Ophthalmic Dispensary treated some 1,119 patients,

and the Eye and Ear Infirmary noted that it had "prescribed for" 8,033 patients, 313 of whom were indoor cases.

32 *8th Annual Report St. Luke's Hospital for the Year Ending... Oct. 18, 1866* (St. Johnland, 1867), pp. 30–31. The rules of the Nursery and Child's Hospital and Infant's Home are printed in *The Medical Register for 1866*, p. 136. The *7th Annual Report* of the Commissioners of Charity (pp. 8–9) prints a list of items made by patients and notes the use of convalescents as oarsmen (p. 83).

33 See the remarks of William Muhlenberg, founder of St. Luke's, on the tragic circumstances of the "incurables" denied treatment. *8th Annual Report St. Luke's Hospital*, pp. 8–9. Thomas Addis Emmett waged a bitter struggle with his board of managers when he sought to treat cancer patients in the Woman's Hospital. Emmett, *Incidents in My Life* (New York, London: Putnam, 1911), pp. 195–196. In 1866, however, the Protestant Episcopal Church did establish the first private "Home for Incurables" at West Farms, an act applauded by the medical profession. *N.Y. Med. J.*, 1866, *3*: 318.

34 Valentine Mott Francis, *A Thesis on Hospital Hygiene for the Degree of Doctor of Medicine in the University of New York. Session 1858–59* (New York, 1859), pp. 194, 203. Since nurses at Bellevue and Charity Hospitals were paid $120 a year, it does not seem likely that the more able and ambitious served in these positions. Commissioners of Charity and Correction, *7th Annual Report*, p. 19.

35 J. Bayley Done, "Report of Department of Infants; Charity Hospital Report," *ibid.*, p. 98. The poor condition of abandoned children when received and the consequent difficulties of trying to raise them on an artificial diet were of course the principal element in creating this mortality. The children were, as well, nursed by the Alms-House's elderly female inhabitants, who cared little for extra duties and saw that they were as transitory as possible.

36 D. B. St. John Roosa, *The Old Hospital and Other Papers* (New York, 1889), p. 232 and *passim*; Emmett, *Incidents in My Life*, pp. 199–201. Particularly illuminating is the story of Abraham Jacobi's bitter squabble with the Board of Lady Managers of the Nursery and Child's Hospital. Jacobi, "In re the Nursery and Child's Hospital. Letter to Mrs. R. H. Lemist, Secretary Board of Managers Nursery and Child's Hospital, New York, October 1870," *Collectanea Jacobi*, VII (New York, 1909), 11–42.

37 Society of the New York Hospital, *The Financial Condition and Restricted Charitable Operations of the Society of the New York Hospital. Majority and Minority Reports ... Presented April 17, 1866* (New York, 1866), p. 8. The Ophthalmic Hospital was incorporated April 21, 1865, "for the purpose of affording facilities for the instruction of medical students in the treatment of all diseases of the eye." James J. Walsh, *History of Medicine in New York* (New York: National Americana Society, 1919), III, 855. Existing hospitals were, moreover, gradually being reorganized in terms of special services and clinics. In the spring of 1866, for example, the Charity Hospital was thus reorganized. "The Island Hospital," *Med. Rec.*, 1866, *1*: 63.

38 Flint, *Principles and Practice*, p. 102.

39 On the persistence of tasting urine to detect sugar, see Edward L. Keyes, "Early history of urology in New York," in *History of Urology*, ed. Bransford Lewis (Baltimore: Williams & Wilkins, 1933), I, 77.

40 *Instructions to the Medical Examiners of the Security Life Assurance and Annuity Company of New York* (New York, 1868); Mutual Life Insurance Company of New York, *Instructions to Medical Examiners*, p. 6. Each year the *Medical Register* listed the medical examiners of the various insurance companies in New York, and the list always included a number of the city's more prominent physicians.

41 E. C. Seguin, "The use of the thermometer in clinical medicine," *Chicago Med. J.* 1866, *23*: 193–201; Seguin, "Clinical thermometry," *Med. Rec.*, 1867, *1*: 516–519. Seguin reported that W. H. Draper and Austin Flint at New York and Bellevue Hospital were the physicians sponsoring the experimental use of the thermometer in their services. Both, it should be noted, were members of the Medical and Surgical Society, which held a meeting in November 1866 at which the thermometer was discussed. Van Ingen, *First One Hundred Years*, p. 73. Austin Flint's *Practice*, which did not discuss thermometry in the first edition of 1866, added three pages (pp. 106–108) on the subject in its second edition, 1867. James J. Walsh noted, however, that "It was well on toward the eighties before the thermometer was generally used by city physicians; it was nearly the nineties before it was generally employed in country practice." *History of Medicine*, I, 258.

42 The very existence of such aids to diagnosis helped, of course, to create specialties. Cf. Louis Elsberg, "Laryngology in America . . . ," *Tr. Am. Laryng. Assn.*, 1879, *1*: 33–35.

43 This is based on the statistics of seven dispensaries which provided totals of the number of prescriptions administered during the year. For 160,156 cases, 305,731 prescriptions were provided.

44 Austin Flint, *Essays on Conservative Medicine and Kindred Topics* (Philadelphia, 1874). Cf. Jacob Bigelow, *Brief Expositions of Rational Medicine* . . .

(Boston, 1858). Flint's conservative medicine was not unlike Bigelow's "rational medicine." A full bibliography of Americans adopting this more sceptical position would include scores of names in addition to the well-known ones of Bigelow and Oliver Wendell Holmes. Particularly influential in the mid-1860s was the English clinician Robert Bentley Todd and his emphasis on "stimulating therapy." *Clinical Lectures on Certain Acute Diseases* (Philadelphia, 1860).

45 The alcohol purchases of Bellevue Hospital in 1866 were staggering, including 1,637 gallons best whiskey, 161 gallons common whiskey, 40 gallons brandy, 260 sherry, 68 port, 20 gin, 134 barrels of ale, 85 cases tarragona wine. Bellevue, significantly enough, on the other hand, ordered no calomel and only five pounds of jalap. Much of the alcohol listed must have found its way into the stomachs of attendants and Tammany politicians — but still the enormous quantities are of significance. "Report of Apothecary, Schedule of Liquors, Wines and Ales, Purchased and Expended," Commissioners of Charities, *7th Annual Report*, p. 25. Medicines are listed on pages 26–29. Despite some historical scepticism as to how routinely anaesthetics were employed at this time, it is worth noting that Bellevue purchased 375 pounds of sulphuric ether and 20 gallons of chloroform during the year.

46 S. D. Gross was particularly acid. "Young Physic," he wrote in 1867, "boasts that he has never seen a lancet, and expresses surprise that such a weapon should ever have been in universal use. . . . He looks with disgust at the conduct of his predecessors, loudly proclaiming against their want of judgment, and like the Pharisees in the Bible, devoutly thanks God that he is not like other men. Scrupulously abstaining from the spilling of blood, he entrenches himself behind his wine, his whiskey, his brandy, his milk-punch, and his beef essence, bids defiance to disease. . . ." *Then and Now*, p. 23. Gross does note as well that emetics of any kind were now rarely given and "drastic cathartics" administered less frequently. Cf. Richard D. Arnold to Henry M. Fuller, March 28, 1868, *Letters of Richard D. Arnold, M.D. 1808–1876 . . .*, ed. Richard Shryock (Papers of the Trinity College Historical Society, XVIII–XIX, Durham: Duke Univ. Press, 1929), pp. 135, 137.

47 This statement is based on a survey of a number of contemporary guides to prescribing and collections of prescriptions, as well as textbooks of materia medica. I have, unfortunately, been unable to find the prescription records of any New York pharmacy or established practitioner in 1866. There does seem to have been some truth in the homoeopathic charge that their influence had been important in turning allopaths toward less severe doses — even toward the coating of their own pills with sugar. William Todd Helmuth, "Annual address," *Proc. Am. Inst. Homoeopathy*, 1866, p. 53.

48 Cf. among others: Charles West, *Lectures on the Diseases of Infancy and Childhood* (Phildelphia, 1866), p. 27. West's text was probably the most popular of the period, the edition cited being the fourth American, from the fifth English edition.

49 *Introductory Address Delivered at the College of Physicians and Surgeons, New York, October 17th, 1864* (New York, 1864), p. 31. Cf. Bigelow, *Brief Expositions*, pp. iv, 29; Field, "Continued fever," pp. 338–339, 341; A. P. Merrill, "Homoeopathy and cholera," *Med. Rec.*, 1866, *1*: 275.

50 Druggists were also expected to have available their own compounds of traditional panaceas. Even the forward-looking Edward Parrish's textbook of pharmacy provided recipes for Dalby's Carminative, Bateman's Pectoral Drops, Opodeldoc, Hooper's Female Pills, Turlington's Balsam of Life, No. 6 Hot Drops (Thomsonian), and Composition Powders (Thomsonian), *A Treatise on Pharmacy. Designed as a Text-Book for the Student, and as a Guide for the Physician and Pharmaceutist* . . . 3rd ed. (Philadelphia, 1867), pp. 824–828.

51 Such covert financial arrangements were particularly embarrassing to ethical relationships between physician and pharmacist. A few physicians went so far as to refuse to visit patients unless they agreed to have their prescriptions filled at a particular pharmacy — the physician receiving, of course, a percentage of the prescription's cost for such devotion. Physicians charged druggists with carelessness in filling prescriptions, druggists physicians with carelessness in writing them (usually in pencil and many on scraps of newspaper). "Medicus," "Physician's prescriptions," *Druggist's Circular*, 1866, *10*: 106; [William Proctor, Jr.], "Percentages on prescriptions," *Am. J. Pharm.*, 1867, *15*: 89–90; Edward Dixon, *Back-Bone* (New York, [c. 1866]), pp. 355–358; J. C. Young, *Druggist's Circular*, 1866, *10*: 129. More ethically oriented pharmacists approved of the East River Medical Association's action. [John H. Maisch], "Prescriptions — whose property are they?," *Am. J. Pharm.*, 1867, *15*: 472–473.

52 Smith, *Doctor in Medicine*, p. 17; F. Stearns, "The pharmaceutical business . . . ," *Proc. Am. Pharm. Assn.*, 1866, pp. 202–203.

53 By the 1870s, it was becoming apparent that New York medicine was beginning to overtake the traditional leadership exerted by Philadelphians. "Is not Philadelphia paling before New York?," Richard Arnold wrote in 1871. "What one of us takes a Boston Journal, high in intellect and medical culture as

Boston is?," *Arnold Letters*, p. 151. For an extremely perceptive analysis of the role of New York in fostering specialization — one paralleling many of the points made in the following passages — see George Rosen, *The Specialization of Medicine with Particular Reference to Ophthalmology* (New York: Froben Press, 1944), pp. 34–38.

54 The logic behind this position was, of course, based upon the emphasis in contemporary etiological thought upon the need to understand the "whole man" and his environment. Cf. [George Shrady], "Specialties and specialists," *Med. Rec.*, 1867, *1*: 525–526; Majority Report, "Report of the Committee on Medical Ethics," *Tr. A.M.A.*, 1866, *17*, esp. pp. 504–506. Compare, however, the completely different orientation exhibited in Henry Bowditch's minority report, *ibid.*, pp. 511–512.

55 In January 1864, for example, the New York Obstetrical Society was organized; in March, the New York Ophthalmological Society. The New York Medico-Legal Society was organized early in 1866 and the New York Dermatological Society in 1869. Walsh, *History of Medicine*, I, 213–214, III, 688, 692. Other specialties, as in diseases of the chest or orthopedic surgery, were generally recognized by other physicians.

56 They also played prominent roles in both the Ophthalmological and Obstetrical Societies. Their influence was, however, not as predominant as in terms of hospital appointments.

57 In medical education and medical publishing, however, Philadelphia was still ahead of New York. The larger city's dominance in the production of specialists would seem to be a result of the larger "substrate" it offered, both in clinical materials and, perhaps more important, prospective paying clients.

58 Emmett recalled his being atypically exclusive in his specialization, giving up all routine obstetrical practice. He remembered as well the hostility with which he was rewarded by other physicians, *Incidents in My Life*, p. 203. The best contemporary defense of specialism which I have seen was composed by New York ophthalmologist Henry D. Noyes, "Specialties in medicine," *Tr. Am. Ophth. Soc.*, 1865, pp. 59–74.

59 Traditional preceptorial responsibilities had, moreover, come to be regarded as a mere formality. [George F. Shrady], "Medical preceptorship," *Med. Rec.*, 1866, *1*: 429–430.

60 The following remarks are based largely on the annual announcements for 1865–66 and 1866–67 of New York's three medical schools, the Medical Department of the University of New York, the Bellevue Hospital Medical College, and the College of Physicians and Surgeons. Writers on medical education, it might be noted, unanimously urged the need for combining clinical instruction with traditional didactic methods. A certain defensive tone was also to be found in writers discussing the opportunities of small town and rural practice, cf. Theophilus Parvin, *The Subjective Utility of Medicine. Introductory Address Delivered before the Class of the Medical Society of Ohio . . . Oct. 6, 1868* (Cincinnati, [1868]), pp. 18–19.

61 The volunteer clinic physicians were younger men, unlike the established practitioners who occupied the dispensaries' consulting positions. On the importance of the dispensaries in provding opportunities for clinical training, see William Ludlum, *Dispensaries. Their Origin, Progress and Efficiency* (New York, 1876), p. 26; Abraham Jacobi, "Address at the twenty-fifth jubilee of the German Dispensary of New York," *Collectanea Jacobi*, VIII (New York, 1909), 62–63.

62 [George H. Shrady], "Clinical instruction," *Med. Rec.*, 1866, *1*: 261–262; [Shrady], "The extension of the lecture term," *ibid.*, pp. 213–214; R. Cresson Stiles, *An Introductory Lecture to a Course of Demonstrative Instruction in Histology and Pathological Anatomy* (New York, 1866), p. 4. Stiles urged that students offer proof before graduation of having attended a "demonstrative" course in auscultation and percussion. The quality of formal clinical instruction did not improve for some time: E. C. Seguin, "Higher medical education in New York. III. The system of clinical teaching in colleges," *Arch. Med.*, 1881, *6*: 57–64.

63 Simon Flexner and James Thomas Flexner, *William Henry Welch and the Heroic Age of American Medicine* (New York: Viking Press, 1941), pp. 58–71.

64 The younger Seguin was probably the most self-conscious and vocal. See, for example, his articles cited earlier on the use of clinical thermometry and his "The aesthesiometer and aesthesiometry" (*Med. Rec.*, 1867, *1*: 510–511), in which he called for the general adoption of the "new instruments of positivism" in clinical medicine and noted at the same time the fall of the French and rise of the German school of medicine in the preceding twenty years.

65 *The Medical Register for 1866*, pp. 67–68, provides a list of journals. The large number of German physicians, many of them comparatively recent arrivals, probably explains this fact; however, their very presence was part of the process in which knowledge and values were transmitted.

66 William Welch, for example, attributed the awakening of his interest in German medicine to the influence of Jacobi. Flexner and Flexner, *Heroic Age*, p. 70. The need to foster research and raise standards in American medicine was a pervasive theme in Jacobi's own addresses. For the reactions of

two other German physicians, see Ernst P. Boas, "A refugee doctor of 1850," *J. Hist. Med.*, 1948, *3*: 79–84; "Aerztliche Zustände in Amerika. Aus New-York," *Wien. med. Presse*, 1866, *7*: 358–359.

67 Among obstetricians and gynecologists in the 1860s, for example, it is difficult to find any prominent teacher and practitioner born in the city. T. Gaillard Thomas, E. R. Peaslee, A. K. Gardner, J. Marion Sims, Thomas Addis Emmett, Emil Noeggerath, Fordyce Barker, J. Lewis Smith, and Abraham Jacobi were all born and raised outside New York. A study comparing medical leadership in New York, Philadelphia, and Boston in this period would be of value.

68 For a particularly illuminating view of the casual ethical standards of the time, see the details of the malpractice suit launched by a Mrs. Walsh against Lewis A. Sayre several years later. Willard Parker and J. W. Carnochan, well established and successful physicians, thought nothing of endorsing the patient's claim — without apparently even bothering to make a thorough examination. *The Alleged Malpractice Suit of Walsh vs. Sayre* (New York, 1870); *Comments of the Medical Press on the Alleged Malpractice Suit of Walsh vs. Sayre* (New York, 1871); Lewis A. Sayre, *Introductory Lecture of 1868–69, at Bellevue Hospital Medical College* (New York, 1869), p. 11. The possibility of science forming the basis of a new system of values, one opposed implicitly to the morally compromising conditions of America's commercially centered medicine, was clear enough to at least some contemporaries. Stiles, *An Introductory Lecture*, p. 9; Smith, *Doctor in Medicine*, pp. 130–131.

Therapeutics

Therapeutics, the means of treating illness, is the core of medical practice. Unfortunately, American historians have paid little attention to this important branch of medical history, giving us only a rough outline of major developments. We do know that prior to the 20th century, with its chemotherapy and antibiotics, regular physicians possessed only a handful of specific remedies, one of the most valuable of which was quinine, used to treat malaria. In the absence of more such therapeutic agents, early 19th-century physicians focused their efforts on restoring the body to its normal state. To accomplish this, they generally resorted to the "heroic" measures — bleeding, purging, and blistering — described by Alex Berman.

The overthrow of heroic therapy during the middle third of the century resulted from a two-front assault: by physicians within the regular profession who were growing skeptical about the efficacy of their treatments, and by irregular practitioners who ridiculed the practice of their rivals. These sectarian physicians, many of whom had M.D.'s, offered the sick a range of alternatives to regular medicine, from infinitesimal pills to pure water. At the close of the century these irregulars, primarily homeopaths and eclectics, constituted an estimated 16 to 24 percent of all American practitioners. By this time, however, their therapies differed little in practice from regular medicine, and the old sectarians soon faded away, leaving the field to newcomers like osteopaths and chiropractors.

Medical therapy, of course, does not necessarily involve a physician, either orthodox or unorthodox. Throughout history many people have chosen to treat themselves, while some have sought help from faith healers, quacks, and others on the fringes of the healing arts. Self-treatment has long been practiced by individuals lacking access to physicians, wanting to save money, or simply embarrassed by the prospect of discussing delicate problems. As Ronald L. Numbers points out, they often turned for advice to a do-it-yourself manual, a friend, or perhaps a patent-medicine peddler. Although the extent of domestic practice is difficult to determine, one survey conducted in Philadelphia shortly after World War I revealed that 21.7 percent of the sick looked after their own health care entirely by themselves, while many others supplemented their physicians' prescriptions with over-the-counter drugs or concoctions of their own making.

Quacks offered still other varieties of therapy, usually secret and expensive. During the middle decades of the 19th century, when licensing laws were nonexistent and anybody could be a "doctor," these greedy pretenders to medical knowledge flourished openly. And even today, as James Harvey Young shows, quackery remains a thriving business, milking hapless citizens of millions of dollars annually for worthless cures.

5

The Heroic Approach in 19th-Century Therapeutics

ALEX BERMAN

I

For medical historians, the therapeutic mayhem perpetrated by American physicians during the first decades of the 19th century is painful but commonplace knowledge. "It is fortunate in that day," wistfully wrote an elderly doctor in 1878, "that we had a hardy, well developed race of men and women, possessing sufficient tenacity of life to not only resist the disease, but the remedies used to combat it." And as an afterthought, he added, "Should this practice again prevail with the badly developed race we now have, the percentage of deaths would be largely increased and few would come safely out of the hands of the doctors."[1]

William Cullen (1710–1790) of Edinburgh, and his pupil, Benjamin Rush (1745–1813) of Philadelphia, were probably most influential in promoting the heroic medication employed during this period. Rush's ruthless application of his theory of disease was characterized by a contemporary critic as "one of the great discoveries . . . which have contributed to the depopulation of the earth."[2]

Dr. Worthington Hooker (1806–1867) of Yale devoted a portion of an essay published in 1857 to an analysis of Cullen's influence on therapy. Hooker's conclusions may be summarized briefly as follows:[3]

(1) Cullen's writings[4] imparted to contemporary medical practice "a more definite and decided character."

(2) Remedies such as calomel, antimony, emetics, purgatives, opiates, as well as bleeding, etc., although previously employed with some restraint, suddenly became more frequently used, and with more abandon.

(3) Cullen criticized Stahl, Boerhaave, Sydenham, Van Swieten, Lieutaud, and others for timidity in therapeutics and for too much trust in the curative powers of nature.

(4) According to Hooker, "The reign of active medication, thus established chiefly by Cullen, reached its culminating point somewhere in the first quarter of this century. It was not introduced by him in full, but was fairly begun, and then was consummated in the course of a few years by those who followed him. This may be very distinctly seen in relation to the use of mercury. Cullen . . . had no idea of the extent to which this remedy was destined to be applied by his successors in the treatment of inflammations and fevers, much less of the common and indiscriminate use of it described by Hamilton"[5] (*Rational Therapeutics*, p. 16).

(5) Finally, Hooker concludes: "During the past twenty-five or thirty years, the reign of active medication has been manifestly declining." (Written in 1857.)

The evidence seems to indicate that what we would call "active medication" today, reached a culminating point later than "somewhere in the first quarter" of the 19th century and that its decline between 1825 and 1857 was considerably slower than implied in the above statements.[6] Vestiges of the heroic approach persisted as late as 1878, as exemplified by the practices of George B. Wood (1797–1879) and his nephew, H. C. Wood (1841–1920), the influential Philadelphia professors. In an article ("The heroic treatment of idiopathic peritonitis," *Boston Med. & Surg. J.*, 1878, *98*:555–560) H. C. Wood wrote:

ALEX BERMAN is Professor Emeritus of History and Historical Studies in Pharmacy, University of Cincinnati, Cincinnati, Ohio.

Reprinted with permission from the *Bulletin of the American Society of Hospital Pharmacists*, 1954, *11*: 320–327.

> I remember my uncle, Dr. George B. Wood, saying that he never lost a case of peritonitis in an adult, and the reason he gave was that he always bled his patients from the arm until they fainted, and then put one hundred leeches on the abdomen. I am proud to say that I am a thorough believer in the same plan of treatment, antiquated as it may appear . . . I have never, you see, had cause to regret having bled my patients copiously. It makes very little difference whether you take the blood from the arm or from the abdomen, provided you draw enough to make a profound impression . . . What is to be done after venesection? I take my stand on the old theory that calomel has power to modify inflammatory action . . . I am, as you see, a most entire believer in the antiphlogistic properties of calomel . . . As peritonitis is an exceedingly severe disease, and means death in ninety-nine out of a hundred cases unless they are treated promptly and efficiently, mercury, to do any good, must be taken in decided doses . . . In connection with the calomel, opium is undeniably of great value . . . The ability to stand large doses of opium in peritonitis is wonderful. In one of my cases, *seventy-five* grains of solid opium were taken daily for five days, and the patient made an excellent recovery . . . After the abdomen has been thoroughly poulticed for two or three days, blisters may be used, provided the temperature of the body has not remained high; that is, a blister may be applied at the end of three days if the temperature has fallen in the meanwhile. Do not put on a small blister. I was talking with my uncle, Dr. George B. Wood, the other evening about this very case, and he said that if he were in my place, he would order a blister ten by ten (inches). I have ordered a blister eight by ten.[7]

Rush, of course, had no monopoly on speculative pathology. His friend, Dr. Edward Miller (1760–1812), whose theory of disease causation resembled the one advanced by Broussais in France much later, made constant use of his lancet. Others were John Esten Cooke (1783–1853) whose obsession with the liver caused him and his pupils to inundate the Mississippi Valley with calomel; Dr. J. A. Gallup (d. 1849) who viewed disease as sthenic and inflammatory, bled without mercy; and Drs. Miner and Tully — Gallup's contemporaries, who had exactly opposite notions of what constituted disease — condemned bloodletting, and pushed calomel and opium to extremes. These gentlemen were subjected to a searching and devastating criticism by Elisha Bartlett in 1844.[8]

In 1844, T. D. Mitchell of Transylvania University openly accused many of his colleagues of killing their patients with lethal doses of calomel.[9] "The English writers who have quoted some accounts of large doses of calomel as employed in India and in this country," stated Mitchell, "have yet to learn what is meant by large doses . . ." Mitchell was scornful of Christison who was only able "to cite the use of this medicine to no greater extent than 840 *grains in eight days* . . ." "What will he say," asked Mitchell, "*of table spoonful doses every hour*, until the patient held, somewhere between the mouth and the rectum, a *pound* of the article? That such doses have been given, is just as susceptible of proof as the fact that calomel is employed at all. I have known it to be prescribed in tea spoonful doses, as if it were calcined magnesia."[10]

One writer, Alexander Means, admitted that calomel had been misused at times; he conceded that it was a powerful remedy, but he indignantly questioned whether physicians should "consent to cower at the outcry of blind prejudice, or ignorant and interested empiricism, and, before the eyes of the living myriads whom it has rescued from the jaws of the grave, deliberately pronounce the blistering curse of Science upon its head, and consign it to the reproach and maledictions of posterity?"[11]

Means left no doubt as to where he stood on the question; his answer was;

> No, never! — Sooner let the fate of the lacerated and engulphed multitudes, who have fallen under the explosive power of uncontrolled steam, and found their winding sheet in the ocean wave, authorize the utter expulsion of this great agent from the civilized world, when ten thousand burning axles are rolling under its impulse, and bearing with the speed of the winds the exchanges of intelligence and commerce to the

> nation. And yet who is prepared for such a national sacrifice? — None. The voice of civilization is the voice of reason, and the world obeys; — hear it: —
> Study more profoundly your science — strengthen your cylinders, — modify your machinery, and increase your circumspection, but, still retain THE MASTODON IN HARNESS, to do the work of an AGE in a YEAR.[12]

The editors of the *New Orleans Medical Journal* referred to Means' article as a "most spirited defense of this once omnipotent, but now much abused medicine." They assured their readers that only "the ignorant steam doctors, whose business it is to pander to the whims and prejudices of the unprofessional community" denied the value of mercurial preparations, and that there was no danger of these remedies becoming obsolete.[13]

The justification for "active" medication was often rationalized on the grounds that powerful methods were very efficacious if employed judiciously, and this is illustrated in the treatment advocated for pulmonary consumption by Dr. Charles W. Wilder, in 1843, before the Massachusetts Medical Society.[14] "Effective means are not wanting when the principle of action is once established. The lancet, the leech, the cupping-glass, the Spanish fly, croton oil, tartarized antimony, ipecacuanha and mercury, are instruments of power and of great utility when skillfully used. Much, however, depends on the time and manner of their use."[15]

Elaborating more fully, he announced that:

> . . . The remedial agents to be relied on are venesection, having strict regard to the effects produced, instead of the quantity of blood abstracted; leeching; cupping; blistering and irritating the surface of the chest with tartar emetic ointment, croton oil and sinapisms, while the pulse and other circumstances of the patient will tolerate them; at the same time we should call to our aid, when the disease is obstinate, tartarized antimony, and give it in sufficient doses, in solution in water to keep up more or less nausea for hours, or even days, as the case may require; giving a gentle emetic, every evening, of ipecacuanha, when no peculiarity of the patient contradicts its use . . .[16]

II

By 1860, the worst features of the heroic practice had disappeared. To be sure, traces of the old therapeutics persisted into the late 1870s; and the abuse of calomel was still widespread at the time of the Civil War. But by and large, physicians no longer thought it necessary to resort to the violent methods mentioned above. This change was described in an 1860 issue of the *Medical and Surgical Reporter* as follows:

> The almost universal abandonment of the lancet, the substitution of milder plans of treatment for those heroic modes, yet in vogue a generation ago, are matters of history. Quinine and iron are now given, where tartar emetic was formerly resorted to; patients are kept upon a nutritious diet where once they were bled, and while formerly the patient was denied water for fear of increasing the fever, he is now put upon brandy in larger or smaller doses. The general tendency of therapeutics is, to use a favorite and expressive clinical phrase, "building up," sustaining and stimulating. That such is the tendency of our day, about this there can be no dispute.[17]

One would like to regard the improvement in therapeutics at this time as being part of the general scientific advance. The facts indicate, however, that scientific considerations played a minor role in demolishing the old heroic practice, and what was called "rational" medication in 1860 was brought about largely by empirical and often irrational factors. Contributing also to the abandonment of the curative measures was the constant barrage of criticism hurled at the regulars by Thomsonian and other sectarian practitioners.

In 1871, the eminent Henry I. Bowditch pleaded in vain for a judicious revival of bloodletting.[18] Deprecating its former indiscriminate use, Bowditch pointed out certain cases where venesection could prove to be of value.[19] "The bleeders have now been so effectually silenced," he announced, "that we have virtually thrown aside, as worse than worthless, one of the most valuable of all therapeutic means which the long experience of the ages has taught us."[20]

Four years later, Dr. Samuel D. Gross made a last-ditch but futile attempt to convince his colleagues[21] of the value of bloodletting. "If, now and then, one is bold enough to bleed," Gross complained, "he is sure to be taken to task about it, if he is not actually denounced as a murderer . . . the lancet is an obsolete instrument, the office of the bleeder has departed, venesection has long been unfashionable, and few of the present generation of medical men would, if called upon, be able to open a vein in a scientific and creditable manner. Bloodletting, as I have already declared, is emphatically, one of the lost arts."[22]

This abandonment of bloodletting as a remedial agent entailed a shift in therapeutic thinking; the early conviction that the disease could be bludgeoned out of the patient gave way to the realization that "building up" and conserving his strength was essential.

In a significant symposium conducted by the Philadelphia County Medical Society in 1860,[23] the reasons for the rapid decline of bloodletting were discussed. The following causes were suggested by various speakers, to account for the disfavor into which this remedy had fallen:

> 1. *Change in type of diseases, and in the constitution of patients.*
> ". . . for many years past, all diseases have been assuming more and more of a typhoid character . . . diseases have become more asthenic, more adynamic in their character or type than formerly, and that, in consequence of this change, they do not tolerate as well bloodletting and other depletory remedies."[24]
>
> 2. *Propaganda activities of Thomsonians, Homeopaths, etc.*
> ". . . Thompsonism and Homeopathy have doubtless had some share; . . . Previous to the advent of the latter, the former had gained a footing in many places, and the people of these sections of country were so imbued with its fallacious teachings as to be hostile to venesection on nearly all occasions."[25]
>
> 3. *Decline of bloodletting on irrational grounds.* Took place "involuntarily and unconsciously. No one can justify it."[26] "It was by no sudden revolution in the fundamental doctrines of therapeutics, that bloodletting lost, in the estimation of the medical profession generally, its prominence as a remedial agent . . . its disuse in many of the cases . . . took place gradually — almost imperceptibly. Not among any particular class of practitioners, nor among those of any particular country or place, but almost universally. The great body of the profession everywhere, and without previous interchange of views, we might almost say, without themselves being always aware of the fact, made bloodletting, to a certain extent, a subordinate remedy, even in diseases . . . in the treatment of which, but a short time before, it had been considered . . . the chief remedy."[27]
>
> 4. *Decline of bloodletting on empirical grounds.*
> (a) *Realization through experience that heroic bloodletting was harmful.* "Bloodletting, unfortunately, like many other good and useful things, has been sadly, in its use abused. It has been . . . unwisely practiced . . ."[28]
> (b) *Empirical substitution of other remedies for bloodletting.*
> "A more widely extended and exact acquaintance with the antiphlogistic powers of various depressing or sedative agents, and their more general use subsequent to, in conjunction with, or to the exclusion of the lancet, cups, or leeches, in cases of inflammatory disease, or the control of which physicians were wont, formerly to confide, solely in free and repeated bleedings, may likewise be included among the causes which have contributed to confine the employment of direct depletion, of late years, within more narrow limits, and to curtail, materially, the extent to which it is carried, and the frequency of its repetition, even in those cases where it is still held to be an important remedy. In cases in which tartarized antimony, opium, veratrum viride, aconite, and other sedative agents have not been made to supersede entirely bloodletting, which in times past was reputed to be, in those cases, the chief and most efficient remedy, it is very certain that their employment has caused the

amount of blood drawn to be greatly restricted, and a repetition of bloodletting a rare exception where it was once almost the universal rule."[29]

5. *Influence of Louis' "Numerical Method."* "Numerical [medical] statistics have been especially appealed to by the opponents of the use of bloodletting."[30]

6. *Greater scientific knowledge.* ". . . more disposed to attribute the limited use of bloodletting to the more accurate and extended knowledge of pathology — the more positive knowledge of the modus operandi of therapeutical agents, possessed by the profession of today, beyond that, which was in the keeping of those of the profession whom we call our immediate predecessors . . ."[31]

7. *Influence of certain authorities.* "By a few of the most distinguished practitioners in Great Britain, and on the Continent of Europe, it has been doubted even whether the abstraction of blood in any disease . . . is in fact necessary . . . Louis, Stokes and several German authorities maintain that bloodletting has little if any control over the progress of the issue of pneumonia; whilst Dr. Hughes Bennett, and others, insist that it is positively injurious in this and all other acute inflammations."[32]

Surprisingly, one important trend contributing to the overthrow of the bleeding and purging system was not discussed at the symposium, or if it was, it was not reported in the *Medical and Surgical Reporter*. This trend was the therapeutic skepticism and reliance on the curative powers of nature, as evinced by a number of physicians, beginning in the late 1830s. Jacob Bigelow's essay[33] on "self-limited" diseases, published in 1835, was influential in this respect as was the paper by John Forbes published in 1846 in the *British and Foreign Medical Review*.[34] An interesting feature of Forbes' article was his thesis that the infinitesimal dosing of Homeopathy had unwittingly vindicated the case for therapeutic skepticism, and that the validity of regular therapeutics was thus by implication at stake. Forbes wrote:

> In finishing our examination of the writings of the Homeopathists, we said, that we did not shrink from admitting and adopting the inferences — however unfavorable to Allopathy — which seemed necessarily to flow from the results of their treatment of diseases. The principal of these inferences have been already stated more than once. It seems necessary, however, to recapitulate the more important of them here.
>
> These are:
>
> 1. That in a large proportion of the cases treated by allopathic physicians, the disease is cured by nature, and not by them.
>
> 2. That in a lesser, but still not a small proportion, the disease is cured by nature, in spite of them; in other words, their interference opposing, instead of assisting the cure.
>
> 3. That, consequently, in a considerable proportion of diseases, it would fare as well, or better, with patients, in the actual condition of the medical art, as more generally practised, if all remedies, at least all active remedies, especially drugs, were abandoned.[35]

Dr. Oliver Wendell Holmes, himself probably the most forceful exponent of this trend, considered that Bigelow's essay had influenced a number of New England physicians.[36] To judge from an address given by Holmes, the trend of "the nature-trusting heresy" had been practiced chiefly in Massachusetts and Boston.[37] He pointed out in the same address that the American pupils of Louis had brought back with them a spirit of skepticism, based on their experiences in Louis' wards, where they had observed that many patients recovered by themselves, with no medication whatever.[38] Fifteen years later, Gross, in his speech referred to earlier, specifically singled out Bigelow's work in Boston, and Forbes' teachings in London as having had a restraining influence on unbridled medication and bloodletting.[39]

The *Medical and Surgical Reporter*, commenting editorially on the symposium of the Philadelphia County Medical Society, expressed the view that there had been essentially two ways of interpreting changes in therapy between 1840 and 1860: one group of physicians was convinced that diseases had become asthenic; another, that physicians had simply acquired a fuller understanding of disease and its treatment, and that there had been no change in the type of diseases. The editor then undertook to explain the "revolution" in therapeutics in terms of social change: factory conditions, the rapid growth of urban populations, and the increased tempo of industrial life had had a marked effect on the physical constitution of man and had caused people to become more susceptible to attack by diseases of debility; hence, they could not withstand the former heroic medication.[40]

Dr. S. D. Gross accused Robert Bentley Todd (1809–1860), Professor of Physiology and General and Morbid Anatomy in King's College, London, of having been the chief proponent of the doctrine of change in disease. According to Gross, Todd had formulated his "absurd" theory as a result of his experience with victims of London factory and slum life who were unable to tolerate depleting remedies.[41]

Whether we, today, view "Toddism" as an interesting rationalization or as a curious theory, the fact remains that a large number of physicians who held this doctrine modified their therapeutics. We must therefore regard this trend as having contributed materially to the downfall of heroic therapy.

As for the other reasons advanced at the Philadelphia symposium to account for the *volte-face* in therapeutic thinking, all appear to possess some validity. The attack on orthodox therapy carried on by the botanics and other medical sects unquestionably aroused public opinion or "public prejudice," as the regulars were inclined to call it. One must also not discount the large number of physicians whom Roberts Bartholow characterized as having "no settled convictions, who are content to drift along, hoping they do good, but whose vaporous therapeutic notions have never crystallized into definite forms."[42] Many of these practitioners gradually abandoned the old methods without being too clear about the reasons. Empirical substitution of various remedies[43] definitely helped to demolish the old practice, and although Louis' numerical method[44] exerted some influence in undermining "active" medication, it is difficult to evaluate other scientific factors, if any, that may have operated in therapeutics prior to 1860.

III

Despite the general transformation and improvement in therapy by the time of the Civil War, many doctors still showed marked preference for calomel, and pushed this remedy to extremes. This situation was dramatically highlighted by Surgeon General Hammond's order in 1863 removing calomel and tartar emetic from the supply table of the army.[45] The Surgeon General indicated that reports from his Medical Inspectors had shown many cases of "profuse salivation" and not infrequently "occurrences of mercurial gangrene" brought on by calomel. As for tartar emetic, Hammond justified its removal on the grounds that this remedy had been abused, was not really needed, and that its presence on the supply table was "a tacit invitation to its use."

The roar of rage with which Hammond's pronouncement was greeted by the majority of regular physicians[46] drowned out the approbation of his supporters and the gleeful applause of the botanics.[47] A group of irate physicians meeting in Cincinnati drew up a resolution denouncing Hammond and expressed the opinion that "the removal of W. A. Hammond from his position as Surgeon General would meet the approbation of the profession, be of advantage to our soldiers and creditable to the Government."[48] On the heels of this blast came several resolutions from the American Medical Association, severely censuring Hammond's action; his order was criticized as an insult to the profession and as a "reckless attempt to cut the Gordian knot of intricate pathology by the exercise of official power."[49]

Woodward reported on the basis of evidence he had gathered that prior to the issuance of Hammond's order, "mercurials were abused in certain quarters, but there is by no means so much of it as seems to be implied by the unlucky circular of May 4."[50] According to Woodward, Hammond's order was never enforced, and it did not have any appreciable influence on the use of mercurials in the army during the war.[51]

The immediate effect of Hammond's circular was three-fold: it whipped up a furious reaction on the part of organized medicine, with the A.M.A. accusing the Surgeon General of having grossly insulted the medical profession and of having maligned two "most invaluable" remedies, mercury and antimony;[52] it bolstered the stand of the botanics who were inveighing against calomel and antimony;[53] and Hammond's position, which had been seriously undermined by a feud with Secretary of War Stanton, became even more precarious.[54]

In the meantime, evidence gained through animal experimentation in Europe slowly accumulated to explode the myth that calomel promoted biliary secretion. The work of H. Nasse (1852), R. A. Koelliker (1853–1854), and F. Mosler (1858) in Germany, and George Scott (1859) in England showed that calomel actually decreased the secretion of bile.[55] This work, not too well known at first, especially in this country, was confirmed by the report to the British Medical Association made by the "Edinburgh Committee" in 1868, under the chairmanship of J. H. Bennett ("Report of Edinburgh Committee on Action of Mercury, Podophylline and Taraxacum on the Biliary Secretion," *The British Medical Journal*, 1868–1869). The findings of this committee, based on experiments with dogs, showed that calomel, blue pill and podophyllin definitely diminished the flow of bile, while taraxacum had no effect on the liver. This report not only scientifically demolished a cherished fable which the regulars had zealously cultivated, but it also delivered a stunning blow to the eclectics who were using podophyllin for the same purpose. Seven years later, William Rutherford of Edinburgh and his associate, M. Vignal, advanced still more evidence to support the conclusions of the "Edinburgh Committee."[56] By this time, calomel had ceased to occupy the prominent position it had so long held in the materia medica, although it has been retained in official pharmaceutical compendia up to the present day.

IV

The conflicting views of Alfred Stillé and Roberts Bartholow vied for acceptance in the 1870s, with the victory of Bartholow pointing the direction which modern therapeutics was to take. Stillé's viewpoint is perhaps best summed up in his own words:

> . . . The domain of therapeutics, is, at the present day, continually trespassed upon by pathology, physiology, and chemistry. Not content with their legitimate province of revealing the changes produced by disease and by medicinal substances in the organism, they presume to dictate what remedies shall be applied, and in what doses and combinations. Their theories are brilliant, attractive and specious, and they seem to satisfy a craving experienced by every reasoning man for an explanation of the phenomena which he witnesses; but, when submitted to the touchstone of experience, they prove to be only counterfeits. They will neither secure the safety of the patient nor afford satisfaction to the physician.[57]

The line of reasoning reflects, of course, the strong influence of the Paris clinical schools the deep faith in empirical observation; the repudiation of theorizing; and, above all, the conviction that therapeutics could not be derived from any of the sciences.[58] Although they helped to demolish the old heroic practice, the brilliant American disciples of Louis also tended to delay the growth of experimental therapeutics and pharmacology in this country.[59]

Bartholow's answer to Stillé was to state that:

> . . . modern physiology has rendered experimental therapeutics possible, and has opened an almost boundless field of research which is being diligently cultivated . . . I cannot but regard it as unfortunate that a writer of Stillé's eminence should occupy such a reactionary position . . . It is obvious that no science of therapeutics can be created out of empirical facts. We are not now in a condition to reject all the contributions to therapeutics made by the empirical method, but a thorough examination of them must be undertaken by the help of the physiological method.[60]

Dr. Bartholow buttressed his position by citing Liebreich's experiments with chloral (1869), Fraser's work with physostigmine, and Brunton's use of amyl nitrite in angina pectoris, as vindicating the physiological method; he also referred to the work of Claude Bernard as demonstrating the validity of animal experimentation to solve problems in therapeutics.

Stillé's views however, were not entirely erroneous. Today we know that clinical evaluation and experience are still the final tests in judging the efficacy of a remedy after it has left the laboratory.

NOTES

1 G. S. B. Hempstead, "Reminiscences of the physicians of the first quarter of the present century, with a review of some features of their practice," *The Cincinnati Lancet and Clinic*, *40*, n.s. *1*, 1878, 54. The worst features of this early 19th-century therapy quickly became the target of violent attack by rising American botanico-medical groups, providing them with powerful means for making converts, and indeed, constituting for them a fundamental *raison d'être*. The activities of these botanic groups were investigated by this writer in a doctoral dissertation entitled "The impact of the nineteenth century botanico-medical movement on American pharmacy and medicine" (Univ. of Wisconsin, 1954). Portions of the first chapter of this dissertation form the basis of the present article.

2 This statement was made by the famous polemicist and pamphleteer, William Cobbett (1763–1835) in *The Rush-light*, New York, Feb. 28, 1800, p. 49. Cited by R. H. Shryock in his article on "Benjamin Rush" in the *Dictionary of American Biography*.

3 Worthington Hooker, *Rational Therapeutics: A Prize Essay* (Publications of the Massachusetts Medical Society, Vol. I, No. 11, Boston, 1857), pp. 157–160.

4 Notably his *Materia Medica* (1772) and his *Practice of Physic* (1784).

5 James Hamilton, the younger (d. 1839), professor of midwifery at the University of Edinburgh, was one of the few men of his day who criticized the universal practice of indiscriminate, massive dosing with calomel. In the introduction to his book, *Observations on the Use and Abuse of Mercurial Medicines in Various Diseases* (1820), he speaks of the dangerous properties of mercury. He states: ". . . for some ages after mercury became an article of the Materia Medica, physicians recommended it only on the most urgent occasions — but within these few years British practitioners seem to have overlooked the necessity for such caution, and to exhibit that medicine with very little scruple" (American edition, 1821).

6 For example, in his work on the history of malaria in the upper Mississippi Valley, Ackerknecht has observed that "the decline of . . . 'active' treatment assumed considerable proportions only in the '50's and even then was slow enough" (E. H. Ackerknecht, *Malaria in the Upper Mississippi Valley* [Baltimore, 1945], p. 118).

7 Cited by J. J. Woodward, Surgeon, U.S.A., in *The Medical & Surgical History of the War of the Rebellion*, Part 2, Vol. I, *Medical History*, p. 687 (1879). A good example of G. B. Wood's reactionary views is to be found in his *Treatise on Therapeutics and Pharmacology or Materia Medica*, 2 vols. (Philadelphia, 1868). He writes on bloodletting: "As an antiphlogistic measure, the loss of blood holds a position far above any other agent; and it is in this capacity, moreover, that it exercises the most beneficial therapeutic influence" (II, 40).

8 Elisha Bartlett, *An Essay on the Philosophy of Medical Science* (Philadelphia, 1844), pp. 224–244.

9 Thos. D. Mitchell, "Calomel considered as a poison," *New Orleans Med. & Surg. J.*, 1844–45, *1*: 28 ff.

10 *Ibid.*, p. 30.

11 Alexander Means, "Calomel — Its chemical characteristics and mineral origin considered, in view of its curative claims," *Southern Med. & Surg. J.*, March, 1845. Cited in the *New Orleans Med. J.*, 1845, *1*: 588.

12 *Ibid.*, p. 589.

13 *Ibid.*, p. 591.

14 Chas. W. Wilder, "Pulmonary consumption, its causes, symptoms & treatment," *Med. Comm. Mass. Med. Soc.*, 7, 2nd series, Vol. III (Boston, 1848). Read at the annual meeting, May 31, 1843.

15 *Ibid.*, p. 116.

16 *Ibid.*, p. 119.

17 *Med. & Surg. Reptr.*, 1860, *5*: 320.

18 Henry I. Bowditch, "Venesection, its former abuse and present neglect" (Publications of the Massachusetts Medical Society, Vol. III, No. 3, Boston, 1871), pp. 223–249.

19 Bowditch recommended venesection in cases where: 1. "the heart . . . becomes distended with blood"; 2. during "very acute pain in any part of the thorax, for example, from inflammation of the pleura, causing orthopnoea and distress"; 3. "in violent acute cephalic symptoms . . . when the head is hot, the face flushed, and the pulse full and hard"; and 4. "in certain cases of threatened miscarriage." *Ibid.*, p. 249.

20 *Ibid.*, p. 223.

21 S. D. Gross, "A discourse on bloodletting considered as a therapeutic agent," *Tr. A.M.A.*, 1875, *26*: 421–433.

22 *Ibid.*, p. 421.

23 *Med. & Surg. Reptr.*, 1860, *3*: 495–521; *4*: 35.

24 *Ibid.*, *3*: 500.

25 *Ibid.*, *3*: 518. For a study of Samuel Thomson (1769–1843) and his followers, see Alex Berman,

"The Thomsonian movement and its relation to American pharmacy and medicine," *Bull. Hist. Med.*, 1951, *25*: 405–428; 519–538.

26 *Med. & Surg. Reptr.*, *4*: 35.

27 *Ibid.*, *3*: 497.

28 *Ibid.*, *3*: 519.

29 *Ibid.*, *3*: 499.

30 *Ibid.*, *4*: 35. The pioneer work in medical statistics of the great French clinician, Louis, is discussed at length by R. H. Shryock, in *The Development of Modern Medicine* (New York, 1947) pp. 157 ff. Louis did not utilize the calculus of probabilities, but only simple arithmetic for his statistical work.

31 *Med. & Surg. Reptr.*, *2*: 521. The view that the abandonment of bloodletting was the result of greater clinical and pathological knowledge was forcefully stated by J. H. Bennett of Edinburgh (e.g., *Edinburgh Med. J.*, 1856, *2*: 769–796), but was strongly denied by W. P. Alison and others (e.g., *Edinburgh Med. J.*, 1856, *2*: 971; 1044–1052).

32 *Med. & Surg. Reptr.*, *3*: 496.

33 Jacob Bigelow, "Discourse on self-limited disease," *Med. Comm. Mass. Med. Soc.* (Boston, 1835). Bigelow defined self-limited disease as follows: ". . . By a self-limited disease, I would be understood to express one which receives limits from its own nature and not from foreign influences; one which, after it has attained foothold in the system, cannot, in the present state of our knowledge, be eradicated, or abridged, by art, — but to which there is due a certain succession of processes, to be completed in a certain time; which time and processes may vary with the constitution and condition of the patient and may tend to death, or recovery, but are not known to be shortened, or greatly changed, by medical treatment . . ." (Discourse on self-limited disease, p. 322).

34 John Forbes, "Homeopathy, allopathy, and 'Young Physic,'" *Brit. & Foreign Med. Rev.*, 1846, *21*: 225–265.

35 *Ibid.*, p. 257.

36 O. W. Holmes, "Currents and counter-currents in medical science," an address delivered before the Massachusetts Medical Society at the annual meeting, May 30, 1860. Bigelow's influence was reflected in the following essays: A. A. Gould, "Search out the secrets of nature," read at the annual meeting of the Massachusetts Medical Society, 1855; W. Hooker, "Rational therapeutics; a Prize Essay," Boston, 1857; and W. J. Walker, "On the treatment of compound and complicated fractures," read at the annual meeting of the Massachusetts Medical Society, 1845.

37 Holmes, "Currents and counter-currents." The Bigelow influence was still active in Massachusetts in 1868. Three prizes were awarded that year to physicians for essays dealing with "the part performed by nature and time in the cure of diseases."

38 *Ibid.*

39 Gross, "Discourse on bloodletting," p. 426.

40 *Med. & Surg. Reptr.*, 1860, *5*: 321. For several years a highly interesting debate raged at Edinburgh with J. H. Bennett and his followers attacking the view that there had been a change in the type of disease and the constitution of patients, and W. P. Alison, Robert Christison, et al., firmly supporting the theory. See *Edinburgh Med. J.*, Vols. *1–5*, 1855–1860.

41 Gross considered "Toddism" as having "exercised the most perverse and baneful effects upon civilized society. Ensconcing itself behind a false position, it has literally enslaved the medical world, entrapping alike the wise and foolish, and sweeping over human life with a force equal to that of the most destructive hurricane" ("Discourse on bloodletting," p. 423). Elsewhere, Gross wrote that he thought "Toddism" was responsible for having "slain millions of human beings by the indiscriminate manner in which it has been employed" (*Autobiography of Samuel Gross, M.D.*, I [Philadelphia, 1887], 380).

42 Roberts Bartholow, *Annual Oration on the Degree of Certainty in Therapeutics* (Baltimore, 1876), p. 2. Bartholow (1831–1904) was a professor at the Medical College of Ohio and the author of a very popular textbook on materia medica and therapeutics.

43 For example, Ackerknecht has shown how quinine which for a time "was only one element in the treatment of malaria, and often the least important" replaced the old prostrating methods when it was empirically observed that large doses of quinine were very effective (*Malaria in the Upper Mississippi Valley*, p. 115). The same is true of other diseases, e.g., the empirical substitution of aconite and veratrum viride as "antiphlogistic" agents in the treatment of "inflammatory affections" in place of bloodletting (Gross, "Discourse on bloodletting," p. 426).

44 See P. Ch. A. Louis, *Researches on the Effects of Bloodletting in Some Inflammatory Diseases and on the Influence of Tartarized Antimony and Vesication in Pneumonitis*. Translated by C. G. Putnam, M.D. With Preface and Appendix by James Jackson, M.D. (Boston, 1836). Louis' "numerical method" had its zealous advocates in this country (Bartlett, Holmes, et al.) and its detractors (Hooker, et al.)

45 The text of Hammond's "Circular No. 6," is reproduced in the *Tr. A.M.A.*, 1864, *14*: 29–33.

46 A detailed, excellent discussion of the entire incident is given by Woodward, *Medical & Surgical History*, pp. 719 ff.

47 *Ibid.*, p. 719. Woodward mentions several regular medical journals that approved Hammond's action. He also cites a letter on file in the Surgeon General's

office, from the Massachusetts Eclectic Medical Society, tendering "heart-felt congratulations to Surgeon General Hammond for the liberal and independent position assumed in this matter."

48 Cited by Woodward, *ibid.*, p. 719.

49 *Tr. A.M.A.*, 1864, *14*: 29–33.

50 Woodward, *Medical & Surgical History*, p. 720.

51 *Ibid.* Although Hammond's order struck calomel from the supply table it did not affect the following mercurial preparations on the list: Hydrargyri chloridum corrosivum; Hydrargyri iodidum flavum; Hydrargyri oxidum rubrum; Hydrargyri pilulae; Hydrargyri unguentum; and Pilulae catharticae compositae. Woodward reports that calomel was available in plentiful supply, with 140,169 ounces of calomel and 488,447 dozen compound cathartic pills issued by the Union army during the war.

52 See report of the Committee on Order No. 6 of the Surgeon General, in *Tr. A.M.A.*, 1864, *14*: 29–33.

53 For a typical botanic reaction to Hammond's order, see the editorial "A home-thrust at regular medicine by the Surgeon General," *Eclectic Med. J.*, 1863, *22*: 294–295.

54 Wm. A. Hammond, *A Statement of the Causes which Led to the Dismissal of Surgeon General William A. Hammond from the Army* . . . (New York, 1864).

55 Woodward, *Medical & Surgical History*, p. 722.

56 W. Rutherford and M. Vignal, "Experiments on the biliary secretion of the dog," *J. Anat. & Physiol*, (1876).

57 Alfred Stillé, *Therapeutics and Materia Medica*. I (Philadelphia, 1874), 31.

58 Stillé had been in close association with two of Louis' students, Gerhard and Pennock, and had himself gone to study in Paris. See E. Bartlett, *An Essay on the Philosophy of Medical Science* (Philadelphia, 1844), and E. H. Ackerknecht, "Elisha Bartlett and the philosophy of the Paris clinical school," *Bull. Hist. Med.*, 1950, *24*: 43–60.

59 According to Krantz and Carr, pharmacology in this country had its beginnings when John J. Abel (1857–1938) was appointed Professor of Pharmacology at the University of Michigan in 1890. (J. C. Krantz and C. J. Carr, *The Pharmacological Principles of Medical Practice* [Baltimore, 1951], p. 9). In France, experimental pharmacology started with Magendie in 1809 (J. Olmsted, *François Magendie* [New York, 1944], p. 44), who was *sui generis*, and his illustrious pupil, Claude Bernard; in Germany it was closely related to the growth of what Ackerknecht has called "laboratory medicine."

60 Bartholow, *Annual Oration*, pp. 12–14.

6

Do-It-Yourself the Sectarian Way

RONALD L. NUMBERS

Among the most ardent American champions of home health care were the medical sectarians who arose in the 19th century to challenge the heroic therapy of the regulars with their seemingly endless rounds of bleedings, blisterings, and purgings. Over the years a multitude of sects appeared, each offering the long-suffering public a surer, safer, and often cheaper way to health. There were botanics and eclectics, homeopaths and hydropaths, movement-curists and mind-curists, and others too numerous to mention. Despite their many differences, they all shared one trait in common: an enthusiasm for the practice of domestic medicine. Why they felt this way, and how they related their domestic activities to other professional goals, are the questions on which I shall focus. In doing so, I shall look at three of the largest and most influential of the 19th-century sects: the Thomsonians, the homeopaths, and the hydropaths.

While many 19th-century domestic medicine books fall under the general heading "botanic," the line between botanic and regular, sectarian and nonsectarian, is often blurred.[1] John Gunn's best-selling *Domestic Medicine*, for example, contains "descriptions of the Medicinal Roots and Herbs of the United States, and how they are to be used in the cure of disease"; yet its tolerance of calomel and bleeding betrays its orthodox origins.[2] Other works on vegetable and Indian medicines were exclusively botanical, but could hardly be called sectarian in the sense of belonging to an exclusive school of medical practice.

The person who turned the root-and-herb tradition into a full-blown medical sect was Samuel Thomson, a New Hampshire farmer who learned much of his botanic medicine at the side of a local female herbalist.[3] Early in his healing career he became convinced that the cause of all disease was cold, and that the only cure was the restoration of the body's natural heat. This he accomplished by steaming, peppering, and puking his patients, with heavy reliance on *lobelia*, an emetic long used by native Americans.[4]

The simplicity of his system made it ideal for domestic use. Not one to ignore the commercial possibilities of his discovery, Thomson in 1806 began selling "Family Rights" to his practice, for which he obtained a patent in 1813. For 20 dollars purchasers enrolled in the Friendly Botanic Society and received a 16-page instruction booklet, *Family Botanic Medicine*. The section on preparing medicines contained various botanical recipes, but with key ingredients left out. Agents filled in the blanks only after buyers pledged themselves to secrecy "under the penalty of forfeiting their word and honor, and all right to the use of the medicine." By the 1820s Thomson had prepared a more substantial volume entitled *New Guide to Health* (often bound with his autobiography), an edition of which appeared in German for the benefit of recent immigrants.[5]

During the 1820s and 1830s Thomsonian agents fanned out from New England through the southern and western United States urging self-reliant Americans to become their own physicians. Almost everywhere they met with success. By 1840 approximately 100,000 Family Rights had been sold, and Thomson estimated that about three million persons had adopted his system. In states as di-

RONALD L. NUMBERS is Associate Professor and Chairman, Department of the History of Medicine, University of Wisconsin, Madison, Wisconsin.

Reprinted with permission from *Medicine Without Doctors: Home Health Care in American History*, edited by G. B. Risse, R. L. Numbers, and J. W. Leavitt (New York: Science History Publications/U.S.A., a division of Neale Watson Academic Publications, Inc., 1977), pp. 49–72.

verse as Ohio and Mississippi perhaps as many as one-half the citizens were curing themselves the Thomsonian way.[6] And as Daniel Drake observed, the devotees of Thomsonianism were not "limited to the vulgar. Respectable and intelligent mechaniks, legislative and judicial officers, both state and federal barristers, ladies, ministers of the gospel, and even some of the medical profession 'who hold the eel of science by the tail' have become its converts and puffers," he wrote.[7]

The brisk sale of Thomson's *New Guide to Health* encouraged other botanics, including several of Thomson's erstwhile friends, to bring out their own domestic manuals. Elias Smith, once Thomson's general agent, offered a *Medical Pocket-Book, Family Physician, and Sick Man's Guide to Health* as "an extensive improvement" over Thomson's work.[8] Horton Howard, for three and a half years Thomson's agent in Ohio, also broke with the master and published a *Domestic Medicine*.[9] And Morris Mattson, after two frustrating years working with Thomson on a revision of the *New Guide to Health*, finally decided to go it alone with an "improved" guide entitled *The American Vegetable Practice*.[10] Other competitors tried to entice potential Thomsonians with offers of books similar in content to the *New Guide* but priced considerably under 20 dollars.[11]

Individuals wishing to practice Thomsonianism at home were not limited to reading books on domestic medicine. They could also subscribe to botanic journals, attend lectures, or correspond directly with Thomsonian practitioners by mail. Among the numerous botanic journals, several were aimed directly at the domestic medicine market. The editor of the Philadelphia-based *Botanic Medical Reformer* declared his intention of making his "sheet a 'HOME PHYSICIAN,' — and to carry to the fireside that knowledge of Medicine which every parent in our land ought to be possessed of."[12] The *Thomsonian Recorder* of Ohio expressed similar sentiments in more picturesque language: "We . . . ardently long to lead our readers away from the rocky cliffs, the miney depths, and the scorching sands of the mineralogical practice, to the fruitful fields, green pastures, and flowery banks of sweetly-gliding streams and grassy fountain sides, to gather roots, and leaves, and blossoms, barks and fruits, for the healing of the nations."[13]

The Thomsonian rallying cry was "Every man his own physician."[14] Unlike many other sectarians, who simply wanted the public to exchange one kind of physician for another, the early Thomsonians seemed genuinely pleased with the prospect of a world without physicians. Given the Jacksonian temper of the times, their slogan had great popular appeal. It reflected both the widespread distrust of elites and the conviction that the head of an American family "should in medicine, as in religion and politics, think and act for himself."[15] It was high time, declared Thomson, for the common man to throw off the oppressive yoke of priests, lawyers, and physicians and assume his rightful place in a truly democratic society.[16]

On a more practical level the Thomsonians argued persuasively that self-medication was safer than being "doctored to death."[17] Again they struck a responsive chord, for Americans in increasing numbers were growing suspicious of the purported benefits of repeated bleedings and calomel dosings. Common people were more likely to place their trust in the healing power of nature and the indigenous remedies that grew around them.[18] They could be sure that their domestically prepared medicines would be "pure, genuine, and unadulterated," unlike those often prepared by apothecaries, or worse yet, their apprentices.[19] Thomsonians frequently commented on the relative safety of their home treatments. "It has been generally remarked," wrote one, "that those families that employ no physicians, in cases of scarlet fever, canker rash, measles, and &c., lose a less number of children, than those who employ them."[20] Another could not recall "a single death from childbed disease" occurring under Thomsonian treatment.[21]

But Thomsonianism offered more than safety. Being your own physician would not only save your life, promised one botanic manual, but your money as well.[22] After the initial outlay of 20 dollars, the Thomsonian family need never worry about exorbitant bills from physicians and apothecaries. This alone, thought Horton Howard, would be sufficient inducement for most people to turn to domestic medicine.[23] The savings often were substantial; one New Hampshire family calculated theirs to be 75 dollars a year.[24]

Another unquestioned benefit of home treatment was convenience. "[T]he physician and the cure are always at hand," stressed one Thomsonian. "You have not to wander in the night to a distance, and the patient dying, to seek a doctor, with the agony pressing on your spirits, that your wife, or child, or friend may be dead on your return."[25] And where there were no physicians at all, domestic medicine was not only convenient but necessary. In the western states especially, which sometimes experienced shortages of physicians and apothecaries, self-treatment could be essential.[26] Here the Thomsonians were at a decided advantage, because, as Philip D. Jordan has noted, "most settlers had to supply themselves with drugs, and herbs were easier to secure than chemical mixtures and compounds."[27]

Finally, being your own physician allowed women to avoid the embarrassment of going to male physicians. By adopting Thomsonianism, wrote Horton Howard, women escaped "the necessity of consulting the other sex, with all its attendant indelicacy and mortification."[28] They also won the freedom to practice medicine in a limited way. Joseph Kett has recently argued that Thomsonianism, with its emphasis on the wife and mother as physician, opened medical practice to women "without forcing a confrontation of the sensitive question of whether a woman should ever treat a man other than her husband."[29]

With every person a physician, professional healers were left with few tasks indeed. Samuel Thomson, who opposed even Thomsonian infirmaries and medical schools, would have given them virtually none. If Thomsonian physicians were available, he argued, then people would no longer see the desirability of learning to treat themselves — and perhaps more important, though he did not mention it, they would no longer find it necessary to purchase his Family Rights.[30] Among orthodox Thomsonians, the sole function of physicians was educational. "The physician, instead of dealing out poison," explained one, "would deal out advice to his fellow men to live according to the dictates of nature."[31] He was not to be concerned about the prospect of losing his practice as home treatment increased. Instead, he was to expect to tire of his work after eight or ten years and "be happy to have the people take the burthen of the practice upon themselves."[32]

Not all Thomsonians, however, accepted such a restricted role for trained doctors. Horton Howard recommended resorting to physicians in cases of serious cuts, punctured arteries, broken bones, or unusual or dangerous diseases; and Simon Abbott of Charleston, South Carolina, thought doctors might prove useful for "surgical operations and diseases which rarely occur."[33] This tolerance toward professionals became more common with the opening, over Thomson's adamant opposition, of botanic medical schools in the late 1830s. Naturally those associated with such institutions viewed domestic medicine in a different light from Thomson: home manuals were not to replace the physician but to supplement his efforts.[34] (This was also the opinion of Wooster Beach, founder of the rival eclectic school of medicine and author of two works on home medicine.[35]) Acrimonious debates over such issues as medical education eventually rent the Thomsonians into hostile camps and precipitated the demise of the movement.

As Thomsonian strength began to wane in the 1840s, a new medical sect, homeopathy, was rising to national prominence.[36] Homeopathy was the invention of a regularly educated German physician, Samuel Hahnemann, who had grown dissatisfied with the heroics of orthodox practice. During the last decade of the 18th century he began constructing an alternate system based in large part upon the healing power of nature and two fundamental principles, the law of similars and the law of infinitesimals. According to the first law, diseases are cured by medicines having the property of producing in healthy persons symptoms similar to those of the disease. An individual suffering from fever, for example, would be treated with a drug known to increase the pulse rate of a person in health. Hahnemann's second law held that medicines are more efficacious the smaller the dose, even as small as dilutions of up to one-millionth of a gram. Though regular practitioners — or allopaths as Hahnemann called them — ridiculed this theory, many patients flourished under homeopathic treatment and they seldom suffered.

Following its appearance in this country in 1825, homeopathy rapidly grew into a major medical sect. By the outbreak of the Civil War there were nearly 2,500 homeopathic physicians, concentrated largely in New England, New York, Pennsylvania, and the Midwest, and hundreds of thousands of devoted followers.[37] Homeopathy's appeal is not difficult to understand. Instead of the bleedings and purgings of the regulars, or the equally rigorous therapy of the Thomsonians, the homeopaths offered pleasant-tasting pills that produced no discomforting side effects. Such medication was particularly suitable for babies and small children. As the orthodox Oliver Wendell Holmes observed, homeopathy "does not offend the palate, and so spares the nursery those scenes of single combat in which infants were wont to yield at length to the pressure of the spoon and the imminence of asphyxia."[38] Perhaps because of its suitability for children, homeopathy won the support of large numbers of American women, who constituted approximately two-thirds of its patrons and who were among its most active propagators. "Many a woman, armed with her little stock of remedies, has converted an entire community," proudly reported the American Institute of Homeopathy.[39]

Central to the home practice of homeopathy was the "domestic kit," which consisted of a case of infinitesimal medicines and a guide. Scores if not hundreds of these were available during the 19th century in a variety of combinations ranging from small pocket cases with tiny guides to large family chests with thick volumes. Often the books appeared in foreign languages as well as in English, and occasionally they included homeopathic treatments for domestic animals.[40]

The first such kit came from the hands of Constantine Hering, a Leipzig-educated physician who settled in Pennsylvania in the early 1830s and who did as much as any man to promote the cause of homeopathy in America. In 1835 he published the first part of *The Homeopathist, or Domestic Physician*, and three years later he completed the second part. These he sold, together with a small mahogany box of medicines, for five dollars (four dollars for the German edition). The box contained small numbered vials filled with "infinitesimal pills," the numbers on the vials corresponding to the numbered remedies in the book. Self-treatment, once a diagnosis was made, was thus reduced simply to taking a No. 8 or a No. 17 pill, or whatever the manual recommended.[41]

Since most homeopaths were, like Hahnemann and Hering, trained physicians, they understandably did not share the Thomsonian enthusiasm for making every man a physician. Besides, many were recent immigrants from Germany, uninfected by Jacksonian democracy. They envisioned only a limited role for domestic practice. Hering, for example, wrote his book not to replace the physician but to assist families in treating minor complaints and to provide medical advice for students, travellers, mariners, and "those living in remote parts of the country." Like virtually all his homeopathic colleagues, he urged his readers to seek qualified medical assistance in serious cases.[42]

Several homeopathic domestic guides pointedly discouraged self-treatment. One warned that since even physicians could not safely treat themselves, ordinary persons should not think they could. George E. Shipman's popular *Homoeopathic Family Guide* cautioned that "No *very* sensible person will ever attempt to treat himself or his family, who can obtain the advice of a well-qualified physician. If those fail too often, who make the study of disease and their remedies the sole business of their lives," wrote Shipman, "what success can they expect, who know little or nothing of either?"[43]

But regardless of their reservations about home treatment, homeopaths were well aware that the domestic kits were one of their most effective weapons in winning converts from the allopaths. The domestic guides, especially in the early days, were seen as "missionaries of truth" preparing the way for the arrival of homeopathic physicians. Thus most homeopaths viewed domestic manuals not as competitors, but "as necessary allies in the great work of reforming the medical state of the world."[44] Even allopaths did not dispute their effectiveness. Many an "impecunious practitioner" has failed to get a case, complained one regular, because of "Dr. Humphreys' book and box that preceded him in the domestic corner."[45]

The homeopaths also derived encouragement from the knowledge that their practice was relatively harmless — certainly safer than "the Old System of Physic," "whose gentlest weapons are lancets and cathartics." Even if the patient took the wrong medicine, there was no need for alarm, wrote Hering, "for Homoeopathic medicine is so prepared that it will help, when it is the right one, but it will not injure should a mistake occur." The very worst possibility would be a slight delay in the healing process.[46] Readers of one manual were assured that "No life was ever lost by homoeopathic medicine used carelessly, or otherwise," a point conceded by sarcastic allopaths. Homeopathy, wrote Dr. Holmes, "gives the ignorant, who have such an inveterate itch for dabbling in physic, a book and a doll's medicine chest, and lets them play doctors and doctresses without fear of having to call in the coroner."[47]

Domestic homeopathy was not, however, without its difficulties, and its advocates were continually devising new ways of facilitating its practice. As in all forms of home treatment, making a correct diagnosis was probably the greatest challenge to the uninitiated, especially if there were a multitude of symptoms. To assist the bewildered domestic practitioner, one enterprising homeopath invented an elaborate but foolproof diagnostic system composed of a small book listing 2,467 symptoms and a pasteboard box filled with 2,467 numbered slips of paper, one per symptom. On each slip appeared the names of 127 remedies, with assigned weights from one to four. Users were instructed to select the slips corresponding to each of their symptoms, line them up in a row, identify the remedies found on every slip, add the weights for each remedy, and take the one with the highest total. In case of a tie, users were to "select from among the symptoms whichever one seems the most peculiar, or important, and take the rating of the remedies in question there given, as your indication for choice."[48]

Frederick Humphreys, mentioned earlier, discovered another method of simplifying home medication. A sometime professor in the Homeopathic Medical College of Pennsylvania, Humphreys broke with Hahnemann's rule of administering only one medicine at a time and instead recommended combinations of medicines for specific diseases, manufactured by his own Specific Homeopathic Medicine Company. Although some uncharitable colleagues called his invention "Homoeopathic quackery," lay homeopaths seem to have thought otherwise. The sale of his two domestic guides, a large one to accompany his more expensive kits and a smaller one for his cheaper cases, was truly phenomenal. By the early 1890s 15,000,000 copies of the latter work had appeared in five languages, 12,000,000 of which had been distributed in the United States. In one year alone he printed 3,000,000 copies.[49]

Despite the safety and popularity of these domestic kits and their acknowledged role in diffusing the principles of homeopathy, a few homeopaths questioned what they saw as an overemphasis on home medical care. John Ellis of Cleveland thought that books on preventive medicine were far more important "than any work on domestic medicine can possibly be," and claimed that his own *Family Homoeopathy* was written primarily to direct attention to his earlier but often ignored work on *The Avoidable Causes of Disease*.[50] *The Family Journal of Homoeopathy*, published by a group of St. Louis physicians, went even further in condemning "domestic practice of every description." "[W]e would prefer a good Allopath to prescribe for us than an ignorant or mongrel Homoeopath," the editors declared.[51]

As the century progressed and homeopathy came to occupy a secure place in American medicine, homeopaths began directing their attention less to the general public and more toward their own profession.[52] The writings of Charles J. Hempel, who authored a *Homoeopathic Domestic Physician* in 1846, reflect this change. After issuing two editions of his home guide, he became increasingly pessimistic about the value of domestic practice and decided, instead of preparing a third edition, to publish a volume on *Homoeopathic Theory and Practice*, "designed both for the public and for students and practitioners."[53]

The domestic guides that continued to appear during the latter part of the century tended to be somewhat less comprehensive than their predecessors and to focus instead on emergency care and minor diseases. There is no longer any need to provide every person with the "knowledge of a physician," wrote one homeopath in 1887, "for the doctor himself is at hand in every village and hamlet of the land, ready at the first summons to give advice and assistance far more valuable than that of any book."[54] This situation did not last long, however, if in fact it ever existed. Within a few decades homeopathy was fast fading from sight, and the question of homeopathic domestic practice had become moot.

To escape the most obvious pitfalls of allopathic practice, the Thomsonians had turned to botanic remedies and the homeopaths to their infinitesimal pills. A third sect, hydropathy, rejected drugs of every variety, whether botanic or mineral, in large or small doses. The hydropaths placed their trust solely in natural cures like fresh air, sunshine, exercise, proper (often vegetarian) diet, and, above all, water, which they used in every conceivable way.[55]

Hydropathy was a mélange of water treatments devised by a Silesian peasant, Vincent Priessnitz, to heal his wounds after accidentally being run over by a wagon. His therapy proved so successful that he opened his home in Graefenberg as a "water cure" and invited his ailing neighbors to submit their bodies to a bewildering variety of baths, packs, and wet bandages. When news of his methods reached the United States in the mid-1840s, it touched off a water-cure craze that continued unabated until the outbreak of the Civil War. Two regularly educated physicians, Joel Shew and Russell T. Trall, opened the first American water-cure establishments in New York City about 1843. A couple of years later Mary Gove (Nichols), an experienced woman health reformer, opened still a third water cure in the city. It was primarily these three pioneers — Shew, Trall, and Nichols — who introduced Americans to the new water system.

Among them they wrote perhaps a dozen volumes for domestic use. Throughout their writings run many of the themes commonly found in sectarian guides: the economy and absolute safety of their practice, the importance of prevention, and the advantages of self-reliance. On the question of making every man a physician, they fell somewhere between the early radical Thomsonians and the more moderate homeopaths. Since all three writers operated commercial water cures, they could hardly deny the value of professional care; yet they realized that relatively few people had access to such establishments or to hydropathic physicians, of which there were never many.[56]

In theory they saw little justification for limiting self-practice. The water treatments themselves were harmless, with the possible exception of the powerful douche, which one author warned should be used "with great caution, and always under the direction of an experienced hydropathic physician."[57] In Shew's opinion, hydropathy was "destined, not only to make the members of communities their own physicians for the most part, but to mitigate, in an unprecedented manner, the extent, the pains, and the perils of disease." The only time when professional assistance might be necessary was in the event of a serious injury, like a skull fracture.[58] Trall's attitude was basically the same. When the people become familiar with the principles of hydropathy and the laws of life and health, he predicted, "they will well-nigh emancipate themselves from all need of doctors of any sort." He thought home practitioners could successfully treat functional problems, which he estimated to be 99 percent of all ailments, but that they would probably need the skill of a trained surgeon for "mechanical injuries, displacements of parts, organic lesions, etc."[59]

Mrs. Nichols, the only nonphysician of the three, looked forward expectantly to the day when the spread of hydropathy would make physicians obsolete. Since a water-cure family seldom needed a physician more than once, she foresaw the end of medical practice outside the home. "Mothers learn to not only cure the disease of their families, but, what is more important, to keep them in health," she wrote in 1849. "The only way a Water Cure physician can live, is by constantly getting new patients, as the old ones are too thoroughly cured, and too well informed, to require further advice. This is a striking advantage to Water Cure patients, if not to Water Cure physicians."[60]

Like Thomsonians, hydropaths placed special emphasis on the role of women as providers and consumers of health care. In an age of few female doctors, roughly one-fifth of professional hydropaths were women.[61] Many water-curists of both sexes actively participated in the antebellum feminist movement, particularly as it related to freeing women from their "clothes-prisons" and from the dominance of male physicians. As part of their effort to effect the latter goal, they prepared domestic manuals instructing women on the care of their own bodies, as well as on the care of their families.[62]

One of the most successful means of popularizing all facets of hydropathy was the *Water-Cure Journal*, first published by Shew in 1845 and later edited by Trall. Beginning with the third volume, Shew promised to include considerable advice on domestic treatment, "thus enabling persons who cannot visit a hydropathic establishment, to prescribe for themselves." Those desiring more specific counsel than that printed in the journal were invited to correspond with the editor directly, on condition that they send a fee in advance.[63] Because of the scarcity of hydropathic physicians, several practitioners, including Mrs. Nichols, resorted to this semi-domestic device.

Numerous letters from *Journal* readers demonstrate the great popularity of domestic hydropathy and the eagerness of home practitioners to relate their experiences. One elderly man from Missouri vividly described his treatment for fever in the following letter to the publishers:

> . . . I put the patient in a hogshead that I keep for bathing. I have him go entirely under water, head and all, for three or four times, keeping his head under each time as long as he can conveniently hold his breath; then let him dabble in it up to the chin until the heat is reduced to the normal temperature, and the patient feels comfortable . . . . When I have no convenience for bathing, and, in fact, sometimes, as a matter of preference, I pour water on the patient's head, instead of bathing; and, surprising as it may seem, this always has the same effect that bathing has . . . . I have the patient lie with the head over the edge or side of the bed, so that the water will not wet the bedding. I then get a bucket of the coldest water . . . . the cure is completed in a few minutes, and it is a permanent cure, and a cure that all persons can perform at home without any inconvenience.[64]

Besides the *Water-Cure Journal* there were a number of lesser hydropathic magazines vying for the public's attention. One of the best of these was the *Laws of Life*, published in Dansville, New York, at Our Home on the Hillside, an unusually successful water cure operated by James Caleb Jackson and a woman associate.[65] During the waning years of the water-cure movement Jackson turned out a steady stream of works on home hydropathy, including a volume on the treatment of sexual disorders (a favorite topic of many health reformers) and a comprehensive and widely read book on *How to Treat the Sick without Medicine*.[66]

In one sense Jackson's most influential work on domestic medicine may have been a short essay on curing diphtheria with water, which appeared in an upstate New York newspaper during a diphtheria epidemic in the winter of 1862–63. Somehow this paper reached Battle Creek, Michigan, and fell into the hands of Ellen G. White, prophetess of the Seventh-day Adventist church and mother of two boys suffering from sore throats and high fevers. Hopefully she applied the recommended fomentations and met "with perfect success."[67] Several months later, during one of her frequent religious trances, God directed her to lead her Adventist followers into the hydropathic fold. As a result of her labors, in 1866 the Adventists opened their own water cure in Battle Creek and began publishing a hydropathic journal called *The Health Reformer*, which featured answers to questions on home water treatments.[68]

Even more important for the future of domestic hydropathy was Mrs. White's influence on her protégé John Harvey Kellogg (of cornflake fame), whom she and her husband assisted with obtaining both hydropathic and regular medical degrees. Kellogg in turn became the most prolific writer on domestic hydropathy — or hydrotherapy as it came to be called — during the late 19th and early 20th centuries, authoring such works as *The Household Manual of Domestic Hygiene, Ladies' Guide in Health and Disease, The Household Monitor of Health*, and *The Home Hand-Book of Domestic Hygiene and Rational Medicine*, which sold nearly a hundred thousand copies during its first 25 years.[69] Kellogg was the last of the major writers of domestic hydropathic guides, but well into the 20th century there appeared an occasional home manual advocating hydrotherapy as the safest of all therapies.[70] These books, however, were largely devoid of sectarian spirit and probably differed more from Shew's and Trall's early handbooks than from the orthodox guides of the day.

The brief look at sectarian domestic medicine reveals something of the extent to which home health care permeated American society during the 19th century. For literally millions of Americans, the sectarian domestic guides served as primary care physicians. While it is true that much of the sectarian literature simply reflected orthodox concerns with cost, convenience, and accessibility of doctors, in many respects the sectarian tradition was unique: in its exploitation of the therapeutic weaknesses of regular medicine, in its more ready acceptance of domestic medicine as a substitute for professional health care, and in its missionary zeal. In view of the effectiveness of domestic medicine in making and holding sectarian converts, it is no exaggeration to say that home health care was the foundation upon which the American medical sects were built.

NOTES

I wish to thank Blanche L. Singer, of the Middleton Medical Library, University of Wisconsin, and Janet Schulze Numbers for their assistance in the preparation of this paper.

1 See Alex Berman, "The impact of the nineteenth century botanico-medical movement on American pharmacy and medicine" (Ph.D. dissertation, Univ. of Wisconsin, 1954), pp. 92–93.

2 John Gunn, *Gunn's Domestic Medicine, or Poor Man's Friend*, 1st rev. ed. (Philadelphia: G. V. Raymond, 1839). On the popularity of Gunn's book, see Madge E. Pickard and R. Carlyle Buley, *The Midwest Pioneer: His Ills, Cures, and Doctors* (New York: Henry Schuman, 1946), p. 93.

3 Berman's unpublished dissertation remains the most thorough treatment of Thomsonianism; but see also Alex Berman, "The Thomsonian movement and its relation to American pharmacy and medicine," *Bull. Hist. Med.*, 1951, *25*: 405–428; 519–538; Pickard and Buley, *The Midwest Pioneer*, Ch. 4, pp. 167–198; Joseh F. Kett, *The Formation of the American Medical Profession: The Role of Institutions, 1780–1860* (New Haven: Yale Univ. Press, 1968), Ch. 4, pp. 97–131; and James Harvey Young, *The Toadstool Millionaires: A Social History of Patent Medicines in America before Federal Regulation* (Princeton: Princeton Univ. Press, 1961), Ch. 4, pp. 44–57.

4 Samuel Thomson, *New Guide to Health; or, Botanic Family Physician*, 2nd ed. (Boston: For the author, 1825), Part 1, pp. 42–45.

5 *Ibid.*, Part 2, p. 4; Samuel Thomson, *Family Botanic Medicine* (Boston: T. G. Bangs, 1819).

6 Berman, "The impact of the nineteenth century botanico-medical movement," pp. 150–152.

7 Daniel Drake, "The people's doctors," *Western J. Med. & Phys. Sci.*, 1829: *407*, quoted *ibid.*, pp. 42–43.

8 Elias Smith, *The Medical Pocket-Book, Family Physician, and Sick Man's Guide to Health* (Boston: Henry Bowen, 1822), p. viii. Four years later Smith published *The American Physician, and Family Assistant* (Boston: E. Bellamy, 1826) as an improvement over his own *Medical Pocket-Book.*

9 Horton Howard, *Howard's Domestic Medicine*, new enlarged ed. (Philadelphia: Duane Rulison, 1866).

10 Morris Mattson, *The American Vegetable Practice, or A New and Improved Guide to Health Designed for the Use of Families* (Boston: Daniel L. Hale, 1841).

11 See, for example, Reuben Chambers, *The Thomsonian Practice of Medicine* (Bethania, Pa., 1842).

12 Editorial, *Botanic Medical Reformer and Home Physician*, May 7, 1840, *1*: 9–10.

13 Preface to Vol. II, *Thomsonian Recorder* (1833): p. v.

14 See Thomson, *New Guide to Health*, Part 1, p. 10. This motto, or variations of it, appears in numerous botanic works on domestic medicine.

15 William Procter, Jr., *Am. J. Pharm.*, 1854, *26*: 570, quoted in Berman, "The impact of the nineteenth century botanico–medical movement," pp. 40–41.

16 Thomson, *New Guide to Health*, Part 2, p. 5.

17 Howard, *Howard's Domestic Medicine*, p. 30.

18 See, for example, Elisha Smith, *The Botanic Physician; Being a Compendium of the Practice of Physic, upon Botanical Principles* (New York: Murphy and Bingham, 1830), p. vi.

19 L. Sperry, *The Botanic Family Physician, or The Secret of Curing Diseases with Vegetable Proportions* (Cornwall, Vt.: By the author, 1843), p. 5.

20 Benjamin Colby, *A Guide to Health: Being an Exposition of the Principles of the Thomsonian System of Practice* (Nashua, N.H.: Charles T. Gill, 1844), p. x.

21 J. W. Comfort, *Thomsonian Practice of Midwifery* (Philadelphia: Aaron Comfort, 1845), p. iii.

22 F. K. Robertson and Silas Wilcox, *The Book of Health, or Thomsonian Theory and Practice of Medicine* (Bennington, Vt.: J. I. C. & A. S. C. Cook, 1843), p. 5.

23 Howard, *Howard's Domestic Medicine*, p. 427.

24 Colby, *A Guide to Health*, p. x.

25 Simon Abbott, *The Southern Botanic Physician* (Charleston: For the author, 1844), p. ix.

26 P. E. Sanborn urged husbands emigrating west to learn the art of midwifery, since "many females suffer and die in some parts of the West, for want of medical skill and attention." Sanborn, *The Sick Man's Friend* (Taunton, Mass.: By the author, 1835), p. 237.

27 Philip D. Jordan, "The eclectic of St. Clairsville," *Ohio State Archaeol. & Hist. Quart.*, October 1947, *56*: 391.

28 Howard, *Howard's Domestic Medicine*, p. 286.

29 Kett, *The Formation of the American Medical Profession*, p. 119.

30 Samuel Thomson, Editorial, *Thomsonian Manual*, Aug. 15, 1836, *1*: 153.

31 Colby, *A Guide to Health*, p. viii.

32 Robertson and Wilcox, *The Book of Health*, p. 19.

33 Howard, *Howard's Domestic Medicine*, pp. 30–32; Abbott, *The Southern Botanic Physician*, p. v.

34 See, for example, Wm. H. Cook, *Woman's Hand-Book of Health: A Guide for the Wife, Mother and Nurse*, 5th

ed. (Cincinnati: Wm. H. Cook, 1871). Cook was Professor of Botany, Therapeutics, and Materia Medica in the Physio-Medical Institute.

35 Wooster Beach, *The American Practice Condensed, or the Family Physician*, 10th ed. (New York: James McAlister, 1847), p. xv. Beach also published *The Family Physician; or The Reformed System of Medicine on Vegetable or Botanical Principles* (New York: By the author, 1842).

36 On homeopathy in America, see Martin Kaufman, *Homeopathy in America: The Rise and Fall of a Medical Heresy* (Baltimore: Johns Hopkins Press, 1971); Harris L. Coulter, *Divided Legacy: A History of the Schism in Medical Thought* (Washington, D.C.: McGrath Publishing Co., 1973), Vol. III; and Kett, *The Formation of the American Medical Profession*, Ch. 5, pp. 132–164.

37 Coulter, *Divided Legacy*, III, 101–110.

38 Oliver Wendell Holmes, "Some more recent views on homoeopathy," *Atlantic Monthly*, December 1857, 187, quoted *ibid.*, p. 114.

39 *Ibid.*, pp. 114–116.

40 See, for example, C. S. and George E. Halsey, *Halsey's Homoeopathic Guide: For Families, Travelers, Missionaries, Pioneers, Miners, Farmers, Stock Raisers, Horse Owners, Dog Fanciers, Poultry Keepers* (Chicago: C. S. and George E. Halsey, 1885). Domestic manuals appear with great frequency in Thomas Lindsley Bradford, *Homoeopathic Bibliography of the United States, from the Year 1825 to the Year 1891, Inclusive* (Philadelphia: Boericke and Tafel, 1892).

41 C. Hering, *The Homoeopathist, or Domestic Physician*, 2 parts (Philadelphia: J. G. Wesselhoeft, 1835, 1838); Coulter, *Divided Legacy*, III, 101–102; Bradford, *Homoeopathic Bibliography*, p. 145.

42 Hering, *The Homoeopathist*, Part 1, pp. 2–3; Part 2, p. 241.

43 Morton M. Eaton, *Eaton's Domestic Practice for Parents and Nurses* (Cincinnati: M. M. Eaton, Jr., and Co., 1882), p. 77; George E. Shipman, *The Homoeopathic Family Guide*, 2nd ed. (Chicago: C. S. Halsey, 1865), p. ix.

44 J. H. Pulte, *Homoeopathic Domestic Physician; Containing the Treatment of Diseases, with Popular Explanations on Anatomy, Physiology, Hygiene, and Hydropathy* (Cincinnati: H. W. Derby and Co., 1850), pp. iv–v. See also E. H. Ruddock, *The Stepping-Stone to Homoeopathy and Health*, ed. Wm. Boericke, new Am. ed. (Philadelphia: Hahnemann Publishing House, 1890), p. 10.

45 Quoted in Coulter, *Divided Legacy*, III, 117.

46 Egbert Guernsey, *The Gentleman's Hand-Book of Homoeopathy; Especially for Travelers, and for Domestic Practice* (Boston: Otis Clapp, 1855), p. iv; Hering, *The Homoeopathist*, Part 1, p. 7; John Epps, *Domestic Homoeopathy*, ed. George W. Cook, 4th Am. ed. (Boston: Otis Clapp, 1849), p. 8.

47 E. R. Ellis, *Homoeopathic Family Guide and Information for the People*, 2nd ed. (Detroit: By the author, 1882), p. ii; Holmes, "Some more recent views on homoeopathy," p. 187, quoted in Coulter, *Divided Legacy*, III, 116.

48 Bradford, *Homoeopathic Bibliography*, pp. 99–100.

49 Frederick Humphreys, *Manual of Specific Homoeopathy* (New York: Humphrey's Specific Homoeopathic Medicine Company, 1869); *Humphreys' Homeopathic Mentor or Family Adviser* (New York: Humphreys' Specific Homeopathic Medicine Company, 1876); Bradford, *Homoeopathic Bibliography*, p. 167. The reference to "Homoeopathic quackery" is from J. S. Douglas, *Practical Homoeopathy for the People*, 15th ed. (Milwaukee: Lewis Sherman, 1894), p. iii.

50 John Ellis, *Personal Experience of a Physician* (Philadelphia: Hahnemann Publishing House, 1892), pp. 85–87.

51 "Domestic Practice. — No. 2," *Family Journal of Homoeopathy*, July 1854, *1*: 105. See also Guernsey's reply to the criticisms against domestic practice: Guernsey, *The Gentleman's Hand-Book of Homoeopathy*, p. iv.

52 "Progress of Homoeopathy," *Homoeopathic Sun*, September 1868, *1*: 12.

53 Charles J. Hempel, *The Homoeopathic Domestic Physician* (New York: Wm. Radde, 1846); Hempel and Jacob Beakley, *Homoeopathic Theory and Practice*, 4th ed. (New York: William Radde, 1868), p. iii.

54 Henry G. Hanchett, *The Elements of Modern Domestic Medicine* (New York: Charles T. Hurlburt, 1887), p. 3.

55 On hydropathy in America, see Harry B. Weiss and Howard R. Kemble, *The Great American Water-Cure Craze: A History of Hydropathy in the United States* (Trenton, N.J.: Past Times Press, 1967); and Marshall Scott Legan, "Hydropathy in America: a nineteenth century panacea," *Bull. Hist. Med.*, 1971, *45*: 267–280.

56 Weiss and Kemble, *The Great American Water-Cure Craze* (p. 44), were able to identify only 241 American hydropathic physicians.

57 David A. Harsha, *The Principles of Hydropathy, or the Invalid's Guide to Health and Happiness* (Albany, N.Y.: E. H. Pease & Co., 1852), p. 41.

58 Joel Shew, *The Hydropathic Family Physician* (New York: Fowler and Wells, 1854), p. iii; Shew, *The Water-Cure Manual: A Popular Work* (New York: Fowlers and Wells, 1855), p. 132. Shew's *Hand-Book of Hydropathy* (New York: Wiley & Putnam, 1844) was probably the first American domestic guide to hydropathy.

R. T. Trall, American preface to William Horsell, *Hydropathy for the People* (New York: Fowlers and Wells, 1855), p. iii; Trall, *The Hydropathic Encyclopedia: A System of Hydropathy and Hygiene* (New York: Fowler and Wells, 1851), I, 295.

Mary S. Gove Nichols, *Experience in Water-Cure: A Familiar Exposition of the Principles and Results of Water Treatment, in the Cure of Acute and Chronic Diseases* (New York: Fowlers and Wells, 1852), p. 10.

Weiss and Kemble, *The Great American Water-Cure Craze*, p. 44.

See, for example, Mary S. Gove, *Lectures to Women on Anatomy and Physiology, with an Appendix on Water Cure* (New York: Harper and Brothers, 1846); and M. Augusta Fairchild, *How to Be Well, or Common-Sense Medical Hygiene* (New York: Fowler & Wells, 1880).

Water-Cure J., Nov. 1, 1846, *2*: 168; *ibid.*, 1848, *6*: 138. An example of how domestic practice supplemented the use of water-cure establishments is found in the diary of Mrs. Angeline Stevens Andrews, 1863–1864 (C. Burton Clark Collection, Heritage Room, Loma Linda University Library).

Abraham Millar to Fowlers and Wells, Nov. 30, 1850, quoted in Trall, *Hydropathic Encyclopedia*, II, 81–82.

According to the editor, Harriet N. Austin, one of the purposes of the journal was to give "directions for the rational and successful treatment of all [disease]"; *Laws of Life*, August 1865, *8*: 127.

James C. Jackson, *The Sexual Organism, and Its Healthful Management* (Boston: B. Leverett Emerson, 1861); Jackson, *How to Treat the Sick without Medicine*, 10th ed. (Dansville, New York: Austin, Jackson & Co., 1880). See also Jackson, *Consumption: How to Prevent It, and How to Cure It* (Boston: B. Leverett Emerson, 1862); and Jackson, *Diptheria* [*sic*]: *Its Causes, Treatment and Cure* (Dansville, N.Y.: Austin, Jackson and Co., 1868).

67 *Advent Review and Sabbath Herald*, Feb. 17, 1863, *21*: 89.

68 H. S. Lay, "To the reader," *Health Reformer*, August 1866, *1*: 8; "Items for the month," *ibid.* January 1867, *1*: 96. On Ellen White and Adventist health reform, see Ronald L. Numbers, *Prophetess of Health: A Study of Ellen G. White* (New York: Harper & Row, 1976).

69 [John Harvey Kellogg], *The Household Manual of Domestic Hygiene, Foods and Drinks, Common Diseases, Accidents and Emergencies, and Useful Hints and Recipes* (Battle Creek: Modern Medicine Publishing Co., 1893); Kellogg, *Ladies' Guide in Health and Disease* (Battle Creek: Modern Medicine Publishing Co., 1893); Kellogg, *The Household Monitor of Health* (Battle Creek: Good Health Publishing Co., 1891); Kellogg, *The Home Hand-Book of Domestic Hygiene and Rational Medicine*, rev. ed. (Battle Creek: Modern Medicine Publishing Co., 1906). The last work was first published in 1880. Kellogg's older half-brother Merritt also wrote domestic manuals; see [M. G. Kellogg], *The Hygienic Family Physician: A Complete Guide for the Preservation of Health, and the Treatment of the Sick without Medicine* (Battle Creek: Health Reformer, 1874); and M. G. Kellogg, *The Bath: Its Use and Application* (Battle Creek: Health Reformer, 1873).

70 See, for example, Newton Evans, Percy T. Magan, and George Thomason, eds., *The Home Physician and Guide to Health* (Mountain View, Calif.: Pacific Press, 1923), and Hubert O. Swartout, *Guide to Health* (Mountain View, Calif.: Pacific Press, 1938).

Sickness and Health in America

READINGS IN THE HISTORY OF MEDICINE AND PUBLIC HEALTH

Edited by Judith Walzer Leavitt and Ronald L. Numbers

THE UNIVERSITY OF WISCONSIN PRESS

Box 1379 Madison, Wisconsin 53701

7

Device Quackery in America

JAMES HARVEY YOUNG

The text for today's lesson is found in the sixth chapter of *Babbitt*, wherein the sage of Sauk Center says: Babbitt "had enormous and poetic admiration, though very little understanding, of all mechanical devices."[1]

This awe, this admiration, this bafflement, which so many of his countrymen have shared with Babbitt, underlie device quackery in America. Even the simplest devices have served, like the Anodyne Necklace, brought from England to the colonies in the mid-18th century. "Children on the very Brink of the Grave, and thought past all Recovery with their Teeth, Fits, Fevers, Convulsions, Hooping and other violent Coughs . . . , who cannot tell what they suffer, nor make known their Pains, any other Way, but by their Cryings, and Moans; have almost miraculously recovered after having worn the famous Anodyne Necklace but one Night's Time."[2] So promised the advertising, although in England Dr. Johnson raised a skeptical eyebrow.[3]

Since then, stretching gadgets have sought to increase height, compressing gadgets to remould breasts, vibrating gadgets to remove weight, fumigating gadgets to cure catarrh, skull-capping gadgets to restore hair. To combat tuberculosis, Medicated Fur Chest Protectors and Waterproof Anti-Consumptive Cork Soles sought public favor.[4] To fight "those ills arising from sedentary habits," an entrepreneur offered a horseback-simulating "Health Jolting Chair."[5]

The main currents of device quackery in American history, however, have flowed from electromagnetism and electricity. This began in the late 18th century amidst public curiosity over such enterprises as Mesmer's therapeutic séances in Paris and Franklin's kite experiments in Philadelphia. Dr. Elisha Perkins, whose intriguing tale Dr. Quen told us two years ago,[6] produced the first widespread mania with his metallic tractors, "gleaned up," said his state medical society in ousting him, "from the miserable remains of animal magnetism." It was Perkins' theory that his small gold and silver points — the first medical device patented under the Constitution — would, when stroked across the body, draw off a noxious electrical "fluid" which accumulated in the tissues and caused disease. "Quack" is too severe a word for Perkins, Dr. Quen concluded, because Perkins believed in the efficacy of his invention to the extent of martyrdom, dying in New York where he went to minister to victims of yellow fever. Perkins did keep the composition of his device a secret and charged for it an exorbitant price.

The harsh word "quack" is a fitting description for most of Perkins' electromagnetic successors, whether they sought to heal by getting bad electricity out of the body or by putting good electricity in. For a century and a half, the magnetic belt has sought to do the latter, mostly, in its many gaudy versions, aiming to restore "vital power" missing from middle-aged males.[7] A "voltaic belt" of 1890 could do much more: besides improving health and posture, it could comb the hair, press the clothes, and promote a luxuriant mustache — all in 30 days.[8] These belts were joined by countless other items of therapeutic apparel circling the human frame: Electro-Magnetic Wrist-Bands, cravats, anklets, elbow pads, necklaces, head-caps, corsets, all sold with claims that their electrical input would heal dread ailments.[9]

As the utility of electricity became more stunningly apparent to Americans during the ongoing industrial revolution, so too did the utility of electricity increase for quacks. Pill-pushers appropri-

---

JAMES HARVEY YOUNG is Professor of History, Emory University, Atlanta, Georgia.

Reprinted with permission from the *Bulletin of the History of Medicine*, 1965, *39*: 154–162.

ated the names of both the telegraph and telephone; and schemers with a modicum of mechanical skill built gadgets of increasing complexity, trafficking on those amazing but mystifying machines which Edison and other inventors were introducing.

One of quackdom's early Edisons was Hercules Sanche, who marketed first the Electropoise and then the Oxydonor.[10] Each was a sealed metal cylinder, and to one end was attached an uninsulated flexible cord ending in a small disc, to be attached to wrist or ankle with an elastic band. "The Electropoise," Sanche said, "supplies the needed amount of electric force to the system, and by its thermal action places the body in condition to absorb oxygen through the lungs and pores." The main difference between the Electropoise and the Oxydonor was that the latter cost 35 dollars instead of 10. As therapeutic agents, Sanche's "gaspipe cures" belonged in the "same class," so a critic put it, "as the left hind foot of a rabbit caught in a graveyard in the dark of the moon." But their commercial success bred countless imitators, one of them the Oxypathor.[11] This gadget merits an honored place in the history of antiquackery, for in 1915, after a long and hotly-contested legal battle, the Post Office Department won a criminal fraud case against its maker, the first victory against a quack device. Devices had not been covered by the 1906 Pure Food and Drugs Law, and the Oxypathor verdict offered the hope of some control over outrageously fraudulent gadgets if promoted by mail.

Do-it-yourself healing, however, though a large-scale enterprise, was to be overshadowed in the mechanical device field by a system wherein practitioners manipulated the gadgets. Reputable medicine, as the 20th century proceeded, turned more and more to diagnostic and therapeutic instruments, and so too did quackery. By 1915, when the Oxypathor met its doom, "the dean of twentieth century charlatans" had already entered upon his fabulous career.[12] He was the renegade San Francisco physician, Albert Abrams. "The spirit of the age," Abrams wrote, "is radio, and we can use radio in diagnosis." To capitalize on public interest in this new manifestation of electricity, Abrams built a series of interlocking machines. Into the first contraption, the dynamizer, he placed a piece of paper containing a few drops of an ailing patient's blood, removed no matter where or when, but only while the patient faced the west. From the dynamizer a wire ran to the rheostatic dynamizer, from that to the vibratory rate rheostat, from that to the measuring rheostat. And from that a wire also extended, ending in an electrode. The use of this Rube Goldberg sequence for diagnosis required the participation of a healthy third party, whom Abrams called the "subject." When the moment came for diagnosis, Abrams, operating in dim light, stripped the subject to the waist, faced him westward, and attached the electrode to his forehead. Then the doctor percussed the subject's abdomen, determining by the various areas of resonance and dullness, what diseases plagued the patient, however distant, whose dried blood lay quietly four machines back up the line.

Abrams' "Electronic Reactions" were superbly sensitive. Not only could his chain of devices detect dread diseases, but their precise location within the body, the sex of the patient, even his religious faith. In time Abrams found that a patient's autograph worked as well as his dried blood, and this permitted excursions into the past. Pepys, Dr. Johnson, Longfellow, and Poe, Abrams reported, all had had syphilis.

Abrams developed a new machine, the oscilloclast, which cured what his other machines detected. The oscilloclast produced vibrations in consonance with the vibratory rates of all known diseases. Applied to a sufferer and set by its operator to produce the proper rate, the force of vibrations shattered and destroyed the ailment. The oscilloclast was not for sale. Abrams would lease it only, for a fancy fee, and the lessee agreed by contract never to open the apparatus.

In fact, the insides were a weird jumble of ohm-meters, rheostats, condensers, and other parts, wired together without rhyme or reason. "They are the kind of device," said the physicist Robert Millikan, "a ten-year-old boy would build to fool an eight-year old." But Abrams' fame expanded and reached a high plateau in 1922 — the year of *Babbitt*'s publication — when another novelist, Upton Sinclair, wrote in a national magazine a paean of praise to Abrams, the glorious medical pioneer. To counter such misguided enthusiasm, the *Scientific American* set a blue-ribbon panel of scientists to work, and the result appeared in twelve long articles published monthly through an entire year. "At best," the scientists concluded, Abrams' scheme "is an illusion. At worst, it is a colossal fraud."

While the series was in midstream, Dr. Abrams, a man of 60, died of pneumonia, leaving a two-million dollar estate. He left also hundreds of machines around the land and a hard corps of disciples, dedicated to his name and system, organized as the Electronic Medical Foundation.

Device quackery preys on the same widespread credulity, fear, and desperation which permit all other forms of quackery to flourish. Gadgets can possess certain kinds of persuasiveness denied to drugs. One is the power to shock. A New York "clinic" of an earlier day treated young men who were led to believe they might be suffering from syphilis or the dire consequences of self-abuse.[13] The patient sat naked upon a sort of toilet throne, his bare back resting against a metal plate, his scrotum suspended in a whirling pool. The plate and pool were linked by wire to a battery. No frightened sufferer could question the rigor of this therapy. Gadgets can appeal to several of the senses. The Violetta, vended as useful in 86 ailments, ranging alphabetically from abscess to writer's cramp, impressed itself simultaneously upon the hearing, seeing, smelling and feeling of its user.[14] A small high-voltage generator, ionizing the air in a hollow glass head, the Violetta buzzed and crackled, produced a bluish glow, exuded ozone, and with its sparks tingled and warmed the skin.

Devices permit quacks to display their customary ambivalence toward orthodox medicine. Relying for impressiveness in part on the alleged kinship of their gadgets to known and respected instruments like the x-ray and the electrocardiograph, quacks also promote their machines at the expense of reputable medicine by boasting of their druglessness. A public uneasy about huge doses of calomel, which might cost them teeth and even jawbones, as in America's "heroic age" of medication, a public disturbed about thalidomide, as in our own day, pays heed to the bragging of the drugless healer. "Electricity," he says — and I am quoting one — ". . . will do more for you than all the drugs ever compounded."[15]

Whatever special advantages device quackery may have, its fundamental force comes from the combination of admiration and incomprehension which Sinclair Lewis noted. Here in the heartland of mechanization, equipment of enormous complexity, with flashing lights and wiggling dials, sends voices through the air, detects and shoots down planes, directs accumulating vehicles through an assembly line, detects errors in an income tax return, guides satellites through outer space. Why not also cure disease?

It was a graduate engineer named Rice who, in 1948, reported to his wife, anguished about a growing lump in her breast: "I [have] found a miracle." The miracle was a Radio Therapeutic Instrument, made and sold by one of Albert Abrams' heirs, a woman utterly devoid of medical training, Ruth Drown of Hollywood.[16] The end of World War II had seen an upsurge of device quackery. Radar and television excited public interest. Onto the market had poured a vast quantity of surplus electrical equipment, easy to get and cheap for fashioning into awesome contrivances. The Food and Drug Administration, ending its war-time responsibilities, was closing in on some of the major areas of drug quackery, using new weapons given it by Congress in 1938, thus prodding some quacks to try machines.

Mrs. Drown's black box, which cost the engineer $423, had nine dials and two protruding wires, ending in electrodes made — shades of Perkins' metallic tractors — each of a different metal. Mrs. Rice spent many hours using the machine in her home in a suburb of Chicago. Even when not giving herself direct treatment, she engaged in what was claimed to be equally efficient therapy, going off to shop while a blotter containing her blood was clamped between the two electrodes of the machine. Despite such diligence, no improvement was detectable; indeed, another lump developed in her breast. From California, Mrs. Drown answered an anxious query: Mrs. Rice's "condition has never been cancerous," she said. The engineer's wife "must realize if she is to get well she must swing her attention on to the work and put every effort forth. . . ." It was hard to pursue therapy more zealously than 24 hours a day, but for three months more the trial went on. Finally, disillusion dawning, Mr. Rice went to the Bureau of Investigation of the American Medical Association. In the presence of its director and agents of the Food and Drug Administration, the engineer witnessed the opening of Mrs. Drown's black box and saw the simple electrical circuit that it contained. The two dissimilar metals, in contact with each other or with the skin, generated a very small voltage which moved the needle on a sensitive microammeter. That was all.

The 1938 Food, Drug, and Cosmetic Act had extended federal controls over device quackery, and this tragic Chicago episode, involving interstate commerce, became the basis for a legal attack on Mrs. Drown which the Food and Drug Administration had long been looking for. Most of Mrs. Drown's sales had been to chiropractors, osteopaths, and M.D.'s, who used the devices in their office practices and were naturally averse to cooperating with the F.D.A. The Rices, unlike most of quackery's chastened victims, permitted their private misfortune to go on public display in federal court.

At the trial, the engineer told his tragic tale. His wife by then was far too ill to testify. Physicists, engineers, and medical scientists pronounced Mrs. Drown's ridiculous machine "perfectly useless." It could do "no conceivable good," said a former chairman of the California Board of Health, and would be "laughable if . . . not so dangerous" in lulling patients to neglect proper treatment until too late.

Mrs. Drown's devoted followers did not agree. "We don't call it 'a box,'" one woman testified. "We call it 'an instrument,' an instrument played by a master artist." And she credited the instrument with saving her from pneumonia when she was in Atlantic City by healing rays aimed in her direction all the way from Hollywood. Its range was even greater. Should she be in a terrible accident, she said, in Moscow, the rays of the machine would penetrate the Iron Curtain, diagnosing the extent of her injuries and producing a cure. Mrs. Drown's device "is not black magic," her champion argued. "It is science." Such was the ardent testimony of faith in Mrs. Drown presented in court by the chairman of the school board for Los Angeles.

Fined $1000 for violating the law,[17] Mrs. Drown was thereafter careful about vending her Radio Therapeutic Instrument across state lines. Several of her gadgets have been used by other local practitioners, and Mrs. Drown herself kept on practicing her pseudohealing art in her own offices, treating through the years an estimated 35,000 suffering men and women.[18]

Albert Abrams had numerous other heirs, and many imitators as well, whose Oscillitrons, Depolarays, Electropads, Neurolinometers, and Radioclasts have awed the ailing and done much mischief.[19] Against their makers the Food and Drug Administration has fought an increasingly vigorous and successful war. On the state level, however, actions against device quackery have been few and far between. The right of a licensed practitioner to determine what therapy is best for his patients is not one to be transgressed lightly, and this legitimate safeguard for the reputable physician has shielded many licensed "quacks."

In March 1962 a landmark decision by a United States Circuit Court of Appeals provided some useful guidance in this delicate zone.[20] The case involved the Ellis Micro-Dynameter, a sort of first cousin to Mrs. Drown's device, sold with claims that it could diagnose some 55 diseases and conditions and guide the practitioner to proper modes of treatment: ". . . the Micro-Dynameter," the judges ruled, "is not safe for use even in the hands of a licensed practitioner. A device whose labeling claims it to be an aid in diagnosing as many diseases as this one, when in fact it is not, is unsafe for use no matter who uses it."

The Micro-Dynameter decision has provided the Food and Drug Administration with a bigger club to swing against the fake machines.[21] It offers encouragement to state authorities too. In California, Mrs. Drown, her daughter, and one other are currently awaiting trial for Grand Theft and Attempted Grand Theft.[22] Pending before the Congress is a bill which, if enacted, would curtail device quackery still more.[23] When Mrs. Drown lost her case in 1951, the burden of proof was on the federal government to show the uselessness of her machine. Many skilled scientists spent scores of hours working with the Radio Therapeutic Instrument so they could testify before a jury that its simple galvanic current could not stop cancer in Mrs. Rice's breast. The proposed law would shift the burden of proof to the gadget's vendor. Unless he could demonstrate the device's therapeutic effectiveness in treating ailments listed in the labeling, he could not put his instrument upon the market.

So Babbitt and the rest of us are better protected than we ever have been, should our awe and perplexity when faced with machines tempt us to the device quack's door. But we still are vulnerable, and hazard is still at hand. "Despite the success we have had in court attacking device quackery," F.D.A. Commissioner Larrick stated recently, "so many fake gadgets are still in the hands of practitioners that if we set all of our inspectors at work on nothing else it would take several years to find and take successful action against all of these devices."[24]

AUTHOR'S POSTSCRIPT

The Medical Device Amendments of 1976, enacted by the Congress after more than a decade of consideration, markedly increase the Food and Drug Administration's ability to control quackery in the device field. Device manufacturers must register and must notify the F.D.A. 90 days prior to marketing a new device; the agency can require evidence of safety and effectiveness before permitting the device to reach the market. As to devices already in the marketplace, the amendments permit the F.D.A. quickly to ban those which are deceptive or hazardous.

NOTES

Read at the 37th annual meeting of the American Association for the History of Medicine, Bethesda and Washington, May 2, 1964.
This paper is based upon research supported by a fellowship from the Social Science Research Council and by Public Health Service Research Grant GM 07199 from the Division of General Medical Sciences.

1 Sinclair Lewis, *Babbitt* (New York: Grosset & Dunlap, 1922), p. 68.

2 *New-York Gaz. revived in the Weekly Post-Boy*, Oct. 17, 1748, cited in Rita S. Gottesman, *Arts and Crafts in New York, 1726–1776* (New York: New York Historical Society, 1938), pp. 287–288.

3 Johnson cited in E. S. Turner, *The Shocking History of Advertising!* (New York: E. P. Dutton & Company, 1953), p. 37.

4 Harcourt, Bradley & Co., New York, to Birchall and Owen, Springfield, Ill., Oct. 3, 1854, in author's possession.

5 Sargent Manufacturing Co., New York, 1887 catalog, State Historical Society of Wisconsin.

6 Jacques M. Quen, "Elisha Perkins, physician, nostrum-vendor, or charlatan?," *Bull. Hist. Med.*, 1963, *37*: 159–166.

7 Gerald Carson, *One for a Man, Two for a Horse* (New York: Doubleday & Company, 1961), pp. 33–35.

8 *Printers' Ink: Fifty Years, 1888–1938* (New York: Printers' Ink Publishing Co., 1938), p. 84.

9 *A Treatise on the Application of John H. Tesch & Co.'s Electro-Magnetic Remedies* (Milwaukee, 1866), in the Rare Book Division of the Library of Congress. Boston Electro-Pathy Institute broadside, 1859, in the American Antiquarian Society.

10 American Medical Association, *Nostrums and Quackery*, 2nd ed. (Chicago: A.M.A. Press, 1912), pp. 295–301.

11 Arthur J. Cramp, *Nostrums and Quackery* (Chicago: A.M.A. Press, 1921), pp. 706–713.

12 Arthur J. Cramp, *Nostrums and Quackery and Pseudo-Medicine* (Chicago: A.M.A. Press, 1936), p. 112. The account of Abrams is based on *ibid.*, pp. 112–114; Albert Abrams folders, A.M.A. Department of Investigation; "Albert Abrams, A.M., M.D., LL.D., F.R.M.S.," an A.M.A. reprint of material on Abrams from various issues of *J.A.M.A.*; Cramp, "The Electronic Reactions of Abrams," *Hygeia*, 1924, *2*: 658–659; the twelve-part *Scient. Am.* series, 1923, *129*: 130, to 1924, *131*: 158–260, 220–222; Nathan Flaxman, "A cardiology anomaly, Albert Abrams (1863–1924)," *Bull. Hist. Med.*, 1953, *27*: 252–268; Morris Fishbein, *The Medical Follies* (New York: Boni & Liveright, 1925), pp. 99–118.

13 Champe Seabury Andrews, *A Century's Criminal Alliance between Quacks and Some Newspapers* (New York: Stettiner Bros., 1905), pp. 7–8, in New York Public Library.

14 Promotional material in Violetta folder, A.M.A. Department of Investigation. The author has a working model in his possession.

15 Cramp, *Nostrums and Quackery* (1921), p. 721.

16 The account of the Ruth Drown case is taken from the Food and Drug Administration's carbon copy of the typewritten transcript of testimony in the case of U.S.A. v. Ruth B. Drown in the District Court in Los Angeles, Sept. 11–24, 1951.

17 Food and Drug Administration, Notices of Judgment under the Federal Food, Drug, and Cosmetic Act, Drugs and Devices, 4029 (issued December 1953). The trial judgment was confirmed in a Court of Appeals, 198 F.2d 999, and a petition for certiorari denied by the Supreme Court.

18 Milton P. Duffy, Chief, Bureau Food and Drug Inspections, California Department of Public Health, to author, Sept. 1, 1964.

19 *Fake Medical Devices, An F.D.A. Report* (Washington, D.C.: Food and Drug Administration, 1963). K. L. Milstead et al., "Quackery in the medical device

field," in *Proceedings, Second National Congress on Medical Quackery* (Oct. 25–26, 1963) (Chicago: A.M.A., 1964), pp. 30–39.

20 U.S.A. vs. Ellis Research Laboratories, Inc., 300 F.2d 550 (1962).

21 Milstead, "Quackery in the medical device field," p. 31.

22 Duffy letter, Sept. 1, 1964.

23 H. R. 6788 introduced in the 88th Congress, 1st session, on June 4, 1963, by Congressman Oren Harris.

24 George P. Larrick to author, April 21, 1964.

Education

America's first medical school opened in Philadelphia in 1765. Prior to that time colonials who wanted to become physicians either studied in Europe or served an apprenticeship with a local practitioner. Even after the advent of formal medical education the apprenticeship remained the primary means of obtaining clinical experience, supplementing the lectures available in schools.

By 1800 Columbia, Harvard, and Dartmouth also had established medical departments, and within a few decades medical schools were flooding the country. Although some continued to affiliate with colleges or universities, most of the new schools were run by private individuals who cared more about profits than pedagogy. The typical mid-century institution had five or six nonsalaried professors, usually physicians, whose income depended on how many lecture tickets they could sell. Each term lasted only three or four months and consisted of perhaps half a dozen courses ranging from anatomy to the theory and practice of medicine. To graduate with an M.D. degree, students attended the same lectures for two terms and — at least in theory — completed an apprenticeship.

Efforts to improve this dismal situation, described by Robert P. Hudson, culminated in Abraham Flexner's 1910 exposé, which hastened the closing of the most wretched schools. The institutions that survived into the 1920s offered a four-year, graded curriculum, usually divided between the basic sciences (e.g., anatomy, physiology, and biochemistry) and practical experience in the clinic or hospital. Unlike times past, when reading and writing were virtually the only skills required for admission, students now had to attend college for at least two years before entering.

As medicine grew more and more complex in the 20th century, medical educators found it increasingly difficult to squeeze into four years all the clinical training a physician or surgeon would need to practice medicine effectively. Thus in the 1910s schools and state licensing boards began requiring an additional year of internship in a hospital. But even this proved insufficient training for some specialties, and by the 1920s and 1930s a number of physicians were continuing to train for several years past the internship in postgraduate residency programs, specializing in fields like ophthalmology, obstetrics, and orthopedic surgery. After World War II it was customary for all but general practitioners to study medicine for about eight years before engaging in independent practice.

Until shortly before the Civil War American medical schools admitted only white males, but this barrier fell under the influence of the ante-bellum abolitionist and feminist movements. Elizabeth Blackwell in 1849 became the first American woman to earn a medical degree, but, as Regina Markell Morantz shows, the entrance of women into the medical profession was not accomplished without a struggle. Nevertheless, women made rapid strides in separate as well as coeducational medical schools during the late 19th century — only to fall back again in the 20th. Few medical schools between 1910 and 1960 enrolled more than 5 percent women and an even smaller percentage of minority students. But once again social ferment forced these schools to re-evaluate their admission policies, and by the mid-1970s almost one-fourth of entering students were women and one-eighth represented various minority groups.

8

Abraham Flexner in Perspective: American Medical Education 1865–1910

ROBERT P. HUDSON

The Flexner report of 1910[1] justifiably stands as a monument in the reform of American medical education. Yet there is much in the report itself to suggest that Flexner's contribution was not so much revolutionary as catalytic to an already evolving process. The present study reassesses Flexner's impact, but only peripherally. The principal aim rather is to sketch in some of the pertinent social and educational trends during the half century between the end of the Civil War and Flexner's genteel thunderbolt.[2]

The Civil War abated only temporarily the spread of proprietary medical schools. This spread, it should be remembered, was malignant less because it produced too many physicians and more because the ensuing competition for students diluted the already limited resources and eroded academic standards.[3] Plumpers for reform who had sounded their monotonous litanies in the quarter century after the founding of the American Medical Association were by 1870 generally pessimistic. They not only appeared to agree with John Shaw Billings that "it does not pay to give a $5000 education to a $5 boy,"[4] but by now they had despaired of doing anything about either education or the boy.

Still defeatism was not universal. A few observers thought they saw glimmers of improvement both in the quality of incoming students and in the educational process itself.[5] These disparate views can be made at least comprehensible. Part of the improvement was purely on paper. Medical school catalogues became increasingly imaginative as competition for students grew ever more heated. The catalogues of around 1880 contained few stipulations which could be described, in the parlance of recent campus radicals, as non-negotiable. Most medical colleges specified, for example, that applicants must have a high school diploma or its "equivalent." Flexner, with characteristic candor, disposed of the equivalent as "a device that concedes the necessity of a standard which it forthwith proceeds to evade."[6]

There can be no serious disagreement with Shryock's conclusion that American medical training remained "relatively inferior" during the two decades following the Civil War.[7] But it was a complex period, one in which entrenched mediocrity and rising reform coexisted. While new schools continued to pop up with the discouraging persistence of dandelions, worthier seeds were sprouting. These early improvements, though they frequently interlocked, can be considered under three headings: admission requirements, medical school curricula, and postgraduate training.

The 35 years before the turn of the century saw something of a revolution in higher education in America. The public, which previously saw little utility in education, began to change its mind. This new attitude was reflected in the state's perception that it had an obligation to make educational opportunities more accessible to the masses. The 1862 Morrill Act not only initiated the land grant university movement, but indirectly gave rise to a new institution, the public high school. These multiplied so rapidly that by 1892 their enrollment surpassed that of the academies.[8] Thus premedical education of improved quality became generally available during the period under consideration.[9] Even though compulsory education reportedly existed in only seven states by 1896,[10] the fact re-

ROBERT P. HUDSON is Professor and Chairman, Department of the History and Philosophy of Medicine, University of Kansas Medical Center, Kansas City, Kansas.

Reprinted with permission from the *Bulletin of the History of Medicine*, 1972, *56*: 545–561.

mains that the opportunity at least for better premedical preparation expanded rapidly in the post-bellum decades.

The question remains — did more students bound for medical studies during this time take advantage of their new opportunities?[11] A precise answer in numerical terms is not possible. There is evidence that students increasingly pursued premedical training of steadily improving quality, and that medical colleges upgraded their entrance requirements both on paper and in fact. But the case should not be overstated. The situation was characterized by a spectrum rather than by uniformity, and most students still received inferior premedical training. The Johns Hopkins required an academic degree from the outset (1893) but by 1906 the Council on Medical Education of the American Medical Association was still recommending only a minimal one year of college for medical school admission.[12]

Still trends slowly pushed toward higher standards. John Rauch, a champion of reform in Illinois, reported that the number of medical colleges exacting certain specified educational requirements for matriculation was 45 in 1882, 114 in 1886, 117 in 1889 and 124 in 1890.[13] Of the 155 schools Flexner surveyed, 16 required two years of college and 6, which demanded only one year, were scheduled to go to a two-year requirement in 1910.[14] Among these 16 schools 1,850 students had satisfied the two-year requirement as of 1908–1909.[15] By way of balance it should be recalled that in 1910 some 50 medical colleges demanded for admission only a high school education or the much abused equivalent.[16]

One of the most significant features of the decades under study was that many aspiring physicians fashioned educational programs superior to those dictated by law or custom. This held true for collegiate preparation as well as medical and postgraduate training. Regarding premedical studies evidence of this is found in an analysis of the 1,513 physicians in the *Dictionary of American Medical Biography* (*D.A.M.B.*) who took their medical training in 19th-century America. A surprising 607 or some 40 percent of these men earned predoctoral degrees before beginning medical studies. Another 430 had education beyond grammar school but short of a degree.[17]

By definition men selected for inclusion in the *D.A.M.B.* are not representative of the general physician population. Still, if properly qualified, the figures have value. For one thing the 1,513 physicians may be more representative than they appear at first glance. In the 19th century America did not produce fifteen hundred physicians who distinguished themselves by scientific or literary contributions to medicine. Deciding just why a given physician was selected for inclusion in the *D.A.M.B.* was imprecise at best, but in this study 531 were included apparently because they achieved excellent reputations in medical practice and nothing more. These men must have differed little from many others who were not selected by editors Kelly and Burrage.

Two other features of the *D.A.M.B.* study apply to the question at hand. The average age at which the 607 men took their predoctoral degree increased from 19.5 years in the first decade to 21.1 in the last. There are several possible explanations for this, but the most reasonable is that as the century progressed these students undertook more college preparatory work or a longer collegiate program or both.

Finally in the *D.A.M.B.* the percentage of men earning a predoctoral degree increased steadily decade by decade. In the seventh decade the figure was 46.9 percent and by the tenth, 63.4. (That is 63.4 percent of all men completing medical training in the tenth decade had earned a predoctoral degree.) In short both the quality of premedical education and the number of men pursuing predoctoral degrees increased as the century progressed. Putting aside the question of representativeness, the *D.A.M.B.* sample was itself improving with time.

The 45 years encompassed in the present study saw a persistent though phlegmatic upgrading of the formal medical curriculum as well. The process involved the teaching of laboratory medicine as well as the length and content of clinical training. Before the Civil War medical studies centered about a preceptorship (nominally three years in length, but steadily diluted in practice during our period) and two lecture courses of some three months duration. The lecture courses were ungraded and the second was identical to the first — tedium compounded. Earlier requirements for Latin and the M.D. thesis were by now defunct, and since students were assessed a diploma fee final examinations rarely took a scalp. Even the rule that medical graduates must be 21 years of age was widely ignored.[18]

Throughout the first four post-bellum decades basic science teaching, with few exceptions, remained the domain of practising physicians. In the earlier decades of the 19th century these men generally had no formal basic training beyond their own medical school experience. This too began changing as the 20th century approached. Laboratory medicine (along with laboratory science generally) was scantily taught prior to the Civil War,[19] but increased thereafter with the period of rapid development beginning between 1890 and 1895.[20] During this time the number of nonmedical graduate students rose "with astonishing speed."[21] These men formed the pool from which specialized basic science teachers eventually came, but by Flexner's time the appointment of Ph.D. teachers in medical schools was still an innovation to be "watched with interest."[22] Widespread support of basic research in America was spurred by the impressive practical successes of German science. The movement was well under way by 1900 and was bound to contribute to the favorable reception accorded Flexner's recommendations.

With a few significant exceptions[23] clinical teaching prior to 1865 took place in the crowded formality of classrooms and amphitheaters. Riesman scored the principal defect of the method when he said of his own experience at Pennsylvania, "It really made no difference what ailed the patient; the professor could use him as text for almost any disease and we would be none the wiser."[24] Even in medical schools with affiliated hospitals the situation could be deceptive. Norwood could justly say of Philadelphia schools, "What appears to be a formidable array of clinical material was in reality not always made available for clinical teaching."[25]

But again improvement was under way. After the Civil War a growing number of medical colleges graded the curriculum[26] and extended its length. Those who opposed stretching the term argued that a six-month session was "preposterous, in violation of all laws of health, physical or mental. . . ."[27] As always in this situation it is difficult to sort out true convictions from the economic incentives that in fact dominated many actions by proprietary professors. In any event the transition was far from painless. The University of Pennsylvania attempted a six-month course of study as early as mid-century, but had to abandon the experiment when competing schools refused to fall in line.[28]

Between 1800 and 1830 the lecture term generally remained at 13 weeks.[29] By 1882, 42 schools reportedly required courses of six months or more and by 1890 the figure was 76.[30] Improvement continued so that by 1910 practically all schools offered four years of graded instruction although the number of months required each year continued to vary.[31]

Despite the many defects of the American M.D. degree program at this time, a physician must have been better prepared for practice by earning a degree than by the simple process of self-ordination. Another bit of positive evidence appears in the *D.A.M.B.* study where the number of men earning medical degrees increased consistently in the three decades after the Civil War.[32]

For the more affluent student of this period two domestic postgraduate experiences were available — house staff training and postgraduate clinics. The latter came on the scene relatively late; the New York Polyclinic, for example, opened its doors in 1882.[33] A few of these clinics flourished, but generally they never attained the prestige of their European counterparts. To Flexner the earlier clinics were nothing more than "undergraduate repair shops,"[34] though this is less an indictment than Flexner may have intended, because a measure of repair was needed. Still the postgraduate clinic was not as important for our purposes as house staff training. The clinics rather quickly settled on imparting the technical skills of a specialty, and were not looked to as a source of broad clinical training.

Insofar as it helped remedy the deficiencies of formal clinical instruction the role of postgraduate hospital training[35] has been underestimated. The situation is inevitable if one thinks only in terms of formal internships and residencies as they exist today. In the pre-Flexnerian period house staff training was arranged more or less informally, and there is evidence that such personal arrangements were not rare. As early as 1914 an internship was made requisite to licensure in Pennsylvania,[36] and in that same year the American Medical Association published its first list of approved internships plus a list of 95 hospitals offering specialty training.[37] Even more striking is the report that a year or two earlier 70 percent of the nation's medical graduates elected an internship.[38] Of the 1,513 physicians in the *D.A.M.B.* sample 248 took some form of house staff training. In the first decade of the 19th century the figure was only 1.6 percent, for the seventh decade, 20.2 percent, and by the last decade, 43.9.[39]

In part the importance of house staff training in improving physician education during this time has been understressed because the movement arose spontaneously and informally with no visible external crusade such as that directed against the undergraduate curriculum by the American Medical Association and others from mid-century on. Hospitals were growing in numbers and practitioners needed resident physicians. At the same time medical graduates were increasingly aware of their inadequate clinical skills. The two needs met quietly in a symbiotic relationship which was well established and which had most of the characteristics of modern house staff training by the time Flexner came along.

The third postgraduate option open to American students was medical training abroad. Remembering that students were under no legal compulsion to undertake such a costly venture, the numbers involved are mildly staggering. Bonner estimated that some fifteen thousand visited Germany and Austria alone in the period 1870–1914.[40] In the *D.A.M.B.* study 372 (24.6 percent of the 1,513 subjects) went abroad within five years after completing their American medical training. Only 14.8 percent did so in the first decade, a figure that rose to 24.6 percent in the seventh decade and 36.6 in the tenth.[41]

It could be argued and correctly that this amazing European exodus merely underscored the inadequacy of clinical opportunities at home. Yet the larger significance is that they *did* go abroad, most of them presumably intent on improving their medical proficiency. Each wave of returning students evangelized a new group which in turn came back impressed with what medical training could and should be like. The influence of these European-trained men in abetting eventual reform is impossible to assess quantitatively, but undoubtedly it was greater than observers appreciated at the time. When the Johns Hopkins University opened a medical school along German lines, J. S. Billings feared it would be many years before the school could hope to graduate a class of 25. The first class graduated only 15, but two years later the figure was 32.[42]

Field points out that 16 of the 28 founding members of the American Physiological Society (1887) were trained in Germany and four others had studied in England or France. The group included a number of men who later led the battle to reform medical education in this country, such names as H. P. Bowditch, W. H. Howell, H. N. Martin, C. S. Minot, William Osler, and William Welch.[43] It is reasonable to conclude that the fifteen thousand or so men who saw German medical education firsthand must have been a powerful, though never organized, influence supporting Flexner's efforts of 1910 and thereafter.

It was Welch who summarized the period by saying "The results were better than the system."[44] He was right, and in part the results were better than the system because an increasing number of students forsook the system to create a system of their own. In assessing the status of American medical education before Flexner it is important to look beyond the extant degree requirements and consider the finished product as well. While the majority continued to settle for the prevailing mediocrity, a growing number of young physicians around the turn of the 20th century voluntarily supplemented their formal medical education with undergraduate collegiate preparation, house staff training, and study abroad. During the same period certain social forces began to be felt, and these too contributed to the catalytic effect of the implacable little schoolmaster from Louisville. Among the external forces were organized medicine, state licensing boards, and the improbable educational experiment made possible by Baltimore businessman Johns Hopkins.

The two principal medical organizations involved were the American Medical Association (A.M.A.) and the Association of American Medical Colleges (A.A.M.C.). From its inception in 1846 to the end of the century the A.M.A. battled for reform with little visible effect. Lacking any legal bite the A.M.A. sought to work by moral suasion alone. A main reason for its failure is found in the structure of the A.M.A. itself. From the outset the A.M.A.'s architects faced an organizational dilemma. If physician-owners of proprietary schools were to be induced to join a national organization which strongly favored educational reform, they would have to be offered greater voter representation than their numbers would dictate. On the other hand, of course, giving the medical schools too large a voice would block any chance for reform. The founders attempted a compromise which was doomed from the beginning. Only about a third of the eligible medical schools were present at the A.M.A.'s organizational convention in 1846.[45] From 1847 to 1852 medical college representation fell from 59 to 39 while medical society membership increased from 178 to 226.[46] The rift grew so wide that in 1853 there was an attempt to eliminate medical college delegates altogether.[47] Thus a town-gown split was all but assured by the A.M.A.'s original constitution, though it is difficult to imagine any scheme that would have satisfied the contending factions. Perceiving that the A.M.A. was essentially powerless, the physician-professors refused to participate and thus were free to ignore the A.M.A.'s exhortations. The best that can be said for the A.M.A. before 1900 is that its monotonous editorial lamentations did keep the matter somewhere in the far reaches of the profession's conscience. So frustrated did matters become in reality that at one time the A.M.A. entertained such now-startling possibilities as federal legislation and a national medical college.[48]

In 1904 the A.M.A. formed a permanent Council on Medical Education and from that point on its voice began to be heard. Staffed originally with a group of outstanding men, the council periodically inspected medical schools and began a rating system of A (worthy), B, and C (hopeless). Their reports were broadcast and the ensuing publicity undoubtedly contributed to the closure or merger of 29 schools between 1906 and Flexner's report[49] four years later.

In 1908 the council helped enlist Carnegie Foundation support for Flexner's survey and made available to him data accumulated from the council's previous investigations.[50] Dr. N. P. Colwell, secretary of the council, accompanied Flexner on several inspection trips, and, although Colwell's reports had to be couched "cautiously and tactfully,"[51] his medical insights must have proved helpful to Flexner. When it came time to write, Flexner, with his independent status, was free to put down with brutal objectivity many of the findings Colwell had felt free only to mutter about.

During the years after 1846 the disabling internecine problems of the A.M.A. became apparent to a small number of reform-minded men in the ranks of medical education itself. Responding to an organizational call on June 2, 1876, representatives from 22 medical colleges met to consider the possibility of reform from within. The following year they organized as the American Medical College Association.[52] Their laudable idealism soon came to grief. In 1880 the A.A.M.C. voted to require three years of medical training with at least six months of each year in a "proper medical college." Within two years ten schools withdrew, including several of the better founding colleges, and the organization collapsed. A successful reorganization took place in 1890 and from then on the pace of reform picked up. By 1896 the renamed Association of American Medical Colleges could report that 55 of the nation's 155 medical colleges were "cooperating," which meant at least nominal adherence to the higher self-imposed standards of A.A.M.C. members.[53] This, it should be recalled, at a time when even catalogue adherence to higher standards placed a school at a real disadvantage in the fierce competition for students.

The overriding importance of the A.A.M.C.'s early years was that at last reform was stirring within the proprietary system itself. Educators themselves now admitted at least that a mess existed. Earlier A.A.M.C. standards, while not always met by member schools themselves, created something of a self-fulfilling prophecy. The fact that a number of schoolmen could now organize for reform finally cracked the solid front presented by proprietary professors for most of the century. As its power and prestige grew the A.A.M.C. demanded a series of higher standards from its member colleges, and in 1905 the Confederation of State Medical Examining and Licensing Boards adopted the A.A.M.C.'s standard curriculum. From this point on the story became one of increasingly effective cooperation between the A.A.M.C., the A.M.A., and a new force, state legislatures, intent upon revitalizing medical practice acts.

During the early 19th century licensure was under some measure of legal control in most states of the Union. Regulatory mechanisms variously involved medical societies, medical schools, and governing boards of universities. Around 1830 licensure laws began to be repealed and by 1850 legislative control of medical licensure was practically nonexistent.[54] The anarchy that characterized American medicine from 1830 to 1875 came about for a number of reasons which cannot be detailed here. In general, abandonment of medicine by the state paralleled the rise of medical sects and indeed in the judgment of Reginald Fitz the spread of Thomsonianism was "the first serious blow to the regulation by the State of the practice of medicine. . . ."[55]

To put the matter perhaps too simply, public dissatisfaction with the heroic therapy of regular physicians coupled with widespread confusion over the conflicting claims of some two dozen different medical sects led legislators to withdraw legal sanctions from all the contending parties. A nadir of sorts was reached in 1838 when Maryland made it legal for any citizen of that state to charge and be paid for medical services.[56]

In medical practice absolute freedom can corrupt as thoroughly as absolute power, and in truth the two become effectively synonymous. N. S. Davis, whose prescience becomes more remarkable with time, resolved at the first convention of the A.M.A. that licensing be placed in the hands of a single independent state board in each state.[57] Not surprisingly the resolution failed and by 1860 editorialists such as Stephen Smith had given up hope for state control and tossed the matter back to the A.M.A.[58] By 1875 the chaos could not be ignored any longer. The process of repeal reversed itself and states began writing new laws controlling licensure and practice. New York was in the vanguard, and the story there in many ways exemplifies the complex seesaw evolution of legislative attempts at controlling medical licensure.[59] By 1894 Fitz reported that all states except New Hampshire and his own Massachusetts had laws regulating medical practice.[60] Although these laws varied in their inherent worthiness as well as the energy with which they were prosecuted, Fitz concluded that "to them, more than any one cause, is due the difference which exists between the condition now [1894] and in 1870."[61]

The state licensing boards created by this new wave of legislation confederated and finally there existed a national organization invested with the power that for years the A.M.A. and A.A.M.C. could only sigh after. To Flexner's eye the state boards of 1910 left much to be desired — their continued loose interpretation of his *bête noire*, the "equivalent," for example — but he wisely perceived that the legal approach held the best hope for reform. "The state boards," he said, "are the instruments through which the reconstruction of medical education will be largely effected."[62]

Viewed in terms of the ground they plowed for Flexner, legislative reforms after 1870 were far more significant than their immediate success in eliminating diploma mills, quacks, and ignorant but sincere sectarians. The new laws reflected a wholly new national attitude. No longer was the scene dominated by fears of class legislation, by the pervasive attitude of *laissez-faire*, or Herbert Spencer's version of social Darwinism which made the patient responsible for his own folly when he chose his physician unwisely.[63] The confused lawlessness of 1830–1870 had by now convinced the populace and their lawmakers that some degree of state regulation was both proper and necessary.

Other factors contributed. Regular medicine emerged as genuinely superior to its sectarian competition, which was handicapped by a simplistic, usually unitarian, approach to disease causation and therapy. Whatever its faults regular medicine retained the capacity for change, a trait that allowed it to accommodate the remarkable advances of European medicine, albeit at times with some chauvinistic delays. The regulars could scarcely claim a jockey's role in medicine's late 19th-century emergence as a science, but at least they backed the right horse. Nationalistic elements remained, but by Flexner's time the profession and the public generally accepted the superiority of German science.

The next step was eminently reasonable. If the fruits of German medical science could be imported into this country, why not the educational system that underpinned it all? Indeed the process had begun as far back as 1876 in the hands of a few visionary men and a Baltimore merchant who was wise enough to avoid all restrictive adjectives when he endowed a new type of American university.[64] The Hopkins' story is too well known to need retelling here.[65] The fact that the Johns Hopkins medical school succeeded almost two decades before the Flexner report testifies that American attitudes toward medical education had changed drastically between 1865 and 1893. True, a number of proprietary schoolmen refused to see the message on the wall, but by 1910 the writing was plainly there.

A final force deserves mention, that of economics. The same free marketplace which originally encouraged the wild growth of medical schools had begun to take its toll. Supply now exceeded valid demand, and as Flexner wryly remarked, "Nothing has perhaps done more to complete the discredit of commercialism than the fact that it has ceased to pay. It is but a short step from an annual deficit to the conclusion that the whole thing is wrong anyway."[66]

Indeed commercialism had ceased to pay. Flexner found that during the single year prior to his report a dozen schools had collapsed and "many more are obviously gasping for breath."[67] Had this attrition rate prevailed consistently it would more than have accounted for the decrease in schools from a 1906 peak of 161 to the 100 or so surviving in 1915.[68]

Thus the tide of reform was running heavy by 1910. Flexner himself observed that "there is no denying that especially in the last fifteen years, substantial progress has been made."[69] Yet none of this need detract from Flexner's renowned contribution.[70] There is no doubt but that his meticulously documented survey shocked the nation and hastened the closing of a number of marginal schools. But that was not his chief bequest. The sorry state of America's medical schools was no secret before 1910. His enduring legacy derived from what he accomplished quietly after the sensation created by his report had subsided. Largely due to Flexner's efforts John D. Rockefeller donated almost fifty million dollars to improve the nation's medical schools through the ministrations of the General Education Board. Within a few years a fine new school was established at the University of Rochester and major overhauls had been financed at schools such as Iowa, Cornell, Vanderbilt, and Washington at St. Louis. Nor did the tide stop there. As Flexner and members of the General Education Board anticipated, state rivalries erupted around the few schools selected for financial assistance.[71] Many of these states, when they failed to secure philanthropic help, took upon themselves the long-neglected fiscal responsibility for training their own physicians. Thus Flexner is properly remembered not so much for the fire he set as for his blueprint of the new structure which was to rise from the ashes.

NOTES

1 A. Flexner, *Medical Education in the United States and Canada* (New York: Carnegie Foundation, 1910).

2 Elements of the story appear in chapters by W. F. Norwood and J. Field in *The History of Medical Education*, ed. C. D. O'Malley. U.C.L.A. Forum Med. Sci. No. 12 (Los Angeles: Univ. of California Press, 1970), pp. 463–499 and 501–530.

3 N. S. Davis calculated that physicians and population had increased *pari passu* in the 35 years prior to 1876. *Contributions to the History of Medical Education and Medical Institutions in the United States of America 1776–1876* (Washington, D.C.: Government Printing Office, 1877), pp. 41–42. Davis makes no mention of men entering practice without degrees. Stern agreed when he estimated one physician for 572 persons in 1860 and one for 578 persons in 1900. B. J. Stern, *American Medical Practice in the Perspectives of a Century* (New York: Commonwealth Fund, 1945), p. 63. Stern is quoting the *Eighth Census* (Washington, D.C., 1860), pp. 670, 677. Flexner, *Medical Education*, p. 14, concurred in Stern's figures, but argued that the ratio was too great. Current thought would tend to support Flexner, but transportation and distribution of physicians would demand a higher ratio for the last part of the 19th century.

4 F. H. Garrison, *John Shaw Billings: A Memoir* (New York: Putnam's, 1915), p. 256.

5 Samuel Chew, generally inclined to the rosy view, said, "A favorable change has already taken place. The number of well educated young men who engage in the study of medicine is every year increasing." *Lectures on Medical Education* (Philadelphia: Lindsay and Blakiston, 1864), p. 136. The bulk of contemporary editorial opinion of course was distinctly pessimistic.

6 Flexner, *Medical Education*, p. 30.

7 R. H. Shryock, "Public relations of the medical profession in Great Britain and the United States: 1600–1870," *Ann. Med. Hist.*, 1930, n.s. *2*: 327.

8 T. R. Sizer, *Secondary Schools at the Turn of the Century* (New Haven: Yale Univ. Press, 1964), p. 4.

9 R. F. Butts summarized the trends in higher American education during the 19th century as follows: growth of large elective curricula, broadening of the traditional B.A. degree, rise of the German ideal of the university, increase in teaching of science and technology, decline of the notion that intellectual discipline could be honed only on the classics, increasing secularism, greater personal freedom for students, and opening college to all classes including women. *A Cultural History of Education* (New York: McGraw-Hill, 1947), pp. 519–521.

Flexner, speaking of the South, which lagged behind the rest of the nation in this regard, described the scene as an educational "renaissance." *Medical Education*, p. 40. He reported some 300,000 students enrolled in public high schools in 1910 and about 120,000 (males) in colleges of the North and West as of 1908, excluding preparatory and professional students. *Ibid.*, p. 42.

10 F. V. N. Painter, *A History of Education* (New York: Appleton, 1898), p. 322.

11 On the negative side McIntire surveyed 222 New Jersey and Pennsylvania physicians in 1882 and found 178 with no collegiate preparation at all. Unfortunately he does not indicate how many of his sample took their medical training before the Civil War. C. McIntire, Jr., *The Percentage of College-Bred Men in the Medical Profession* (Philadelphia: American Academy of Medicine, 1883), pp. 3–6.

12 M. Fishbein, *A History of the American Medical Association: 1847–1947* (Philadelphia: Saunders, 1947), p. 243.

13 J. H. Rauch, *Report on Medical Education, Medical Colleges and the Regulation of the Practice of Medicine in the United States and Canada 1765–1890* (Springfield: Illinois State Board of Health, 1890), pp. iii–iv.

14 Flexner, *Medical Education*, p. 28.

15 *Ibid.*, p. 46

16 *Ibid.*, p. 29.

17 H. A. Kelly and W. L. Burrage, eds., *Dictionary of American Medical Biography* (New York: Appleton, 1928). The study is by R. P. Hudson, "Patterns of medical education in nineteenth century America" (Unpublished essay for the M.A. degree, The Johns Hopkins University, 1966). The section dealing with premedical education is on pp. 23–34. This study will be referred to several times in the present paper, so a *caveat* is in order. The *D.A.M.B.* analysis is essentially statistical. This demanded the employment of certain arbitrary definitions and categories which are carefully spelled out in the essay. These should be consulted firsthand before any figures or conclusions from the study are used. The analysis included the reasons individuals were included in the *D.A.M.B.*, patterns of premedical, medical, and postgraduate education decade by decade, patterns of age, the influence of economic factors, effects of father's occupation and marriage, and educational patterns of the various specialities.

18 W. F. Norwood, *Medical Education in the United States Before the Civil War* (Philadelphia: Univ. of Pennsylvania Press, 1944), p. 406, states that the requirement for an attained age of 21 "seems to have been the only general regulation that was not grossly violated at some time during the decades covered by this survey." However the *D.A.M.B.* study revealed that 100 of the 1,513 men earned the M.D. degree before the age of 21. Hudson, "Patterns of medical education," p. 46. See also H. B. Shafer, *The American Medical Profession 1783 to 1850* (New York: Columbia Univ. Press, 1936), p. 82, and the implication of Daniel Drake's plea in *Practical Essay on Medical Education and the Medical Profession in the United States, 1832* (as reprinted in Baltimore by the Johns Hopkins Press, 1952), p. 57.

19 R. Hofstadter and C. D. Hardy, *The Development and Scope of Higher Education in the United States* (New York: Columbia Univ. Press, 1952), p. 20. The authors refer to W. P. Rogers, *Andrew D. White and the Modern University* (Ithaca: Cornell Univ. Press, 1942), pp. 23–29, and D. J. Struik, *Yankee Science in the Making* (Boston: Little Brown, 1948), chs. VI, X.

20 This is the estimate of R. M. Pearce, "An analysis of the medical group in Cattell's Thousand Leading Men of Science," *Science*, 1915, n.s. *42*: 264. Flexner dated the beginning of improved laboratory teaching at 1878, when Francis Delafield and William H. Welch opened clinical laboratories at the College of Physicians and Surgeons (N.Y.) and Bellevue Hospital Medical College respectively. *Medical Education*, p. 11.

21 Figures given are 198 in 1871, 2,382 in 1890 and 9,370 in 1910. Hofstadter and Hardy, *Development and Scope of Higher Education*, p. 64.

22 Flexner, *Medical Education*, p. 72.

23 Probably because of its French connections New Orleans apparently had a genuine go at bedside teaching as early as the 1850s. Speaking of his New Orleans School of Medicine in 1857, D. W. Brickell said flatly, "Six, out of ten, of us give *daily* bed-side instruction in the great Charity Hospital. . . ." *New Orleans Med. News & Hosp. Gaz.*, December 1857, *4*: 601. See also A. E. Fossier, "History of medical education, in New Orleans from its birth to the Civil War," *Ann. Med. Hist.*, 1934, n.s. *6*: 432. For the French influence see R. Matas, *The Rudolph Matas History of Medicine in Louisiana*, ed. J. Duffy (Louisiana State Univ. Press, 1962), II, 237–268.

Norwood appears to accept the New Orleans claim. *Medical Education . . . Before the Civil War*, p. 370.

Abraham Jacobi reportedly initiated bedside pediatrics teaching in New York in 1862. *The American Pediatric Society 1888–1938* (Privately printed, 1938), p. 4. According to Shryock, Jacob Da Costa began bedside teaching at Jefferson around 1870. "Medicine in Philadelphia during the nineteenth century," *Bull. Soc. Med. Hist. Chicago*, 1948, *6*: 70. On the other hand, Osler maintained that as of 1890 there was "not a single medical clinic worth the name in the United States." W. Osler, "The coming of age of internal medicine in America," *International Clinics*, 1915, *4*: 3.

24 D. Riesman, "Clinical teaching in America with some remarks on early medical schools," *Tr. Coll. Physicians Phila.*, 1939, 3rd series, 7: 109.

25 Norwood, *Medical Education . . . Before the Civil War*, p. 107.

26 Credit for the first graded curriculum is difficult to assign. To be answered the question must be put with precision. Who first advocated grading the curriculum? Where was it first attempted? Was it optional or required? Where did it first take hold? See F. C. Waite, "Advent of the graded curriculum in American medical colleges," *J. Assn. Am. Med. Colls.*, 1950, *25*: 315–322.

27 Quoted by Brickell, *New Orleans Med. News & Hosp. Gaz.*, December 1857, *4*: 599.

28 J. Carson, *A History of the Medical Department of the University of Pennsylvania* (Philadelphia: Lindsay and Blakiston, 1869), p. 172.

29 Shafer, *American Medical Profession*, p. 51.

30 Rauch, *Report on Medical Education*, p. iv.

31 Flexner, *Medical Education*, pp. 10–11.

32 In the *D.A.M.B.* sample (n. 17) subjects were categorized as degreed, nondegreed, and delayed, meaning the man earned a degree but only after he had begun medical practice. Forty-eight were delayed, and 68 nondegreed. The remaining 1,397 earned medical degrees before practising. In the first decade only 55.7 percent earned the M.D. Figures for the last four decades were 96.0, 99.4, 100, and 100 respectively. All figures excluded honorary and *ad eundem* degrees. Hudson, "Patterns of medical education," p. 53.

At the other extreme Norwood states that two-thirds to three-fourths of medical school matriculates did not remain to take the degree, implying that they entered practice without ever earning the M.D. *Medical Education . . . Before the Civil War*, p. 432. This estimate strikes me as too dismal. It was based on a "sampling of school circulars and catalogues and contemporary literature." The use of catalogues and circulars for this purpose is particularly precarious, since many students wisely took the second lecture course at a different school from the first. Such students would appear in successive catalogues as dropouts rather than transfers.

33 T. E. Keys, "Historical aspects of graduate medical education," *J. Med. Educ.*, 1955, *30*: 260. As Keys makes clear, this was not the first attempt at graduate medical education in America.

34 Flexner, *Medical Education*, p. 174. Flexner summarizes postgraduate schools as of 1910 on pp. 174–177.

35 House staff training is used here to cover all hospital-based clinical training taken after the medical degree. So used, the term must be approached with caution, because terminology describing hospital training shared the general educational confusion of the time. See, for example, *Graduate Medical Education* (Chicago: Univ. of Chicago Press, 1940), p. 98. The terms "resident" and "resident physician" have a tortuous history dating back at least 125 years. *Ibid.*, p. 97. The earliest hospital training programs centered around medical students who were called resident students. They were outgrowths of the indenturing practice such as that initiated in 1773 at Pennsylvania Hospital. Beginning in 1820 at City Almshouse of Philadelphia, house pupils were required to pay a fee and were dignified by the title of house physician or house surgeon. By 1823 a candidate for this position had to be a medical graduate. Norwood, *Medical Education . . . Before the Civil War*, p. 49. The following year the same held true of Pennsylvania Hospital, and a similar evolution occurred elsewhere. T. Morton and F. Woodbury, *The History of the Pennsylvania Hospital 1751–1895* (Philadelphia: Times Printing House, 1895), p. 480.

For most of the 19th century "interns" were medical students, the equivalent of the early hospital pupils. To illustrate, in 1880 the Board of Trustees of Charity Hospital in New Orleans decided that interns must have one year of medical study before appointment. A. E. Fossier, "The Charity Hospital of Louisiana," reprinted from *New Orleans Med. & Surg. J.*, May–October 1923, *75–76*: 38. As applicants for the position of intern gradually were required to be physicians, hospital pupils came to be known as externs, and in 1892 we find the two working side by side "without any official friction." *Ibid.*, p. 43. The Philadelphia and New Orleans examples are not offered as precise for other geographical situations, but rather to provide illustrations of the confusion that followed the evolution of hospital training positions.

The term "internship" reportedly first appeared about the time of the Civil War. *Graduate Medical Education*, p. 31. The word gained distinction only slowly and did not achieve its modern meaning until about 1914. From the end of the Civil War to the end of the century, however, "intern" continued to be used interchangeably with "resident" and "resident physician." Today's highly standardized residency program was patterned on the German system and formalized by William Halsted at the Johns Hopkins at the beginning of the 20th century. See W. S. Halsted, "The training of the surgeon." *Johns Hopkins Hosp. Bull.*, 1904, *15*: 271 ff. The current use of the word "resident" followed.

36 Fishbein, *A History of the American Medical Association*, p. 899.

37 *Ibid.*, p. 899–900.

38 *Ibid.*, p. 899. The source of this figure is not given and it is difficult to know if the year referred to is 1912 or 1913.

39 Hudson, "Patterns of medical education," p. 108.

40 T. N. Bonner, *American Doctors and German Universities* (Lincoln: Univ. of Nebraska Press, 1963), p. 23.

41 Hudson, "Patterns of medical education," p. 88. The five-year limitation was imposed in an attempt to eliminate the large number of physicians who toured Europe after years of successful practice.

42 Flexner, *Medical Education*, p. 46.

43 O'Malley, *History of Medical Education*, p. 504. Field apparently surveyed the founders' biographies in W. J. Meek, W. H. Howell, and C. W. Greene, *History of the American Physiological Society semicentennial 1887–1937* (Baltimore, 1938).

44 Flexner, *Medical Education*, p. 10, quotes Welch, "Development of American medicine," *Columbia Univ. Quart. Suppl.*, December 1907.

45 N. S. Davis, *History of the American Medical Association* (Philadelphia: Lippincott, 1855), p. 37.

46 *Ibid.*, p. 117.

47 *Ibid.*, p. 115.

48 Dr. William Baldwin, president of the newly formed Association of American Medical Editors, suggested federal legislation in an address to the A.M.A. in 1869. Fishbein, *A History of the American Medical Association*, p. 79. A resolution supporting the establishment of a national school of medicine was introduced at the 1870 meeting of the A.M.A. (*Tr. A.M.A.*, 1870, *21*: 37–39), and the idea was revived in his presidential address of 1876 by J. Marion Sims. *Ibid.*, 1876, *27*: 94–95.

49 See O'Malley, *History of Medical Education*, pp. 507–508. Of 140 schools visited by the Council on Medical Education and reported to the A.A.M.C. in 1910, 68 were rated A, 38 B, and 34 C. D. F. Smiley, "History of the Association of American Medical Colleges, 1876–1956," *J. Med. Educ.*, 1957, *32*: 520.

50 H. S. Pritchett in Flexner, *Medical Education*, p. viii.

51 A. Flexner, *An Autobiography* (New York: Simon and Schuster, 1960), p. 74.

52 This story can be found in Smiley, "History of the Association of American Medical Colleges."

53 In the earlier years the A.A.M.C. had difficulty mounting a vigorous leadership role. Their higher standards usually were adopted only after a number of schools had led the way. In 1900 premedical requirements were upgraded, but the A.A.M.C. did not insist that member colleges require three years of collegiate preparation until 1952. *Ibid.*, p. 523. By 1904 66 member schools reported a required four-year medical curriculum with terms ranging from six to nine months. *Ibid.*, p. 518.

54 R. H. Fitz, "The legislative control of medical practice," *Med. Comm. Mass. Med. Soc.*, 1894, *16*: 306–307. Fitz's account is perhaps the best to come from the contemporary scene. To his mind, laws regulating medical practice were unpopular because (1) they were considered class legislation, (2) legislators suspected the motives of regular physicians, (3) the populace believed every person had a right to choose his own medical attendant, and (4) regular physicians themselves objected, out of a belief that the very act of regulating irregulars would exert a protective influence upon them. *Ibid.*, pp. 282 ff.

55 *Ibid.*, pp. 301–306. Fitz saw Thomsonianism as paving the way for homeopathy, "which proved to be the more effectual agent in annulling the licensing of physicians."

56 *Ibid.*, p. 306.

57 Davis, *History of the American Medical Association*, p. 35.

58 "What shall be our title?" *Am. Med. Times*, July 28, 1860, p. 63. The editorial is unsigned, but in a personal communication Gert Brieger expressed his conviction that Smith was the author.

59 J. B. Bardo, "A history of the legal regulation of medical practice in New York State," *Bull. N.Y. Acad. Med.*, 1967, *43*: 924–940. Bardo's narrative is revealing in that it shows the difficulties encountered in efforts at regulating licensure when neither the state, the medical schools, nor the profession had clear-cut legal backing. In 1684 New York law prohibited medical practice without the "consent of those skillful" in it. In 1760 specified magistrates were empowered to examine and license, and in 1797 the magistrates could license by endorsing a preceptor's certificate. An 1806 law made the medical profession responsible through state and local medical societies. Three years later the University of

the State of New York could authorize colleges to issue the M.D. degree, which was then a license to practice as well. By 1872 the Regents could appoint a board of examiners, which again made licensure a state function. In 1880 medical societies were divested of any licensing function, and by 1890 the M.D. degree no longer conferred automatic licensure, which was now solely in the Regents' hands. To insure professional input, Boards of Medical Examiners were created, one each for regular practitioners, homeopaths, and eclectics. In 1893 existing laws were brought together as part of a Public Health Law and in 1907 the three separate boards were made one. At no point in this long evolution did enforcement of a law necessarily follow its enactment.

60 Fitz, "Legislative control," pp. 294, 313.

61 *Ibid.*, p. 315.

62 Flexner, *Medical Education*, pp. 167–173.

63 Spencer is quoted as saying, "Unpitying as it looks, it is best to let the foolish man suffer the appointed penalty of his foolishness. For the pain — he must bear it as well as he can; for the experience — he must treasure it up and act more rationally in the future." *Social Statics*, 1851, p. 373, quoted in Fitz, "Legislative control," p. 284.

64 A. Flexner, *Daniel Coit Gilman: Creator of the American Type of University* (New York: Harcourt, Brace, 1946), p. 35.

65 *Ibid.*, and especially R. H. Shryock, *The Unique Influence of the Johns Hopkins University on American Medicine* (Copenhagen: Munksgaard, 1953).

66 Flexner, *Medical Education*, p. 11.

67 *Ibid.*

68 The figures are from *The General Education Board* (New York: General Education Board, 1915), p. 161.

69 Flexner, *Medical Education*, p. 10.

70 In some current circles it has become fashionable to criticize Flexner for the nationwide adoption of the Hopkins' plan — for what has come to be called the tyranny of the four-year lockstep curriculum. This is akin to holding Galen responsible for the 1500 years his doctrines influenced medical thought after his death. Worse, it ignores Flexner's own unequivocal caveat, "In the course of the next thirty years needs will develop of which we here take no account. As we cannot foretell them, we shall not endeavor to meet them." *Medical Education*, p. 143.

71 This story is told in Flexner, *An Autobiography*. See esp. pp. 178 ff.

9

The "Connecting Link": The Case for the Woman Doctor in 19th-Century America

REGINA MARKELL MORANTZ

Little more than a decade before the Civil War, Elizabeth Blackwell, daughter of a prominent reform-minded family, achieved notoriety by becoming the first woman to earn a medical diploma in the United States. Soon after she received her degree in 1849, Geneva Medical College, a small regular institution in upstate New York, closed its doors to women. Undaunted, women continued to seek medical training. Within two years, three female students at the eclectic Central Medical College in Syracuse — the first coeducational medical school in the country — gained medical licenses.

In Philadelphia a group of Quakers led by Dr. Joseph Longshore pledged themselves to teach women medicine and established the Woman's (originally Female) Medical College of Pennsylvania in 1850. The following year eight women graduated in the first class. A Boston school, founded originally by Samuel Gregory in 1848 to train women as midwives, gained a Massachusetts charter in 1856 as the New England Female Medical College. Here Marie Zakrzewska, former medical associate of Elizabeth Blackwell, early female graduate of the Cleveland Medical College, and the influential founder of the New England Hospital for Women and Children, came to teach in 1859.

Meanwhile, in New York the Homeopathic New York Medical College for Women, established in 1863 by still another early graduate, Clemence Lozier, enjoyed such success that by the end of the decade it had matriculated approximately 100 women. Five years later Elizabeth Blackwell, now joined in practice by her sister Emily, also a graduate of Cleveland, opened the Women's Medical College of the New York Infirmary.

By 1870 a handful of medical schools, both orthodox and sectarian, accepted women on a regular basis. In fact, over 300 women had already graduated, though mostly from sectarian institutions. Several of these women founded dispensaries in New York, Boston, and Philadelphia to offer needed clinical training to the increasing numbers of female colleagues. Of course, opportunities for women in medicine remained circumscribed, for throughout the century the majority of institutions barred them from attendance. Nevertheless, the ranks of female physicians grew: by 1900 their numbers reached an estimated 7,387.[1]

Women entered the medical profession as part of a broader 19th-century movement toward self-determination in which all reformist women, from conservative social feminists to radical suffrage advocates, played a significant part. Like many members of their sex, women doctors sought to examine and redefine the concept of womanhood to fit the changing demands of a complex, industrializing society. Furthermore, the move to educate women in medicine grew out of the antebellum health reform crusade. Abolitionists, peace advocates, temperance reformers, and women's righters participated in the drive to improve the nation's health, and middle-class women were particularly active in health and dietary reform in these years.[2]

Indeed, medicine attracted more women votaries in the 19th century than any other profession except teaching. Female physicians took seriously their role in health education. For many, medical training appeared the logical outcome of their

REGINA MARKELL MORANTZ is Assistant Professor of History, University of Kansas, Lawrence, Kansas.

prior interest in health issues. Borrowing arguments from the health reformers, they emphasized the importance of giving information on hygiene and physiology to all women. Women's new and central role in family life made systematic knowledge imperative. Female physicians, as teachers and clinicians concerned with such issues, would be essential to improving the health and nurturing the expertise of all women.

Although they remained a small minority, women doctors were conspicuous because they violated 19th-century norms of female behavior. Consequently they became the focus of a vigorous controversy over women's proper role in and relationship to public and private health. Whereas amateur female instructors of physiology could be dismissed as objects of public ridicule, professionally trained women doctors were entirely another matter. By the end of the 1860s protests against them mounted from within the profession, forcing them and their supporters to refine and elaborate an ideology to defend their cause.

The arguments with which they chose to justify themselves revealed women physicians both as ideological innovators and as daughters of their century. Sharing this role with other women of their generation who sought an expansion of their activities, their ideas fell well within the mainstream of feminist thinking. Their ideology served a dual purpose. As self-explanation it enabled them to convey to the world what they hoped to accomplish and why. By their use of ideas they attempted to place themselves in cultural and historical perspective. Yet their ideology also exerted a powerful influence on the way they perceived reality, shaping that perception and giving it meaning within the context of Victorian values.

This essay examines the means by which women physicians justified their role in the 19th-century health revolution. Because their arguments deviated only slightly from those of others favoring a more active place for women in society, such an investigation illustrates how similar groups of 19th-century women came to grips with their culture. The reasoning of women physicians was often brilliant and effective, and their practical work extremely important. Yet their ties to 19th-century values also impaired their vision. Only a handful of them understood the ways in which a self-limiting conception of their potential contribution hampered their progress within the profession.

I

The opponents of medical education for women deserve attention first because their objections fixed the context of the debate. Women doctors remained sensitive to criticism, realizing that professional opposition reached far beyond ideology in its implications, sharply curtailing their opportunities to study and practice.

Most doctors were traditionalists who shared the same ambivalence towards women's role that dominated 19th-century American culture. Placing women on a pedestal and cementing them firmly within the confines of the home, they justified an emotional preference for sequestered women by making them the moral guardians of society and the repositories of virtue. Fearing that women who sought professional training would avoid their childrearing responsibilities, they reminded their colleagues in overworked metaphors that "the hand that rocks the cradle rules the world." Woman, argued a spokesman, held "to her bosom the embryo race, the pledge of mutual love." Her mission was not the pursuit of science, but "to rear the offspring and ever fan the flame of piety, patriotism and love upon the sacred altar of her home."[3]

Rational legitimation of the female role often veiled less rational preferences: the home represented for 19th-century Americans a refuge from an immoral and often brutalizing world. A woman who dared to move beyond her sphere was "a monstrosity," an "intellectual and moral hermaphrodite." Nevertheless, insisted Dr. Paul de Lacy Baker, women controlled society, government, and civilization through the "home influence." Home was

> the place of rest and refuge for man, weary and worn by manual labor, or exhausted by care and mental toil. Thither he turns him from the trials and dangers, the temptations and seductions, the embarrassments and failures of life, to the one spot beneath all the skies where hope and comfort come out to meet him and drive back the demons of despair that pursue him from the outside world. There the sweet enchantress that rules and cheers his home supports his sink-

> ing spirits, reanimates his self-respect, confirms his manly resolves and sustains his personal honor.[4]

While revering the purity and repose of the home, doctors, like other Victorians, feared the animal in man and dwelt on the significance of female moral superiority in curbing man's most brutal instincts. Woman's venturing out into the world would bode ill for civilization, for women kept men respectable. In copying men, they ran the risk of demoralizing both sexes. Men, confessed Dr. J. S. Weatherly to his colleagues, were "little less than brutes," and "where men are bestialized, women suffer untold wrongs." Woman's great strength and safety, he concluded, was in the institution of marriage, and "everything she does to lessen men's respect and love for her, weakens it, and makes her rights more precarious; for without the home influence which marriage brings, men will become selfish and brutal; and then away go women's rights."[5]

Traditionalists also worried that teaching women the mysteries of the human body would affront female modesty. "Improper exposures" would destroy the delicacy and refinement that constituted women's primary charms. Men recoiled at the thought of exposing young women to the "blood and agony" of the dissecting room, where "ghastly" rituals were performed.[6]

Despite the popularity of this defense of female delicacy, traditionalists compromised their case when they admitted that women's ready sympathy made them excellent nurses. Praising Florence Nightingale's achievements in the Crimea, they credited them primarily to her ignorance of scientific medicine. Medical education, they argued, would surely have hardened her heart, leaving her bereft of softness and empathy.[7]

Supporters of female education quickly discovered, however, that respect for Victorian delicacy could work in their favor. Was the mother who nursed her family at the bedside ever shielded from the indelicacies of the human body? they asked. Furthermore, if the issue was female modesty, then why should men — even medical men — ever be allowed to treat women? As the use of pelvic examinations became part of ordinary practice, male physicians posed a greater threat to feminine delicacy than women practitioners. Indeed, many supporters of medical training for women were conservative champions of female modesty.[8] Though the arguments of these supporters were extremely persuasive within the context of Victorian values, traditionalist physicians continued throughout the century to object to training women on the grounds of Victorian delicacy.

Some male physicians alleged other unsuitable character traits against women besides their innocence. Many agreed that Nature had limited the capacity of women's intellect. They were impulsive and irrational, unable to do mathematics, and deficient in judgment and courage. Their passivity of mind and weakness of body left them powerless to practice surgery. And if these disadvantages were not enough, there remained the enigmatic side of the female temperament. Dependent, "nervous," and "excitable," women, "as all medical men know," were subject to hysteria over which they had no control. "Hysteria," regretted J. S. Weatherly, M.D., "is second Nature to them."[9]

Because at least some women physicians in the 19th century received inferior training, doctors often mistook poor preparation for innate ignorance. On this point critics were most disingenuous. The issue became particularly controversial as local and national medical societies began to debate the admission of female members in the 1870s and 1880s. Though circular, the reasoning seemed incontrovertible — at least for a time. First-rate regular medical schools barred women from attendance. Meanwhile opponents unfairly stigmatized the women's medical colleges as either irregular or of poor quality. While denying them access to the kind of education they could approve, critics held their alleged inferior training against them, often refusing to consult with women physicians and ostracizing male practitioners who did. The final irony was that a fair number of medical women received excellent training in the 19th century. A comparative study of curriculum and clinical offerings in several 19th-century medical schools suggests that the women who earned their diplomas from the New York Infirmary and the Woman's Medical College of Pennsylvania were exposed to a vigorous, demanding, and comparatively progressive course of study.[10] Self-conscious of their need for proper preparation, other women sought postgraduate training in Europe.

Probably much of the grumbling over inferior

training arose out of disgust for the multiplication of proprietary schools in the 1830s and 1840s and the resulting sharp increase in the number of practitioners. Some physicians complained of the possibility of increased economic competition if women were admitted to study. Such concern dissipated toward the end of the century when women doctors appeared to segregate themselves in certain specialties. What remains most striking about this objection, however, is that it took for granted not only women's ability to practice medicine, but also their ready acceptance by the public.[11]

Rejecting many of the preceding arguments, an increasingly influential group of medical men preferred instead to take a more scientific posture. Rallying around Harvard professor E. H. Clarke's book *Sex in Education: A Fair Chance for Girls*, published in 1873, they based their case against women entirely on the predominating negative influence of their biology. When they chose to emphasize the debilitating and still mysterious effects of menstruation, traditionalists were indeed effective. Physicians knew little about the influence of women's periodicity, and the culture treated menstruation as a disease.[12] Reasoning that only rest could help women counteract the weakness resulting from the loss of blood, complete bedrest was commonly prescribed. Thus even if opponents appeared willing to concede women's intellectual equality — and many were prepared to do so — women's biological disabilities seemed insurmountable.[13] Since menstruation incapacitated women for a week out of every month, could they ever be depended on in medical emergencies?

Female physicians helped to dispel doubts about the effects of menstruation in their own professional lives. A few investigated the problem scientifically. Outraged by the influence of E. H. Clarke's book, the feminist community in Boston cast about for a woman doctor with the proper credentials to call its thesis into question. In 1874 women gained a public forum when Harvard announced that the topic for its celebrated Boylston Essay would be the effects of menstruation on women. Writing to Dr. Mary Putnam Jacobi in 1874, C. Alice Baker urged her to take up the "good work," and "win credit for all women, while winning for yourself the Boylston Medical Prize for 1876." Jacobi met the challenge; and her pioneering essay, "The Question of Rest for Women During Menstruation," which, to the opposition's chagrin, won the esteemed prize, was exemplary in its modern statistical methodology. Her conclusion, that there existed "nothing in the nature of menstruation to imply the necessity, or even the desirability, of rest for women whose nutrition is really normal," directly challenged conservative medical opinion.[14] Despite widespread respect for her paper, it failed to convince many physicians, and the debate continued into the 20th century.

In the realm of emotion, of course, apologists for women's sphere needed to be neither scientific nor consistent; they offered arguments for female inferiority, vulnerability, and dependence alongside claims for their moral superiority and responsibility. After all it was they who molded the life of future generations and spent tireless hours tending the sick long after the physician had retired from his daily rounds. Nineteenth-century society never did come to terms with this Manichean image of women, at least not until female physicians and other social feminists exploited the contradictions in the ideal and forced a reconciliation of the two extremes. In the process they created a new image for their sex and a broader definition of woman's sphere.

II

Women physicians argued within the context of the shared values of 19th-century culture. They and their male supporters took seriously the idea of their moral superiority and their ability as natural healers, embracing 19th-century definitions of feminine qualities intact. With intelligence and skill they made Victorian ideology yield to them and used these notions to justify seeking medical education.

One example of their subtle use of the value structure has already been noted: their reversal of the "delicacy" argument. Defending the "propriety of entrusting feminine life to feminine hands," they denounced exclusive male attendance to women's ailments as an outrage against female modesty pernicious to the "social and moral welfare of society."[15] Elizabeth Blackwell called it an "unnatural and monstrous arrangement" that women had "no resort but to men, in those diseases peculiar to themselves." Were the "methods of modern medicine quietly received and passively submitted to," she claimed, "it would indicate a terrible deficiency in some of the most important elements of womanly character." Here medical science clashed with morality, in the demand that to preserve morality women be taught science.[16]

Female physicians did not quarrel with the concept of separate spheres for men and women, though they meant something quite different from their opponents when they spoke of "woman's sphere." They sought an altogether novel definition of "femaleness." Examining the ethical implications of scientific methods for medicine and society, they claimed for women the task of integrating Science and Morality.

A glance at the titles of the popular health manuals of the period reveals the pervasiveness of the concept of Woman as Healer.[17] In response to these widespread assumptions traditionalists had glorified women's abilities as nurses, while denying them the right to become physicians. Supporters of medical training for women were outraged by such logic. "Is not Woman man's Superior?" asked Dr. J. P. Chesney of Missouri. "It is an idea extremely paradoxical," he continued, "to suppose that woman, the fairest and best of God's handiwork, and practical medicine, a calling little less sacred than the holy ministry itself, should, when united, become a loathsome abomination . . . from which virtue must stand widely aloof." If the traditionalists' own logic were applied consistently, he noted, "men would long ago have been banished from obstetrics."[18]

Zealously cataloguing women's past contributions to healing, supporters of female medical education argued that women needed the tools of modern medicine. Women *would* attend in the sickroom, and instinct and sympathy were not sufficient as advances in medical therapeutics rendered folk medicine ineffective. "It has begun to occur to people," observed Dr. Emmeline Cleveland of the Woman's Medical College of Pennsylvania in 1859, "that perhaps the fullest performance of her own home duties" required of woman "a more extended and systematic education . . . especially in those departments of science and literature which have practical bearing upon the lives and health of the community."[19]

Women doctors and their allies frequently echoed Victorian sentimentality over womanly attributes. Like their opponents they constantly connected womanhood with the guardianship of home and children. Women were morally superior to men, claimed Elizabeth Blackwell, because of the "spiritual power of maternity." The true physician, male or female, she argued, "must possess the essential qualities of maternity."[20]

Medical training was necessary for scientific motherhood. Ignorance of her own body and poor training in child management were taking their toll on American mothers and offspring alike. "What higher trust could be dedicated to the wife and mother," asked Dr. Joseph Longshore in his introductory lecture to the first class at the Woman's Medical College of Pennsylvania, "then guardianship of the health of the household?" His colleague Emmeline Cleveland, a brilliant gynecological surgeon, affirmed the necessity of giving to all women knowledge of the human body. She reminded her students that their high vocation was "as nature's appointed guardians of childhood and youth," that as mothers and teachers they would "become the conservators of public health and in an eminent degree responsible for the physical and moral evils which afflict society."[21]

Medical women like Cleveland intended to play a central role in the elevation of their sisters. As science was brought to bear on domestic life, women physicians would become the "connecting link" between the science of the medical profession and the everyday life of women.[22] To accomplish this purpose, each of the female medical schools offered courses in physiology and hygiene to nonmatriculants, who were often mothers and teachers hoping to gain knowledge in health education.

When critics charged that medical training was wasted on women who would eventually marry and have children, female physicians responded by pointing out that medical knowledge was important for any woman, even if the skills acquired would not be used to practice. Competence in medicine made women better mothers. Others were bolder, displaying the temerity that helped to expand society's conception of woman's role: they saw no necessary conflict between motherhood and general practice. This recognition of the possibility of combining marriage and career marked a radical departure from 19th-century thinking.

"A woman can love and respect her family just as much if not more," asserted Dr. Georgiana Glenn, "when she feels that she is supporting herself and adding to their comfort and happiness." Dr. Mary Putnam Jacobi agreed. Conceding that marriage complicated professional life, she nevertheless felt that "the increased vigor and vitality accruing to healthy women from the bearing and possession of children, a good deal more than compensates for the difficulties involved in caring for them, when professional duties replace the more usual ones, of sewing, cooking, etc."[23]

The social Darwinism of the post-Civil War period enabled traditionalists to reiterate their prejudices with the finality of scientific truth. Little changed in the controversy over female physicians besides the language of the debate. Scientific rationalism predominated by the 1880s, with evolution and eugenics mustered in defense of both sides. Critics of women doctors made pessimistic pronouncements that female higher education would be biologically destructive of the race.[24] Female physicians countered with measured optimism. They depicted themselves as living examples of the transition to higher life forms. Yet they also remained suspicious of prevailing trends, especially the frivolous pursuits of leisured women. Warning that the increased leisure accruing from technological advances demanded that women be given noble work to do, they urged society to check the notorious aimlessness of the civilized woman's life. Women's boredom was notorious: "For one case of breakdown from overwork among women," quipped Dr. Ruffin Coleman, "there are a score from ennui and sheer inanation from doing nothing."[25]

Along with most American scientists of the period, physicians accepted the neo-Lamarckian concept of the inheritance of acquired characteristics. Women doctors drew the logical object lesson: if mental as well as physical characteristics were inherited, the race would steadily improve only if women could uplift themselves. Their arguments remained a warning as well as a prophecy: Hold back your women — your mothers — and you retard the race.[26]

Medical women also insisted that they had special contributions to make to the profession. Feminization could enhance the practice of medicine, which concentrated on the eradication of suffering. Association with female colleagues would "exert a beneficial influence on the male." Combining the best of masculine and feminine attributes should raise medical practice to its highest level.

Occasionally supporters carried the implications of this reasoning even further. Female physicians expected to challenge heroic therapeutics directly. As the "handmaids of nature," women would place greater value on the "natural system of curing diseases . . . in contradistinction to the pharmaceutical." They would promote a "generally milder and less energetic mode of practice." "The Past," claimed the health reformer Mary Gove Nichols, "with the lancet, and poison, and operative surgery, did not insult woman by asking her to become a physician; and the Past has not asked her to become a hangman, general, or jailer. We may well excuse all believers in Allopathy, if they judge woman unfit for the profession."

Many women physicians did spurn heroic medicine. The husband of Hannah Longshore, the first female physician to establish a practice in Philadelphia, recorded the following in a biographical sketch of his wife:

> The Woman's Medical College claimed to be an entirely regular or old school institution and its faculty had a testimony to bear against homeopathy and eclecticism or in any irregularity of its graduates from the established old school practice. But many of its alumni [*sic*] discovered that the growing aversion to large doses of strong and disagreeable medicine among the more liberal and progressive elements in society and that many intelligent women had become tinctured with the heresy of Homeopathy and gave a preference to the physician who would prescribe or administer their milder and pleasant remedies, and especially for the children who would take their medicines voluntarily. This discovery led the woman doctor to an investigation of their remedies and theories of therapeutics and to partial adoption of their remedies and methods of treatment. This conformity to the demands for mild remedies gave the women doctors access to many families whose views were in accord with the reform movements that rec-

> ognized the growing interest in enlarging the sphere of woman. The woman doctors who saw that the door was opening for this reform of regular practice and prepared themselves accordingly were the first to get into successful business.

Marie Zakrzewska, who, as founder of the New England Hospital for Women and Children in Boston, earned the respect of even the most stubborn members of the male opposition, also remained skeptical of heroic dosing. In a letter to Elizabeth Blackwell she confessed that her whole success in practice was based on the cautious use of medicine, "often used as Placebos in infinitesemal forms." "In fact," she wrote, "I have the reputation among my large clientele, men, women, and children as giving hardly any medicine but teaching people how to keep well without it. This subject is a large theme and I am thankful from the innermost of my emotions . . . that nobody has ever been injured, if not relieved by my prescriptions."[27]

In keeping with this interest in prevention rather than cure, friends claimed that women physicians would become zealous advocates of public health and social morality. Emmeline Cleveland noted that women were naturally altruistic, while Elizabeth Blackwell expected her female colleagues to provide the "onward impulse" in seeing to it that human beings were "well born, well nourished, and well educated." Dr. Sarah Adamson Dolley urged women doctors to bring to the profession their "moral power." "Educated medical women," wrote Dr. Eliza Mosher, of the University of Michigan, "touch humanity in a manner different from men; by virtue of their womanhood, their interest in children, in girls and young women, both moral and otherwise, in homes and in society." Most of their male supporters agreed. Dr. James J. Walsh admitted that men did not recognize their social duties as readily as women. "Therefore," he confessed, "I have always welcomed the coming into the medical profession of that leaven of tender humanity that women represent."[28]

III

It is possible to claim that women doctors made their arguments, not necessarily because they believed them, but because they sensed the pervasiveness of traditional ideas about woman's sphere. Their rhetoric, as well as that of other feminists, has been interpreted as a calculated and well-planned offensive designed to challenge 19th-century assumptions with familiar ideas. Yet women physicians sincerely believed that they were different from men and that they had their own special contribution to make to society. Of course many of them realized the expediency of their case, especially because it did not wholly challenge traditional assumptions. Yet the desire to educate women in medicine remained part of 19th-century social feminism, a movement with roots in ante-bellum reform and nurtured in an atmosphere of perfectionist concern with the revival of moral values. Female physicians were not the only group of women to seek a broadening of women's role by expanding the notion of separate spheres.

Certainly many women chose a career in medicine for more private reasons than the belief in their own special female abilities. Many probably saw medical practice as a lucrative means of self support. But whatever their personal motives, such women belonged to a movement that justified itself in larger terms, and they gained their self-image from the social context in which they acted. After wishing the New York Infirmary graduating class of 1899 financial success — "we are always glad to hear of a woman's making money" — Dean Emily Blackwell urged her students to remember that "there are other kinds of success that . . . we hope you will always consider far higher prizes." These, she continued, were "the consciousness of doing good work in your own line, of being of use to others, of exerting an influence for right in all social and professional questions." Readily conceding that her students "doubtless all entered upon medical study from individual motives," she hoped that they had learned "that the work of every woman physician, her character and influence, her success or failure, tells upon all, and helps or hinders those who work around her or come after her."

Forty years earlier, a younger Emily Blackwell confided similar sentiments to her diary when she thanked God that she was only 25 and not yet too old to commence a life's labor full of "great deeds." Newly decided on a medical career, she prayed that at life's close God would grant her the ability to look back on a "woman's work done for thee and my fellows." Opportunities were then appearing for women to live a "heroic life," and Emily desperately wished to avail herself of them.[29]

Victorian ideology, then, was not entirely repressive to women. On the contrary, courageous individuals hoping to move out of the home could use the ideology for their own ends, and in a way consistent with their acceptance of prevailing values. The glorification of woman's moral power was their most potent weapon. Taking refuge in the concept of female superiority, they provided future generations of women with an imperfect but essential stepping stone on the route to sexual equality.

While both sides in the debate claimed to be seeking moral progress and civilization's advancement, female physicians, in their commitment to using women's abilities systematically and scientifically, diverged fundamentally from their conservative opponents. Women doctors hoped to reform society by feminizing it, a task which required the professionalization of "womanhood." Acknowledging that their goals required a broader interpretation of woman's sphere, they felt this a small price to pay for a morally righteous and civilized America.

Nineteenth-century women doctors never drifted out of touch with the mainstream of Victorian ideology. As proponents of the gradual expansion of women's role, they perceived gradual change to be the only kind the public would tolerate. Slowly they succeeded in creating a positive image for the female physician. A minority proved that wives and mothers could handle a professional career. Their inevitable interaction with male colleagues eventually convinced many critics that women could be competent doctors and still maintain their femininity.

Female physicians confined themselves to feminine specialties — obstetrics and gynecology in the 19th century, pediatrics, public health, teaching, and counseling later on. Such specialization was not due solely to resistance from male professionals, although women doctors occasionally blamed discrimination. Women practitioners gravitated to these specialties because they were conscious of their "special" abilities. They concerned themselves with the health problems of women and children because they hoped to raise the moral tone of society through the improvement of family life.

Doubtless for some unmarried women physicians, the practice of obstetrics or pediatrics gave them vicarious fulfillment from an intimate involvement in the primary events of the female life cycle, while freeing them from traditional Victorian marriage. Recently, historians have explored the female support systems that existed throughout the 19th century.[30] Many women physicians gravitated to feminine specialties — in fact, to medicine itself — out of a desire to perpetuate these support systems. Mothers, they argued, would more readily discuss their problems with women doctors because male physicians did not have "the patience to deal with the anxieties, ignorance, and frequent terrors of women who are often overwhelmed by some misunderstood condition in themselves or in their children." During the sensitive period of gestation, a woman needed someone whom she could approach "without reserve," and from whom she could get "a woman's sympathy." "Being women as well as physicians," acknowledged Dr. Florence B. Sherbon, president of the Iowa State Society of Medical Women, "we share with our sex in the actual and potential motherhood of the race. Being women we make common cause with all women. . . . And being women and mothers, our first and closest and dearest interest is the child. . . ."[31]

Such arguments naturally had limitations. Confining themselves to women's concerns circumscribed women physicians' professional influence. A few even willingly advocated an informal curtailment of their medical role, hoping to gain support by taking themselves out of competition with men.[32] But the more perceptive disdained this approach. Such women converted early to the modern and empirical world of professional medicine, and their first love was science. Often uneasy in the moralistic world of their medical sisters, they exhibited a toughness and clarity of vision which set them apart from those women who used medicine primarily as a moral platform. Physicians like Mary Putnam Jacobi and Marie Zakrzewska insisted from the beginning that medical women need be of superior mettle. Fearing that specialization in diseases of women and children would mean a loss of grounding in general medicine, they warned that women would be justly relegated to the position of second-class professionals. Eventually their performance even within their specialty would become second-rate. If women were to succeed in medicine, they asserted, they had to be thoroughly trained.[33] Despite their predictions, specializing remained popular throughout the 19th century and into the next because it provided advantages in blunting the resentment of male colleagues.

The emphasis female physicians placed on the mother's child-rearing responsibility also reflected and reinforced social values which would present future problems. As more married women entered the work force, acute ideological conflicts arose to hamper the development of alternative methods of child-rearing. When Charlotte Perkins Gilman proposed to professionalize child care at the turn of the century, she was virtually ignored. Even more revealing is the intensity of the conflict over child care centers that emerged within the federal government during World War II, a time when married women were entering the work force in large numbers and government facilities were a palpable necessity.[34]

While stressing women's peculiar adaptability to medicine, women doctors perpetuated an exaggerated concept of womanhood, rendering their arguments inapplicable to other, less obviously "feminine" pursuits. Dr. Frances Emily White attributed women's great success in medicine compared with other professions to a "peculiar fitness" for the work and the lack elsewhere "of equal opportunities for the exercise of those qualities that have become specialized in women."[35] Pursuits like teaching and nursing fit the pattern well, but law did not. Though women lawyers chose to justify their interests in a similar fashion, it was harder for them to claim that their work was an extension of women's natural sphere, and, indeed, few women preferred law to medicine in the 19th and early 20th centuries. All the reasons for this disparity remain complex, but the "natural sphere" argument did exhibit vexing limitations as women moved out of the home and into the world.[36]

A few perceptive individuals struggled uncomfortably with the implications of such reasoning. The journalist Helen Watterson, for example, denounced the woman movement's emphasis on "woman's qualities." Mary Putnam Jacobi quipped that "recently emancipated people are always bores, until they themselves have forgotten all about their emancipation." And Marie Zakrzewska frowned on women who chose medicine out of female "sympathy." The only motives the profession permitted its votaries, she maintained, were "an inborn taste and talent for medicine, and an earnest desire and love of scientific investigation."[37]

The brilliant Jacobi sensed the psychological disadvantages that hampered women physicians from attaining equal status within the profession. Society was still against them, impairing both their own confidence and that of other women in them. Because society refused to judge medical women by their achievements, women doctors were in danger of setting lower standards for themselves. In the 19th century any woman who ventured beyond the domestic role was considered an anomaly. Jacobi insistently urged her students to measure themselves by the highest standards of professional excellence. Mediocre women doctors, she warned, would doom their cause.

Jacobi, forever impatient with the deficiencies of the women's medical schools, tolerated no compromises in quality because of their disadvantaged position. Her tough-mindedness remained a source of inspiration to those who occasionally lost sight of the larger goal. Still the courage and conviction of the early generations of medical women are beyond reproach. In the face of strenuous opposition they pressed for the right of women to study medicine as part of a redefinition of woman's role in a reformed industrial society. Although their goals remained circumscribed by a particular cultural vision, these pioneers effected real changes in their own lives and in the lives of many women around them. They did so without *radical* ideological innovation. Paving the way for the future by their deeds, they failed to understand that true equality between the sexes could not come if women remained confined to a "sphere," no matter how expansively it was defined. Nineteenth-century women doctors passed on a large legacy of unfinished business to their daughters and granddaughters. They left future generations of women to struggle with the implications of Mary Putnam Jacobi's prophetic warning, "if you cannot learn to act without masters, you evidently will never become the real equals of those who do."[38]

NOTES

1 The last statistic is taken from a survey done by W. C. Hunt, statistician, of Washington, D.C., reprinted in H. Scott Turner, "History of women in medicine," *Los Angeles J. Eclectic Med.*, 1905, *2*: 125. The number of male physicians in the United States in 1900 is in dispute. Census records set the figure at 132,002, the A.M.A. at 119,749. See U.S. Bureau of the Census, *Historical Statistics of the United States: Colonial Times to 1970* (Washington, D.C., 1975), Part 1, pp. 75–76.

2 See William B. Walker, "The health reform movement in the United States, 1830–1870" (Ph.D. dissertation, Johns Hopkins Univ., 1955); John Blake, "Health Reform," in *The Rise of Adventism: Religion and Society in Mid-Nineteenth Century America*, ed. Edwin S. Gaustad (New York, 1975), pp. 30–49. For health reform and women see Regina Markell Morantz, "Nineteenth century health reform and women: a program of self-help," in *Medicine Without Doctors: Home Health Care in American History*, ed. G. Risse, R. Numbers, and J. Leavitt (New York, 1977), pp. 73–93, and "Making women modern: middle class women and health reform in nineteenth century America," *J. Soc. Hist.*, 1977, *10*: 490–507.

3 W. W. Parker, M.D., "Women's place in the Christian world: superior morally, inferior mentally to man — not qualified for medicine or law — the contrariety and harmony of the sexes," *Tr. Med. Soc. St. Va.*, 1892, pp. 86–107.

4 Paul de Lacy Baker, "Shall women be admitted into the medical profession?" *Tr. Med. Assn. St. Ala.*, 1880, *33*: 191–206. See also Julien Picot, "Shall women practice medicine?" *North Carolina Med. J.* 1885, *16*: 10–21; N. Williams, "A dissertation on female physicians," read before the Clay, Lysander and Schroeppel (N.Y.) Medical Association, *Boston Med. & Surg. J.*, 1850, *43*: 69–75; J. F. Ziegler, "Woman's sphere," Presidential address to the Medical Society of Pennsylvania, *Tr. Med. Soc. St. Penn.*, 1882, *14*: 25–38; Joseph Spaeth, "The study of medicine by women," *Richmond & Louisville Med. J.*, 1873, *16*: 40–56; *Men and Women Medical Students and the Woman Movement* (Philadelphia, 1869), *passim.*

5 J. S. Weatherly, "Woman: her rights and her wrongs," *Tr. Med. Assn. St. Ala.*, 1872, *24*: 63–80. For a reversal of the argument, defending female medical education as a step *up* from primitive brutality, see Edwin Fussell, *Valedictory Address to the Students of the Female Medical College of Pennsylvania* (Philadelphia, 1857), pp. 5–6.

6 Reynell Coates, *Introductory Lecture to the Class of the Female Medical Cclege of Pennsylvania* (Philadelphia, 1861), pp. 3–4. See also articles cited in n. 4 and n. 5. "Female physicians," *Boston Med. & Surg. J.*, 1856, *54*: 169–174, and "Female practitioners of medicine," *Boston Med. & Surg. J.*, 1867, *76*: 272–274.

7 Medical women, of course, claimed just the reverse. See Weatherly, "Woman: her rights," p. 76; Sophia Jex-Blake, *Medical Women: Two Essays* (Edinburgh, 1872), p. 36; J. P. Chesney, "Woman as a physician," *Richmond & Louisville Med. J.*, 1871, *11*: 6.

8 Samuel Gregory, who founded the New England Female Medical College, was one of those concerned primarily with the improprieties of male accoucheurs.

9 Weatherly, "Woman: her rights," p. 75.

10 See Martin Kaufman, "The admission of women to 19th-century American medical societies," *Bull. Hist. Med.*, 1976, *50*: 251–260. The assessment I give here of the quality of medical education at the women's medical colleges is based on my own preliminary research. Although the majority of male physicians opposed the medical education of women, female physicians had many prominent male supporters who were loyal and enthusiastic. These included Henry I. Bowditch and James Chadwick in Boston; Steven Smith and Abraham Jacobi in New York; Hiram Corson, Henry Hartshorne, and later Alfred Stillé in Philadelphia; and William Byford and I. N. Danforth in Chicago.

11 *Boston Med. & Surg. J.*, 1884, *111*: 90; 1849, *40*: 505; 1873, *89*: 23. "The practice of midwifery by females — by one of the class," *Boston Med. & Surg. J.*, 1849, *41*: 59–61; Coates, *Introductory Lecture*, pp. 3–4; D. W. Graham, "The demand for medically educated women," *J.A.M.A.*, 1886, *6*: 479.

12 Carroll Smith-Rosenberg, "Puberty to menopause: the cycle of femininity," in *Clio's Consciousness Raised*, ed. M. Hartman and L. Banner (New York, 1974), pp. 1–22. The debate over premenstrual tension and the related effects of woman's cycle on her psyche still goes on in medical circles. See K. J. and R. J. Lennane, "Alleged psychogenic disorders in women — a possible manifestation of sexual prejudice," *New Eng. J. Med.*, Feb. 8, 1973, *290*: 288–292.

13 "Female physicians," p. 169; Horatio Storer, "The fitness of women to practice medicine," *J. Gynec. Soc. Boston*, 1870, *2*: 266–267; "Female practitioners of medicine," pp. 272–274; E. H. Clarke, *Sex In Education: Or A Fair Chance for the Girls* (Boston, 1873); Lawrence Irwell, "The competition of the sexes and its results," read before the American Association for the Advancement of Science, August 1896, *Am. Medico-Surg. Bull.*, 1896, *10*: 316–320.

14 Mary Putnam Jacobi, *The Question of Rest for Women*

During Menstruation (New York, 1877), p. 227. See also C. Alice Baker to Mary Putnam Jacobi, Nov. 7, 1874, Jacobi MSS, Schlesinger Library, Radcliffe. For studies by other women doctors see Elizabeth R. Thelberg, physician at Vassar, "College education as a factor in the physical life of women," Alumnae Association of the Woman's Medical College of Pennsylvania, *Transactions*, 1899, pp. 73–87; Elizabeth C. Underhill, resident physician at Mt. Holyoke, "The effect of college life on the health of women students," *Woman's Med. J.*, 1913, *22*: 31–33; Clelia Duel Mosher, "Normal menstruation and some factors modifying it," *Johns Hopkins Hosp. Bull.*, 1901, *12*: 178–179.

15 George Gregory, *Medical Morals* (New York, 1852), pp. 5, 20; Rev. William Hosmer, *Appeal to Husbands and Wives in Favor of Female Physicians* (New York, 1853), pp. 3–24; Thomas Ewell, *Letters to Ladies Detailing Important Information Concerning Themselves and Infants* (Philadelphia, 1817), pp. 23–27.

16 Elizabeth Blackwell, *Address on the Medical Education of Women* (New York, 1856), pp. 8–9.

17 For example, G. Fenning, *Every Mother's Book: or the Child's Best Doctor, Being a Complete Course of Directions for the Medical Management of Mothers and Children* (New York, n.d.), or D. Wark, *The Practical Home Doctor for Women* (New York, 1882).

18 Chesney, "Woman as a physician," p. 4.

19 Emmeline Cleveland, *Introductory Lecture to the Class of the Female Medical College of Pennsylvania* (Philadelphia, 1859), p. 7.

20 Elizabeth Blackwell, "Criticism of Gronlund's Cooperative Commonwealth; Chapter X–Woman," given before the Fellowship of New Life, n.d., pp. 9–10; *The Influence of Women in the Profession of Medicine* (London, 1889), p. 11; "Anatomy," Lecture Notes, n.d., all in Blackwell MSS, Library of Congress.

21 Joseph Longshore, *Introductory Lecture to the Class of the Female Medical College of Pennsylvania* (Philadelphia, 1859), p. 11. Joseph Longshore, *The Practical Importance of Female Medical Education* (Philadelphia, 1853), p. 6; Female Medical College of Pennsylvania, "Appeal to the Corporators," Medical College of Pennsylvania Archives [hereafter cited as M.C.P]; Ann Preston, *Valedictory Address to the Graduating Class of the Female Medical College of Pennsylvania* (Philadelphia, 1858), pp. 9–10.

22 Elizabeth and Emily Blackwell, *Medicine as a Profession for Women* (New York, 1860), pp. 8–9; Richard C. Cabot, "Women in medicine," *J.A.M.A.*, 1915, *65*: 9–17; Cora B. Lattia, "Public health education among women," *N.Y. St. J. Med.*, 1913, *13*: 12–17; "Appeal to the Corporators."

23 Georgiana Glenn, "Are women as capable of becoming physicians as men," *The Clinic*, 1875, *9*: 243–245; Jacobi, "Inaugural Address," Women's Medical College of the New York Infirmary, *Chicago Med. J. & Exam.*, 1881, *42*: 580.

24 A. Lapthorn Smith, "Higher education of women and race suicide," *Popular Science Monthly*, 1905, *66*: 466–473; A. Lapthorn Smith, "What civilization is doing for the human female," *Tr. Southern Surg. & Gynec. Assn.*, 1889, *2*: 352–360; F. W. Van Dyke, "Higher education as the cause of physical decay in women," *Med. Rec.*, 1905, *67*: 296–298; William Goodell, R. Gaillard Thomas, M. Allen Starr, J. J. Putnam, "Symposium on the co-education of the sexes," *Med. News, N.Y.*, 1889, *55*: 667–672; J. T. Clegg, "Some of the ailments of woman due to her higher development in the scale of evolution," *Texas Hlth. J.*, 1890–91, *3*: 57–59; A. J. C. Skene, *Education and Culture as Related to the Health and Diseases of Women* (Detroit, 1889), p. 39.

25 Elizabeth and Emily Blackwell, *Medicine as a Profession*, p. 4; Henry Hartshorne, *Valedictory Address to the Graduating Class of the Woman's Medical College of Pennsylvania* (Philadelphia, 1872), pp. 13–14; Louise Fiske-Byron, "Woman and nature," *N.Y. Med. J*, 1887, *66*: 627–628. For Ruffin Coleman's remark see "Woman's relation to higher education and the professions as viewed from physiological and other stand points," *Tr. Med. Assn. St. Ala.*, 1889, *42*: 233–247.

26 Emily Blackwell made this argument even before social Darwinism came into vogue: "Mankind," she confided to her diary, "will never be what they should be until women are nobler." Diary, June 4, 1852, p. 83, Blackwell MSS, Library of Congress. See also *J. Hyg. & Herald Hlth.*, 1894, *44*: 236; J. G. Kiernan, "Mental advance in woman and race suicide," *Alienist and Neurologist*, 1910, *30*: 594–599; Elizabeth Blackwell, *Pioneer Work in Opening the Medical Profession to Women* (New York, 1895), p. 253.

27 Samuel Gregory, "Female physicians," *The Living Age*, 1862, *73*: 243–249; Mary Gove Nichols, "Woman the physician," *Water-Cure J.*, 1851, *12*: 3; Thomas Longshore's manuscript is in the M.C.P. Archives, p. 106. See also Marie Zakrzewska to Elizabeth Blackwell, March 21, 1891, Blackwell MSS, Schlesinger Library.

28 Blackwell, *Pioneer Work*, p. 253; Emmeline Cleveland, *Valedictory Address to the Graduating Class of the Woman's Medical College of Pennsylvania* (Philadelphia, 1874), p. 3; Eliza Mosher, "The value of organization — what it has done for women," *Woman's Med. J.*, 1916, *26*: 1–4; James J. Walsh, "Women in the medical world," *N.Y. Med. J.*, 1912, *96*: 1324–1328.

29 Emily Blackwell, "Address at the Thirty-first Annual

Commencement of the Women's Medical College of the New York Infirmary," May 25, 1899, printed in *Final Catalogue* (New York, 1899). Also Emily Blackwell, Diary, October 1851, p. 47. Rarely until after 1900 does one come across the argument that medicine is enriching from the standpoint of personal development. It is primarily society which is to benefit; individuals gain *because* they are aiding society.

30 Carroll Smith-Rosenberg, "The female world of love and ritual: women and sexuality in nineteenth century America," *Signs*, Autumn 1975, *1*: 1–29.

31 Margaret Vaupel Clark, "Medical women's contribution to the education of mothers," *Woman's Med. J.*, 1915, *25*: 126–128; Glenn, "Are women as capable," pp. 243–245; "The woman physician and her special obligation and opportunity," *Woman's Med. J.*, 1915, *25*: 74–79. Numerous women doctors gave public health lectures.

32 For use of the argument see J. Stainbeck Wilson, "Female medical education," *Southern Med. & Surg. J.*, 1854, *10*: 1–17; Emmeline Cleveland, *Valedictory Address to the Graduating Class of the Female Medical College of Pennsylvania* (Philadelphia, 1858), p. 10; Clark, "Medical women's contribution," pp. 126–128; Harriet Williams, "Women in medicine," *Texas Med. News*, 1903, *12*: 613–615.

33 See Jacobi, "Inaugural address," pp. 561–585.

34 Elizabeth Blackwell, for example, opposed public child care. Her belief was that parents as well as children suffered: "Neither can parental responsibility be wisely devolved upon the creche, the nursery, the school and the workshop. . . . No social arrangements must ever be allowed to destroy the essential education which is given to the parent by the children." "Criticism of Gronlund," p. 11. For government ambivalence see William Chafe, *The American Woman* (New York, 1972), pp. 159–172.

35 Frances Emily White, "The American medical woman," *Med. News, N.Y.*, 1895, *67*: 123–128.

36 An interesting example of how conservative this type of argument can be is provided by the situation in India and Pakistan. There "purdah," the seclusion of women, still exists. Yet similar arguments for training a core of professional women to administer to an exclusively female clientele are extremely popular. See Hanna Papenek, "Purdah in Pakistan: seclusion and modern occupations for women," *Journal of Marriage and the Family*, August 1971, pp. 517–530.

37 Helen Watterson, "Woman's excitement over 'Woman'," *Forum*, 1893, *16*: 75–85; Mary Putnam Jacobi, "An address delivered at the Commencement of the Women's Medical College of the New York Infirmary, May 30, 1883," *Arch. Med.*, 1883, *10*: 59–71; Marie Zakrzewska, *Introductory Lecture Before the New England Medical College* (Boston, 1859), pp. 3–26; C. L. Franklin, "Women and medicine," *The Nation*, 1891, *52*: 131.

38 Jacobi, "Commencement address," p. 70.

Image and Income

Medicine today is the most trusted and envied of all professions. But, as John Duffy explains, this was not always so. During the first three hundred years of our country's history the practice of medicine ranked low in professional status. The prestige of physicians reached its nadir in the middle third of the 19th century, with the proliferation of low-quality medical schools, the fragmentation of the profession into quarreling sects, and the repeal of laws regulating the practice of medicine. Of course, there was always great diversity within the profession, and some physicians enjoyed considerable affluence and respect. But for the profession as a whole, there seems to have been little regard.

The status of physicians improved markedly during the latter part of the century, as medicine grew more scientific, efficacious, and restrictive. By 1900 most states had enacted licensing laws to exclude incompetents from inflicting themselves on the public. Nevertheless, other occupations, like law, business, and even the ministry, continued to attract the best and brightest students.

The relatively low income of physicians undoubtedly contributed to medicine's lack of appeal. Although a handful of 19th-century physicians acquired small fortunes, a large percentage of medical-school graduates eventually abandoned medicine to seek greener fields elsewhere. As late as 1913 the American Medical Association estimated that only about 10 percent of physicians in the United States were earning "a comfortable income." The tax records of Wisconsin for the next year lend credence to this statement. Fewer than 60 percent of the state's practitioners earned enough even to be eligible for taxes, and among those who had to pay, the average earnings were $1,488 a year, compared to $3,581 for bankers and capitalists, $2,810 for manufacturers, and $2,567 for lawyers.

The financial advantages of medicine did not become apparent until the time of World War II. As Ronald L. Numbers argues, health insurance—first voluntary, then government-sponsored—played a crucial role in elevating the income of physicians. By the mid-1970s the average American doctor worked approximately 58 hours a week and earned more than $50,000 a year. With increased income came high status, especially in certain specialties, like thoracic surgery and neurosurgery. Among physicians, general practitioners and physiatrists benefitted the least.

Despite frequent complaints about the high costs and poor quality of medical care in the United States, most Americans have nothing but praise for their own physicians. This apparent paradox is illustrated by a recent survey that found 85 percent of the respondents satisfied with their own doctors, but only 60 percent who thought the quality of medical care in America was good or excellent. Among the young, many of whom fought desperately for a chance to become physicians, no profession held greater promise.

10

The Changing Image of the American Physician

JOHN DUFFY

The high status that American physicians enjoy in present-day society is largely a product of two factors, the broad application of science and technology to medicine and the advancing standard of living which has created a steadily increasing demand for medical services. This fortunate situation is of quite recent origin. Indeed, the 20th century was at hand before the art of medicine successfully united with science and technology to provide a sound basis for the profession. During much of American history, practitioners of medicine had relatively low status.

In the colonial period, the most immediate problem arose from the acute shortage of properly trained medical men. While a great many Americans who trace their genealogy discover that their forefathers were aristocrats, nonetheless, the majority of settlers to the New World came from the lower economic groups. Physicians in 17th- and 18th-century Europe were trained in universities, a fact which virtually guaranteed that they came from an upper-middle-class background. Their clientele was usually well-to-do, and once a physician's practice was established, he could live an exceedingly comfortable life. Under these circumstances, university-trained practitioners had little to gain by migrating. Moreover, aside from the hardships and danger involved in settling in the New World, the fluidity of American society made it impossible to maintain the sharp distinction between physicians, surgeons, and apothecaries which characterized the British and European medical systems. In America, patients expected their doctors to diagnose, to perform any necessary surgery, and often to provide drugs. The result was that relatively few well-educated doctors were to be found in the colonies.

By the 18th century, as the population increased and substantial towns developed, an apprenticeship system had emerged which helped to fill the gap. Even so, the growing population was constantly short of medical care. Since nature abhors a vacuum, there was no dearth of medical practitioners, for a host of minister-physicians, empirics, and quacks assumed responsibility for tending to the physical needs of the people. The most able group were the minister-physicians. Medical training in universities was primarily a matter of reading — indeed, the phrase "to read Medicine" was used down to the end of the 19th century — and local ministers, the best educated men in the community, frequently were well versed in medical literature. Cotton Mather, the Boston divine generally considered the epitome of Puritanism, represented the best of this tradition. He participated in an autopsy of one of his infant children and wrote on a number of medical matters with remarkable perception.

During the 18th century the Society for the Propagation of the Gospel in Foreign Parts, a missionary society dedicated to carrying the Anglican faith throughout the British Empire, sent approximately 300 missionaries to the American colonies. Some of these men were indignant when they discovered their congregations seeking physical as well as spiritual solace, but most rejoiced on discovering that medicine gave them an entrée to the community. One wrote in 1716: "My little Knowledge in Physick has given me a great Opportunity of conversing with Men by which I have done that which by preaching I could not have done."[1] A few

---

JOHN DUFFY is Priscilla Alden Burke Professor of History, University of Maryland, College Park, Maryland.

Reprinted with permission from the *Journal of the American Medical Association*, 1967, *200*: 136–140.

years later the Reverend John Miln, who found many prospective church members being lured away by the diverse sects flourishing in the province of New York, reported that the "Practice of Physick in which thank God I have had good success has been a great means of preserving the Church in these times of madness."[2]

The greater number of those who attempted to prescribe for the colonists, however, were empirics and outright quacks. The former practiced a mixture of folk medicine and the orthodox therapy of bleeding, blistering, vomiting, purging, and sweating. Since the rugged depletive therapy of the orthodox practitioners was almost as likely to kill as to cure, the empirics probably did not do much more harm than the regular physicians. The quacks and charlatans, however, who were reported to abound like locusts, were another matter, and it was this group which was undoubtedly responsible for bringing the entire medical profession into disfavor.

Whatever the case, 18th-century Americans were dubious of the medical profession. William Byrd wrote from Virginia in 1706: "Here be some men indeed that are call'd Doctors; but they are generally discarded Surgeons of Ships, that know nothing above very common Remedys."[3] John Oldmixon, author of a contemporary history of the British Empire, declared that the Virginians "have but few Doctors among them, and they reckon it among their Blessings, fancying the Number of their Diseases would increase with that of their Physicians."[4] William Douglass, a Scottish M.D. who arrived in New England early in the 18th century, asked a local doctor for the standard method of practice. He was informed that "their practice was very uniform, bleeding, vomiting, blistering, purging, Anodyne, &c. If the Illness continued, there was *repetendi*, and finally *murderandi*." The New England practitioners, Douglass said, "follow Sydenham too much in giving paregoricks, after catharticks, which is playing fast and loose." So many quacks and poorly trained doctors abounded, he declared, that there was often "more danger from the physician, than from the distemper." He added the consoling thought that occasionally "nature gets the better of the doctor, and the patient recovers."[5]

This same universal suspicion of medical practitioners is reflected in colonial newspapers and other historical records. A colleague reporting the death of the Reverend Mr. William Urquhart in 1709 wrote: "This Gentleman had the misfortune to take Physick of a pretended Phisitian [*sic*] which work't so violently that it gave him 100 vomits and as many stools, brought the Convulsions on him, which soon carryed him off, and caused him to purge till he was Interr'd."[6] In 1733 the New-York *Gazette* matter-of-factly related how the wife of a local silversmith had fallen ill, requiring the services of a physician. On seeing the patient, the doctor "appointed her a portion of Physick; after the receiving of which, she fell to vomiting to such a degree" that she died two days later.[7] A satirical article in a 1786 newspaper told of a young man suffering from a slight fever who was persuaded to seek the services of a physician. The latter proceeded to give him the full "heroic" treatment, which led to his death. Commenting upon the current medical care, the editor concluded that if the patient "dies after all this treatment, which it is fifty to one if he does not, he has had everything done for him that could be done; with which his friends are satisfied — mourn as usual — all is well, and nobody blamed."[8]

Even among better-educated individuals, who presumably were more selective in their choice of physicians, the same underlying distrust of medical practitioners existed. Cadwallader Colden, who later became a leading political figure in the Province, had originally come to New York to practice medicine. Despairing of his profession, he soon turned to politics. In 1720 he wrote a long letter to Governor Robert Hunter in which he discussed the difficulties confronting the profession. Comparing the backwardness of medicine with the advances in astronomy, Colden ascribed the latter's success to the support it had received both from the gentlemen of leisure and from public funds. In the case of physic, he said, "The Hopes of sordid Gain" have encouraged "Men Ignorant of all the Sciences" to intrude themselves into the profession. As a result, "the Art is become in many places Contemptible," and intelligent and learned men "have been deterr'd from enquireing into this Science."[9]

In 1764 John Watts of New York was requested

to help a young British physician obtain a position as lecturer in anatomy. He replied that there were few medical students in New York and no available medical lectureships, adding, "besides we have so many of the Faculty allready destroying his Majestys good Subjects, that in the humor people are, they had rather one half were hangd that are allready practicing, than breed up a New Swarm."[10] Three years later, Dr. Peter Middleton, an able New York doctor, deplored the fact that competition from quacks and empirics had compelled even respectable physicians to prescribe popular nostrums and secret cures or else to find their practice sadly limited. "Such being the state of physic here," he wrote, "what wonder is it that this city should be pestered in so remarkable a manner with the needy outcasts of other places, in the character of doctors; or that this profession of all others, should be the receptacle and resource for the refuse of every other trade and employment?"[11] A young Philadelphian who had been sent abroad for his medical training informed his father in 1764 that he had no desire to return home. "Indeed the Prospects of Practicing in Philadelphia at best, are not very tempting." Fees are so low, he said, that it "is a severe piece of Drudgery" for a physician just "to maintain his family Genteelly."[12]

The 19th century saw little improvement in the public image of the profession. Chemistry, physics, biology, and the other sciences were making remarkable strides, but medicine was still preoccupied with theorizing. Among the more thoughtful physicians, old theories were denounced and new ones hotly debated, but the average practitioner continued to bleed and purge, blister and vomit, much as his predecessors had done for generations. To the public, it seemed that the current medical theories, instead of determining medical practice, were designed to justify the existing forms of therapy. Moreover, the new scientific attitude permeating society made the literate public and the better physicians suspicious of all grandiose concepts. Nonetheless, reflective physicians like Dr. Benjamin Rush, who urged his students to maintain a skeptical viewpoint but did not follow his own precepts, could not resist the temptation to modify old theories and issue the results as brave new ideas.

The great epidemic diseases which had confronted physicians since the earliest days still remained as mysterious as ever. Every medical theory quickly gained a school of adherents, and the resulting quarrels between the many schools of thought literally tore the profession apart. The more dogmatic theorists were not content to denounce opposing concepts but with equal bitterness denounced their advocates. Clashes over particular forms of treatment added to the confusion, and in the southern states, at least, personal vilification reached a point where medical men resorted to fists, knives, pistols, and shotguns to settle their professional differences. To add further to the difficulties of the profession, nearly all orthodox physicians, although disagreeing upon the philosophical basis of medicine and differing considerably in their practice, accepted the precepts of Benjamin Rush and other advocates of what was called "heroic" medicine. As mentioned earlier, bleeding, purging, vomiting, sweating, and blistering represented a standard approach to all ills. Convinced that the body could replace its entire blood supply within 24 hours and that calomel, if administered in large enough doses, was bound to bring salutory results, the orthodox profession plied the lancet and mercurials to an unbelievable extent.

Medical journals are replete with articles urging the profession to act decisively and firmly in times of crisis. Dr. M. L. Haynie, writing in the *Medical Repository* in 1813 on the treatment of tropical fevers, typified the school of thought which maintained that desperate diseases required desperate remedies. In fevers, he noted, the pulse is either unusually full and strong or apparently weak. In either case, bleeding was required to ease the heart and the arteries. Since prostration was a concomitant of the disorder, stimulants were "the only anchor of hope; and mercury affords one, the most *uniform and immediate* in its effect, as well as the most lasting." "A few grains (the quantity is not dangerous), introduced into the system," he continued, "will excite a pulse *fuller, stronger*, and more *durable* than any other stimulus I have ever used in similar cases." He proportioned the dosage to the violence of the disease and had given, in extreme cases, as much as 200 grains or a tablespoonful at a dose! He then epitomized the attitude of the heroic school of medicine when he declared: "It is but trifling with the life of a man, to give him less of a remedy than his disease calls for."[13]

The appearance of homeopaths, Thomsonians, hydropaths, and other irregulars further confused the medical picture. The wrangling between these groups and the regular physicians was well aired in newspapers, pamphlets, and legislative halls, until the public came to view medical practitioners with either complete cynicism or amused contempt.

From all sections of the country came caustic remarks about the medical profession. A New York newspaper declared in 1819 that the difference between philosophers and doctors is "that the conceits and absurdities of philosophers, are generally harmless; whereas those of physicians may draw along with them the most serious and fatal calamities." The journal then attacked the tendency of poorly educated doctors to hide their ignorance behind a facade of meaningless jargon: "The experience and common sense of mankind will not surrender themselves, to any profession of bewildering words, however confidently and imposingly pronounced."[14] An even more damning comment came from a New York health officer, Dr. Peter S. Townsend. In 1822 he advocated the establishment in New York City of a board of health consisting of distinguished citizens. The majority of the members should be laymen, he said, since if the board was "exclusively made up of medical gentlemen there is too much reason to fear that their different opinions might lead, as too often happens, to interminable disputes, and to most disastrous consequences."[15]

In 1839 the editor of the New Orleans *Courier*, in reporting that two Thomsonian practitioners were being tried in New York for the deaths of four smallpox patients under their care, commented bitterly: "This is a good commencement, and one which should be extended to others of the medical profession, who, though they treat differently, [have] as many lives to answer for as any of the Thomsonian practitioners."[16] One Philadelphia editor a few years later denounced the "poisoning and surgical butchery" which he said was common in medical practice, while another one referred to the entire medical profession as "a stupendous humbug."[17] After quoting several physicians with opposing views on the subject of yellow fever, the New Orleans *Daily Delta* editorialized in 1859: "But it is the fate of the medical profession to differ — so much so, that if their medicines disagreed with patients half as much, as they disagree with one another, their practice would be more deadly than any of the diseases which it is their business to treat." The editor softened his remarks by adding, "Fortunately, however, the honest zeal of most of them to preserve human life, keeps pace with their rage for destroying each other's theories, though, perhaps, not rewarded with proportionate success."[18] Not surprisingly, the editor of the *Cincinnati Medical Observer* wrote about this time: "It has become fashionable to speak of the Medical Profession as a body of jealous, quarrelsome men, whose chief delight is in the annoyance and ridicule of each other,"[19] and the *Medical & Surgical Reporter* carried a letter to the editor entitled "To What Cause Are We to Attribute the Diminished Respectability of the Medical Profession in the Estimation of the American Public?"[20]

In truth, the public image of the profession had declined as the 19th century advanced. The striking advances in science, industry, and technology during these years only accentuated the lack of progress in medical practice, causing the profession to experience an increasing sense of frustration, and the public to become even more contemptuous. An examination of the Pittsburgh newspapers clearly shows the changing attitude towards orthodox medicine. In the late 18th and early 19th centuries, articles in the Pittsburgh *Gazette* and *The Commonwealth* spoke highly of the local physicians.[21,22] The editor of the *Gazette* reported with pride the opening of the Medical School of Transylvania University in 1819 and commented that American students no longer needed to go to London or Edinburgh for their medical training.[23] Visitors to Pittsburgh in these early years also were struck by the high esteem in which the profession was held. One traveler who visited the city around 1810 described its four practitioners as men "of considerable practice, experience, and reputation."[24] Forty years later, news items reflecting discredit on the doctors were appearing in the newspaper columns. An article in the *Daily Gazette* on June 14, 1849, entitled "Disgraceful," related how a young man had returned from a trip to his home near Pittsburgh suffering from diarrhea. Suspecting cholera, two local physicians had refused to attend him and a third had made only a slight pretense of giving aid.[25] Another news story told how a soldier had been found critically injured near a railroad trestle late one night. Although several physicians had been called, they all refused help, and it was not until the following morning, when it was too late, that the man received medical aid.[26]

A major factor in detracting from the physician's image in the mid-19th century was the bitter public struggle between the homeopaths, aided by the hydropaths, botanists, and other irregulars, and the orthodox profession. The moderate treatment provided by irregulars gained them strong public support, and efforts by the newly organized American Medical Association to limit practice to those holding degrees from orthodox medical schools brought a strong public reaction. A small-town Louisiana newspaper in 1847 expressed satisfaction at the appearance of a New Orleans medical journal and expressed the hope that its editors would permit a full discussion of the merits of all schools of medical thought, allopathy (orthodox medicine), homeopathy, hydropathy, neuropathy, and Thomsonianism. "There is truth in all those systems," its editor declared, "and the time is coming when we will have a new and perfect *Medical Science*." Emphasizing the need for a scientific approach to medicine, he asserted that there "is just as much uncertainty and confusion among medical men as among Theologians and Politicians."[27] An eastern journal in 1855 suggested that the "public will act as an umpire" in the quarrels between the regulars and irregulars. Its decision, the paper added with tongue in cheek, would be reached, "after a careful perusal of the undertaker's bills."[28]

The mid-century was a period when equalitarianism and Jacksonian democracy had reached its peak. Attempts to regulate the practice of physic were denounced by legislators and newspaper editors as incompatible with individual freedom and as attempts to create monopolies — a word which at that time had all the connotations of socialism today. A Pittsburgh newspaper editor declared: "The idea that a single school of medicine shall regulate and control the practice is repugnant to every idea of free government and smacks too much of imperialism and class legislation to be tolerated." The "true Democratic principle," he continued, guaranteed the right of any individual to freely select his physician. Apropos the clash between the homeopaths and the regulars, he stated firmly: "If any portion of the community, and in many localities opinion is about equally divided, prefer the Homeopathic treatment, there is no earthly power that may justly deprive them of their right."[29]

The old saying that it is always darkest before dawn was never better exemplified than in the case of American medicine in the mid-19th century. In the course of the next 50 years, the accumulated effect of broad advances in the biological and physical sciences suddenly and profoundly affected the whole field of medicine. Other major developments which improved both the status and public image of the physician were the formation of the American Medical Association and the rising standards in medical education.

Following the American Revolution, the ties with England and Europe were understandably loosened, and Americans were reluctant to seek medical training abroad. As of 1800, only four medical schools were in existence to supply America's growing need for doctors. To fill the vacuum, a host of proprietary medical schools appeared after 1820. Most of these schools were informally organized by groups of physicians and surgeons seeking both prestige and financial gain. Few of them provided clinical or laboratory facilities, and most had virtually no requirements for admission. Competition for students, even among the better schools, tended to keep standards at a low level. A student in the Medical Department of the University of Tennessee wrote to his family in 1860: "When I think of the short time required of students to prepare for the profession . . . I am astonished at the cupidity of the medical professors." He went on to say that the American Medical Association was appealing to schools to lengthen their courses, but, he said, "none will take the step for they know they will lose students." Several members of his class had transferred to medical schools in Georgia, he added, and were graduated in the spring, thus obtaining their medical degrees in less than one year.[30]

This deplorable situation was a prime factor in pointing up the need for a national medical organization. Two major objectives of the founders of the American Medical Association were to reform and improve medical education and to promote a sense of professional unity. In both cases, the struggle was not an easy one, but by the advent of the 20th century the main battles had been won. The fight against the homeopaths in the early years saw many setbacks and antagonized a large section of the public. Yet it undoubtedly helped to unify the profession, and eventually even the public realized that well-trained practitioners were essential to sound medical care. The opposition from the homeopaths also helped in the establishment of a code of professional ethics. In seeking to win public and legislative approval for licensure acts, members of state and local medical associations recognized that they could ill afford to air their professional quarrels publicly.

By the early 20th century the American medical profession had established a strong and effective organization; the level of medical education had moved up sharply and was to see equally rapid gains in the immediate future; the lag between medicine and the other scientific and technological areas had disappeared; and the position of the American physician had never been so high. To appreciate the discoveries in physics and chemistry requires a high degree of sophistication, but the seeming miracles performed by medicine and surgery in the 20th century were apparent to all. By the mid-20th century, the American physician and surgeon, the man in white, literally symbolized all of the great strides in human knowledge. Since mankind often reacts better to adversity than to success, the new status of the American physician carries with it a heavy burden of responsibility. Economic success, a frequent corollary of high status, often engenders complacency and in many subtle ways influences moral judgments. For the past hundred years American physicians have demonstrated an ability to live up to their professional obligations. Their status in American society today requires an even greater obligation to live up to their social responsibilities.

NOTES

Read before the Society of Medical History of Chicago, Oct. 19, 1966.

1 Mr. Lucas to Secretary, Newberry, New England, July 24, 1716, Society for the Propagation of the Gospel in Foreign Parts, mss, series A, vol. 11 and 12, film p. 311.

2 John Miln to Secretary, Monmouth County, N.Y., June 18, 1744, Society for the Propagation of the Gospel in Foreign Parts, mss, series B, vol. 12, p. 23, film pp. 77–80.

3 William Byrd to Sir Hans Sloane, Virginia, April 20, 1706, *William & Mary Coll. Quart.*, series 2, 1921, *1*: 186.

4 J. Oldmixon, *The British Empire in America* (London: J. Brotherton, J. Clarke, etc. 1741), I, 429.

5 W. Douglass, *A Summary, Historical and Political, of the First Planting, Progressive Improvements, and Present State of the British Settlements in North America* (London: R. & J. Dodsley, 1760), II, 351–352.

6 Mr. Bradford to Secretary, New York, Sept. 12, 1709, Society for the Propagation of the Gospel in Foreign Parts, mss, series A, vol. 5, No. 53, film pp. 141–150.

7 New-York *Gazette*, Jan. 7–14, 1733.

8 *Daily Advertiser* (New York), March 4, 1786.

9 S. Jarcho, "Obstacles to the progress of medicine in colonial New York: the letter of Cadwallader Colden to Governor Robert Hunter (1720), *Bull. Hist. Med.*, 1962, *36*: 459–461.

10 Letter Book of John Watts, New-York Historical Society *Collections*, 1928, *61*: 254–255.

11 J. J. Walsh, *History of the Medical Society of the State of New York* (Brooklyn: Eagle Press, 1907), p. 33.

12 Thomas Ruston to Job Ruston, Edinburgh, Sept. 30, 1764, in Thomas Ruston Papers, Library of Congress.

13 M. L. Haynie, "Observations on the fever of tropical climates, and the use of mercury as a remedy," *Medical Repository*, n. s., 1813, *1*: 218–220.

14 New York *Evening Post*, Sept. 9, 1819.

15 P. S. Townsend, *An Account of the Yellow Fever, as It Prevailed in the City of New York, in the Summer and Autumn of 1822* (New York: O. Halsted, 1823), p. 235.

16 New Orleans *Courier*, Jan. 22, 1839.

17 Philadelphia *City Item*, Nov. 6, 1858, quoted in R. H. Shryock, *Medicine in America: Historical Essays* (Baltimore: Johns Hopkins Press, 1966), pp. 150–151.

18 New Orleans *Daily Delta*, April 17, 1859.

19 *Cincinnati Medical Observer*, 1857, *2*: 129.

20 *Med. & Surg. Reptr.*, n.s., 1858, *1*: 141–143.

21 Pittsburgh *Gazette*, Aug. 26, 1780, reprinted in *Register of Pennsylvania*, 1831, *7*: 348.

22 *The Commonwealth* (Pittsburgh), Dec. 23, 1807.

23 Pittsburgh *Gazette*, Oct. 22, 1819.
24 F. Cuming, *Sketches of a Tour to the Western Country...* (Pittsburgh: Cramer, Spear & Eichbaum, 1810), p. 71.
25 Pittsburgh *Gazette*, June 14, 1849.
26 Pittsburgh *Gazette*, Feb. 6, 1864.
27 *Planters' Banner* (St. Mary's Parish, Louisiana), July 15, 1847.
28 *United States Democratic Review*, 1855, *35*: 263, quoted in Shryock, *Medicine in America*, p. 172.
29 Pittsburgh *Daily Post*, Feb. 20, 1875.
30 Charles James Johnson to Louisa Butler McCrindell, Nashville, Tennessee, Nov. 1, 1860, in Johnson Letters and Family Correspondence, 1860–1862, Louisiana State University Department of Archives, Baton Rouge.

11

The Third Party: Health Insurance in America

RONALD L. NUMBERS

> No third party must be permitted to come between the patient and his physician in any medical matter.
>
> *American Medical Association, 1934*[1]

American medicine in the 19th century was essentially a two-party system: patients and physicians. Medical practice was relatively simple, and doctors — out of economic necessity more than to preserve an intimate physician-patient relationship — personally collected their bills. Most practitioners billed their patients annually or semi-annually, although those with office practices usually insisted on immediate payment.[2] They were not, however, always free to charge what they pleased. In many communities local medical societies established schedules of minimum fees and instructed members never to undercut their colleagues.[3] There was little objection to providing free care for the poor — or to overcharging the wealthy — but generally the American medical profession preferred fixed fees to the so-called "sliding scale."[4] When hospitals began to mushroom late in the century, they, too, charged patients directly according to fixed prices.

But even in the 19th century a small, but undetermined, number of Americans carried some insurance against sickness through an employer, fraternal order, trade union, or commercial insurance company. Most of these early plans, however, were designed primarily to provide income protection, with perhaps a fixed cash benefit for medical expenses; few provided medical care, and those that did, like the plans sponsored by remotely located lumber and mining companies, generally contracted with physicians at the lowest possible prices. This type of "contract" practice restricted the patient's choice of physician, allegedly commercialized the practice of medicine, sometimes resulted in shoddy medical care — and always elicited the opposition of organized medicine.[5] During the latter half of the century the American Medical Association (A.M.A.) repeatedly condemned arrangements that provided unlimited medical service for a fixed yearly sum and urged the profession to maintain "the old relations of perfect freedom between physicians and patients, with separate compensation for each separate service."[6]

Widespread interest in health insurance did not develop in the United States until the 1910s, and then the issue was compulsory, not voluntary, health insurance. During the late 19th and early 20th centuries rising costs and increased demands for medical care had prompted many European nations, beginning with Germamy in 1883, to provide industrial workers with compulsory health insurance.[7] Americans, however, paid little attention to these foreign experiments before 1911, when the British parliament passed a National Insurance Act.

Inspired by developments abroad and the spirit of Progressive reform at home, the American Association for Labor Legislation in 1912 created a Committee on Social Insurance to prepare a model bill for introduction in state legislatures.[8] By the fall of 1915 this committee had completed a tentative draft and was laying plans for an extensive legislative campaign. Its bill required the participa-

---

RONALD L. NUMBERS is Associate Professor and Chairman, Department of the History of Medicine, University of Wisconsin, Madison, Wisconsin.

tion of virtually all manual laborers earning $100 a month or less, provided both income protection and complete medical care, and divided the payment of premiums among the state, the employer, and the employee.[9]

The medical profession's initial response to this proposal bordered on enthusiasm. Three progressive physicians — Alexander Lambert, Isaac M. Rubinow, and S. S. Goldwater — had served on the drafting committee, and for a brief period after the turn of the century organized medicine was in a reform-minded mood. Upon receiving a copy of the A.A.L.L.'s bill, Frederick R. Green, secretary of the A.M.A.'s Council on Health and Public Instruction, informed the bill's sponsors that their plan for compulsory health insurance was

> exactly in line with the views that I have held for a long time regarding the methods which should be followed in securing public health legislation. . . . Your plans are so entirely in line with our own that I want to be of every possible assistance.

Specifically, Green wanted to give the A.A.L.L. "the assistance and backing of the American Medical Association in some official way," and he proposed setting up an A.M.A. Committee on Social Insurance to cooperate with the A.A.L.L. in working out the medical provisions of the bill.[10] As a result of his efforts, the A.M.A. Board of Trustees early in 1916 appointed a three-man committee, with Lambert as chairman. He, in turn, hired Rubinow as executive secretary and set up committee headquarters in the same building with the A.A.L.L.

The *Journal of the American Medical Association* hailed the appearance of the model bill as "the inauguration of a great movement which ought to result in an improvement in the health of the industrial population and improve the conditions for medical service among the wage earners."[11] In the editor's opinion, "No other social movement in modern economic development is so pregnant with benefit to the public."[12] At the A.M.A.'s annual session in June 1916, President Rupert Blue called compulsory health insurance "the next step in social legislation,"[13] and Lambert, as chairman of the Committee on Social Insurance, presented a report that stopped just short of endorsing the measure.[14]

Physician support at the state level was similarly strong. In 1916 the state medical societies of both Pennsylvania and Wisconsin formally approved the principle of compulsory health insurance, and the Council of the Medical Society of the State of New York did likewise.[15] Reasons for favoring health insurance varied from physician to physician. According to the *Journal of the American Medical Association*, the most convincing argument was "the failure of many persons in this country at present to receive medical care";[16] but the average practitioner, who earned less than $2,000 a year, was probably more impressed by the prospect of a fixed income and no outstanding bills.[17] Besides, the coming of health insurance appeared inevitable, and most doctors preferred cooperating to fighting. "Whether one likes it or not," wrote the editor of the *Medical Record*,

> social health insurance is bound to come sooner or later, and it behooves the medical profession to meet this condition with dignity. . . . Blind condemnation will lead nowhere and may bring about a repetition of the humiliating experiences suffered by the medical profession in some of the European countries.[18]

By early 1917, however, medical opinion was beginning to shift, especially in New York, where the A.A.L.L. was concentrating its efforts. One after another of the county medical societies voted against compulsory health insurance, until finally the council of the state society rescinded its earlier endorsement.[19] Both friends and foes of the proposed legislation agreed on one point: the medical profession's chief objection was monetary in nature. As the exasperated secretary of the A.A.L.L. saw it, the "crux of the whole problem" was that physicians were constantly hearing the lie that the model bill would limit them to 25¢ a visit or about $1,200 a year.[20] "If you boil this health insurance matter down, it seems to be a question of the remuneration of the doctor," observed one New York physician, who believed that 99 out of 100 physicians had taken up the practice of medicine primarily "as a means of earning a livelihood."[21] Another New York practitioner, who opposed the A.A.L.L.'s bill, described all other objections besides payment as "merely camouflage for this one crucial thought." Medical opposition would melt away, he predicted, if adequate compensation were guaranteed.[22]

The medical profession was, of course, not alone in opposing compulsory health insurance. Commercial insurance companies, which would have been excluded from any participation, were especially critical; and some labor leaders, like Samuel Gompers, preferred higher wages to paternalistic social legislation.[23]

America's entry into World War I in April 1917 not only interrupted the campaign for compulsory health insurance, but touched off an epidemic of anti-German hysteria. Patriotic citizens lashed out at anything that smacked of Germany, including health insurance, which was reputed to have been "made in Germany." As the war progressed, Americans in increasing numbers began referring to compulsory health insurance as an "un-American" device that would lead to the "Prussianization of America."[24]

Shortly before the close of the war California voters, in the only referendum on compulsory health insurance, soundly defeated the measure by a vote of 358,324 to 133,858 and dampened the hopes of insurance advocates.[25] Their spirits revived briefly in the spring of 1919, when the New York State Senate passed a revised version of the model bill, but the bill subsequently died in the Assembly. By 1920 even the A.A.L.L. was rapidly losing interest in an obviously lost cause.

As the prospects for passage of the model bill declined, the stridency of anti-insurance doctors increased. "*Compulsory Health Insurance*," declared one Brooklyn physician, "is an Un-American, Unsafe, Uneconomic, Unscientific, Unfair and Unscrupulous type of Legislation [supported by] Paid Professional Philanthropists, busybody Social Workers, Misguided Clergymen and Hysterical women."[26] In 1919 he and other critics launched a campaign to have the A.M.A.'s House of Delegates officially condemn compulsory health insurance. They failed on their first attempt, but the following year the delegates overwhelmingly approved a resolution stating

> That the American Medical Association declares its opposition to the institution of any plan embodying the system of compulsory contributory insurance against illness, or any other plan of compulsory insurance which provides for medical service to be rendered contributors or their dependents, provided, controlled, or regulated by any state or the Federal Government.[27]

This repudiation of compulsory health insurance was not, as one writer has suggested, the result of "an abdication of responsibility by the scientific and academic leaders of American medicine."[28] Nor was it primarily the product of a rank-and-file takeover by conservative physicians disgruntled with liberal leaders.[29] The doctors who rejected health insurance in 1920 were by and large the same ones who had welcomed — or at least accepted — it only four years earlier. Frederick Green, the person most responsible for the A.M.A.'s early support of compulsory health insurance, was by 1921 describing it as an "economically, socially and scientifically unsound" proposition favored only by "radicals."[30] And his experience was not atypical.

Many factors no doubt contributed to such changes of heart. Opportunism undoubtedly motived some, and the political climate surely affected the attitudes of others. But more important, it seems, was the growing conviction that compulsory health insurance would lower the incomes of physicians rather than raise them, as many practitioners had earlier believed. With each legislative defeat of the model bill, the coming of compulsory health insurance seemed less and less inevitable, and the self-confidence of the profession grew correspondingly. "[T]his Health Insurance agitation has been good for us," concluded one prominent New York physician as the debate drew to a close. "If it goes no farther it will have brought us more firmly together than any other thing which has ever come to us."[31]

An additional factor affecting the medical profession's attitude toward compulsory health insurance was its recent experience with workmen's compensation, which was probably the most common form of health insurance in America from the 1910s to the 1940s. Beginning in 1911 many states passed laws making employers legally responsible for on-the-job injuries, but few of the early compensation acts provided comprehensive medical benefits. During the war, however, most states added such provisions or liberalized existing ones, giving American doctors their first taste of social insurance. For many, it was not pleasant. Employers often took out accident insurance with commercial companies, which either contracted with physicians to care for the injured or paid local practitioners according to an arbitrary fee schedule.[32] Neither arrangement pleased the medical profession, which complained that the abuses resulting from such practices "were akin to mayhem and murder."[33] It was evident from this experience, reported the A.M.A., that "pus and politics go together."[34]

In 1925 the New York State Medical Society reported that health insurance "is a dead issue in the United States. . . . It is not conceivable that any serious effort will again be made to subsidize medicine as the hand-maiden of the public."[35] The victorious New York physicians had every reason to be confident, but they failed to reckon with economic disaster. The Great Depression invalidated many assumptions about American society and threatened the financial security of both hospitals and physicians. Between 1929 and 1930 hospital receipts per patient declined from $236.12 to $59.26, and occupancy rates fell from 71.28 percent to 64.12 percent.[36] As the Depression continued, income from endowments and contributions decreased by nearly two-thirds, and the charity load almost quadrupled.[37] Particularly hard hit were the private voluntary hospitals, which had been expanding six times faster than the population.[38] The net income of physicians during the first year of the Depression dropped 17 percent, with general practitioners suffering the biggest losses. In some regions, particularly the cotton-growing states, collections from patients fell 50 percent, and the situation grew worse as the Depression continued.[39]

In response to this disaster, several hospitals began experimenting with insurance. Although not the first, the most influential of these experiments was the Baylor University Hospital plan, often described as the "father" of the Blue Cross movement. In December 1929 Baylor Vice-President Justin F. Kimball, former superintendent of the Dallas public schools, enrolled 1,250 public school teachers, who paid 50¢ a month for a maximum of 21 days of hospital care, an arrangement consciously modeled after the prepayment plans used in the lumber and railroad industries.[40] The success of single-hospital insurance at Baylor and other places soon led to the development of multiple-hospital plans that included all hospitals in a given area. The first of these appeared in Sacramento, California, in 1932, and by 1937, when the American Hospital Association began approving such programs, there were 26 in operation with 608,365 participating members.[41]

The motives behind these early endeavors are difficult to determine. In two recent studies of Blue Cross, for example, Odin W. Anderson stresses the altruistic spirit of the pioneers, while Sylvia Law emphasizes their economic interests.[42] There is, as one might expect, some evidence for both interpretations. Voluntary hospital insurance, said Michael M. Davis in 1931, has "the double aim of furnishing a new and broader base of support for hospitals and of helping small income people to meet their big sickness bills."[43] Economic concerns are, however, easier to document than altruism. It is significant that although financially disinterested civic organizations occasionally contributed funds to establish hospital insurance programs, "In most cases the initiative and main drive for the starting of the various plans came from the hospitals of the community — from hospital administrators and trustees."[44] In his 1932 survey of prepayment plans Pierce Williams concluded that hospitals had promoted insurance primarily "to put their finances on a sound basis."[45]

Physician reaction to these early experiments in hospital insurance was mixed. Those affected the most seemed pleased. A physician associated with a Grinnell, Iowa, plan described the attitude of local practitioners as "very cordial,"[46] and Kimball reported that Dallas doctors appreciated both the increased availability of hospital care for their patients and the fact that insurance got "the patient's hospital bill out of the way of the doctor's personal collections."[47] The A.M.A., however, was openly antagonistic, characterizing prepayment plans "as being economically unsound, unethical and inimical to the public interests."[48] According to the director of the Association's Bureau of Medical Economics, such schemes were largely "a result of 'tactics of desperation,' in which hard-pressed hospitals are seeking 'any port in a storm.'"[49] The A.M.A.'s solution to the problem of financing health care was "to save for sickness."[50]

Despite these negative pronouncements, health insurance continued to grow — especially after the publication in 1932 of the final report of the Committee on the Costs of Medical Care. This group of 45 to 50 prominent Americans drawn from the fields of medicine, public health, and the social sciences set out in 1927 to ascertain the medical needs of the American people and the resources available to meet them. Ray Lyman Wilbur, a former president of the A.M.A., served as chairman, and over half of the members were physicians. At the end of five years of exhaustive study, funded by several philanthropic organizations, a majority of the committee, including the chairman, modestly recommended the adoption of group practice and voluntary health insurance as the best means of solving the nation's health care problems.[51]

But even this was too radical for eight of the physicians on the committee, who, with one other member, prepared a minority report denouncing "the thoroughly discredited method of voluntary insurance" as being more objectionable than compulsory health insurance. Health insurance, said the minority, would inevitably lead to the

> solicitation of patients, destructive competition among professional groups, inferior medical service, loss of personal relationship of patient and physician, and demoralization of the profession. It is clear that all such schemes are contrary to sound policy and that the shortest road to the commercialization of the practice of medicine is through the supposedly rosy path of insurance.

The dissenting doctors did, however, favor action to alleviate the financial plight of the medical profession, caused in part by having to provide free care to the poor. Thus they recommended that the government relieve physicians of this unfair "burden" by assuming financial responsibility for the care of the indigent. The results of such a plan, they said, "would be far reaching." In particular, the income of physicians would increase and young doctors would find it easier to begin the practice of medicine.[52]

Although some state medical societies (including those in Alabama and Massachusetts) endorsed the majority report,[53] and although more of the committee's physicians had voted with the majority than with the minority, the A.M.A.'s House of Delegates declared that the minority report represented "the collective opinion of the medical profession." Group practice and health insurance, said the delegates, "would be inimical to the best interests of all concerned."[54] Morris Fishbein, the outspoken editor of the association's *Journal*, characteristically reduced the issue to "Americanism versus sovietism for the American people."[55] "The alinement is clear," he wrote,

> on the one side the forces representing the great foundations, public health officialdom, social theory — even socialism and communism — inciting to revolution; on the other side, the organized medical profession of this country urging an orderly evolution guided by controlled experimentation.[56]

The alignment may have seemed clear in 1932, but a revival of interest in compulsory health insurance soon blurred it. In 1934, President Franklin D. Roosevelt appointed a Committee on Economic Security to draft legislation for a social security program, which, everyone assumed, would include health insurance. Pressure from organized medicine, however, forced the President to drop health care from the bill he sent to Congress in 1935. Undaunted, progressive members of his administration continued to agitate for compulsory health insurance and in 1938 held a National Health Conference in Washington. This event aroused great popular interest in a government-sponsored health program, resulting the next year in Senator Robert F. Wagner's introduction of a bill to provide medical assistance for the poor, primarily through federal grants to the states.[57]

In view of these developments, the A.M.A. reversed its position on voluntary health insurance, hoping that such action would quiet demands for a compulsory system. In 1937 the House of Delegates approved group hospitalization plans that confined "their benefits strictly to the facilities ordinarily provided by hospitals; viz., hospital room, bed, board, nursing, routine drugs."[58] A short time later the association began taking credit for promoting the growth of hospitalization insurance, which it had so bitterly opposed only a few years before.[59]

At the same time it was giving its blessing to hospitalization insurance, the A.M.A. was working out a physician-controlled plan to provide medical care insurance. In 1934 the House of Delegates took a tentative step in that direction by agreeing on ten principles to govern "the conduct of any social experiments." These included complete physician control of medical services, free choice of physician, the inclusion of all qualified practitioners, and the exclusion of persons living above the "comfort level." The delegates stopped short of endorsing health insurance and made a point of emphasizing the traditional view that medical costs "should be borne by the patient if able to pay at the time the service is rendered."[60]

In February 1935, shortly after the Committee on Economic Security reported to the President, the House of Delegates met in special session — the first since World War I — to reaffirm its opposition to "all forms of compulsory sickness insurance." Recognizing the need to offer an alternative to government-sponsored insurance, the delegates encouraged "local medical organizations to establish plans for the provision of adequate medical service for all of the people . . . by voluntary budgeting to meet the costs of illness."[61] The language was vague, but the intention was clearly to foster the creation of society-controlled medical insurance plans.

In the aftermath of the National Health Conference of 1938 the A.M.A. called a second special session on insurance. This time the House of Delegates approved the development of "cash indemnity insurance plans" for low-income groups, controlled by local medical societies.[62] By offering cash benefits instead of service benefits, physicians hoped to retain their freedom to charge fees higher than the insurance benefits whenever it seemed appropriate.[63] In 1942, to meet competition from commercial insurance companies, the A.M.A. took the final step of approving medical service plans.[64]

By the late 1930s a number of local medical societies, particularly in the Northwest, had already organized "medical service bureaus" offering medical care for a fixed amount per year.[65] In 1939 the California Medical Association, in an effort to stave off compulsory health insurance, established the first statewide medical service plan.[66] Seven years later, when the A.M.A. created Associated Medical Care Plans, the precursor of Blue Shield, there were 43 medical society plans with a combined enrollment of three million members.[67] In most places coverage was limited to low-income families, who would otherwise have been among the least able to pay physicians' fees.

The threat of "socialized medicine" was no doubt the most compelling reason why organized medicine decided to embrace health insurance. As the demand for compulsory health insurance grew, more and more physicians came to see voluntary plans as their "only telling answer to federalization and regimentation."[68] "[I]t is better to inaugurate a voluntary payment plan," advised the secretary of the State Medical Society of Wisconsin, "rather than wait for a state controlled compulsory plan."[69]

But fear of compulsory health insurance was not the only reason why the medical profession changed its mind. By the late 1930s many physicians were also discerning potential benefits in health insurance.[70] A 1938 Gallup poll showed that nearly three-fourths of American doctors favored voluntary medical insurance, and over half were confident that it would increase their incomes.[71] Health insurance, predicted one Milwaukee physician, "would do away with the uncollectible accounts. . . . It would offer to the physician an opportunity of earning a living commensurate with the value of the service that he performs."[72] Furthermore, by paying for expensive services like x-rays and laboratory tests, it would enable doctors to practice a better quality of medicine.[73]

Once the profession recognized these possible benefits, it sought absolute control over medical service plans. In many states physicians won the right to monopolize medical care insurance through special enabling acts, which critics ironically regarded as "un-American."[74] In other places organized medicine tried to discourage physicians from participating in nonsociety plans by threatening expulsion and the denial of hospital privileges. In 1938 such heavy-handed tactics brought the A.M.A. an indictment (and eventual conviction) for violation of antitrust laws.[75]

Despite a genuine concern for the welfare of their patients, doctors did not embrace health insurance primarily to assist the public in obtaining better medical care. In fact, throughout the 1930s spokesmen for organized medicine repeatedly denied that health care in America was inadequate and attributed the good health of Americans to "the present system of medical practice," that is, to the traditional two-party system.[76] The physicians of Massachusetts may, as they claimed, have supported a medical service plan in recognition of "a problem in the distribution of the cost of decent medical care." But even in that progressive state competition from consumer cooperatives was just as important.[77]

Proudly displaying the medical profession's stamp of approval, health insurance entered a period of unprecedented growth (see Fig. 1). By 1952 over half of all Americans had purchased some health insurance, and prepayment plans were being described as "the medical success story of the past 15 years."[78] Behind this growth was consumer demand, especially from labor unions, which after the war began bargaining for health insurance to meet rapidly rising medical costs that were making the prospect of sickness the "principal worry" of industrial workers. Following a 1948 Supreme Court ruling that health insurance benefits could be included in collective bargaining, "the engine of the voluntary health insurance movement," to use Raymond Munts's metaphor, moved out under a full head of steam. Within a period of three months the steel industry alone signed 236 contracts for group health insurance, and auto workers were not far behind.[79]

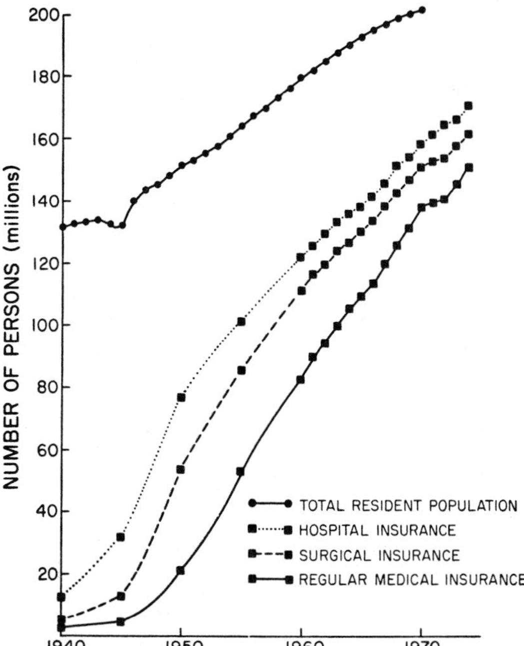

Fig. 1: Growth of health insurance in the United States. Sources: *Source Book of Health Insurance Data, 1975–76* (New York: Health Insurance Institute, 1976), p. 22; U.S. Bureau of the Census, *Historical Statistics of the United States: Colonial Times to 1970* (Washington, D.C.: Government Printing Office, 1975), Part 1, p. 8.

Growth statistics, however, do not tell the whole story. Although most Americans did have some health insurance by mid-century, coverage remained spotty. In 1952 insurance benefits paid only 15 percent of all private expenditures for health care (see Fig. 2). Besides, the persons most likely to be insured were employed workers living in urban, industrial areas, while the unemployed, the poor, the rural, the aged, and the chronically ill — those who needed it the most — went uninsured.[80]

With voluntary plans failing to protect so many Americans, the perennial debate over compulsory health insurance flared up again. Encouraged by organized labor, the Social Security Board in 1943 drafted a bill — named after its congressional sponsors, Senators Robert Wagner and James Murray and Representative John Dingell — providing health insurance to all persons paying social security taxes, as well as to their families. The time, however, was inauspicious. World War II was diverting the nation's attention to other issues, and without the President's active support the bill died quietly in committee.[81]

Two years later, with the war over and Harry S. Truman in the White House, prospects for passage appeared much brighter. Since his days as a county judge in Missouri, Truman had been concerned about the health needs of the poor, and within a few weeks of assuming the presidency he decided to lend his support to the health insurance campaign. Following a strategy session with the President, Wagner, Murray, and Dingell reintroduced their bill, this time adding dental and nursing care to the proposed benefits.[82]

These developments terrified the A.M.A., which viewed the Wagner-Murray-Dingell bill as the first step toward a totalitarian state, where American doctors would become "clock watchers and slaves of a system."[83] To head off passage of such legislation, the A.M.A. in 1946 began backing a substitute bill, sponsored by Senator Robert A. Taft, which authorized federal grants to the states to

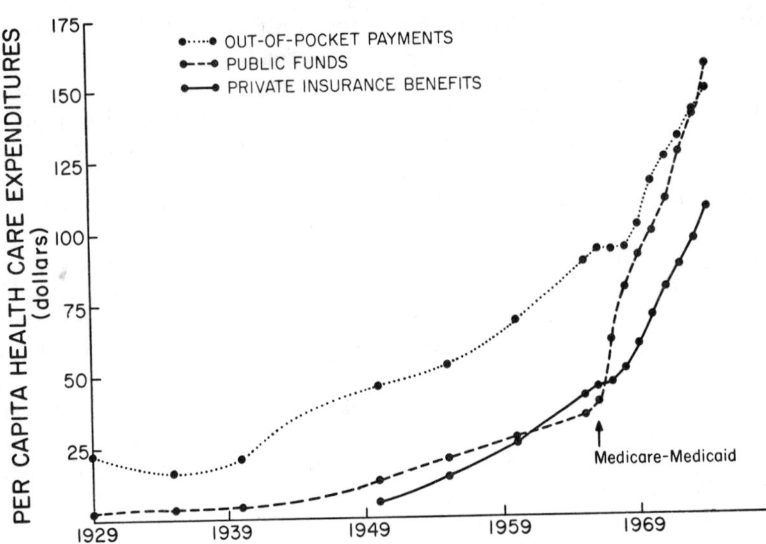

Fig. 2: Sources of health-care expenditures in the United States. Source: Nancy L. Worthington, "National health expenditures, 1929–74," *Social Security Bulletin*, February 1975, *38*: 16.

subsidize private health insurance for the indigent.[84]

The basic problem, as the Association's spokesman Morris Fishbein defined it, was one of "public relations." The medical profession had "to convince the American people that a voluntary sickness insurance system . . . is better for the American people than a federally controlled compulsory sickness insurance system."[85] Actually, most Americans needed little convincing. A 1946 Gallup poll showed that only 12 percent of the public favored extending social security to include health insurance, and more individuals thought the Wagner-Murray-Dingell proposal would have a negative effect on health care than believed that it would be beneficial.[86]

Truman's surprise victory in 1948, at the close of a campaign that featured health insurance as a major issue, convinced the A.M.A. that it was time to declare all-out war. Shortly after the election returns were in, the House of Delegates voted to assess each member $25 to raise a war chest for combatting socialized medicine, which was defined as "a system of medical administration by which the government promises or attempts to provide for the medical needs of the entire population or a large part thereof."[87] Within a year $2,250,000 had been raised, and the public relations firm of Whitaker and Baxter was putting it to effective use in an effort to "educate" the American people.[88] The showdown came in 1950 when organized medicine won a stunning victory in the off-year elections, forcing many candidates to renounce their earlier support of compulsory health insurance and defeating "nearly 90 percent" of those who refused to back down.[89]

Throughout this controversy representatives of organized medicine insisted that the country did not need compulsory health insurance, just as they had insisted in the early 1930s that voluntary insurance was unnecessary. "There is no health emergency in this country," said a complacent A.M.A. president in 1952. "The health of the American people has never been better."[90] If some individuals could not afford proper medical care, it was probably the result of self-indulgence rather than genuine need:

> Since one out of every four persons in the United States has a motor car, one out of two a radio, and since our people find funds available for such substances as liquors and tobacco in amounts almost as great as the total bill for medical care, one cannot but refer to the priorities and to the lack of suitable education which makes people choose to spend their money for such items rather than for the securing of medical care.[91]

What Americans needed, said the doctors, was more voluntary insurance, which had worked out so well that most physicians by the early 1950s no longer thought coverage should be restricted to low-income groups.[92] The financial and political benefits of health insurance were so great, the medical profession jealously protected it. When rumors began circulating that some surgeons were doubling their fees to insured patients, the A.M.A. called for an immediate crackdown. "Voluntary prepayment plans are the medical profession's greatest bulwark against the socialization of medicine," said one official. "This program must not be jeopardized by avaricious physicians."[93]

The election of a Republican administration in 1952 effectively ended the debate over compulsory health insurance, and organized medicine breathed a sigh of relief. "As far as the medical profession is concerned," wrote the A.M.A. president, "there is general agreement that we are in less danger of socialization than for a number of years. . . . We have been given the opportunity to solve the problems of health in a truly American way."[94] The "American way," it went without saying, was the way of voluntary health insurance.

The Eisenhower years indeed proved to be tranquil ones for the medical profession. Encouraged by their physicians and by the constantly rising costs of medical care, an increasing number of Americans purchased health insurance, until by the early 1960s nearly three-fourths of all American families had some coverage (see Fig. 1). Still, this paid for only 27 percent of their medical bills, and many citizens, especially the poor and the elderly, had no protection at all.[95]

This problem led Representative Aime Forand in the late 1960s to reopen the debate over compulsory health insurance with a proposal limiting coverage to social security beneficiaries. In 1960 Senator John F. Kennedy introduced a similar measure in the Senate.[96] To organized medicine, even such restricted coverage amounted to "creeping socialism,"[97] and the A.M.A. would have none of it. The association's "strongest objection" continued to be that "it is unnecessary and would lower the quality of care rendered," the same argument it had been using since the 1910s. Its only concession was to approve a government plan providing assistance to "the indigent or near indigent," which would benefit physicians as much as the poor.[98] Thus in 1960 Congress, with A.M.A. approval, passed the Kerr-Mills amendment to the Social Security Act, granting federal assistance to the states to meet the health needs of the indigent and the elderly who qualified as "medically indigent."

If the medical profession hoped to forestall the coming of compulsory health insurance by this small compromise, Senator Kennedy's election to the presidency that fall soon convinced them otherwise. Upon occupying the White House, he immediately began laying plans to extend health insurance protection to all persons on social security, whether "medically indigent" or not. The A.M.A. denounced his plans as a "cruel hoax" that would disrupt the doctor-patient relationship, interfere with the free choice of physician, impose centralized control, and — worst of all — undermine the financial incentive to practice medicine. They would not only endanger the quality of medical care, but would discourage the best young people from entering the field.[99] Despite these ominous predictions, Congress in 1965 voted to include health insurance as a social security benefit (Medicare) and to provide for the indigent through grants to the states (Medicaid). Thus, after 50 years of debate, compulsory health insurance finally came to America.

In 1967, just two years after the passage of Medicare, third parties for the first time paid more than half of the nation's medical bills.[100] Many Americans continued to be without health insurance coverage, but seldom by choice.[101] Although critics frequently attacked the insurance business, no one advocated returning to a two-party system. In the opinion of one observer, the acceptance of health insurance was a phenomenon "without parallel in contemporary American life."[102] Prepayment plans benefitted both providers and consumers of medical care, but especially the providers.

Hospitals, the pioneers of voluntary health insurance, profited from the start. In 1947 Louis Reed reported that hospital administrators agreed unanimously that insurance plans had reduced their volume of free care and increased revenues.[103] In the years between 1939 and 1951 the amount of charity care provided by Philadelphia hospitals, for example, fell from 60 percent to 24 percent.[104] Later, in the 1960s and 1970s, the windfall from Medicare and Medicaid enabled many hospitals to improve — or at least to expand — their facilities.

Health insurance also proved advantageous to physicians, especially financially. In the period following the development of medical service plans, their incomes climbed dramatically (see Fig. 3); and, according to some analysts, the "most significant factor" contributing to this increase was third-party payments, which rose from 15.5 percent to nearly 50 percent of physicians' incomes in the two decades between 1950 and 1969.[105] Proving a cause-and-effect relationship is difficult, but the testimony of physicians themselves supports this view. In 1957, for example, over half of the doctors in Michigan reported increased incomes as a result of prepaid medical care, with smalltown physicians and general practitioners registering the greatest gains. The most frequently cited explanations were better bill collecting and more patients.[106]

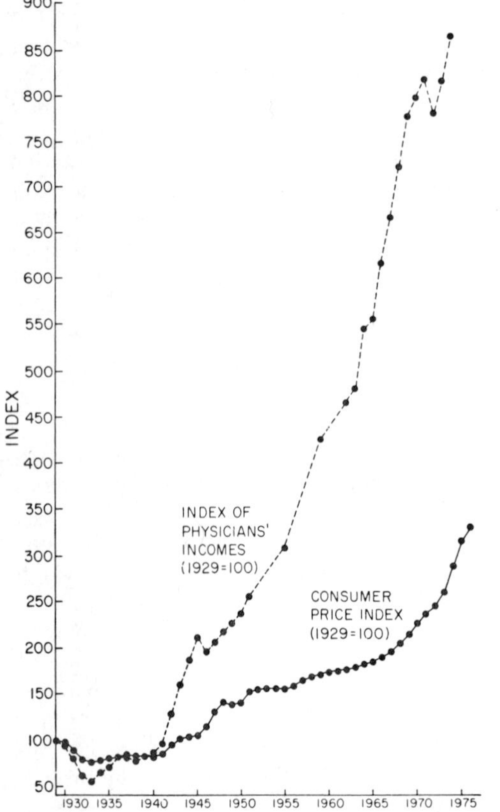

Fig. 3: The income of American physicians, 1929–1975. Sources: U.S. Bureau of the Census, *Historical Statistics of the United States: Colonial Times to 1970* (Washington, D.C.: Government Printing Office, 1975), Part 1, pp. 175–176, 210–211; U.S. Bureau of the Census, *Statistical Abstract of the United States, 1975* (Washington, D.C.: Government Printing Office, 1975), p. 77; *Medical Economics*, Oct. 24, 1960, *37*: 40, and Nov. 10, 1975, *52*: 184; U.S. Bureau of Labor Statistics, *Consumer Price Index*, 1971–76. Graph prepared by Lawrence D. Lynch.

Certainly there can be little doubt that Medicare and Medicaid benefitted the medical profession handsomely. In fact, Robert and Rosemary Stevens concluded that "it seemed to be the physicians who gained the most."[107] After complaining for years that compulsory health insurance would beggar the profession and reduce the financial incentive to practice medicine, physicians discovered the results to be just the opposite. In the first year under Medicare the rate of increase in physician fees more than doubled (from 3.8 percent to 7.8 percent), while the rate of increase of the Consumer Price Index only rose from 2.0 percent to 3.3 percent.[108] A 1970 Senate Finance Committee investigation turned up at least 4,300 individual physicians who had received $25,000 or more from Medicare in 1968, and 68 of these had gotten over $100,000 each. Although most of this money was earned fairly, reports of questionable practices abounded. Some physicians allegedly saw patients more often than necessary, billed for care never given, and on occasion even resorted to the notorious "gang visit," charging $300 or $400 for one cursory sweep through a hospital ward or nursing home.[109] Such flagrant abuses prompted the president of one local medical society to warn his colleagues "to quit strangling the goose that can lay those golden eggs."[110]

Compared with the relatively tangible benefits of health insurance for hospitals and physicians, those to patients are more difficult to calculate. Prepayment plans undeniably gave Americans greater access to medical care than ever before, eased the financial strain of paying medical bills, and brought peace of mind to millions of policyholders. A grateful public showed its appreciation by buying increasingly comprehensive coverage. But it is not certain that they enjoyed better health for it. On the one hand, there are studies showing that "those who were eligible for Medicaid were likely to have better health than similar groups who were not."[111] But other studies indicate that although Medicare apparently encouraged more expensive types of treatment, like surgery rather than radiation for breast cancer, recovery rates remained roughly the same.[112]

Under health insurance from 1941 to 1970, life expectancy at birth in America did increase from 64.8 years to 70.9 years.[113] But again it is hard to determine how much — if any — of this should be credited to improved medical care, much less to the way in which it was financed. By the early 1970s even organized medicine was downplaying the ability of the medical profession to prolong life and preserve health. As Max H. Parrott of the A.M.A. testified in 1971, choice of life-style had become as important as medical care in determining the nation's health: "No matter how drastic a change is made in our medical care system, no matter how massive a program of national health insurance is undertaken, no matter what sort of system evolves, many of the really significant, underlying causes of ill health will remain largely unaffected."[114] In a society in which heart disease, cancer, accidents, and cirrhosis of the liver all ranked among the top ten killers,[115] it was indeed unrealistic to expect health insurance to cure the nation's ills.

NOTES

1 Minutes of the 85th annual session, June 11–15, 1934, *J.A.M.A.*, 1934, *102*: 2200.

2 D. W. Cathell, *The Physician Himself and What He Should Add to His Scientific Acquirements*, 3rd ed. (Baltimore: Cushings & Bailey, 1883), pp. 16, 175–176; Charles E. Rosenberg, "The practice of medicine in New York a century ago," *Bull. Hist. Med.*, 1967, *41*: 229–230. [See pp. 55–74 in this book.]

3 George Rosen, *Fees and Fee Bills: Some Economic Aspects of Medical Practice in Nineteenth Century America* (Supplement No. 6, *Bull. Hist. Med.*; Baltimore: Johns Hopkins Press, 1946).

4 Jeffrey Lionel Berlant, *Profession and Monopoly: A Study of Medicine in the United States and Great Britain* (Berkeley: Univ. of California Press, 1975), pp. 101–102.

5 Pierce Williams, *The Purchase of Medical Care through Fixed Periodic Payment* (New York: National Bureau of Economic Research, 1932); Jerome L. Schwartz, "Early history of prepaid medical care plans," *Bull. Hist. Med.*, 1965, *39*: 450–475.

6 *1846–1958 Digest of Official Actions: American Medical Association* (Chicago: A.M.A., 1959), pp. 121–122.

7 For a summary of the European experience, see Richard Harrison Shryock, *The Development of Modern Medicine* (New York: Hafner Publishing Co., 1969), pp. 381–402.

8 This account of the first American debate over compulsory health insurance is based on Ronald L. Numbers, *Almost Persuaded: American Physicians and Compulsory Health Insurance, 1912–1920* (Baltimore: Johns Hopkins Univ. Press, 1978).

9 *Health Insurance: Standards and Tentative Draft of an Act* (New York: American Association for Labor Legislation, 1916).

10 F. R. Green to J. B. Andrews, Nov. 11, 1915, A.A.L.L. Papers, Cornell University.

11 "Industrial insurance," *J.A.M.A.*, 1916, *66*: 433.

12 "Cooperation in social insurance investigation," *ibid.*, pp. 1469–1470.

13 Rupert Blue, "Some of the larger problems of the medical profession," *ibid.*, p. 1901.

14 Report of the Committee on Social Insurance, *ibid.*, 1951–1985.

15 Proceedings of the Medical Society of the State of Pennsylvania, Sept. 18–21, 1916, *Penn. Med. J.*, 1916, *20*: 135, 143; Proceedings of the House of Delegates, State Medical Society of Wisconsin, Oct. 5, 1916, *Wis. Med. J.*, 1916, *15*: 288; Minutes of the Council, Medical Society of the State of New York, Dec. 9, 1916, *N.Y. St. J. Med.*, 1917, *17*: 47–48.

16 "Social insurance in California," *J.A.M.A.*, 1915, *65*: 1560.

17 Income statistics are scarce for this period, but a 1915 survey of physicians and surgeons in Richmond, Virginia, showed that "the very large proportion of physicians were earning less than $2,000," and income tax records for Wisconsin in 1914 indicate that the average income of taxed physicians was $1,488. Committee on Social Insurance, *Statistics Regarding the Medical Profession* (Social Insurance Series Pamphlet No. 7; Chicago: A.M.A., n.d.), pp. 81, 87.

18 "Opposition to the Health Insurance Bill," *Med. Rec.*, 1916, *89*: 424.

19 Report of the Committee on Legislation, *N.Y. St. J. Med.*, 1917, *17*: 234.

20 J. B. Andrews to New York Members of the A.A.L.L., Nov. 3, 1919, A.A.L.L. Papers.

21 "A Symposium on compulsory health insurance presented before the Medical Society of the County of Kings, Oct. 21, 1919," *Long Island Med.*

J., 1919, *13*: 434. George W. Kosmak made the statement.

22 M. Schulman to J. B. Andrews, Feb. 22, 1919, A.A.L.L. Papers.

23 See Gompers' testimony before the *Commission to Study Social Insurance and Unemployment: Hearings before the Committee on Labor, House of Representatives, 64th Congress, First Session, on H. J. Res. 159, April 6 and 11, 1916* (Washington, D.C.: Government Printing Office, 1918), p. 129.

24 See Roy Lubove, *The Struggle for Social Security, 1900–1935* (Cambridge, Mass.: Harvard Univ. Press, 1968), pp. 66–90.

25 On the California debate, see Arthur J. Viseltear, "Compulsory health insurance in California, 1915–18," *J. Hist. Med.*, 1969, *24*: 151–182.

26 "A Symposium on compulsory health insurance," p. 445. John J. A. O'Reilly made the statement.

27 Minutes of the House of Delegates, *J.A.M.A.*, 1920, *74*: 1319.

28 John Gordon Freymann, "Leadership in American medicine: a matter of personal responsibility," *New Eng. J. Med.*, 1964, *270*: 710–715.

29 Elton Rayack, *Professional Power and American Medicine: The Economics of the American Medical Association* (Cleveland: World Publishing Co., 1967), pp. 143–146. For a similar view, see Carleton B. Chapman and John M. Talmadge, "The evolution of the right to health concept in the United States," *Pharos*, 1971, *34*: 39.

30 Frederick R. Green, "The social responsibilities of modern medicine," *Tr. Med. Soc. St. N.C.*, 1921, pp. 401–403.

31 Henry Lyle Winter, "Social insurance," *N.Y. St. J. Med.*, 1920, *20*: 20.

32 On the early history of workmen's compensation in America, see Harry Weiss, "The development of workmen's compensation legislation in the United States" (Ph.D. dissertation, Univ. of Wisconsin, 1933); and Lubove, *The Struggle for Social Security*, pp. 45–65.

33 Bureau of Medical Economics, *An Introduction to Medical Economics* (Chicago: A.M.A., 1935), p. 80.

34 Committee on Social Insurance, *Workmen's Compensation Laws* (Social Insurance Series Pamphlet No. 1; Chicago: A.M.A., [1915]), p. 60.

35 Report of the Committee on Medical Economics, *N.Y. St. J. Med.*, 1925, *25*: 789.

36 Sylvia A. Law, *Blue Cross: What Went Wrong?*, 2nd ed. (New Haven: Yale Univ. Press, 1976), p. 6. According to *J.A.M.A.*, the percentage of occupied beds in nongovernmental hospitals declined from 64.6 percent to 63.2 percent between 1929 and 1930. "Hospital service in the United States," *J.A.M.A.*, 1933, *100*: 892.

37 J. T. Richardson, *The Origin and Development of Group Hospitalization in the United States, 1890–1940* (Univ of Missouri Studies, Vol. XX, No. 3; Columbia: Univ. of Missouri, 1945), p. 12.

38 "Hospital service in the United States," pp. 892–894.

39 Maurice Leven, *The Incomes of Physicians: An Economic and Statistical Analysis* (Committee on the Costs of Medical Care, Publication No. 24; Chicago: Univ. of Chicago Press, 1932), pp. 76–81. The fraction of California doctors earning less than $6,000 a year rose from approximately one-half in 1929 to three-fourths in 1933. Arthur J. Viseltear, "Compulsory health insurance in California, 1934–1935," *Am. J. Public Hlth.*, 1971, *61*: 2117.

40 J. F. Kimball, "Group hospitalization," *Tr. Am. Hosp. Assn.*, 1931, *33*: 667–668; J. F. Kimball, "Prepayment plan of hospital care," *American Hospital Association Bulletin*, 1934, *8*: 42–47; Odin W. Anderson, *Blue Cross Since 1929: Accountability and the Public Trust* (Cambridge, Mass.: Ballinger Publishing Co., 1975), pp. 18–19.

41 Louis S. Reed, *Blue Cross and Medical Service Plans* (Washington, D.C.: Government Printing Office, 1947), pp. 10–12.

42 Anderson, *Blue Cross Since 1929*, pp. 29–44; Law, *Blue Cross*, pp. 6–8. Anderson quotes one pioneer, J. Douglas Colman, as saying that "All this notion that it was going to solve the financial problems of hospitals was farthest from their [the Blue Cross founders'] minds." But Colman himself became involved with prepayment plans because hospitals might have to close without them. "An interview with J. Douglas Colman," *Hospitals*, 1965, *39*: 45–46.

43 Michael M. Davis, "Effects of health insurance on hospitals abroad," *Tr. Am. Hosp. Assn.*, 1931, *33*: 585. At the same meeting where Davis read this paper, the president of the A.H.A. called for insurance as a partial answer to the problem of decreasing occupancy rates; *ibid.*, pp. 195–197.

44 Reed, *Blue Cross and Medical Service Plans*, pp. 13–14.

45 Williams, *The Purchase of Medical Care*, p. 219.

46 Letter from E. E. Harris, Dec. 10, 1930, quoted *ibid.*, p. 238.

47 Kimball, "Prepayment plan of hospital care," p. 45.

48 *1846–1958 Digest of Official Actions*, p. 313.

49 R. G. Leland, "Prepayment plans for hospital care," *J.A.M.A.*, 1933, *100*: 871. For similar expressions, see the address of President-Elect Dean Lewis, Minutes of the 84th annual session, June 12–16, 1933, *ibid.*, p. 2021; and the editorial "Hospital insurance and medical care," *ibid.*, p. 973.

50 *1846–1958 Digest of Official Actions*, p. 313.

51 *Medical Care for the American People: The Final Report of the Committee on the Costs of Medical Care* (Committee on the Costs of Medical Care, Publication No. 28; Chicago: Univ. of Chicago Press, 1932), pp. v–viii, 120.

52 *Ibid.*, pp. 164–65, 171–72. The committee's study of the incomes of physicians revealed that "the average volume of free work furnished by physicians throughout the country is only 5 percent of the total." Leven, *The Incomes of Physicians*, p. 66.

53 Oliver Garceau, *The Political Life of the American Medical Association* (Hamden, Conn.: Archon Books, 1961), p. 138.

54 Minutes of the 84th annual session, June 12–16, 1933, p. 48.

55 "The Report of the Committee on the Costs of Medical Care," *J.A.M.A.*, 1932, *99*: 2035.

56 *Ibid.*, p. 1952.

57 The fullest account of this second debate over compulsory health insurance is Daniel S. Hirshfield, *The Lost Reform: The Campaign for Compulsory Health Insurance in the United States from 1932 to 1943* (Cambridge, Mass.: Harvard Univ. Press, 1970). But see also Roy Lubove, "The New Deal and National Health," *Current History*, August, 1963, *45*: 77–86, 117; Edwin E. Witte, *The Development of the Social Security Act* (Madison: Univ. of Wisconsin Press, 1962); Arthur J. Altmeyer, *The Formative Years of Social Security* (Madison: Univ. of Wisconsin Press, 1966); and James G. Burrow, *AMA: Voice of American Medicine* (Baltimore: Johns Hopkins Press, 1963), pp. 185–252.

58 Minutes of the 88th annual session, June 7–11, 1937, *J.A.M.A.*, 1937, *108*: 2219.

59 Minutes of the special session, Sept. 16–17, 1938, *ibid.*, 1938, *111*: 1193.

60 Minutes of the 85th annual session, June 11–15, 1934, *ibid.*, 1934, *102*: 2199–2201.

61 Minutes of the special session, Feb. 15–16, 1935, *ibid.*, 1935, *104*: 751.

62 Minutes of the special session, Sept. 16–17, 1938, *ibid.*, 1938, *111*: 1216; *1846–1958 Digest of Official Actions*, pp. 321–322. At this session black physicians representing the National Medical Association pledged to join the struggle against compulsory health insurance, even though it might not be in the best interest of their race. *J.A.M.A.*, 1938, *111*: 1211–1212.

63 Nathan Sinai, Odin W. Anderson, and Melvin L. Dollar, *Health Insurance in the United States* (New York: Commonwealth Fund, 1946), pp. 64–65.

64 Minutes of the 93rd annual session, June 8–12, 1942, *J.A.M.A.*, 1942, *119*: 728.

65 Reed, *Blue Cross and Medical Service Plans*, pp. 136–146.

66 Viseltear, "Compulsory health insurance in California, 1934–1935," pp. 2115–2126; Arthur J. Viseltear, "The California Medical-Economic Survey: Paul A. Dodd versus the California Medical Association," *Bull. Hist. Med.*, 1970, *44*: 151. Although the second debate over compulsory health insurance took place primarily on the national level, many compulsory health insurance bills were also introduced in state legislatures. See Carl W. Strow and Gerhard Hirschfeld, "Health insurance," *J.A.M.A.*, 1945, *128*: 871.

67 Anderson, *Blue Cross Since 1929*, p. 54.

68 R. L. Novy, "In retrospect: changing attitude of the medical profession," *J. Mich. St. Med. Soc.*, 1950, *49*: 708. See also George Farrell, "Development of voluntary nonprofit medical care insurance plans," *N.Y. St. J. Med.*, 1957, *57*: 560–564.

69 J. G. Crownhart, "The economic status of medicine," *Wis. Med. J.*, 1934, *33*: 230. I wish to thank Jennifer Latham for her assistance in locating this and other documents relating to health insurance in Wisconsin.

70 E. Minihan and T. Levi develop this point in their unpublished paper, "The political economy of health care financing: the foundation for medical care in Wisconsin" (April 1975), pp. 22–23.

71 George H. Gallup, *The Gallup Poll: Public Opinion, 1935–1971* (New York: Random House, 1972), I, 107.

72 James C. Sargent, "Shall medicine be socialized?" *Wis. Med. J.*, 1933, *32*: 562. See also Donald K. Freedman and Elinor B. Harvey, "Development of voluntary health insurance in the United States," *N.Y. St. J. Med.*, 1940, *40*: 1704.

73 Reed, *Blue Cross and Medical Service Plans*, p. 230.

74 "Wisconsin Cooperative Association assails State Medical Society," *Wis. Med. J.*, 1946, *45*: 3.

75 *The United States of America, Appellants, vs. The American Medical Association . . . Appellees* (Chicago: A.M.A., 1941).

76 Minutes of the 90th annual session, May 15–19, 1939, *J.A.M.A.*, 1939, *112*: 2295–2296. See also the comments of President-Elect J. H. J. Upham, Minutes of the 88th annual session, June 7–11, 1937, *ibid.*, 1937, *108*: 2132.

77 James C. McCann, "Medical service plans," *ibid.*, 1942, *120*: 1318.

78 President's Commission on the Health Needs of the Nation, *Building America's Health* (Washington, D.C.: Government Printing Office, [1952]), I, 43; II, 257.

79 Raymond Munts, *Bargaining for Health: Labor Un-*

ions, Health Insurance, and Medical Care (Madison: Univ. of Wisconsin Press, 1967), pp. 10–12, 49, 250. See also Frank G. Dickinson, "The trend toward labor health and welfare programs," *J.A.M.A.*, 1947, *133*: 1285–1286.

80 President's Commission on the Health Needs of the Nation, *Building America's Health*, I, 43; II, 253–254; Reed, *Blue Cross and Medical Service Plans*, pp. 28, 119; Sinai, Anderson, and Dollar, *Health Insurance in the United States*, pp. 57–58, 73; Odin W. Anderson and Jacob J. Feldman, *Family Medical Costs and Voluntary Health Insurance: A Nationwide Survey* (New York: McGraw-Hill Book Co., 1956), pp. 14–20.

81 Altmeyer, *The Formative Years of Social Security*, p. 146; Peter A. Corning, *The Evolution of Medicare: From Idea to Law* (Washington, D.C.: Government Printing Office, 1969), pp. 53–55.

82 Monte Mac Poen, "The Truman administration and national health insurance" (Ph.D. dissertation, Univ. of Missouri, 1967), pp. 54–63.

83 "The President's national health program and the new Wagner bill," *J.A.M.A.*, 1945, *129*: 950–953. See also "Senator Wagner's comments," *ibid.*, 1945, *128*: 667–668.

84 Burrow, *AMA*, p. 347.

85 Morris Fishbein, "The public relations of American medicine," *J.A.M.A.*, 1946, *130*: 511.

86 Gallup, *The Gallup Poll*, I, 578. See also *ibid.*, II, 801–804, 862–863, 886.

87 *1846–1958 Digest of Official Actions*, p. 331; Minutes of the interim session, Nov. 30–Dec. 1, 1948, *J.A.M.A.*, 1948, *138*: 1241; "A call to action against nationalization of medicine," *ibid.*, pp. 1098–1099; "Reply by officers and trustees," *ibid.*, 1949, *139*: 532. A.M.A. officers later referred to this action as "American Medicine's Declaration of Independence"; Report of Co-ordinating Committee, *ibid.*, 1951, *147*: 1692.

88 Burrow, *AMA*, pp. 361–364.

89 R. Cragin Lewis, "New power at the polls," *Medical Economics*, January 1951, *28*: 76.

90 John W. Cline, "The president's page: a special message," *J.A.M.A.*, 1952, *148*: 208.

91 "A call to action against nationalization of medicine," *ibid.*, 1948, *138*: 1098. This comment was made in response to the Federal Security Administrator's statement that millions of Americans could not afford proper medical care. See Oscar R. Ewing, *The Nation's Health: A Report to the President* (September, 1948).

92 Odin W. Anderson, *The Uneasy Equilibrium: Private and Public Financing of Health Services in the United States, 1875–1965* (New Haven: College & Univ. Press, 1968), p. 140.

93 Cline, "The president's page: a special message," p. 1036.

94 Louis H. Bauer, "The president's page," *J.A.M.A.*, 1952, *150*: 1675.

95 Ronald Andersen and Odin W. Anderson, *A Decade of Health Services: Social Survey Trends in Use and Expenditure* (Chicago: Univ. of Chicago Press, 1967), pp. 75, 109, 153. See also Ethel Shanas, *The Health of Older People: A Social Survey* (Cambridge, Mass.: Harvard Univ. Press, 1962).

96 On the events leading up to Medicare, see Max J. Skidmore, *Medicare and the American Rhetoric of Reconciliation* (University: Univ. of Alabama Press, 1970), pp. 75–95.

97 J. H. Houghton, "President's message to the House of Delegates," *Wis. Med. J.*, 1965, *64*: 208.

98 "New drive for compulsory health insurance," *J.A.M.A.*, 1960, *172*: 344–345. See also Edward R. Annis, "House of Delegates report," *ibid.*, 1963, *185*: 202.

99 Donovan F. Ward, "Are 200,000 doctors wrong?" *ibid.*, 1965, *191*: 661–663; *The Case against the King-Anderson Bill (H.R. 3820)* (Chicago: A.M.A., 1963), pp. 17, 118–119.

100 Nancy L. Worthington, "National health expenditures, 1929–74," *Social Security Bull.*, February 1975, *38*: 13–14.

101 Estimates of the number of uninsured in the early 1970s varied between 17 and 41 million; see Marjorie Smith Mueller, "Private health insurance in 1973: a review of coverage, enrollment, and financial experience," *ibid.*, p. 21. The likelihood of having health insurance corresponded directly with income. Over 90 percent of families earning above $10,000 in 1970 carried hospital insurance, for example, while less than 40 percent of families with incomes under $3,000 had it. Cambridge Research Institute, *Trends Affecting the U.S. Health Care System* (DHEW Publication No. HRA 76-14503; Washington, D.C.: Government Printing Office, 1976), p. 188.

102 President's Commission on the Health Needs of the Nation, *Building America's Health*, IV, 43.

103 Reed, *Blue Cross and Medical Service Plans*, p. 230.

104 President's Commission on the Health Needs of the Nation, *Building America's Health*, V, 390–391.

105 John Krizay and Andrew Wilson, *The Patient as Consumer: Health Care Financing in the United States* (Lexington, Mass.: Lexington Books, 1974), p. 111. During the 1960s physicians' incomes increased faster than those of other professionals, including chief accountants, attorneys, chemists, and engineers. *Ibid.*, p. 109.

106 *An Opinion Study of Prepaid Medical Care Coverage in Michigan* (Michigan State Med. Soc., 1957), p. 140.

107 Robert Stevens and Rosemary Stevens, *Welfare Medicine in America: A Case Study of Medicaid* (New York: The Free Press, 1974), p. 191. "One unforeseen result of Medicare and Medicaid," say the Stevenses, "was that in formalizing the system of doctors' charges by developing profiles of the 'usual and customary' fees prevailing in each area, some physicians became aware of what others were charging. Quite clearly, there was some 'standardizing-up' . . . ." *Ibid.*, p. 194.

108 Theodore R. Marmor, *The Politics of Medicare* (London: Routledge & Kegan Paul, 1970), p. 89.

109 *Medicare and Medicaid: Problems, Issues, and Alternatives*, Report of the Staff to the Committee on Finance, U.S. Senate (Washington, D.C.: Government Printing Office, 1970), pp. 9–10, 13.

110 Quoted in Stevens and Stevens, *Welfare Medicine in America*, p. 197.

111 *Ibid.*, p. 202.

112 Victor R. Fuchs, *Who Shall Live? Health, Economics, and Social Change* (New York: Basic Books, 1974), pp. 94–95.

113 U.S. Bureau of the Census, *Historical Statistics of the United States: Colonial Times to 1970* (Washington, D.C.: Government Printing Office, 1975), Part 1, p. 55. The great gains came before the 1960s; between 1961 and 1970 life expectancy only increased from 70.2 to 70.9, and actually decreased slightly for black males.

114 *National Health Insurance Proposals: Hearings before the Committee on Ways and Means, House of Representatives, Ninety-Second Congress, First Session on the Subject of National Health Insurance Proposals, Oct.–Nov., 1971* (Washington, D.C.: Government Printing Office, 1972), p. 1950.

115 Monroe Lerner and Odin W. Anderson, *Health Progress in the United States, 1900–1960* (Chicago: Univ. of Chicago Press, 1963), p. 16.

Institutions

The hospital, so central to health care today, assumed little importance in American medical history until the late 19th century. Except for the almshouses and pest houses found in the large towns along the Atlantic seaboard, there were no hospitals in the British colonies of North America until 1751, when Benjamin Franklin and his Philadelphia friends founded the Pennsylvania Hospital. Modeled after the voluntary hospitals of England, this institution admitted both the mentally and physically ill and accepted those who could pay as well as those who could not.

Because of the nation's predominantly rural population and the social attitudes described by Morris J. Vogel, the idea of hospitals caught on slowly in America. Physicians throughout the 19th century continued to treat most of their patients at home and even to perform surgery there. As late as 1873 there were fewer than 200 hospitals in the United States, about a third of which were for the mentally ill. Yet only 50 years later the number of hospitals was approaching 7,000. This rapid growth resulted as much from the social changes associated with urbanization as from advances in medical technology, like aseptic surgery and x-rays.

Mental hospitals in America date from 1773, when the colony of Virginia opened an institution in Williamsburg "for persons of insane and disordered minds." However, it was not until 50 years later, with the founding of the Worcester State Lunatic Hospital in Massachusetts, that public asylum-building began in earnest. By 1860, 28 of the 33 states had one or more mental hospitals, thanks in large part to the efforts of Dorothea Dix and other reformers. Although founded with the best intentions, these asylums soon degenerated into custodial institutions offering little treatment and even less chance of a cure.

For the urban poor in the 19th century, the most important medical institution was not the hospital but the dispensary, whose various functions are described by Charles E. Rosenberg. As the popularity of the dispensary declined in the early 20th century, the neighborhood health center arose to take its place. This new institution, which George Rosen defines as "an organization which provides, promotes and coordinates needed medical service and related social service for a specified district," flourished until the late 1930s. Following a three-decade hiatus it reappeared in the mid-1960s as part of President Lyndon B. Johnson's "war on poverty." Funded by the Office of Economic Opportunity and the Public Health Service, comprehensive health centers provided medical care and advice to millions of poor Americans from Watts in Los Angeles to Mound Bayou, Mississippi, often with startling results. In some primarily black southern communities such centers helped to reduce infant mortality by nearly 40 percent in only four years. Nevertheless, the problem of providing adequate medical care for the poor, both rural and urban, remains a pressing national concern.

12

Social Class and Medical Care in 19th-Century America: The Rise and Fall of the Dispensary

CHARLES E. ROSENBERG

To most mid-20th-century physicians, the term "dispensary" evokes the image of a hectic hospital pharmacy. To his mid-19th-century counterpart, it was both the primary means for providing the urban poor with medical care and a vital link in the prevailing system of medical education. These institutions had an effective life-span of roughly a hundred years. Founded in the closing decades of the 18th century, American dispensaries increased in scale and number throughout the 19th century and remained significant providers of health care well into the 20th century. By the 1920s, however, the dispensaries were on the road to extinction, increasingly submerged in the outpatient departments of urban hospitals. Historians have found the dispensary of little interest; even those contemporary medical activists seeking a usable past for experiments in the delivery of medical care, are hardly aware of their existence.[1] Yet a study of the dispensary illustrates not only an important aspect of medicine and philanthropy in the 19th-century city — but the social logic implicit in their rise and fall underlines permanently significant relationships between general social needs and values and the narrower world of medical men and ideas.

The dispensary was invented in late 18th-century England; it was an autonomous, free-standing institution, created in the hope of providing an alternative to the hospital in providing medical care for the urban poor. Like most such benevolent innovations, it was soon copied by socially conscious Americans; dispensaries were established in 1786 at Philadelphia, 1791 at New York, 1796 at Boston, and at Baltimore in 1800. Their growth was at first very slow. No additional dispensaries were established until 1816, when the managers of the Philadelphia Dispensary helped establish two new dispensaries, the Northern and Southern, to serve their city's rapidly developing fringes.[2] New Yorkers established the Northern Dispensary in 1827, the Eastern in 1832, the DeMilt in 1851, and North-Western in 1852. By 1874 there were 29 dispensaries in New York, by 1877, 33 in Philadelphia. Their growth was equally impressive in terms of number of patients treated; in New York, for example, the city's dispensaries treated 134,069 patients in 1860, roughly 180,000 in 1866, 213,000 in 1874 and 876,000 in 1900.[3]

The dispensaries shared certain organizational characteristics. Almost all had a central building — with the prominent exception of Boston which had none until the 1850s — and usually employed one full-time employee, an apothecary or house-physician who acted as steward, performed minor surgery, often vaccinated and pulled teeth — as well as prescribing for some patients. (Though most dispensaries limited their aid to prescriptions written by their own staff physicians, a few would fill prescriptions for the indigent patients of any regular physician.)[4] By mid-century the house-physicianship had in the larger dispensaries evolved into two separate positions, resident physician and druggist-apothecary. Most dispensaries also appointed younger physicians who visited patients too ill to attend the dispensary. Such "district visiting" was the principal task of the Philadelphia Dispensary when founded in 1786, remained the sole activity of the Boston Dispensary until 1856 — and was continued by almost all urban dispensaries until the end of the 19th century, though the

Charles E. Rosenberg is Professor of History at the University of Pennsylvania, Philadelphia, Pennsylvania.

Reprinted with permission from the *Journal of the History of Medicine*, 1974, *29*: 32–54.

treatment of ambulatory patients grew proportionately more prominent in all. The dispensaries also appointed attending and consulting staffs from among their community's established practitioners, the attending staff treating patients well enough to visit the dispensary, the consulting staff serving a largely honorary role.

The dispensaries were shoe-string operations. Most, with the exception of those in New York which enjoyed state and city subventions, were supported by private contributions and the often-voluntary services of local physicians.[5] As late as the 1870s and 1880s — when a dispensary might treat over 25,000 patients a year — budgets of four or five thousand dollars were still common and annual reports vied in reporting how little had been spent for prescriptions — an average of under five cents per prescription was common. The Boston Dispensary and Philadelphia Dispensary gradually accumulated some endowment funds, though most others remained financially marginal. All, however, were sensitive to cyclical economic shifts, for contributions declined in periods of depression while patient pressure increased proportionately. As a result of the economy's downturn in 1857, for example, New York's Eastern Dispensary reported an increase of 22 percent in cases over 1858 and 42 percent over 1856.[6] A useful index to the shaky financial condition of many of the dispensaries was their frequent practice of renting a portion of their building to commercial tenants; such income often constituted a substantial portion of the institution's budget and could not be given up even when the dispensary needed room for expansion.[7]

Some of the dispensaries published detailed statistics of the numbers and kinds of ailments treated by their physicians; thus we can begin to reconstruct their everyday responsibilities. Most cases were, of course, relatively minor — for example, bronchitis, colds, or dyspepsia — and rarely were the numbers of deaths equal to more than 2 or 3 percent of the patients treated. Consistently enough, the number of female patients was always greater than that of males, in some instances as much as two to one; working men, that is, had necessarily to tolerate disease symptoms of far greater intensity before feeling able to consult a physician. In those cases serious enough to be treated at home by visiting physicians sex ratios tended to be more nearly equal. (It was not until the end of the century that dispensaries began to consider evening hours for workers.) Although the general level of mortality among all dispensary patients was low, mortality among patients treated in their homes approached the 10 or 11 percent normal for hospitals at the beginning of the century. Such death rates were particularly discouraging, for the district physician never treated many intractable cases. Chronic and degenerative ailments brought incapacity and eventual alms-house incarceration; these cases never found their way into the dispensary's mortality statistics. The dispensaries also performed minor surgery, treating fractures, contusions and lacerations — as well as casual if frequent dentistry, essentially the "indiscriminate extirpation" of offending teeth.[8]

The dispensaries also played an important public health role in providing vaccination for the poor and vaccine matter for the use of private practitioners. From a purely demographic point of view, indeed, vaccination was the most important function performed by the dispensaries. The dispensaries not only made vaccination available without cost, but some mounted door-to-door vaccination programs in their city's tenement districts. In periods of intense demand, most frequently at the outset or threat of a smallpox epidemic, the dispensaries were able to supply large amounts of vaccine matter at short notice. In the opening months of the Civil War for example, the New York Dispensary provided vaccine matter for all the state's recruits.[9]

Despite ventures into surgery, dentistry, and vaccination, dispensary therapeutics were generally synonymous with the writing of prescriptions; dispensaries dispensed. Throughout the first three-quarters of the 19th century, the phrase "prescribing for" was generally synonymous with seeing a patient; busy dispensary physicians could hardly be expected to do more than compose hasty and routine prescriptions. (Dispensary managers tended by mid-century to demand the use of formularies limited in both cost and variety; later in the century some dispensaries were charged with filling prescriptions by number, the dispensing physician being constrained by an abbreviated list of numbered and preformulated prescriptions.)[10] In this routine and exclusive dependence on drug therapy lay the principal difference between the care provided the urban poor and that paid for by the middle class. Physicians in private practice relied consistently in their therapeutics upon adjusting the regimen of their patients, especially in chronic ills; such injunctions were hardly appropriate in dispensary practice. The city poor could not very well vary their diet, take up horse-back riding, visit the seaside, or voyage to the West Indies.

Not surprisingly, the dispensaries tended to develop ties both formal and informal with other urban charities — in New York, for example, with the Commissioners of Emigration, Association for Improving the Condition of the Poor, and Children's Aid Society; in Philadelphia with the Board of Guardians for the Poor.[11] Dispensary physicians were in this sense *de facto* social workers. In New York, for example, a note from the dispensary physician was necessary if the commissioners were to issue a ration of coal; thus a mid-century whimsy referred to "coal fever" — an illness which struck suddenly during cold weather in the city's tenements.[12] In the post-Civil War decades, efforts to provide such physical amenities became somewhat more organized; dispensary physicians continued to work with existing philanthropic agencies and began as well to establish their own auxiliaries in hopes of providing food and nursing in deserving cases. In Philadelphia, the Lying-in and Nurse Charity, and the Lying-In Department of the Northern Dispensary had provided some nursing service since the 1830s, while others had paid occasionally for nursing in selected cases since the opening years of the century. In a more contemporary idiom, the Instructive Visiting Nurse Service of the Boston Dispensary began in the 1880s to aid the dispensary's district physicians in their work, not only nursing, but educating the poor in hygiene and diet. In Boston and New York, diet kitchen associations provided nourishing food for patients bearing a dispensary physician's requisition. By 1883, the New York Diet Kitchen Association operated three kitchens in cooperation with the dispensaries and had fed 7,699 patients, filling 53,893 separate requisitions from dispensary physicians during the year.[13]

Another trend marking the 19th-century evolution of the dispensaries, reflecting and paralleling a more general development within the medical profession, was their internal reorganization along specialty lines. As early as 1826, the New York Dispensary reorganized itself, dividing patients treated at the dispensary into "classes" according to the nature of their ailment. Pioneering dispensaries for diseases of the eye and ear had come into being as early as the 1820s. By mid-century, the need for specialty differentiation was unquestioned. When the Brooklyn Dispensary opened in 1847, for example, it announced that patients would be distributed among the following classes: women and children, heart, lungs and throat, skin and vaccination, head and digestive organs, eye and ear, surgery and unclassified diseases. In the second-half of the century, specialty designations became increasingly narrow and gradually closer to modern categories; nervous and genito-urinary diseases were, for example, among the most frequently created of such departments in the late 1870s and early 1880s. By 1905, the forward-looking Boston Dispensary boasted these impressively varied out-patient clinics: surgical, general medical, children, skin, nervous system, nose and throat, women, eye and ear, genito-urinary, and x-ray.[14] An important related late-19th-century trend was the increasingly frequent establishment of specialized dispensaries, institutions that treated only particular ailments or ailments of particular organs.

These in brief outline were the chief characteristics which marked the growth of the dispensaries between the end of the 18th and last decades of the 19th centuries. Why did the founders and managers of our pioneer dispensaries find them so plausible a response to social need? What factors led to their initial adoption and subsequent growth?

In their appeals for public support, dispensary founders and supporters left abundant records of their conscious motives. Most prominent in the last years of the 18th and opening decades of the 19th centuries was a traditional sense of stewardship. "It is enough for us," as one physician-philanthropist put it, "to be assured that the poor are always with us, and that they are exposed to disease."

> Benevolence [he continued] is not that passive feeling which can be satisfied with doing no injury to our neighbor, or rest contented with mere good wishes for his well-being when he needs our assistance.

The poor, as a prominent New York clergyman explained the need for supporting the dispensary's work, "have feelings as well as we; they are bone of our bone and flesh of our flesh; men of like passions with ourselves."[15] Such sentiments remained deeply felt and were explicitly articulated throughout the first half of the century.

Other, more mundane, motives always coexisted with such humanitarian appeals. One was the familiar mercantilist contention that maintaining the health of the poor would not only save the tax dollars implied by the almshouse or hospital care of chronically-ill workers, but would aid the economy more generally by helping maintain the labor force at optimum efficiency. (These appeals assumed, of course, the ability of the dispensary physicians to diagnose ills at a stage when they might still respond to available treatment.) A related argument urged the dispensaries' function as first-line of defense against epidemic disease; though such ills ordinarily began and reached epidemic proportions among the poor, once established they might attack even the comfortable and well-to-do. No household could feel immune when servants and artisans moved easily from the world of their betters to that of tenement-dwelling friends and families.[16] These arguments soon hardened into rhetorical formulae and were ritually intoned throughout the first two-thirds of the century. Thus, for example, a mid-century dispensary spokesman could, in appealing for support, argue that:[17]

> The political economist will find here cheapness and utility combined. The statesman will discover the greatest good of the greatest number combined promoted. The city official will find his sanitary police materially assisted. The heads of families will soon find how much the lives and health of their household are cared for and secured. The tax-payer will see his burthens diminished. The benevolent will have opened to his view in the Dispensary and its kindred and associated charities the widest field for the exercise of good will towards man; and the Christian will find a new proof of the truth that they do not love God less who love mankind more.

Finally, and matter-of-factly, their advocates always contended that dispensaries would serve as much-needed schools of clinical medicine.

But to catalogue the arguments of managers and fund-raisers is not precisely to explain the logic of their commitment. Why did the dispensaries grow so rapidly? Obviously because they worked, worked that is in terms of particular social realities and expectations. At least four such factors help explain the evolution of the dispensary in 19th-century America. First, they were entirely functional in terms of the internal organization of the medical profession. Second, they were entirely consistent with available therapeutic modalities. Third, they were effectively scaled to the needs of a small and comparatively homogeneous community; once established they became indispensable as urban growth dramatically increased their client constituency. Fourth, the dispensaries made sense in terms of their founders' expectations of the roles to be played both by government and private citizens.

Most fundamental was the relationship between the dispensary and the world of medical education and status. Without the initiative and voluntary support of the medical profession dispensaries would not have been created nor could they have survived. Physicians formed the core-group in the formation of almost every American dispensary from the end of the 18th to the beginning of the 20th centuries.[18]

In the first third of the 19th century, when formal clinical training could not be said to exist outside that presumed in the preceptorial relationship, the dispensary helped fill an important pedagogical void. Not only could visiting and attending physicians themselves accumulate experience and reputation while more firmly establishing their private practice — but they could use their dispensary appointment as a means of providing case materials for their apprentices. Thus Benjamin Rush could recommend Drs. Wistar and Griffits as preceptors since both held dispensary positions, "where a young man will see more practice in a month than with most private physicians in a year." Almost from the first years of the dispensaries, indeed, critics often charged that students and apprentices were allowed to treat the poor. (In Philadelphia, for example, such complaints found their way into newspapers as early as 1791.)[19] In the second quarter of the 19th century, as the preceptorial system grew less significant, the role of the dispensaries in clinical training grew even more prominent; mid-century medical schools vied actively in establishing dispensaries for the benefit of their students.

Most significantly, dispensary physicianships served as a step in the career pattern of elite physicians. Despite the complaints of articulate mid-century critics as to the wretched state of medical education and practice, even a cursory analysis of the profession's structure indicates the existence of a well-defined elite, largely urban, often European-trained, and almost always enjoying the benefits of hospital and dispensary experience. It was just such ambitious young practitioners who served as dispensary visiting and attending physicians while they accumulated experience and gradually made the contacts so important to later success — contacts, it should be emphasized, with older established physicians at least as much as with prospective patients.[20] (Prestigious and largely honorary consulting physicianships were normally reserved, in dispensaries as in hospitals, for a community's most influential and respected physicians.) Contemporaries never questioned the dispensary's teaching function. The trustees of the New York Dispensary admitted, for example, in 1854 that their institution served as "a practical school for physicians," but, they contended, it was a perfectly defensible policy: "for, by this system, these Physicians must become accomplished practitioners, by the time the growth of their private practice shall oblige them to resign their posts at the Dispensary." With the growing importance of specialization as prerequisite to intellectual status and economic success after mid-century, the increasingly specialized dispensaries served as *de facto* residency programs, allowing ambitious — and often well-connected — young men to accumulate experience and reputation. Though formal statements by medical spokesmen uniformly disowned "exclusive" specialism until long after the Civil War, devotion to a pragmatic specialism was established much earlier in America's cities. In 1839, for example, the editor of the *Boston Medical & Surgical Journal* remarked, in commenting on the specialty organization of New York's Northern Dispensary, that "such is manifestly the tendency in our times, in the great cities, and it is the only way of becoming eminently qualified for rendering the best professional services — to learn to do one thing as well as it can be done."[21]

If the dispensary made excellent sense in terms of the institutional needs of American medicine, it was equally consistent with the technological means available — both at the end of the 18th century, and through the first half of the 19th. Beyond the stethoscope — not routinely applied before mid-century — no special aids to diagnosis were available to any physician, no therapeutics beyond bleeding, cupping, and administration of drugs. Surgery was ordinarily limited, for rich and poor alike, to the treatment of lacerations and fractures, the reduction of occasional dislocations, the lancing of boils and abscesses. Dispensaries seemed, for many decades into the 19th century, fully able to provide both adequate care for the poor and adequate training for their attendants.

The dispensaries seemed equally appropriate to the needs of a small and relatively homogeneous community. The world of the late 18th century assumed — even if it did not necessarily practice — face-to-face interaction between members of different social classes, interactions structured by customary relations of deference and stewardship. This social world-view is concretely illustrated in the acceptance by the dispensaries' founding generation of the contributor recommendation as basis for patient referrals. A certificate of recommendation was necessary, that is, before the dispensary would undertake treatment of a particular patient. This followed English hospital and dispensary practice. As the century progressed, however, the dispensaries which maintained the practice sometimes found it a cause of conflict between medical staff and lay managers. By-laws specified the privileges of recommendation accompanying each contributing membership; a typical arrangement was that which in exchange for a five dollar annual subscription offered the right to recommend two patients at any one time during the year. A 50 dollar subscription typically brought the same privilege for life. Similarly, early dispensary by-laws indicate that members of the boards of managers were expected to play an active and often personal role; the New York Dispensary, for example, created a trustees' committee to accompany visiting physicians on their rounds once a month.[22]

Equally revelatory of the world-view shared by the pious and benevolent Americans who founded the dispensaries, was their assumption that a crucial difference separated the dispensary from the hospital patient; the dispensary patients would be drawn from among the worthy poor, hardworking and able to support themselves, except in periods of sickness or general unemployment. Such worthy poor might also include widows, orphans, and the handicapped. The lying-in department of Philadelphia's Northern Dispensary declared in 1835, for example, that it could aid only married women of respectable character, "such as require no aid when in health." Financial support for the dispensary would, the argument followed, keep such honest folk from alms-house residence and morally-contaminating contact with those abandoned souls who were its natural inmates. Dispensary spokesmen tirelessly repeated these stylized categories by way of argument even as experience indicated that this neat and comforting ideological distinction failed to reflect reality. In 1830, a physician of the Boston Dispensary could complain indignantly that persons of the "most depraved and abandoned character frequently apply who think they have a right of choice between the Alms-House and the Dispensary." As late as 1869, the Philadelphia Dispensary could still explain that:[23]

> The principal object of this institution is to afford medical relief to the worthy (not the lowest class of) poor, in those cases where removal to a hospital would for any approved reason be ineligible. . . . In a thrifty population like our own, it is the exception . . . where removal to a hospital should be considered eligible.

The dispensaries were founded and grew, finally, because they were entirely consistent with the assumptions of most Americans in regard to the responsibilities of government and appropriate forms and functions of the public institutions which embodied such responsibilities. The prostitute, the drunkard, the lunatic and cripple were the city's responsibility — social subject matter for the alms-house or city physician. The dispensary, on the other hand, represented an appropriate response of humane and thoughtful Americans to the needs of hard-working fellow citizens, a response demanded both by Christian benevolence and community-oriented prudence; it was a form of social intervention limited, conservative and spiritually rewarding. In the second third of the 19th century, as demographic realities shifted inexorably, this traditional view still served to justify the now-expanded work of the dispensaries — and at the same time to avoid systematic analysis of the changing nature and social condition of the constituency they served. It was only very slowly, and only in the minds of a minority of those associated with dispensary work, that it became clear that many of their city's honest and industrious laboring men were unable to pay for medical care even in times of prosperity.

The dispensary continued to change throughout the second half of the 19th century. We have already referred to their increase in numbers and degree of specialization. Equally significant was expansion of the dispensary form under new kinds of auspices. First, most urban — and even some small town — medical schools anxious to compete for students, established their own dispensaries so as to offer "clinical material" for their embryo physicians. Second, hospitals not only increased in number in the last third of the century, they also began to provide more outpatient care, in some localities duplicating services already offered by dispensaries. In Philadelphia with its flourishing medical schools the rivalry between hospitals and dispensaries emerged as early as 1845.[24] In certain areas outpatient facilities competed for patients, medical school clinics in particular advertising in newspapers and posting handbills. All these events were correlated, of course, with a growing demand within the medical profession for clinical training at every level, for the possession of attending and consulting physicianships, for the accumulation of specialty credentials. At the end of the century, finally, a growing public health movement used the by now familiar dispensary form to shape and deliver medical care and would-be prophylactic measures in slum areas — most conspicuously in the identification and treatment of tuberculosis.

Underlying these developments were a series of parallel changes, first in the scale of the human problems the dispensaries faced, second in the intellectual tools and social organization of the medical profession. First in time came an absolute increase in the numbers and shift in the social origins of those urban Americans calling upon the dispensary. Secondly, in terms of chronology if not significance, were shifts within the world of medicine which made the dispensary increasingly marginal in the priorities of medical men. One need hardly demonstrate the significance to medical practice of increasing specialization, the germ theory and antisepsis, the development of modern surgery, x-ray and clinical laboratory methods, the increasing centrality of the hospital; the way in which demographic and social changes reshaped the dispensaries is perhaps less familiar.

Whatever degree there had been in the original vision of a community bound by common ties of assumption and identity, this unifying vision corresponded less and less to reality as the 19th century progressed. The accustomed social distance between physician and charity patient seemed increasingly unbridgeable. A practical measure of this increasing social distance — and one which correlates with population and immigration statistics — was the growing disquietude of dispensary physicians in contemplating their patients. As early as 1828, New York's Northern Dispensary asked contributors to sympathize with their staff physicians'

> . . . great sacrifices of feeling and comfort, which they must necessarily make, by being forced into daily and hourly association with the miserable and degraded of our species, loathsome from disease, and often still more so by those disgusting habits which go to the utter extinction of decency in all its forms.

The traditional system in which dispensary patients or their messengers called first upon contributors seeking a recommendation and then upon visiting physicians at their regular homes or offices also showed signs of strain. In Boston, where the dispensary's lay managers had long opposed the establishment of a "central office," a major factor helping to overcome this reluctance in the 1850s was the unwillingness of district physicians to have their offices used by so "ignorant and degraded a class." "It is undesirable," as Henry J. Bigelow explained it, "for most physicians to receive at their own apartments the class of applicants who now form the mass of dispensary patients."[25]

The patients who seemed most familiar, closest to the physicians' own experience were those most capable of evoking sympathy and understanding; thus the plight of those fallen in fortune, of the genteel widow, of the orphaned child of good parents were those which touched visiting physicians most deeply.

> It is not infrequently that we witness much feeling manifested by those who have been able to employ their own physicians and purchase their own medicines, when through reverses of fortune they have for the first time applied for assistance from the Institution; such constitute the most interesting portion of our patients.

Other patients were far less interesting.[26]

There were, of course, the venereal and alcoholic; but these had always existed and their existence had always implied a certain conflict between morals and medical care. Far more unsettling by the 1840s were the new immigrants who streamed into America's cities and soon constituted a disproportionate part of the dispensary's clientele. By the early 1850s it was not uncommon for an absolute majority of a particular institution's patients to have been born in Ireland; in the districts of individual visiting physicians over 90 percent of those treated might be foreign born. Not surprisingly, the 1840s and 1850s saw dispensary administrators and trustees pointing again and again to the immigrant as they sought to explain the difficulties of their work and their ever increasing financial need.[27]

It was not only the numbers and the poverty, but the alienness of the immigrants which intensified the differences between them and their would-be medical attendants. It must be recalled that the desirability of dispensary appointments guaranteed their being filled by young physicians of at least middle class background — thus insuring as well a maximum social distance between physician and patient. As early as 1831, for example, Boston Dispensary visiting physicians, dismayed by the conditions they encountered, elected to survey the economic and moral status of their patients. In that age of temperance and pietism, it was only to have been expected that the district physicians found intemperance to be the most important single cause of disease in their patients — and intemperance to be most common among the foreign born. The Irish seemed particularly undesirable, filthy, drunken, generally inhospitable to middle-class standards of behavior. "Upon their habits — their mode of life," a dispensary physician explained in 1850, "depend the frequency and violence of disease. This I am fearful will continue to be the case, since no form of legislation can reach them, or force them to change their habits for those more conducive to cleanliness and health." "Deserving American poor," another Boston Dispensary physician complained, were "often deterred from seeking aid because they shrink from seeming to place themselves on a level with the degraded classes among the Irish."[28] The unfamiliar attitudes and habits of these patients often added to their troublesomeness; they ignored hygienic advice and often defied the physician's simplest requests. The Irish, for example, considered it dangerous to have lymph removed from the lesion of an individual vaccinated for smallpox; thus they refused to return to the dispensary after the required week to have the lesion checked (and to supply the lymph so useful in helping balance the dispensary's budget).[29] Later immigrant groups brought their peculiar beliefs and problems of communication; Jews and Italians replaced the Irish as objects of the dispensary physician's frustration and disdain.

A good many dispensary physicians were, of course, sympathetic to their patients, and in some cases not only sympathetic but convinced that environmental causes contributed to their clients' chronic ill-health. Yet even those individual physicians whose personal convictions made them most sensitive to the deprivation of their city's slum-dwellers, shared the ambivalence and even hostility of their peers. The same mid-century physicians, that is, who denounced basement dwellings, exploitative landlords, rotting meat and adulterated milk — shared a distaste for the intemperance, imprudence, filth, and apparent sexual immorality of those victimized by such conditions. One of the harsher dispensary critics of mid-century tenement conditions could, for example, contend that:

> . . . there is much squalor and other evidences of poverty which might be remedied had the patients more pride in cleanliness and more ambition to be doing well in the world.

As another mid-century physician explained, his patients' degradation and ignorance called "not for pity alone, but for the greatest exercise of patience and forbearance."[30]

A concern with social realities was, moreover, supported by and consistent with mid-19th-century etiological assumptions. Both acute and constitutional ills were seen as related closely to an individual's powers of resistance — itself a product of interaction between constitution and environment. And the conditions encountered by dispensary physicians were exactly those which seemed to lower resistance and hence increase the incidence and virulence of disease. Thus a dispensary physician could note casually that scarlet fever was particularly virulent one year, since it proved as fatal to the rich as to the poor. Similarly, a pioneer ophthalmologist could urge the need for ophthalmological dispensaries because of the relationship between poverty and diseases of the eye:

> The sickly hue, and the toil worn features of these poor people are but the results of constitutional derangements . . . and as clearly reveal the inseparable union between the health of the body and the health of the eye, as between poverty and disease.

Throughout the century articulate dispensary spokesmen were aware of the need to provide food and clothing for their patients, convinced that medicines could be of only marginal help when patients had to return to work before their complete recovery, while their homes had no adequate heat, their tables only impure and decaying food. "No persons can more readily appreciate than we," as one put it, "the utter uselessness of drugs, if there is no possibility of nourishing and warming the patient."[31]

The attitudes of mid and late 19th-century physicians can best be described in terms not of hostility, but of ambivalence — and perhaps most importantly an ambivalence characterized by a world-view which related disease and morals alike to general social conditions. Both morality and morbidity were seen as resultants of the interactions between environmental circumstance and culpable moral decisions. This mixture of social concern, moralism, meliorism and deep seated antipathy was clearly apparent by mid-century and marked the writings of most dispensary spokesmen until the end of the century; it could not prove the basis of a long-lived commitment to the dispensary and the necessity of its peculiar social function.

Nevertheless, a handful of articulate spokesmen for the dispensary did elaborate a characteristic point of view by the century's end, in which disease was seen not only as related inextricably to environment, but which emphasized the dispensary's capacity to reach out into the homes of the sick poor, so as to deal with problems more fundamental than the symptoms which brought the patient to their attention. The ability of the dispensary to relate to the community surrounding it became in the arguments of such dispensary defenders an indispensable aspect of a socially adequate medical care system. Visiting physicians and nurses could simply not be replaced by a hospital outpatient department. Advocates of this higher dispensary calling argued again and again that one could not simply treat a patient's symptoms and do nothing about an environment which had much to do with causing those very symptoms. Such ideas were implemented perhaps most fully in the tuberculosis dispensaries created so widely in the first decade of the 20th century.[32]

Such would-be rationalizers of American medicine as Edward Corwin, S. S. Goldwater, Richard Cabot, and Michael Davis contended that the dispensary could, in addition to supplying primary treatment for the indigent, supplement the necessarily unfinished work of the general practitioner in those numerous cases where the patient could not afford a specialist's consultation or expensive x-rays and laboratory tests. The dispensary could, that is, serve a vast urban constituency able perhaps to afford the services of a general practitioner but unable to manage the cost of more extended or elaborate medical care. And such occasions increased steadily as the profession's ability to understand and even cure increased. Yet even as they urged such prudent considerations, these advocates of social medicine were well aware of the threat posed to the independence and ultimately to the existence of the dispensary by rapid changes in medical ideas, techniques, and institutional forms.

These arguments were consistent as well with the motivations and social assumptions of the contemporary settlement-house movement and other pioneer social welfare advocates. The settlement houses were often involved in dispensary-like programs themselves. But in a precisely timed irony, the dispensary as a viable independent institution was dying just as its most self-conscious advocates were formulating these brave contentions.

How did this come about? The dispensaries could hardly be said to have lost their social function; we have become quite conscious in recent years that their function is still not being adequately fulfilled. In retrospect, however, their dissolution was inevitable. By the 1920s, most significantly, the dispensary had become as marginal to the needs of the medical profession as it had been central in the first two-thirds of the 19th century. A century of work in the city's slums, a growing — if always somewhat ambiguous — awareness of the relationship between health and environment, the conscious commitment of a small leadership group to the need for working in that human environment — all proved ultimately of little importance.

As hospital-centered interne and residency programs became a normal part of medical education — following inclusion of clinical training in the undergraduate years — it was inevitable that those elite physicians who would in earlier generations have been anxious to receive a dispensary appointment would now prefer hospital posts. Not only had hospitals increased greatly in number, but they contained beds, laboratory and x-ray facilities, and a cluster of appropriately trained specialists. The hospital's increasingly exclusive claims to practice the best, indeed the only adequate medicine seemed to grow more and more plausible. When, for example, in 1922 the Managers of the Philadelphia Dispensary decided to merge with the Pennsylvania Hospital, they explained that they had "found it practically impossible for an independent dispensary, unassociated with the facilities and specialists of a large modern hospital, to render the public adequate service."[33]

As the intellectual and institutional aspects of medicine changed, economic pressures also pointed toward the centralized and capital-intensive logic of the hospital. Expensive laboratory facilities, x-rays, modern operating rooms all demanded the investment of unprecedently large sums of money. The routine low-budget dosing which characterized the independent 19th-century dispensary seemed no longer a real option; dispensary boards had to face a growing and embarrassing asymmetry between their limited resources and the demands of high quality medical care. The hospital outpatient department seemed to many medical men a substantial and inevitable improvement over its predecessor institution. The growing tendency in the 20th century for medical schools to forge strong hospital ties only increased the centrality of the hospital.

Shorn of its relevance to the career needs of aspiring physicians, the dispensary was left with the clearly residual function of providing public health — charity — medical care, in itself a low-status occupation throughout the 19th century. Dispensary appointments had brought prestige and clinical opportunities in generations during which there were few other badges of status or roads to the acquisition of clinical skills; by the end of the century, there were other, more prestigious options for the ambitious young physician. Positions as municipal "out-door physicians" had a comparatively low status throughout the 19th century. The dominion of fee for service medicine remained essentially unchallenged by the liberal critics of the Progressive generation. Those ambitious young men incapable of remaining content with the mere accumulation of fees were — as the 20th century advanced — ordinarily attracted not by social medicine but increasingly by the "higher" and certainly less ambiguous demands of research; and even clinical investigation seemed in its most demanding forms to have little place in the dispensary.

If the dispensary had lost much of its appeal for the medical elite by the end of the 19th century, it had lost whatever goodwill it had had in the mind of the average practitioner decades earlier. There had always been occasional complaints in regard to the dispensaries intervening unfairly to compete with private physicians for a limited supply of paying patients. From the earliest years of their operation, American dispensaries had warned that their services were only for "such as are really necessitous." None however chose to investigate systematically the means of their patients until after the Civil War. Until the 1870s, criticism was comparatively muted; throughout the last third of the century, however, and into the 20th, the dispensaries were widely attacked as purveyors of ill-considered charity to the unworthy. The more constructive critics sought to find alternatives, the most popular — in addition to simply demanding a small fee — being the provident dispensary, a species of prepaid health plan which had proven workable in some areas in England. In city after city, local practitioners called meetings and commissioned reports predictably concluding that a goodly portion of those using dispensary services were quite capable of paying a private physician's fees.[34] Americans found it difficult to understand the social configuration of the society in which they lived; only abuse by those in fact capable of paying medical bills could possibly explain the vast numbers who utilized dispensary services. To doubt this was to assume that large numbers of worthy and hard-working Americans were indeed too poor to pay for even minimally adequate medical care.[35]

Physicians were often unwilling to refer their paying patients — even if the payment were only 25 or 50 cents — to the more specialized facilities of neighboring dispensaries. As late as 1914 the director of Pennsylvania's tuberculosis program charged that local practitioners refused to refer patients in the early stages of the disease, unwilling to relinquish treatment until such working-people were too deteriorated to work — and pay. Attacks on the dispensary system were generally supported as well by the charity organization movement which, in city after city, attacked dispensary medicine as an excellent example of that undiscriminating alms-giving which served only to demoralize its recipients. (It should be noted that the majority of empirical studies of dispensary patients completed between the 1870s and World War I indicated that most dispensary patients were not in fact able to pay for medical care.)[36]

By the last quarter of the 19th century the dispensary patient no longer fit into that same vision of an ordered social universe which had guided and inspired the efforts of those benevolent Americans who had founded the first dispensaries a century earlier. Those older views of community and stewardship implied in the contributor-sponsorship system had faded by mid-century, paralleling changes in the environmental reality of America's cities. Similarly, it would have been hardly plausible to argue that New York or Boston tenement-dwellers should be visited in their homes so as to spare them the indignity of hospitalization. The constituency of both hospital and dispensary had changed. By the closing years of the 19th century, the dispensary had very clearly become the provider of charity medicine for a class who — if indeed worthy of such charity — were sharply differentiated from paying patients and who ordinarily lived in a section of the city removed physically from that of contributors, physicians, and private patients. Before mid-century and especially in the first quarter of the 19th century, dispensary managers still sought to enforce requirements that visiting physicians actually reside in the district they served — a natural enough sentiment in the 18th century but impracticable in post-bellum America.[37] The arguments employed by the end of the century to attract contributions had become almost exclusively prudential, appealing little either to explicitly religious convictions or to a feeling of identity with those at risk. Fund-raising circulars emphasized instead the need to avert crime, pauperism and prostitution.

Positive support for the dispensaries was, on the other hand, shaky indeed; aside from the support implicit in the inertia developed by all institutions, only a small group of socially-active physicians and proto-social-welfare activists defended the dispensaries as a positive good. Many social workers, as we have indicated, evinced little affection for an institution which seemed to embody so casual and unscientific an approach to philanthropy. Even the oldest dispensaries did not survive as independent institutions past the early 1920s.

Historians have devoted little attention to the dispensary. Yet as our contemporaries begin to concern themselves with the delivery of medical care this neglect may end; for the dispensary provides such would-be reformers with a potentially usable past. The dispensary did at first provide a flexible, informal, and locally oriented framework for the delivery of public medicine. But the analogy to contemporary problems is limited; the flexibility and informality of the dispensary were a result of medicine's still primitive tools, its local orientation a consequence of the contributors being in some sense — or assuming themselves to be — part of the community served by the dispensary. Such conditions ceased to exist well before the end of the 19th century. And even within its own frame of reference, the 19th-century dispensary provided second-class, routine, episodic medicine, was a victim of shabby budgets, and even in its earliest decades marked by unquestioned distance between physician and patient. (A distance *perhaps* made tolerable by traditional attitudes of hierarchy and deference.)

Yet despite these imperfections, the death of the dispensary and the transfer of its functions and client constituency to general hospitals has not been an unqualified success. And though the history of the rise and fall of the dispensary provides no explicit program for contemporary medicine, it does underline a simple moral: any plan for the reordering of medical care must be based on the accommodation of at least three different factors. One is felt social need, felt, that is, by those with power to change social policy. A second factor is general social values and assumptions as they shape the world-view and thus help define the options available to such decision-makers. Third, there are the needs of the medical profession, needs expressed in the career decisions of particular physicians and needs defined by medicine's intellectual tools and institutional forms. Without a strong commitment to government intervention in health matters — a commitment impossible without an appropriate change in general social values — factors internal to the world of medicine have determined most forcefully the specific forms in which medical care has been provided for the American people. Thus the rise and fall of the dispensary; it was doomed neither by policy nor conspiracy but by a steadily shifting configuration of medical perceptions and priorities.

NOTES

1 The most valuable study of the dispensary is still that by Michael M. Davis, Jr., and Andrew R. Warner, *Dispensaries. Their Management and Development* (New York, 1918). The most useful account of the early years of any single dispensary is [William Lawrence], *A History of the Boston Dispensary* (Boston, 1859). For an example of contemporary interest, see George Rosen, "The first neighborhood health center movement — its rise and fall," *Am. J. Public Hlth.*, 1971, *61*: 1620–1637. [See pp. 185–199 in this book.]

2 Philadelphia Dispensary, Minutebook, 18, June 25, 1816, Archives of the Pennsylvania Hospital, Philadelphia (Hereafter A.P.H.). Cf. "Brief history of the Southern Dispensary," Southern Dispensary, *81st Annual Report* (Philadelphia, 1898), pp. 6–10.

3 Charles E. Rosenberg, "The practice of medicine in New York a century ago," *Bull Hist. Med.*, 1967, *41*: 223–253, p. 236 [see pp. 55–74 in this book]; F. B. Kirkbride, *The Dispensary Problem in Philadelphia. A Report made to the Hospital Association of Philadelphia, October 28, 1903* (Philadelphia, 1903). By 1900, Davis and Warner, *Dispensaries*, p. 10, estimated that there were roughly 100 dispensaries in the United States, 75 general and 25 special.

4 As late as 1899, the City of Baltimore still compensated the Baltimore Dispensary when it filled prescriptions for the indigent patients of any legal practitioner. Baltimore General Dispensary, *Character, By-Laws. &c. . . . Revised 1899* (Baltimore, 1899), p. 14.

5 New York's Eastern Dispensary reported in 1857 that the city's donation to the New York Dispensary had been set at $1000 in 1827. As other dispensaries were founded, these too received the same subvention. *23rd Annual Report, 1856* (New York, 1857), p. 19.

6 Eastern Dispensary (New York), *25th Annual Report, 1858* (New York, 1859), pp. 16–17. The panics of 1857, 1873, and 1893, as well as the Civil War years, all represented such periods of stress for the dispensaries. New York's North-Eastern Dispensary, for example, was so pressed by the Panic of 1873 that it could not even publish annual reports in 1874 and 1875. *15th Annual Report, 1876* (New York, 1877), p. 6.

7 As late as 1891, Philadelphia's Northern Dispensary bemoaned the fact that they could still not afford to stop renting their second floor, despite their establishment of five new specialty clinics and consequent need for space. Northern Dispensary, *74th Annual Report, 1891* (Philadelphia, 1892), p. 9. As early as 1803, the Philadelphia Dispensary was happy to rent its basement to a commercial tenant. Minutes, Dec. 12, 1803. The typical pattern was illustrated clearly by the New York Dispensary's decision in 1868 to build a four-story building, the basement, first, third, and fourth levels being rented, only the second used by the dispensary itself. *77th Annual Report, 1868* (New York, 1869), p. 12.

8 Eastern Dispensary (New York), *23rd Annual Report, 1856*, p. 22; S. L. Abbott to G. F. Thayer, April 6, 1844, Chronological File, Boston Dispensary Archives, New England Medical Center, Boston. (Hereinafter B.D.A.) The phrase describing the dispensary's casual dentistry is from New York Dispensary, *81st Annual Report, 1870* (New York, 1871), p. 17.

9 For a convenient summary of early vaccination work by the dispensaries, see DeMilt Dispensary (New York), *25th Annual Report, 1875* (1876), pp. 20–22. For the role of the dispensaries in the Civil War, see New York Dispensary, *72nd Annual Report, 1862* (New York, 1863), pp. 9–10; Eastern Dispensary (New York), *28th Annual Report, 1861* (New York, 1862), pp. 23–25. Though the poor were normally uninterested in vaccination, the threat of epidemics often created a sudden upsurge of interest; in one case, indeed, the New York Dispensary could refer to a "vaccination riot" on their premises. *76th Annual Report, 1865* (New York, 1865), p. 20. Many of the dispensaries were financially dependent on their sale of vaccine matter.

10 George Gould, "Abuse of a great charity," *Med. News, N.Y.*, 1890, *57*: 534–539; Medical College of the Pacific, Faculty Minutes, Jan. 29, 1878, July 22, 1881, Lane Medical Library, Stanford University. New York's Eastern Dispensary was so lacking in funds that its patients were given neither bottles nor printed instructions: "The patients universally bring a bottle or tea-cup to receive and hold the medicine." *28th Annual Report, 1861*, p. 14. There were only occasional conflicts between physicians and lay managers in regard to such cutting of corners. A revealing incident of this kind shook the Boston Dispensary in 1844 when the managers sought to compel their visiting physicians to employ scarification and bleeding instead of the far more expensive leeches. The physicians argued not only that the leeches had a different physiological effect — but that they had well-nigh banished more painful modes of bloodletting from private practice. G. T. Thayer to Visiting Physicians, Feb. 8, 1844; S. L. Abbott et al. to Thayer, April 6, 1844; S. L. Abbott et al. to President and Managers [February 1844], B.D.A.

11 For an example of such ties in a particular dispensary, see DeMilt Dispensary, *2nd Annual Report, 1852–53* (New York, 1853), p. 12; *4th Annual Report, 1855* (New York, 1856), pp. 10–11.

12 Eastern Dispensary (New York), *32nd Annual Report, 1865* (New York, 1866), p. 14.

13 New York Diet Kitchen Association, *11th Annual Report, 1883* (New York, 1884), p. 5. On nursing, see, for example, Philadelphia Dispensary, Minutes, Feb. 15, 1853, Oct. 17, 1854, A.P.H.

14 Brooklyn Dispensary, *Trustees's Report. April, 1847* (New York, 1847), p. 8; Boston Dispensary, *108th Annual Report* (Boston, 1905), pp. 10–12. For the crediting of the New York Dispensary with this particular first, see DeMilt Dispensary, *25th Annual Report, 1875*, p. 19n.

15 John G. Coffin, *An Address delivered before the Contributors of the Boston Dispensary, . . . October 21, 1813* (Boston, 1813), pp. 6, 15; John B. Romeyn, *The Good Samaritan: A Sermon, delivered in the Presbyterian Church, in Cedar-street, New York, . . . for the Benefit of the New York Dispensary* (New York, 1810), p. 16.

16 "Servants," one board of managers argued at mid-century, "who have relations and friends in the lower walks of life, and who are in the habit of visiting them, often in company with the children of their employers, would be subject to more danger than they are now exposed." DeMilt Dispensary, *3rd Annual Report, 1853–54* (New York, 1854), p. 10.

17 DeMilt Dispensary, *5th Annual Report, 1855–56* (New York, 1856), p. 11.

18 For typical examples later in the century, see Central Dispensary and Emergency Hospital of the District of Columbia, *24th Annual Report . . . Including an Historical Sketch of the Institution* (Washington, D.C., 1894), pp. 8–10; Camden City Dispensary, *26th Annual Report, 1892–93* (Camden, N.J., 1893), pp. 6–9.

19 Rush to John Dickinson, Oct. 4, 1791, *Letters of Benjamin Rush*, ed. L. H. Butterfield (Princeton, N.J., 1951), I, 610; Philadelphia *Dunlap's American Daily Advertiser*, Aug. 16, 18, 1791; Minutes, Philadelphia Dispensary, Aug. 26, 1791. Cf. [Lawrence], *History of Boston Dispensary*, pp. 90–91, 98–99. Another dispensary noted at the mid-century that they had "often been accused, as being rather the schools, where the young and inexperienced might find patients to their hands, than benevolent institutions where sufferings might be allayed and diseases cured." DeMilt Dispensary, *2nd Annual Report, 1852–53*, p. 8.

20 Surviving archives of the Boston Dispensary, for example, indicate in letters of recommendation for district physicians the pattern we have suggested: The Bigelows, James Jackson, and Oliver Wendell Holmes recommend and are recommended. Successful candidates had frequently studied in Europe and the Tremont Medical School or served as house physicians at the Massachusetts General Hospital. Cf. James Jackson to Board of Managers, Aug. 3, 1831; O. W. Holmes to William Gray, Sept. 3, 1845, or see letters in 1836 file from John Collins Warren, Jacob Bigelow, and George Hayward recommending O. W. Holmes as a visiting physician. B.D.A.

21 New York Dispensary, *Annual Report, 1854* (New York, 1855), p. 9. A year later, the same dispensary contended that their staff members "in a few years, hope to be the eminent physicians of New York, and it is their right to expect, and of the community to require, that the unequaled advantages, to be found here, should be freely offered them." *Annual Report, 1855* (New York, 1856), p. 10. *Boston Med. & Surg. J.*, 1839, *20*: 351.

22 New York (City) Dispensary, *Charter and By-Laws . . .* (New York, 1814), p. 8. Another indication of the social assumptions of the generation which created the dispensaries was their concern over whether servants and apprentices were appropriate patients. John Bard argued in New York that servants should indeed be treated, but not at their place of work — which would have compelled "gentlemen to visit the servants of families in which they had no acquaintance with the Masters or Mistresses." *A Letter from Dr. John Bard . . . to the Author of Thoughts on the Dispensary . . .* (New York, 1791), p. 20. See the entry for July 17, 1786 in the Minutes of the Philadelphia Dispensary for the question of treating apprentices.

23 Philadelphia Northern Dispensary, Philadelphia Lying-In Hospital, "Rules and Regulations, Adopted November 4, 1835," Historical Collections, College of Physicians of Philadelphia; [?] to Board of Managers, Oct. 1, 1830, B.D.A.; *Rules of the Philadelphia Dispensary with the Annual Report for 1869* (Philadelphia, 1870), p. 10. As late as 1879, the organizers of a specialized New York dispensary contended that they appealed to those patients able to pay a small fee and thus "saved the necessary associations of a public, free dispensary." *Report of the East Side Infirmary for Fistula and other Diseases of the Rectum* (New York, 1879), p. 5. Cf. Pittsburgh Free Dispensary, *3rd Annual Report, 1875* (Pittsburgh, 1876), p. 9.

24 Philadelphia Dispensary, Minutes, Dec. 26, 1845, A.P.H.

25 Northern Dispensary (New York), *1st Annual Report, 1828* (New York, 1828), cont. p. 10; DeMilt Dispensary, *2nd Annual Report, 1853*, p. 12; Bigelow to D. D. Slade, Aug. 22, 1855, B.D.A. Cf. D. D. Slade to My Dear Sir [William Lawrence], Sept. 3, 1855,

B.D.A.; [Lawrence,] *History of the Boston Dispensary*, pp. 178–180.

26 Northern Dispensary (Philadelphia), *Annual Report, 1847* (Philadelphia, 1848), p. 10. Such sentiments were familiar ones. A "Contributor" to the Boston Dispensary explained in 1819 that its appropriate clients were those "many persons . . . who have been reduced from a state of competence to one little short of poverty, who while blessed with health, can, by industry, support themselves, but when attacked by sickness, and laid upon a bed of illness, find it impossible to pay the physician and apothecary." *New-England Palladium and Commercial Advertiser*, Jan. 12, 1819. The earliest rules of both Philadelphia and Boston dispensaries emphasized their wish to comfort "those who have seen better days . . . without being humiliated." Boston Dispensary, *Institution of . . . 1817* (Boston, 1817), p. 7.

27 In the New York Dispensary, for example, in 1853, of 7,188 patients treated, 1,582 were born in the United States and 4,886 in Ireland. At the Philadelphia Dispensary in 1857, 1,906 were born in the United States, 3,649 in Ireland. New York Dispensary, *64th Annual Report, 1853* (New York, 1854), p. 12; Philadelphia Dispensary, *Rules . . . with Annual Report for 1857* (Philadelphia, 1858), p. 14. Some dispensaries would not allow venereal cases to be treated, some imposed a special fee, while still others allowed individual physicians to decide whether they would treat such errant souls.

28 Luther Parks, Jr., to Board of Managers, June 10, 1850, B.D.A. Referring to the Irish, another dispensary physician explained: "Upon their habits, — and mode of life, depend the frequency and violence of disease. This I am fearful will continue to be the case, since no form of legislation can reach them, or force them to change their habits for those more conducive to cleanliness and health." Charles W. Moore to Board of Managers, April 1, 1857, B.D.A. On the temperance question, see, for example, J. B. S. Jackson to Board of Managers, Oct. 8, 1853, B.D.A.

29 New York Dispensary, *64th Annual Report, 1853*, p. 10; New York Dispensary, *72nd Annual Report, 1862*, p. 20. When, in an effort to solve this problem New York's dispensaries initiated a small deposit to be refunded when the patient returned to have the vaccination checked, these intractable — and seemingly ungrateful — patients chose to regard it as a payment absolving them of any responsibility to the institution.

30 J. Trenor, Jr., physician to middle district, Eastern Dispensary (New York), *25th Annual Report, 1858*, p. 32; New York Dispensary, *Annual Report, 1837* (New York, 1838), p. 7.

31 Edward Reynolds, *An Address at the Dedication of the New Building of the Massachusetts Eye and Ear Infirmary, July 3, 1850* (Boston, 1850), p. 15; Mission Hospital and Dispensary for Women and Children, *2nd Annual Report, 1876* (Philadelphia, 1877), p. 10. The scarlet fever reference was by William Bibbins, DeMilt Dispensary, *6th Annual Report, 1856–57* (New York, 1857), p. 17.

32 For useful descriptions of the tuberculosis clinics, see, for example, F. Elisabeth Crowell, *The Work of New York's Tuberculosis Clinics . . .* (New York, 1910); Louis Hamman, "A brief report of the first two years' work in the Phipps Dispensary for tuberculosis of the Johns Hopkins Hospital," *Johns Hopkins Hosp. Bull.*, 1907, *18*: 293–297. For samples of the more positive defense of the dispensary and its appropriate role, see: S. S. Goldwater, "Dispensary ideals: with a plan for dispensary reform . . . ," *Am. J. Med. Sci.*, 1907, n.s. *134*: 313–335; Richard Cabot, "Why should hospitals neglect the care of chronic curable disease in out-patients?" *St. Paul Med. J.*, 1908, *10*: 110–120; Cabot, "Out-patient work. The most important and most neglected part of medical service," *J.A.M.A.*, 1912, *59*: 1688–1689; Good Samaritan Dispensary (New York), *29th Annual Report, 1919* (New York, 1920), p. 8. The most complete statement of a positive dispensary program is to be found in Davis and Warner, *Dispensaries*.

33 Philadelphia Dispensary, Minutes, Jan. 8, 1923, A.P.H. At the end of the 19th century, for example, the Boston Dispensary began a search for beds; it seemed a necessity if bright young men were to be kept on the staff. *Report of the Dinner given to the Board of Managers of the Boston Dispensary by the Staff of Physicians . . . January 25th, 1909* [Boston, 1909], p. 13. Once allied with a hospital, the dispensary had invariably a lower status. Francis R. Packard charged in 1903 that hospitals would casually spend two or three hundred dollars for new surgical instruments yet balk at ten or fifteen for the dispensary. F. B. Kirkbride, *Dispensary Problem in Philadelphia*, p. 21.

34 Probably most significant is the tone of this debate. It was the ordinary practitioner who generally resented the way in which dispensaries with their elite house staffs attracted cases which might otherwise have remained in the hands of private practitioners. Discussions of "dispensary abuse" also served to express the resentment of many practitioners against the monopolization of hospital and dispensary posts by a minority of well-connected physicians. In its

report on charity abuse, for example, the Medical Association of the District of Columbia also urged limited tenure in hospital staff appointments and access to hospital privileges for all "reputable members of the profession." *Report of the Special Committee . . . on the Hospital and Dispensary Abuse in the City of Washington* (Washington, D.C., 1896), pp. 15–16.

35 [William Lawrence], *Medical Relief to the Poor. September, 1877* (Boston, 1877), pp. 3–4; James Keiser, "The abuses in hospital and dispensary practice in Reading," *National Hospital Record*, 1899.

36 Albert P. Francine, "The state tuberculosis dispensaries," *Penn. Med. J.*, 1914, *17*: 940. See Davis and Warner, *Dispensaries*, pp. 42–58, for a brief discussion of patient eligibility.

37 G. F. Thayer to William Gray, April 12, 1838, B.D.A.

13

Patrons, Practitioners, and Patients: The Voluntary Hospital in Mid-Victorian Boston

MORRIS J. VOGEL

The hospital of the immediate post-Civil War period differed little in some respects from its colonial and early 19th-century predecessor. It treated the same socially marginal constituency that American hospitals had always served. Its patients were the poor and those without roots in the community; dependence as much as disease still distinguished them from the public at large. Yet in some other respects the hospital of this era displayed concerns that were typically Victorian — concerns that shaped the transition of the institution into the hospital as we know it.

The general hospital of the 1870s was likely to be a charity, linking the voluntary efforts of doctors and donors in providing free medical care for those without any suitable alternative. For a hospital to exist, doctors had to be willing to provide gratuitous medical service for the sick poor while feeling sufficiently remunerated that they eagerly sought hospital positions. Donors had to be willing to support an institution that they themselves were never likely to use.

Traditionally, Boston's physicians had provided free care for the sick poor who had sought them out. Self-consciously advancing their claim to be professionals rather than businessmen, medical practitioners recognized a responsibility not to refuse advice or treatment to those who could not pay.[1] But in the hospitals and dispensaries organized up to the very end of the 19th century, many physicians went well beyond their professional obligations and actively made themselves available to patients who could not, and in most instances were forbidden to, pay any fee. Not only did doctors seek duties in such institutions, but often actually founded them, as in the case of inexpensively operated dispensaries, providing only outpatient care. In the case of hospitals, doctors shared leading roles in organizing them with those who provided financial backing.[2]

Hospital and dispensary staff members were part of the city's medical and social elite. They were close in social origins to the donors who supported Boston's voluntary Protestant hospitals, if not directly related to them.[3] This background was part of the reason for their hospital work. The gratuitous treatment they rendered hospital patients was in the same tradition of stewardship as the charitable donations that supported voluntary hospitals.

But free medical treatment was much more than a charitable obligation. As a further consequence of social position, hospital practitioners had professional qualifications and interests that set them apart from their less fortunate medical brethren. In a period when locally available medical training was not advanced, men who later became associated with the city's hospitals were more likely than others to have enjoyed a European medical education after initial training in Boston. Once established in Boston, these upper-class doctors were more likely to assume positions in medical school faculties. And, though conservatives of their own class and background sometimes opposed specialization and even certain imported innovations, young physicians returning from Europe in the second half of the 19th century embraced speciali-

---

MORRIS J. VOGEL is Assistant Professor of History, Temple University, Philadelphia, Pennsylvania.

Reprinted with permission from *Victorian America*, ed. Daniel Walker Howe (Philadelphia: University of Pennsylvania Press, 1976), pp. 121–138.

zation and the increasing scientific content of medicine more readily than Boston doctors less privileged by birth and social standing.[4]

Hospital positions furnished these upper-class doctors with the clinics that were becoming increasingly necessary for medical school teaching. Teaching brought financial benefits, as former students referred difficult cases to former professors for paying consultations. A hospital position also enabled a medical man to see and treat numbers of special cases, comparatively rare in private practice, and so develop a reputation that would itself be remunerative. Thus, though hospital patients did not pay fees to hospital practitioners, these men received what contemporaries referred to as "certain well-understood advantages."[5]

Hospital physicians earned their livelihoods in the care of well-to-do private patients who paid for the knowledge gained in hospital work. Private practice remained the norm. And because the 19th-century hospital was not the center of the doctor's work world, the few hours he put in there each day during his term of perhaps three months each year did not represent income lost.

Economic motives led nonelite doctors to complain about the abuse of charity they perceived in the medical care offered without fee in hospitals. They saw their natural clientele — the poor and working classes — drained off to the hospitals.[6] When the nature of the hospital patient population changed in the 1890s and in the first decade of the 20th century, complaints about abuse came from a new quarter — from doctors who treated the well-to-do patients beginning to enter hospitals at the turn of the century.[7] These complaints were a significant force in leading the hospital away from its purely charitable organization. But until late in the 19th century, Boston's hospitals, whether municipally or voluntarily supported, were charities.

In part, the wealthy supported these institutions because of their connections with the physicians who staffed them. Amos Lawrence, the mercantile prince, underwrote the entire cost of a children's hospital under the charge of his son, Dr. William R. Lawrence.[8] The staffing of South Boston's Roman Catholic Carney Hospital by Back Bay physicians brought in financial contributions from their friends and families.[9]

In part, too, the wealthy supported these institutions because enlightened selfishness led them to share certain of the physicians' goals. The knowledge and experience doctors gained in treating the poor "raised the standard of medical attainments"; hospital and dispensary practice thus "proved a blessing to rich and poor alike."[10] The Children's Hospital appealed "to all those who have children of their own," reminding them that they had a "double interest" in the institution; "not only on account of the great benefit it will confer on its little inmates, but also because of the advantages it offers for the study of special diseases by which their own offspring may be afflicted."[11] The *Boston Evening Transcript* warned the fortunate that their own well-being depended on the continued well-being of hospitals:

> The aids which society distributes to the hospitals are amply restored by the hospitals to society. . . . Mainly in these institutions the experience and insight, the methods of observation and treatment, the scientific research, are evolved which become employed for the general health of the country. . . . If we could imagine the hospitals abolished, the general death rate in all private practice would be increased.[12]

However, the "double interest" remained a divided interest, for the more fortunate classes did not expect to make direct use of the general hospital in the 1870s. Home care remained the norm. Accident victims, for example, though they might be injured outside the home, were likely to be brought home and cared for there. Speaking in 1864 at the dedication of the Boston City Hospital, its president, Thomas C. Amory, Jr., acknowledged that it was unlikely that hospitalization would replace the ideal of home care. Amory gave an example of what he regarded as a futile attempt to remove the prejudice against hospital care:

> One of our former governors . . . meeting with an accident in the street from which he narrowly escaped with his life, insisted, in order to remove this prejudice, upon being carried to the [Massachusetts General] Hospital. His example may have had its effect. But we doubt if many of our own people, born in Boston, when tolerably comfortable

> at home, will go, when ill, among strangers to be cured.[13]

When Amory himself was run down by a streetcar in 1886, "a doctor was called and the injured gentleman was removed to his home in a carriage."[14]

The pattern of care obtaining at local railroad accidents is revealing.[15] When a commuter train crashed near Roslindale in 1887, 24 passengers were killed and 14 hospitalized. But most of the nearly 100 victims were taken to their homes.

> The fact that the accident occurred in the midst of a settled suburban district, and that nobody upon the train was more than five miles away from home, made it possible to transport the dead and injured, so far as it was practicable under the circumstances, directly to their homes, and many were so taken.[16]

The severity of their injuries did not separate those hospitalized from those brought home. Only two of the six admitted to the Boston City Hospital were listed as seriously injured, and only one of eight at the Massachusetts General. Of the cases brought to their own homes, a doctor making 55 home visits the day after the wreck reported nine patients in dangerous condition.[17]

The hospital offered patients no medical advantages not available in the home; actually hospital treatment in the 1870s added the risks of sepsis or "hospitalism." The fact that the hospital offered no special medical benefits reinforced a resistance to hospitalization that stemmed from the role of the home as the traditional setting for those undergoing illness and from a negative image of the hospital. That image derived from the actual danger of hospitalism and the traditional identification of the hospital with the pesthole and almshouse. Thus even when home care was unavailable, hospital care was sometimes shunned.

The well-to-do might make use of a hospital in what were labeled peculiar circumstances. This category included individuals away from home because they were from out of town, and old people living alone. For these potential patients, limited separate facilities existed at both the Massachusetts General and Boston City Hospitals.[18]

Even the sick poor would avoid the hospital if possible. One of the stated advantages of a dispensary was that outpatient care sidestepped the "dread" which the prospect of hospitalization evoked among many of the poor.[19] The city's two diet kitchens, founded in the 1870s, supplied home meals for dispensary patients too sick or poor to secure their own food.[20] The truly unfortunate shared with that minority of the prosperous classes who used the institution the problem of an inadequate or nonexistent home. The Boston Lying-in Hospital received some of its cases from dispensary physicians "who suddenly found themselves called upon to attend some poor woman in quarters utterly unfit for such purposes."[21]

The hospital offered shelter and attention to the sick poor. It replaced comfortless homes "in close courts, narrow alleys, damp cellars or filthy apartments, which the sunshine never enters, nor fresh air purifies." It made up for the absence of "natural protectors" for those without families. It provided relief for "helpless people, who would suffer tenfold more from neglect and ill treatment than they now suffer from disease, were it not for the shelter and care of the hospitals."[22] Indeed the role of hospital was defined in terms of the services it offered the sick and injured victims of a catalog of social ills.

The statistics of hospital use reflected these concerns. An analysis of nativity and occupation shows that patients treated at the Massachusetts General and Boston City Hospital in the 1870s were not a cross-section of the population.

Hospital annual reports listed the occupations admitted; these occupations may be organized according to the socioeconomic classification in Stephan Thernstrom's *The Other Bostonians* and then compared with Thernstrom's observations about the occupational structure of the city.[23] Male patients at the city's two major hospitals were divided into four categories: white-collar, skilled blue-collar, semi-skilled and service, and unskilled and menial. Such an analysis shows occupations with high socioeconomic status were underrepresented among hospital patients in 1870 and 1880, while those with low status were overrepresented.

At the Massachusetts General in 1870, 16.9 percent of the classifiable male patients were in white-collar occupations, while in 1880 that figure was 18.1 percent. In the city population, 32 percent of males were white-collar in 1880. Skilled blue-collar workers accounted for 41.9 percent of Massachusetts General patients in 1870 and 19.4 percent in 1880, while they provided 36 percent of the general male population in 1880. Among patients, 14.2 percent and 11.1 percent were in semi-skilled occupations in 1870 and 1880 respectively, while the city population contained 17 percent in that category in 1880. The unskilled accounted for 26.9 percent (1870) and 51.4 percent (1880) of the patient population and 15 percent of the city population in 1880.[24]

Much the same pattern prevailed at the Boston City Hospital. The largest single occupational category among patients was laborer, consisting of 524 of 1,419 men admitted in 1870/1871 and 792 of 2,696 in 1880/1881. Patients in white-collar occupations totaled 8.2 percent of the hospital's male admissions in 1870/1871 and 10.5 percent in 1880/1881. Skilled blue-collar workers accounted for 36.3 percent of Boston City patients in 1870/1871 and 31.6 percent in 1880/1881. Workers in semi-skilled and service occupations made up 11.8 percent of City Hospital patients in 1870/1871 and 21.7 percent in 1880/1881. As at the Massachusetts General, unskilled (including laborers) and menial workers — 43.5 percent and 36.1 percent — were disproportionately over-represented.[25]

Unfortunately, the listing of many women patients as simply wives or widows, and the absence of a satisfactory analysis of the female occupational structure, makes a comparison of female patients with the general female population more difficult. But the fact that nearly half the female patients admitted to both hospitals in the 1870s were identified as domestics reinforces the conclusion based on male employment patterns that hospital patients were drawn disproportionately from among the lower classes.[26]

Though the absolute and relative numbers undergoing hospitalization continued to increase in the 1870s as they had since the city's first hospital opened in 1821, the hospital's constituency remained largely the same, with the greater number of patients coming from an expanded lower class. The continued use of the institution by the stricken and helpless poor served to associate it with the almshouse and reinforced the negative image of the hospital held by society at large. Its image as a refuge for the unfortunate was further heightened by the fact that its patients were not just poor but, after the beginning of large-scale immigration at mid-century, largely foreign born. The Massachusetts General trustees had at first resisted allowing the Irish to enter the hospital as patients, claiming that "the admission of such patients creates in the minds of our citizens a prejudice against the Hospital, making them unwilling to enter it, — and thus tends directly to lower the general standing and character of its inmates." Feeling "the excess of foreigners among the patients" to be a bane, they had advised the admitting physician to use "the utmost vigilance," but found that "some such admissions must unavoidably take place." Hospital rules directed that all cases of sudden accident were to be admitted, thus bypassing the screening procedure; a very large proportion of accident cases was Irish. In time, the Massachusetts General trustees, "moved by a sense of duty and humanity," opened their wards to the foreign-born.[27]

In 1865, the hospital accepted 628 foreign as against 571 native-born patients. In 1870, the totals showed 718 foreign and 584 Americans, and in 1875 the figures were 1,042 and 799 respectively. The Irish made up the largest segment of the foreign-born population, maintaining at least a majority throughout the 1870s, with those born in the Canadian provinces second.[28] From the opening of the Boston City Hospital in 1864, a majority of its patients was foreign born. In 1865, 647 of its patients were born abroad and 459 in the United States, and in 1870/1871, 1,635 were foreign and 761 native-born. The foreign-born numbered 2,187 and native Americans 993 in 1875/1876. Throughout the period, Irish patients alone outnumbered the native-born.[29]

Just as Irish immigrants tarnished the image of the general hospital, so did the kind of women it cared for taint the image of the lying-in hospital. Maternity care would be among the last reasons causing the comfortable classes to enter hospitals. In the late 19th century women still considered childbirth a natural function, something that could, and should, be performed in the simplest and poorest home.[30] The hospital offered no specialized medical paraphernalia or contrivances, but instead threatened contagion, puerperal fever, and high maternal mortality. Generally, only the most desperate women entered hospitals to have their children. And perhaps the major cause of this desperation was illegitimacy. Small lying-ins, often no more than a few rooms in a tenement or boarding house, kept by midwives or the unscrupulous and untrained, served those seeking "to hide their shame" or having absolutely no alternative. These lying-ins, and the baby farms that sometimes accompanied them, were seen as accessories to vice and degradation, and as adjuncts to brothels. Lying-ins were the first hospitals needing licenses to operate in Massachusetts (1876), but the enforcement problems of the Boston Board of Health suggest that more lying-ins were operated without sanction of law than with it.[31]

Licensed and respectable lying-ins did exist, and did leave records, but their patients, too, were "unfortunate women." Cases included in the first volume of the maternity records of the New England Hospital for Women and Children, covering one-and-one-half years in the early 1870s, list 61 married and 57 unmarried mothers. Over 50 percent of the more than 1,300 mothers delivered in the 1870s at the Boston Lying-in were unmarried. And at St. Mary's Lying-in Hospital, only 20 of 550 patients cared for in the decade from 1874 to 1884 were married.[32] The lying-in hospitals of the period reaffirmed the notion that hospitals were institutions especially for the poor and desperate, and the illegitimacy intimately associated with them added the stigma of immorality.

The hospital was perceived as the kind of place all but the desperate would want to avoid. Yet, although it dealt primarily with the poor, its very nature — the omnipresence of death within its walls — imbued its concerns with a powerful attraction. The community at large was curious as to what went on inside it. This desire to know was heightened by the relative newness of the institution; though its history could be traced back to antiquity, hospitals began to emerge in numbers in Boston and the rest of the nation only after the Civil War. Finally, the curiosity as to what went on within hospitals derived from the fact that even the fortunate individual could not be certain that he would not someday be hospitalized.

Horror was a common response to such a prospect. Joseph Chamberlin, for many years the *Transcript's* "Listener,"[33] reacted strongly after visiting a hospitalized friend:

> If it should fall to the Listener's lot to be called upon to go in sickness to the very best of [hospitals], he would say, "Better a straw cot in an attic at home, with the clumsiest of unprofessional attendance, than the best private room in this place." . . . [T]here is something about the all-pervading presence of Sickness, with a large S, this atmosphere of death, either just expected or just escaped, and all of this amiable perfunctoriness of nursing and medical attendance, that is simply horrible. The hospital . . . gives one sickness to think about morning, noon and night.[34]

A visitor might be acutely discomforted by the unnatural concentration of disease and death. But for the patient the environment was threatening:

> The doctors visit you incessantly, and, in spite of their courtesy, you feel as if you were not exactly an ailing human being, but merely a "case" that was being read as one reads a novel which is interesting enough, no doubt, but which is expected to develop a much more interesting phase, to wit, the catastrophe, at almost any moment. And then the grim disquieting presence of all these people like you in the ward around you![35]

The hospital reaffirmed the patient's mortality, but denied his humanity.

Chamberlin told the story of a patient hospitalized for an operation. After surgery, she was put to bed. She lived through a night punctuated by the "wailing and crying" of fellow patients, the death "in dreadful agony" of a neighboring patient, and the quiet but quick, and therefore ghostly, movement of attendants. It was terrifying: "Why it was like being dead and conscious of it!" The next day was quiet, but "spent in anticipating the coming of such another night, was almost as terrible." This particular hospital stay was cut short when a physician inquired "whether I had not any friend to whom I could go," found she had and "made immediate arrangements to have me taken away." Clearly, this patient and many of her contemporaries shared Chamberlin's conclusion: "What a matter for infinite sorrow it is that there should be homes in the world so dismal, so unhealthy, so ill attended, that their inmates are better off in the public wards of the hospital, when they are sick, than they are at home."[36]

Because the hospital was a strange and frightening place, the public welcomed reassurance from the informed. This might take the form of a newspaper article giving the generic history of the hospital and thus implying that it was not simply a modern aberration but an old institution that had proved its value in the past.[37] Or it might take the form of a correspondent's story of a hospital visit or a patient's description of his hospital stay.

Chamberlin's story was idiosyncratic: more common in the Boston press were counterphobic presentations that were almost uniformly formulaic. These addressed fears based on ignorance and substituted for them informed chronicles which denied the presence of death, disease, and pain in the hospital. Insanity, for example, was not mentioned in an extensive account of an insane asylum, though beautiful flowers and homelike accommodations in cottages were.[38] The smallpox hospital emerged from another narrative as a delightful place, serving wonderful food and providing comfortable beds, while smallpox itself, it was concluded, much improved the system.[39] For those hospitals which depended on the beneficence of the public to operate, reassurances that all was well within served a double function in that they encouraged contributions as well as disarmed anxieties.

Boston's City Hospital was supported as a municipal service, but the hospital tradition in Boston, as in the rest of the United States, had been set by the voluntary hospitals, with groups of private individuals undertaking the care of the sick poor as a public trust.[40] The Massachusetts General Hospital and Children's Hospital formed part of the complex of Boston's Protestant charities that owed their founding and existence, at least in part, to the religious doctrine of stewardship. Social and economic inequalities were legitimized by the notion that God meant for them to exist. But the elect, whose heavenly salvation was generally already demonstrated by their earthly riches, held their wealth only as God's trustees. With their wealth came the obligation to aid the less fortunate. The poor provided their economic betters the opportunity, the privilege actually, of spending God's wealth in a way that continually reemphasized their own chosen state.

The Children's Hospital was founded in 1869. It was intended for the poor, for "the little waifs who crowd our poorer streets." In its early years the institution stressed its spiritual role. Making their first annual report, the trustees stated that the institution would provide its patients "Christian nurture."[41] Sickness provided an opportunity for spiritual healing; the philosophy of the Children's Hospital reflected that of a local newspaper, which editorially downgraded the function of hospitals in furnishing medical treatment while commending them for giving patients the best gifts of all, "wrought through a ministry of sorrow."[42] The theological language in which all this was expressed was largely a carry-over from an earlier time; religious terminology provided a familiar and convenient vocabulary. Soon, society would no longer justify the hospital in traditional religious terms. One can already sense the beginning of a shift in the hospital's mission during Victorian times, from succoring the sick poor as its role in God's order, to denying that man had to accept God's diseases. Within a generation, this would give the hospital a drastically altered justification. But in the 1870s, these religious terms still symbolized real moral and social concerns.

The Children's Hospital defined its role in terms of the "moral benefit" it offered its patients. Socially, these benefits translated into a program of uplift and social control which it was hoped would help cope with the masses of threatening and increasingly alien poor crowding into the city. The trustees had expected that most of their patients would come from the poorest classes of the community. They found that many came "from the very lowest; from abodes of drunkeness, and vice in almost every form, where the most depressing and corrupting influences were acting both on the body and mind."[43] Hospitalization provided an opportunity to separate these children, at a most impressionable time in their lives, from corrupting influences that, if otherwise permitted to proceed unchecked, could perpetuate an impoverished and vicious class, permanently threatening society.

When a child entered, the hospital first decontaminated its new charge. "On their entrance they are immediately placed in a refreshing bath and clothed in the clean robes of the hospital." Uniform red flannel jackets replaced streetclothes.[44] The decontamination process went deeper; new influences were substituted for old in the hope that, in the few weeks it had, the institution could "help the child-soul to lift itself out of the mud in which it had been born, to assert its native purity in spite of unfortunate surroundings."[45]

Since treatment was not purely medical, the hospital did not restrict its practitioners to the medical profession. The entire Christian community was invited to participate in the healing process, to visit patients and encourage them "by word or counsel."[46] The hospital's first nurses were Episcopalian nuns. Their strength lay less in medical training than in the "Christian nurture" they provided patients. Sister Letitia was a model of this style of charity untainted by medical pretension. "Though enfeebled by disease of the lungs, which she knew must soon terminate her life, yet entirely forgetful of self," she continued nursing — all the while, of course, subjecting her charges to tuberculosis — until she died.[47]

The trustees wanted "to bring [their young patients] under the influence of order, purity and kindness." Among the means employed were tender nursing, books, pictures, "little works of art," and "the visits and attentions of the kind and cultivated."[48] Middle- and upper-class children outside the hospital were encouraged to undertake the painting, as wall decorations, of inspirational mottos that would "cultivate the devotional feelings" of the little sufferers inside. The fortunate who supported the hospital were encouraged to visit the children in its wards at any time of the day, to speak with them, provide role models, and in general to furnish that cultivated influence which the children of the poor had missed.[49] At the same time, parents having children in the hospital were severely restricted in the hours they could see their own children. The original parents' visiting hour allowed one relative at a time between eleven and twelve o'clock on weekdays only, raising difficulties for working fathers (or mothers) who wished to visit. Later, parent visiting was further restricted to the hour between eleven and twelve on Monday, Wednesday, and Friday only.[50] The trustees hoped that this regimen would change the children by "quickening their intellects, refining their manners, and encouraging and softening their hearts."[51]

Supporters of the institution hoped that a different child would leave the hospital than had entered it.[52] Children would leave having been "carefully taught cleanliness of habit, purity of thought and word" and with as much attention "paid to their moral training as can be found in any cultivated family," but the benefits of the hospital would not stop there:

> Think what a widespreading influence this becomes when the children return to their homes. . . . Even among the better class of poor people, the children soon notice the discomforts of careless, untidy habits, and are quick to compare such with the "so much better" at the hospital. In the joy of the child's homecoming, the parents are ready to gratify it by trying the new ways, and all unconsciously rise a little in the social scale by so doing.[53]

"In this wise," the hospital's founder wrote, the institution would "commence the education of the poorer classes."[54]

Even if the child did not go home and improve his family, he himself would be changed by the hospital in a way that would benefit society. The affluent and cultivated were told that they could not tell the difference between their own children and those within the hospital, even though the latter might be immigrant children from the North End. One visitor noted that "the faces of the children quickly lost the expression which we commonly meet in our little street Arabs, and become once more human and civilized."[55] Their hearts softened by kindness, mistrust and hostility evaporated from their faces and they no longer appeared as threatening as they had on the streets.

The hospital promised other far-reaching improvements. The health and strength gained during a hospital stay would not only aid the children, by enabling them to grow into "better men and women," but society as a whole — having escaped childhood invalidism, those healthier adults could support themselves. A promotional article mentioned the institution's success in educating its charges, even implying that it taught some how to read.[56] A hospital stay could help prepare a child for a socially desirable role in adult life.

These perceptions were colored, of course, by expectation. No doubt they express more than actually happened in the hospital in the way of having the children of the poor fulfill the fantasies of the rich. Further, these social expectations were less than the full rationale for the institution. The Children's Hospital was founded by physicians, in part for the sorts of professional reasons earlier suggested. At the same time, however, the founding physicians were responsible for much of this socially oriented promotional rhetoric. There is no reason to believe these doctors did not take their own language seriously. They were members of a social class as well as of a professional group, and shared the didactic concerns typical of Victorian culture.

The Massachusetts General Hospital, a secularly oriented Protestant hospital in the same sense as the Children's Hospital, also began with the mission of uplifting its patients. When founded, it had been intended for native American patients, and had offered to tide them over a bad time and send them on their way having meanwhile reinforced their view of a basically good society in which they could lead good lives.[57] But after the hospital had been overwhelmed by unappealing and apparently intractable and unimprovable adult immigrants, it gave up this aspect of its role. By the 1870s, its literature no longer expressed concern for the character of its patients, and the hospital continued to care for the sick poor with a diminished concern about what it was doing for its patients in a nonphysical sense. The hospital kept the support of its donors for a variety of reasons, the chief (probably) being an inertia in which benefactions served as a quiet reaffirmation of stewardship. An obligation to keep the hospital going because it served the needs of medical practitioners was recognized. Finally, the fact that the McLean Asylum for the Insane was a branch of Massachusetts General and served the upper classes in a very direct way maintained their interest in the corporation. Since the asylum generally met its operating expenses from patient revenues, the contributions it generated helped support the hospital.

Yet the loss of reforming zeal brought no relaxation of discipline within Massachusetts General; if anything, it reinforced it. The "influence of order" which pervaded the Children's Hospital furthered that institution's resocialization of its young patients. Order was a concern in Massachusetts General, too, but there it was a reflection of social reality, not part of a vision of social change. Many of the hospital's patients were not bedridden, but able to move around the wards and grounds, and expected to be able to leave the institution to walk about the city or enjoy the carriage rides into the countryside furnished by the Young Men's Christian Union. The hospital treated people new to urban life (through the 1870s the percentage of its patients born in Boston never approached 10 percent) and to the demands of institutional living. To help maintain discipline, its grounds were surrounded by a high wall and an always guarded gate through which patients and visitors had to pass.[58] Patients needed signed passes to leave and reenter the hospital, and visitors were carefully screened.[59] This discipline was maintained for internal reasons; rather than reform a patient who misbehaved, the hospital expelled him.[60]

In one sense, Massachusetts General helped keep order in the general community. Like other hospitals, it functioned as a guarantor of social stability, or as one supporter of the Children's Hospital put it, "There is a practical side to this charity, which may commend it to thoughtful men." Hospitals provided the working classes with evidence that the wealthy were aware of their responsibilities: "the only sure way to reconcile labor to capital is to show the laborer by actual deeds that the rich man regards himself as the steward of the Master."[61] Until workmen's compensation went into effect, corporations, especially railroads and street railways, underwrote free beds at the Massachusetts General to which they sent employees injured on the job. These accident-prone enterprises provided a paternalisic form of insurance, absolved themselves of responsibility to their injured employees, and attempted to defuse issues that might otherwise build up workers' grievances.[62]

Concern for social order was apparent in the community's support of hospitals in general. One observer noted that "the hospitals act as a kind of insurance system for the laboring classes. They take the risks incidental to their position the more cheerfully, because they know that if injured they are assured of a special provision for their need in our hospitals."[63] Similar reasoning was used to elicit support for the Children's Hospital. Were it not there, or were it unable to admit a suffering child, there would be no telling what even the most respectable worker, distraught over his inability to secure aid for his child, might do. "It is under such circumstances the iron enters a man's soul, and he is ready for a 'strike' or any other desperate remedy that promises better times and money with which to provide good nursing and delicacies for his suffering children." A mother, turned down when applying for admission for her sick child, might go "fiercely on her way, ripe for any evil deed. . . ." But assured that the hospital would care for their sick children, the poor would respond with gratitude rather than violence.[64]

Beside acting as a guarantor of social stability, the hospital was perceived by some as contributing to community prosperity, both through the more tractable labor force it ensured and through the fact that the health of the population was directly translatable into material wealth. In encouraging support for the city's voluntary hospitals, the *Transcript* editorially assured "those who look into the matter [that they would] see that our hospitals are among the very bases of national health and prosperity, and the working of these institutions is, therefore, a matter of general interest and public importance."[65] The hospital thus served much the same function as the public school, to which it was sometimes likened by those arguing that the institution served the entire community and those needing it should use it as a guaranteed right with any cost borne by the community. But of course only a minority fully appreciated all the functions of a hospital; Boston's City Registrar complained that too many of those "by mere fortuitous circumstance different situated" had yet to learn that "the material condition of the whole community is involved in this subject."[66]

Though hospital treatment of the poor protected the established order and added to the wealth of the community, the people for whom it was intended were made to feel recipients of charity and reminded repeatedly that they were enjoying a privilege and their gratitude was expected in return. This attitude was embodied in law. In one case, a man treated gratuitously sued the Massachusetts General Hospital, claiming his broken leg was set improperly. The courts held that even if he had been treated incompetently and negligently, he was not entitled to recover because the institution was a charity.[67] In another case, a woman charity patient operated on at the Free Hospital for Women sued, claiming her operation was not successful. During the course of protracted litigation, "A Friend to our Charities" wrote the *Transcript* complaining that such hospital malpractice suits arose because "there are some patients so wholly devoid of ordinary gratitude for favors to which they had not a shadow of a claim, as to make their benefactors suffer by reason of their very kindness." When a verdict for the hospital was finally returned, the *Transcript's* headline, "A Victory for Charity," translated the jury's decision into a reaffirmation of the status of the hospital, though only meaning to imply that money given hospitals would not be drained by lawsuits.[68]

It is from this background that the modern hospital emerged. Changes in social attitudes and medical practice — products of social change and scientific progress — have reshaped the institution. But the hospital that was transformed by these forces was itself a shaping force, a product of its own past. It has influenced medical organization and the kind of medical care available. The hospital now cares for patients of all classes, but it is not a classless institution. The hospital allows physicians to practice the best medicine available, but its clinical setting sometimes discourages the human component of caring. And while government financing and third party payment have redistributed the burden of hospital support throughout society, the institution has often remained unresponsive to the mass of its patients. Finally, the hospital has not evolved toward any foreordained perfection. It is no more the ideal form of medical organization today than it was of social consideration for the poor in the second half of the 19th century.

NOTES

1 See, in this regard, the career of George Cheyne Shattuck (1813–1893), Shattuck Papers, Massachusetts Historical Society.

2 Nathaniel I. Bowditch, *A History of the Massachusetts General Hospital*, 2nd ed. (Boston: The Bowditch Fund, 1872), p. 3; "A statement made by four physicians . . ." (Boston: 1869), in "Papers and Clippings" (hereafter P.&C.), a scrapbook kept by Dr. F. H. Brown about the Children's Hospital, 1869–1879, in the Countway Library, Boston; For the Dispensary for Skin Diseases and the Dispensary for Diseases of the Nervous System, *Boston Med. & Surg. J.*, 1872, *86*: 81, 82; 1872, *87*: 58; F. H. Brown, *Medical Register for the Cities of Boston, Cambridge, Charlestown, and Chelsea* (Boston: J. Wilson & Son, 1873), n.p.

3 Morris J. Vogel, "Boston's hospitals, 1870–1930: a social history" (Ph.D. dissertation, Univ. of Chicago, 1974), pp. 147–150.

4 James Clarke White, *Sketches from My Life, 1833–1913* (Cambridge, Mass.: Riverside Press, 1914), pp. 267–271.

5 *Boston Med. & Surg. J.*, 1882, *107*: 455. See also Henry J. Bigelow, "Fees in hospitals," *Boston Med. & Surg. J.*, 1889, *120*: 378. Bigelow noted: "It has been said, with truth, that these hospital offices would command a considerable premium in money from the best class of practitioners were they annually put up at auction." An annual report of the Boston Dispensary discussed why doctors served: "It is not to be supposed that the motives of the attending physicians have been wholly foreign from considerations of personal advantage. They have doubtless been actuated by the hope of professional improvement and the prospect of building up an honest fame, as well as by the desires of fulfilling the benevolent intentions of this charity." Quoted in *Boston Med. & Surg. J.*, 1882, *106*: 137.

6 *Boston J. Hlth.*, March 1886, *1*: 100.

7 *Boston Med. & Surg. J.*, 1905, *152*: 295–320.

8 Bowditch, *M.G.H. History*, p. 415.

9 Carney Hospital, *Annual Reports*, 1879–1889.

10 Boston Dispensary, *Annual Report*, quoted in *Boston Med. & Surg. J.*, 1882, *106*: 137.

11 Children's Hospital, *Appeal*, 1869, in P.&C.

12 *Boston Evening Transcript*, April 20, 1881.

13 Boston, *Proceedings at the Dedication of the City Hospital* (Boston: J. E. Farwell, 1865), p. 58.

14 *Boston Evening Transcript*, June 10, 1886.

15 Detailed sources exist for who used hospitals, but since there is no reliable census of accident and illness, it is difficult to deduce what proportion of any different category of sickness or injury was hospitalized and what was not. Catastrophes, like train wrecks, can provide a rough idea. The pattern derived, while inconclusive, is reaffirmed by an examination of actual hospital use in the period.

16 *Boston Evening Transcript*, March 14, 1887.

17 *Boston Evening Transcript*, March 14, 17, 1887; *Boston Med. & Surg. J.*, 1887, *116*: 268. Another "frightful disaster" with the same general pattern occurred with the wreck of an excursion train on the Old Colony Railroad, *Transcript*, Oct. 9, 10, 1878. There was a different pattern after a crash on the Eastern Railroad in Revere. A greater proportion of the injured were hospitalized; probably because an express Pullman was involved, many of the survivors were from out of town. *Transcript*, Aug. 28, 1871.

18 M.G.H., *60th Annual Report, 1873*, p. 9; George H. M. Rowe (superintendent, B.C.H.) to John Pratt (superintendent, M.G.H.), March 7, 1894, in M.G.H. archives, Phillips House file.

19 *Boston Med. & Surg. J.*, 1872, *86*: 81, 82.

20 North End Diet Kitchen founded 1874; South End Diet Kitchen a short time later. *Boston Evening Transcript*, Oct. 20, 1874; Nov. 9, 1875; Dec. 2, 1878.

21 Boston Lying-in Hospital, *Annual Report for 1881*, quoted in *Boston Med. & Surg. J.*, 1882, *106*: 462.

22 Children's Hospital, *Appeal*, 1869, in P.&C.; *Boston Evening Transcript*, Oct. 28, 1876; April 1, 1881; Nov. 17, 1883.

23 Thernstrom does not classify census data for 1870 into these socioeconomic categories, so hospital figures for both 1870 and 1880 are compared to data for the general population derived from the 1880 census. Since Thernstrom finds very little change in the city's occupational structure from 1880 to 1920, this is not unreasonable. Stephan Thernstrom, *The Other Bostonians: Poverty and Progress in the American Metropolis, 1880–1970* (Cambridge, Mass.: Harvard Univ. Press, 1973), pp. 50, 51, 289–302.

24 The category of skilled workers in both 1870 and 1880 consisted entirely of Massachusetts General patients listed as "mechanics." This is an ambiguous term and appears to have been applied differently in 1870 and 1880. The number of patients in this category fell from 291 in 1870 to 219 in 1880. Over the same years there was a large jump in laborers (the whole of the unskilled category) from 187 to 580. This suggests that mechanics were not all skilled workers in 1870 and that their 41.9 percent of the male population over-represents skilled workers among the hospital's patients. At the same time, the figure of 26.9 percent may undercount the proportion of hospital patients who were unskilled in 1870. The M.G.H. admitted 780 males (85 un-

classified, all minors) in 1870 and 1,363 (235 unclassified) in 1880. Computed from M.G.H., *Annual Reports*.

25 Computed from B.C.H., *Annual Reports*.

26 Computed from M.G.H. and B.C.H., *Annual Reports*.

27 M.G.H., "The Report of a [trustees'] Committee on the Financial Condition of the M.G.H., February 16, 1865." The trustees dated their financial difficulties from the change from "the industrious classes of our native population," many of whom had paid something toward their board, to the foreign-born, who dramatically increased the numbers treated free. The trustees' committee recommended carefully restricting the number of nonpaying patients (read foreign-born) and segregating them in a distinct section of the hospital, so that the institution could get back to serving "the classes for whose advantage it was established." The trustees rejected that suggestion, apparently because of the urging of the medical staff which feared that decreasing the numbers of the really poor would hurt medical education. M.G.H. Trustees [printed letter], April 1, 1865, both in Countway Library; Bowditch, *M.G.H. History*, p. 454.

28 Computed from M.G.H., *Annual Reports*. In 1870, the United States Census listed 35.1 percent of Boston's population as foreign born.

29 Computed from B.C.H., *Annual Reports*.

30 Frances E. Kobrin, "The American midwife controversy: a crisis of professionalization," *Bull. Hist. Med.*, 1966, *40*: 350–363. [See pp. 217–225 in this book.]

31 Boston, Board of Health, *Annual Report for 1879*, p. 20.

32 New England Hospital for Women and Children, MSS Maternity Records, Vol. 1, in Countway Library; Computed from Boston Lying-in Hospital, *Annual Report for 1930*, p. 58; for St. Mary's, *Boston Med. & Surg. J.*, 1884, *110*: 363, 364.

33 Joseph Edgar Chamberlin, *The Boston Transcript: A History of its First Hundred Years* (Boston: Houghton Mifflin Co., 1930), p. 165.

34 *Boston Evening Transcript*, Feb. 24, 1888.

35 *Ibid.*

36 *Ibid.*

37 E.g., a long feature article, "The origin of hospitals," *ibid.*, July 13, 1886.

38 *Ibid.*, July 10, 1885. This account is of the McLean Asylum, a branch of the M.G.H.

39 *Ibid.*, Nov. 29, 1881.

40 Odin Anderson, *The Uneasy Equilibrium: Public and Private Financing of Health Services in the United States, 1875–1965* (New Haven: College and Univ. Press, 1968), p. 29.

41 Children's Hospital, *1st Annual Report, 1869*, p. 10.

42 *Boston Evening Transcript*, April 20, 1881.

43 Children's Hospital, *3rd Annual Report, 1871*, pp. 7, 8.

44 Charlestown *Chronicle*, Nov. 11, 1871; Boston *Post*, March 1, 1872; both in P.&C.

45 "The Children's Hospital: what 'Fireside' thinks about it," *Boston Evening Transcript*, Jan. 22, 1879.

46 Children's Hospital, *1st Annual Report, 1869*, p. 13; *3rd Annual Report, 1871*, pp. 8–10.

47 Children's Hospital, *8th Annual Report, 1876*, p. 8. It is perhaps unfair to draw so sharp a distinction between medicine and charity in this case. Koch's work was yet to come, and there was no hard medical knowledge of the transmission of tuberculosis.

48 Children's Hospital, *Appeal*, 1869, in P.&C.; Children's Hospital, *1st Annual Report, 1869*, p. 13.

49 Children's Hospital, *3rd Annual Report, 1871*, p. 10; *5th Annual Report, 1873*, p. 9. Young readers of the *Christian Register* were invited to come with their mothers to visit "the dear little occupants." *Christian Register*, May 8, 1869, June 5, 1869; in P.&C.

50 Children's Hospital, *1st Annual Report, 1869*, back cover; *15th Annual Report, 1883*, p. 9.

51 Children's Hospital, *1st Annual Report, 1869*, p. 13.

52 Boston *Post*, March 1, 1872, in P.&C.

53 "Fireside," *Boston Evening Transcript*, Jan. 22, 1879.

54 *Boston Med. & Surg. J.*, 1870, *83*: 140, 141, editorial; the hospital's founder doubled as the editor of the *Journal*.

55 Boston *Sunday Times*, Dec. 29, 1872, in P.&C.; letter to the editor, "My visit to the Children's Hospital," by "A Lady," *Boston Evening Transcript*, Feb. 22, 1875.

56 Boston *Post*, March 1, 1872, in P.&C.; Children's Hospital, *7th Annual Report, 1875*, p. 13.

57 Drs. James Jackson and John C. Warren, "Circular letter," [1810], in Bowditch, *M.G.H. History*, pp. 3–9.

58 Grace W. Myers, *History of the Massachusetts General Hospital: June, 1872 to December, 1900* (Boston: Griffith-Stillings Press, 1929), p. 12.

59 Dr. D. B. St. John Roosa described the visitors lining up at the gate for the twice weekly visiting hour at the New York Hospital, and how visitors were searched before entering. *The Old Hospital and Other Papers* 2nd ed. (New York: W. Wood & Co., 1889), p. 12.

60 E.g., M.G.H. Trustees MSS Records, Aug. 3, 1877, in M.G.H. archives.

61 "Fireside," *Boston Evening Transcript*, Jan. 22, 1879.

62 M.G.H., *Annual Reports, 1870–1910*.

63 *Boston Evening Transcript*, April 20, 1881.

64 Children's Hospital, *7th Annual Report, 1875*, p. 7; *Boston Evening Transcript*, Jan. 22, 1879; a letter

from a grateful parent, *Transcript*, Feb. 29 [*sic*], 1874.

65 Registrar's Report of the City of Boston, quoted in *Boston Med. & Surg. J.*, 1871, *85*: 83; *Boston Evening Transcript*, April 20, 1881.

66 Letter to the editor, *Boston Evening Transcript*, Feb. 29, 1888; Registrar's Report, in *Boston Med. & Surg. J.*, 1871, *85*: 84.

67 McDonald vs. M.G.H., 120 Mass. 432, in E. B. Callander, "Torts of hospitals," *Am. Law Rev.*, 1881, *15*: 640; *Boston Evening Transcript*, July 12, 1875.

68 Stogdale vs. Baker, reported in *Boston Evening Transcript*, Nov. 21, 1885, Dec. 12, 1887, Jan. 5, 1888.

14

The First Neighborhood Health Center Movement — Its Rise and Fall

GEORGE ROSEN

INTRODUCTION

Among aspects of urban life in modern times which have been regarded as conducive to social disease and decay, the connection between poverty and ill-health has long been recognized as a major focus of community concern and action. Awareness of the widespread prevalence of disease among the poor and of the inadequacy of the health care available to them has at various times motivated efforts to improve their health by providing more effective medical care. Historically, such concern has expressed itself in the creation of programs and facilities ranging from the dispensaries of the 18th century to the current neighborhood health centers.

Indeed, the latter grew out of a recognition that existing arrangements and programs in the United States were not satisfactorily meeting the complex health needs of the poor.[1] As a result, the neighborhood health center has been developed to remedy this situation by providing "a one-door facility, in which virtually all ambulatory health services are available; close coordination with other community resources; professional staff of high quality; and intensive participation by and involvement of the population to be served."[2] In these terms, the current wave of neighborhood health centers has been viewed by some as having brought forth a new institutional form. Yet neither the concept of providing health services on a local basis, nor the creation of facilities to deliver such care, nor the stated objectives of the neighborhood center are essentially new. The concept of a community health center providing service on a neighborhood basis, and its embodiment in organizational forms provided the core for a widespread movement which developed in the United States during the second and third decades of this century, reached its peak during the 30s, and then declined. Since the circumstances out of which this movement grew, the objectives at which it aimed, and the organizational forms it assumed are not unlike those characteristic of the neighborhood health center movement, an examination of the earlier movement may perhaps throw some light on the future possibilities of current trends.

URBANISM, IMMIGRATION, AND HEALTH

The roots of the health center movement, which began around 1910, are to be found in the changes which occurred in American society during the preceding decades. From 1860 to 1910 the urban portion of the population rose from 19 to 45 percent of the total, due in large measure to a flood of immigrants which poured into the cities and industrial towns where workers were in demand.[3] From about 1880 the majority of the immigrants came from southern and eastern Europe where they had left the backward, wretched circumstances of countryside and hamlet to seek a better life in the New World.[4] Some were skilled workers and craftsmen, a category which was largest among Jewish immigrants, of whom thousands entered the needle trades. A certain number of Italian immigrants also possessed skills adaptable to urban conditions, and some, particularly women, took jobs in the garment industry. Others entered service occupations or set up as shopkeepers or

---

George Rosen (1910–1977), distinguished pioneer in the social history of medicine, was Professor of the History of Medicine, and Epidemiology and Public Health, Yale University.

Reprinted with permission from the *American Journal of Public Health*, 1971, *61*: 1620–1635.

peddlers. As early as 1890, for example, most fruit peddlers and bootblacks in New York City were Italian, and not much later Italians were already heavily represented among waiters, barbers and shoemakers. Most immigrants, however, were unskilled and had to accept poorly paid jobs performing heavy manual work. But even those who were skilled worked excessively long hours for low wages under unhealthful conditions. Frequently they worked for their compatriots, often converting their dwellings into sweatshops.

Separated from the native Americans by language and custom, the immigrants crowded together in segregated neighborhoods where mutual aid and understanding were available. These neighborhoods were a geographic expression of the immigrants' endeavor to maintain their identity by living within a cultural environment in which they had roots, and from which they might make contact with and learn about the unfamiliar American world in which they found themselves. To the native American, however, the areas where these impoverished aliens congregated were loathsome, sickening slums whose denizens challenged and threatened the fabric of his social and psychological order. As early as 1883 Henry George, anticipating the end of the public domain viewed the flooding immigrant tide with alarm and asked "What in a few years are we to do for a dumping ground? Will it make our difficulties the less that our human garbage can vote?"[5] George was not alone in his opinion, which was echoed with numerous variations in succeeding decades. Robert A. Woods, a leading Boston social worker of the period, recoiled from the "unspeakable degraded standard of life" of the immigrants, while his collaborator Joseph Lee was amazed that this "human rubbish" produced a "number of physically, mentally and morally efficient citizens."[6]

The revulsion and dismay expressed in such statements are related to two reactions to the immigrants which clashed in principle but in practice tended to blend in various, sometimes ambiguous ways. One was a reaction to the differing lifestyles and values of the immigrants, comprising feelings of contempt, distrust and fear, as well as a sense that the alien masses were inferior and a menace. General antiforeign attitudes, views of foreigners as unruly and dangerous were refracted through specific ethnic or national stereotypes to which unfavorable characteristics and qualities were attributed.[7] This attitude found its more unsophisticated expression in the tendency to single out "wops," "sheenies," "polacks," "bohunks" or some other group as inherently criminal, avaricious or subversive.

But even those Americans who were sympathetic to the foreign-born were not completely exempt from the influence of the current stereotypes. In the early 1900s, the distinguished physician, Richard Cabot, examining his reactions to foreign-born patients at the Massachusetts General Hospital, noted that "the chances are ten to one that I shall look out of my eyes and see, *not* Abraham Cohen, but *a Jew* . . . I do not see *this* man at all. I merge him in the hazy background of the average Jew. But," he went on, "if I am a little less blind than usual to-day . . . I may notice something in the way his hand lies on his knee, something that is queer, unexpected. That hand- . . . it's a muscular hand, it's a prehensile hand; and whoever saw a Salem Street Jew with a muscular hand before? . . . I saw *him*. Yet he was no more real than the thousands of others whom I had seen and forgotten, — forgotten because I never saw *them*, but only their ghostly outline, their generic type, the racial background out of which they emerged."[8]

Cabot's self-analysis is an aspect of the other reaction to the immigrants, an aspect of an endeavor to come into close enough contact with them to learn about them as people, to begin to understand the stresses and strains to which they were exposed in an alien environment. This tendency appeared most prominently with the establishment of social settlements in the 1890s in the poorest sections of Chicago, New York, and other cities. Since these sections, the slums, were also overwhelmingly the foreign quarters, most of those with whom settlement dwellers worked were immigrants. The settlement workers soon became aware of the deep gulf which separated the poor immigrants from the larger society in which they lived, but to which they did not belong. Recognizing the need for social integration of the newer immigration with the older America, they set themselves the task, as Lillian Wald put it, of "fusing these people who come to us from the Old World Civilization into . . . a real brotherhood among men."[9]

For the most part, the settlements approached this task in practical, concrete terms. Recognizing that the influences to which the immigrants were subjected, and the treatment which they received after arrival, resulted in exploitation and neglect, they endeavored to prevent or repair the damage by turning to social action and dealing with specific problems such as economic exploitation, overcrowded and decrepit housing, destitution, broken homes, crime, alcoholism, prostitution and ill-health. The settlement dwellers worked largely on a local basis, directing their efforts and programs specifically at immigrant needs, at the needs of an oppressed minority. In so doing, they planted the seeds of a national social welfare program but their immediate concern was the neighborhood. This positive interest in the welfare of the immigrant poor went hand-in-hand with a desire to work with them, as well as for them, and also with a growing awareness that by accepting the cultural heritage and enhancing their self-respect, the slum dwellers were more likely to become involved in solving or ameliorating the problems of their group and their neighborhood.[10]

The great importance of health problems within this complex context was well-recognized. In 1909, Edward T. Devine,[11] a leading social worker, noted not only that "ill health is perhaps the most constant of the attendants of poverty," but he went on to emphasize that "An inquiry into the physical condition of the members of the families that ask for aid . . . clearly indicates that whether it be the first cause or merely a complication from the effect of other causes, physical disability is at any rate a very serious disabling condition at the time of application in three-fourths . . . of all the families that come under the care of the Charity Organization Society, who are probably in no degree exceptional among families in need of charitable aid."[12]

Activities in New York and Chicago also are indicative of the importance attached to health work among the poor immigrants. In 1893, Lillian D. Wald and Mary Brewster opened the Nurses' Settlement on Henry Street in New York in order to bring the benefits of public health nursing to an entire neighborhood. The Henry Street Settlement developed an organized community service intended to prevent disease, as well as to help the sick. As its program grew, involvement in studies of health and social welfare extended the influence of Henry Street far beyond the locality.[13]

Also in 1893, four years after Jane Addams opened Hull House, a public dispensary was organized at the settlement in Chicago. It was open every day from three to four in the afternoon and from seven to eight in the evening. There was also a physician in residence at Hull House, and another doctor who lived nearby helped out. A nurse from the Visiting Nurses' Association was stationed at the settlement, and received her orders there. In addition, various studies and programs were undertaken to improve health conditions in the neighborhood where the settlement was located. These involved improvement of housing and garbage collection, combatting cocaine addiction among minors, regulation of midwifery, studies of tuberculosis in relation to overcrowding, and of typhoid fever and poor sanitation.[14]

Thus, throughout the last decades of the 19th century and the early years of this century, the growing cities of the United States were increasingly confronted by the problems of poverty, crime, disease, and other attendant ills of the slums, problems most often associated with immigration.[15] The inescapable fact of these urban problems, plus a growing conviction of the need for social change led to a broad movement of reform dedicated to the eradication of demonstrable social ills and the realization of conditions for a better life through planned social action. From this standpoint campaigns were mounted to deal with a wide range of problems: poverty and dependency, tenement house reform, sweatshops, prostitution, juvenile delinquency, and others among which ill health was prominent as a cause or a consequence.[16]

COORDINATING HEALTH WORK

While these changes were taking place, the work of Pasteur, Koch, and their contemporaries had been answering some of the pertinent questions concerning the causation and prevention of communicable diseases, and this knowledge was being applied in public health programs. As a result, by the end of the first decade of this century, there was a solid basis for the control of a number of infectious diseases and throughout succeeding decades advances along this line continued.[17]

Alongside these trends, a shift was beginning to take place in the concept and orientation of community health action, a shift of attention from the environment to the individual. As health authorities and others became aware of noxious influences, other than those emanating from the physical environment, as activities in connection with maternal and child health, industrial hygiene, tuberculosis, venereal disease, and mental ill-health developed, public health expanded. As new areas of concern became a part of public health, new programs developed and new personnel were trained to execute them.[18] Increasing expansion of the scope of community health work created problems for official and voluntary health agencies. As more and more special programs, operated by separate personnel and often through special agencies, came into being, it also became increasingly clear that better ways of organizing and administering health work were needed.[19] It was recognized that there was a need for the coordination of hitherto separated agencies, facilities and services, many of which were concerned with the same population. Even within a single agency (such as a large urban health department), duplication of effort and lack of coordination among its constituent units were found both wasteful, inefficient and irritating to the people who needed the services. In 1914, S. S. Goldwater, the Health Commissioner of New York City, observed that "Various bureaus send their representatives into the same house, which results in undue expenditure of time and energy and in annoyance to the individual citizens."[20] A similar point of view was expressed by Charles F. Wilinsky in Boston. ". . . Gaps in the programs," he said, "duplication and consequent waste, frequent inefficiencies and misunderstandings, could not help but lead to the conclusion that there was a great need for better coordination and correlation, more efficient organization, and more harmonious understanding between those agencies concerned with the public health and with the amelioration of human suffering." He went on to add "that the fault of public health administration in large cities particularly was due to the fact that it was too far removed from the people it attempted to serve."[21]

Wilinsky's last remark touches on another factor which reinforced the tendency to develop local health work, namely, recognition that effective application of health programs, especially among the poor and the foreign-born, required an approach to the people on their own ground, in their neighborhood. By locating a service in the section where they lived, one avoided the necessity of drawing these people away from familiar streets and landmarks. Strangeness and distance, as well as language barriers and long waiting periods, were serious limiting factors in the use of health facilities such as dispensaries and hospitals.[22] As Michael M. Davis pointed out, long waits were particularly important for mothers, "when children must either be brought along or left at home in the care of a busy neighbor, or of children too young to take the responsibility."[23] Moreover, "the mother in her home, seldom, if ever, getting out to gatherings of any sort, is the hardest member of the immigrant group to reach, and often the slowest to give up her racial habits; yet in her position as homekeeper she has most to do with the health of her family. Taking our health work into her neighborhood is the surest way to get acquainted with her."[24]

Nevertheless, even such a localization of health and social services was not enough as long as the prospective users, the consumers, confronted a multiplicity of uncoordinated agencies in a situation where they were Alices in a Wonderland of confusing community resources. About the time of World War I, in East Harlem, in New York City, for example, there were many clinics, dispensaries, and district offices of welfare agencies, but the ordinary citizen had only the vaguest idea of what they did, what services they provided. Nor did he have any more precise notion of the service he needed. "He might be in trouble of some kind," wrote Homer Folks, "his health failing, or one of the children backward at school, or running afoul of the police, or the family just could not make ends meet. He needed assistance badly, somewhere, from somebody, but just what sort of help, or where to go to find it, or whether it could be had, were vague uncertainties. . . . Possibly he remembered having seen a sign somewhere in the locality or someone had told him that somebody had said that someone had been helped from an office on the north side of 116th Street near First Avenue. If of an optimistic and pioneering type, he bravely started on a voyage of discovery of what we call the social resources of the community.

"If his courage were strong, and his health not too bad, the needy person might persevere and by making the rounds, calling, on one office and clinic after another, and being referred from one agency to another, he might finally arrive at the place where he should have gone in the first instance for real help for his particular trouble." The consequences of this situation were frequently deplorable; ". . . the fact of not knowing just what was needed, nor just where to go, resulted on the part of the less enterprising, in not going anywhere. And, going nowhere and doing nothing meant that things went from bad to worse."[25]

An implicit consequence of this statement is that health and welfare agencies should, as far as possible, be brought together, perhaps under one roof. As settlement workers had already recognized, the problems for which poor people needed help were usually neither simple nor single and had no easy solutions. More often than not their health and social problems were closely linked, so that those endeavoring to solve them had to establish the closest possible collaboration. This point was explicitly underscored by Robert A. Woods. "The local health center," he wrote, "gathers under one head a group of services which in greater or lesser degree have been undertaken in the past by the settlement. In all their technical phases the settlement clearly and unquestionably must be ready to pass them over to the health center. It is however, equally clear — and this the promoters of the health centers do not always appreciate — that all the values of acquaintance and influence which the settlement has in its various organizations — must continue to be of indispensable importance to any sort of comprehensive local health campaign."[26] With this comment Woods touched upon another important dimension, the sociopsychological. Unless geographic localization and administrative coordination were complemented by social organization of the neighborhood with active participation of the population served, the fullest benefits of localized services would not be achieved. What was needed was a democratic educational process involving local people on an organized basis.

This aspect was most fully developed by Wilbur C. Phillips and his wife Elsie Cole Phillips.[27] The initial source for his idea of a community health plan was his experience as secretary of the New York Milk Committee established in 1907 by the Association for Improving the Condition of the Poor.[28] The objective of the committee was to reduce infant mortality in New York City by improving its milk supply, and seeing that babies received clean milk. Phillips undertook to achieve this aim by establishing infant milk depots throughout the city. This in itself was not new; the philanthropist Nathan Strauss had begun to establish a system of milk stations in 1893.[29] However, Phillips soon recognized that distribution of milk was not enough. Stimulated by the work of Pierre Budin, Professor of Obstetrics at Paris who, in 1892, established a system of infant consultation centers, and based on his own experience, by 1909, Phillips had developed a concept of the milk depot as a "centre of influence for child life" where babies could receive medical examinations, where mothers could be taught how to keep their babies well, and from which would "radiate the influences of education and social betterment."[30]

THE FIRST HEALTH CENTERS, 1910–1919

In 1911, this idea was expanded by Phillips in a Polish district of Milwaukee into a demonstration center for maternal and child care on a broad democratic basis using a so-called "block plan."[31] After resigning from the New York Milk Committee in 1910, he left for Milwaukee where implementation of his idea appeared feasible. Milwaukee had a high infant mortality, and seemed ready to deal with such problems in terms of basic social change, since it had recently elected a Socialist administration to office, the first large American city to do so. Phillips was then a member of the Socialist Party, having joined because as he says, "I knew at that time no other way of registering my opinion that poverty could and should be abolished — and that it could not be abolished through charity. But first, as the Socialists preached, came education — getting wider and wider numbers of people to understand the root causes of poverty and the way to remove them."[32]

In May 1911, at the instigation of Phillips, a nonpartisan Child Welfare Commission was appointed of which he became secretary. Its objective was to investigate the causes of infant mortality, and to formulate and carry out a plan of child welfare work from the standpoint of the entire community. By the end of the year the studies had been completed and a child health program based on a system of preventive health centers was proposed. This program was to be carried out by the municipality through its health department which would direct the work of social organization, promotion and education that was regarded as absolutely essential for the development of the child health program, and which the Phillipses had been doing. As a demonstration, they set up a child health station in a Polish area, comprising 33 city blocks with a population of 16,000 people and between 350 to 400 mothers and babies. The medical staff to provide the preventive consultations was selected by the physicians of the district, who also agreed on a fixed fee of two dollars to be paid each doctor for his period at the clinic. Cooperation of midwives and other local people was obtained. An unprecedented degree of support was obtained from the mothers by the creation of block committees headed by a block worker for each of the blocks in the demonstration area. This was the germ of the social unit idea which Phillips was then to try to implement in Cincinnati.

This was in the spring of 1912, but by June of that year, Wilbur Phillips and his wife were on their way to New York. Their activities had been upset by a change in the municipal administration. The Child Welfare Commission was terminated, and the child health program was limited to its purely medical aspects as part of a health department activity. But the idea of an "Educational Health Center" had been formulated, an idea which was to provide the basis for the Social Unit Organization, which in 1917 took form under Phillips' leadership in the Mohawk-Brighton district of Cincinnati. This was undertaken as a demonstration of the National Social Unit Organization created by Phillips in 1916, with headquarters in New York City. The purpose of this group was "to promote the type of democratic community organization through which the citizenship as a whole can participate directly in the control of community affairs, while at the same time making constant use of the highest technical skill available."[33]

After some deliberation, the Mohawk-Brighton district of Cincinnati was chosen for the purpose of carrying out a "social unit" community experiment on a large scale, and funds were made available by the national organization for a period of three years, with a certain proportion of the budget to be raised in Cincinnati. This city was chosen in large measure because Courtenay Dinwiddie, secretary of the Cincinnati Anti-Tuberculosis League (realizing the importance of community organization) worked hard to have the demonstration there. The league had developed plans in 1917 for a neighborhood health center through which its aims might be attained, and now felt that the Social Unit Plan was capable of achieving even more than their initial goals.

The demonstration was carried out in a neighborhood of some 15,000 inhabitants, of whom between 5 and 10 percent were recent immigrants.[34] The area was divided into 31 "blocks" of approximately 500 people each, and in each block, the residents over 18 years of age elected a council. This council elected a block worker who represented the residents of the block on the Citizens' Council of the unit. Her duties were to visit the families in her section, keep them in touch with the unit, and to bring specific problems they had to the proper department of the organization. The block worker was paid four dollars a week for the time lost from her household activities. Just as the Citizens' Council represented the people of the district, an Occupational Council secured the interest and cooperation of the various occupational and professional groups in the district, while the doctors, nurses, and social workers had their groups for the consideration of problems involved in their work. The Occupational Council was a neighborhood planning body working with other groups in the city. No new activities were undertaken until they had been endorsed by the people of the district through their representatives on the various councils. Most of the health and welfare agencies in Cincinnati, not only the Anti-Tuberculosis League, but also the Associated Charities, the Better Housing League and the Humane Society, cooperated with the Social Unit Organization.

The Cincinnati Social Unit demonstration was an experiment in applied democracy with health as its focal point. The health activities carried on included antepartum care, well child care for infants and preschool children, antituberculosis work, dental examination of school children, nursing service, medical care during the influenza epidemic of 1918, and periodic examination of adults. In short, beginning with health as a field of activity, Phillips and his coworkers endeavored to develop a consciously self-governing local unit in the midst of a large city. This enterprise was one of the most seminal experiments in social organization for health in the United States. It offered a vision of a community in which citizens working together as members of a vitally cooperating group sought the common welfare rationally and intelligently. It also raised profound political and social questions which are still unresolved. Can such a vision be realized in the heart of a large urban center? Can its inhabitants become truly conscious of mutual interests and be, in some degree, self-governing? Do such aims require a stable population, and how can such stability be maintained?

The Cincinnati experiment answered some but not all the questions. Opposition to it developed from the Director of Public Welfare, the newly elected mayor, a local medical society and various conservatives who charged that the Social Unit demonstration was a Red plot, a not uncommon occurrence in the supercharged patriotic atmosphere at the end of World War I. Although an investigation of the charges showed that they were unfounded, and a referendum within the Mohawk-Brighton district revealed a strong sentiment for the demonstration, the municipal administration withdrew its support, the funds that had been pledged were not forthcoming, and by 1920 the Social Unit demonstration was over. Without political and economic leverage, the inhabitants of the district could hardly make their wants felt. Phillips had not adequately established a financial basis nor had there been adequate time to create a political power base. The demonstration raised questions but provided only partial or ambiguous answers.

Meanwhile, efforts had been made elsewhere to provide health services to a definite population on a local basis. In 1912, William C. White, a physician and medical director of the Tuberculosis League of Pittsburgh, tried such an approach to tuberculosis control. As his model, he took the district system of the public schools. "In the educational field," he said, "there has gradually developed a knowledge of the equipment necessary for a given population, and this equipment has been apportioned so as to be readily accessible to those whom it is to serve. The management of these units is centered in a legally constituted governing body which also controls the expenditure of funds collected by taxation. The same form of control is applicable to tuberculosis and other health problems."[35] However, White's scheme lasted only six months. That year also saw an effort in Philadelphia by Samuel M. Hamill, a physician, to apply the same idea to child health work creating a basis for a growing program. Broader and more enduring efforts were also undertaken in New York, Boston, and Buffalo.

In 1913, the New York Milk Committee established a health center on the lower West Side of Manhattan to serve a district populated largely by Syrians and Irish-Americans, where housing was poor and medical resources were limited.[36] The Bowling Green Neighborhood Association composed of local residents and outside specialists was formed to administer the center which provided chiefly antepartum and infant care. Neighborhood associations composed of voluntary groups of citizens were not new in New York City and many of them had worked with the Health Department in one way or another.[37]

S. S. Goldwater, Health Commissioner of New York, was aware of these developments and in September 1914 formulated a plan to apply the principle of localization to health administration in order to see how far the work of the department could "be improved by the substitution of a system of local or district administration for the present purely functional administrations."[38] To answer this question an experimental health district was established by January 1915 on the lower East Side of Manhattan in an area populated almost entirely by Jews.[39] The district comprised a highly congested area of 21 blocks housing 25,000 people. The staff comprised a part-time district health officer in full charge of local administration, a part-time medical inspector who was responsible for medical inspection of preschool and school children as well as the infants' milk station, three nurses and one nurses' assistant, a food inspector and a sanitary inspector, both part-time. The basic principles underlying district work were coordination of health department functions, local administration in terms of local needs, and establishment of a community spirit. In accordance with the latter point, the health officer of the district was a Jewish physician who understood the people, their language, backgrounds and characteristics.

The experiment proved so satisfactory that on May 1, 1916, it was extended by Haven Emerson, (Health Commissioner from 1915 to 1917), to Queens, where four health districts were opened (Long Island City, Flushing, Ridgewood, and Jamaica). In 1916, there was also created within the Health Department a Division of Health Districts under the Deputy Commissioner of Health, and in 1917 the district health officers were placed on a full-time basis.[40] Unfortunately, at this time, there was a change in the city government, and the new administration slipped smoothly back into the established rut of the *status quo ante*. Among other actions, it halted the plans to extend district health administration to other parts of the city, and it was not until more than 12 years later that district health centers were established on a more solid basis in New York. Nevertheless, experience had been gained for such a program, and some advantages to be derived from decentralized public health administration were demonstrated. For example, as a consequence of the coordination of services, it was possible to serve families more efficiently, with all services rendered to a family provided by a single nurse. This led to the introduction of a Family Record Card which contained a continuous history of the family as far as Health Department services were concerned. However, this abortive attempt to apply the principle of local administration to health work in New York City brought forth a problem which was to plague the revived district system in 1930s, namely, the division of responsibility and the relationships between the district health officers and the chiefs of the central functional bureaus of the department.

During this period, health departments and private health and welfare agencies in a number of American cities and towns undertook to coordinate their activities on a localized basis and to develop neighborhood health centers and programs. In 1916, on the initiative of Charles F. Wilinsky, Deputy Health Commissioner of Boston (who has been referred to above), the Blossom Street Health Unit was opened in the West End, one of the most congested sections of the city.[41] The objective was to provide a local center from which agencies engaged in health and welfare work could serve a geographically defined population. Among the agencies included in the center were the Consumptives Hospital Department, the Instructive District Nursing Association, the Milk and Baby Hygiene Association, the visiting physician of the Boston Dispensary, and the Hebrew Federated Charities. Later additions were clinics for dental care and mental health counseling. Eventually, Boston had eight centers, each serving a population of 50,000. This expansion was assisted by a bequest by George Robert White of six million dollars to the city of Boston for this purpose.

Similar developments occurred in other large cities. Beginning with one experimental station in 1914, Buffalo developed a citywide system of district services. By 1920 there were seven districts of 26,000 to 91,000 population (average about 75,000) with a center in each. The system represented a cooperative arrangement between the Department of Health and the Department of Hospitals and Dispensaries. Arrangements and proceedings were also worked out to govern relationships with private medical and social agencies. Basically this system was intended for the poor people of the city, and the districts were correlated with the existing tracts covered by the Charity Organization Society.[42]

HEALTH CENTERS SPREAD

As C.-E. A. Winslow noted in 1919, "The most striking and typical development of the public health movement of the present day is the health center."[43] World War I had emphasized the possibilities of coordinated effort in achieving results, as well as the importance of health, and these lessons were not lost on community leaders. When the war ended, health centers and demonstrations financed by foundations, voluntary health agencies, or other social welfare organizations, as well as by local governments were established in many parts of the United States. A decision by the American Red Cross at the end of the war to further the establishment of health centers gave additional impetus to this trend.[44] Local chapters undertook to create health centers, and more generally such facilities became the fashion in community health work.

The scope of this development is evident from the following figures obtained by the Red Cross during the latter part of 1919 in a survey of existing and planned health centers.[45] The report showed that as of January 1, 1920, there were 72 centers in 49 communities, of which seven cities had more than one center. In addition to the existing centers, 33 centers were being proposed or planned in 28 other communities. An analysis of the existing and proposed centers showed that at the time of the report, 33 were administered entirely by public authorities, 27 were under private control, and 16 were under combined public and private control. The Red Cross was involved in 19 instances. There was considerable variation in the work and aims of the existing health centers. In 40 communities with health centers in operation, 37 contained clinics of some type, 34 carried on visiting nursing, 29 did child welfare work, and 27 did anti-tuberculosis work. Twenty-two had venereal disease clinics, 14 had dental clinics, and 11 had eye, ear, nose and throat clinics. Only 10 had laboratories, and 9 had milk stations.

The succeeding decades witnessed a further development of health centers and districting of health services. In 1930, a subcommittee on health centers collected information for the White House Conference on Child Health and Protection. It obtained data for 1,511 major and minor health centers throughout the United States. Eighty percent had been established since 1910. Of the total number, 725 were operated by private agencies, 729 by county or municipal health departments, and a small number by the Red Cross, hospitals, tuberculosis associations, case-work agencies and the like. In nearly half these centers, the principal support came from public funds, while supplementary aid came through community chests, or from private funds.

As is not infrequently the case when a professional development or trend is in "fashion," the name by which it is designated acquires an aura of approval, and is used to describe activities and enterprises that differ widely, so that they may share some of the aura. This was also the fate of the health center concept, and is in part responsible for its decline. As one observer put it in 1921, "We find it used as a name for child welfare stations, tuberculosis dispensaries, venereal disease clinics, out-patient departments of hospitals, settlement houses, and substations of local health departments."[46] The Red Cross concept of a health center was that of an institution which could be locally operated with a minimum of outside direction and with an emphasis on its function as an educational, informational facility. "Functionally, the health center is an institution through which the community may get in touch with all health promoting agencies and with the health problems of local and of national importance."[47] Administratively, however, the Red Cross view was that the health center should be under the combined guidance and control of all the local health agencies.

Michael M. Davis, writing in 1927, defined the health center more definitely and related it more specifically to health care, both preventive and curative. "Observation of a large number of health centers," he said, "leads to an indication of two factors which all those studied appeared to present: first, the selection of a definite district, or of a population unit, with the aim of serving all therein who need the services offered; second, coordination of services within this area, embracing both the facilities furnished by the health center itself and those provided by other agencies. A definition might therefore be stated as follows: A health center is an organization which provides, promotes and coordinates needed medical service and related social service for a specified district."[48] Davis also emphasized that there were still many unanswered questions concerning policy, objectives, organization, administration and evaluation of health centers. For example, he asked, "How far is organization of the people of a district themselves a practical means of promoting the services at the center, and of advancing health education throughout the district? Experience shows great value in a loose local organization of agencies interested in medical or health work, in education, especially public and parochial schools, and neighborhood and recreational bodies. On the other hand, the attempt to organize the people of a district into a local council, with or without block workers, has generally yielded little result in proportion to the effort expended. The reasons for this difficulty lie deep in the characteristics of American neighborhood life, whether among native or foreign born."[49]

Meanwhile, significant district health programs were created and developed in a number of

American communities. It is obviously impossible to discuss those developments in detail, but several selected examples can indicate some of their characteristics. In New York City a program of district health administration was developed after 1929, and a group of health centers was opened beginning with one in rented quarters in central Harlem. Actually, this program grew out of two demonstrations in the 1920s. The East Harlem Health Center was initiated in 1920 by the New York County chapter of the Red Cross, and was opened in November 1921. The demonstration was planned as a three-year project involving the cooperation of the Health Department and 21 voluntary agencies, and was described as a "department store of health and welfare,"[50] where clients could find under one roof almost all the health and welfare services needed. Throughout the decade the Health Center continued to develop, and eventually became one of the municipal district health units. While East Harlem was the first general health center, the Bellevue-Yorkville Health Demonstration, organized in 1924 and opened to the public in 1926, led eventually to the adoption by New York City of the principle of district health administration.[51] Financed by the Milbank Memorial Fund and the Health Department, the demonstration was carried on for ten years in cooperation with a very large number of participating official and voluntary agencies.[52] With the example of two health centers in operation, and under pressure from leaders in the private health and welfare field, the Health Department developed a citywide plan of district administration, with a health center building in each district serving as a local headquarters for both private health and welfare agencies and for the field activities of the department. In 1934, under the administration of Fiorello H. La Guardia, the city embarked on a program of districting which has had its ups and down over the years — but is still in existence at present. Owing to changing policies and intramural conflicts the potential of this system was never fully realized.

Plans initially started by William H. Welch in Baltimore in the 20s eventuated in 1932 in the establishment of the Eastern Health District as a cooperative endeavor of the Baltimore City Health Department, the Johns Hopkins School of Hygiene and Public Health, as well as several voluntary agencies. This district has made possible the intensive study of public health problems and has provided a field laboratory for the testing of new administrative procedures and for the training of personnel. A second district was organized in 1935.

The district health center, coordinating hitherto separated clinics and services, was inaugurated to replace centralized control of particular services. Generally, the health center has been a branch or unit of a local health department or some other official health agency. Except for such diseases as tuberculosis, venereal diseases and a few other conditions considered as public health problems, most medical care concerned with diagnosis and therapy remained outside the sphere of activity of health centers, which emphasized prevention. Far-sighted leaders in the health field realized that the health center concept might be employed to improve the organization and provision of medical care, issues which had come to the forefront of public attention at the same time as the health center. The Social Unit experiment in Cincinnati had touched on this problem, as did J. L. Pomeroy, the County Health Officer of Los Angeles, in his ambitious program undertaken in 1919.[53] In his centers, Pomeroy originally included clinics staffed by physicians, nurses and social workers to provide preventive and curative services on an ambulatory basis. The clinics were available to the poor whose eligibility was established by a means test. Due largely to the complaints of physicians that medical care was being given to patients who should go to private practitioners, by 1935 this work had, for the most part been turned over to the Welfare Department and the county general hospital. This attempt foundered on the slogan that undeserving individuals were abusing the service intended only for the indigent, a theme which has been played with variations for about one hundred years.[54]

The most imaginative approach was made by Hermann Biggs in 1920 when he endeavored to deal with health service for rural areas in New York State.[55] As Commissioner of Health, he proposed the establishment of local health centers to include one or more of the following elements: hospital, clinics (for tuberculosis, venereal diseases, prenatal and child care, mental illness, dental care, and general medical care), laboratories, public health nursing, and district health administration.

Such centers could be established in any county with the approval of the State Health Commissioner. The proposal was permissive and not mandatory in any of its details. In addition to coordinating public health services, these centers were intended "to encourage and provide facilities for an annual medical examination to detect physical defects and disease"; and "to provide for the residents of rural districts, for industrial workers and all others in need of such service, scientific medical and surgical treatment, hospital and dispensary facilities and nursing care at a cost within their means or, if necessary, free." State aid in the form of 50 percent cash grants for buildings, a cash allowance for the treatment of patients unable to pay, together with certain allowances toward maintenance, were to be furnished to all communities fulfilling the requirements of the State Health Department. While a large number of community organizations supported these proposals, the Sage-Machold Bill which embodied this health center program, was defeated in the New York legislature. The whole concept was ahead of public opinion, and especially of opinion in the medical profession.

Biggs had realized that the next step in the development of community health services required a coalescence of preventive and curative medicine. Since 1920, this seminal concept has evolved in several directions. Among these the idea of comprehensive group practice coupled with prepayment, as exemplified by the Kaiser-Permanente Foundation and the Health Insurance Plan of Greater New York, has been demonstrated as practicable. Another approach was promoted by Joseph W. Mountin, of the U.S. Public Health Service, based on his belief that hospitals and health departments must eventually combine or coordinate their facilities and resources to provide a comprehensive health service for the communities they serve. As part of such a plan, he proposed to correlate the health center with the general hospital in the community.

After 1946, following the passage of the Hill-Burton Act, there was a renewal of the earlier interest in the role of the health center. A proponent of the idea who tied it to regionalization was John B. Grant of the Rockefeller Foundation. In fact, in 1949, he pointed out that the health center of the future had not yet been established.[56] Nevertheless, such centers did not really take hold after the 1940s.

WHY DID THE HEALTH CENTER MOVEMENT DECLINE?

The concept of a local health center had developed largely in response to the circumstances and the needs of the urban poor, particularly the immigrants. From the time of World War I, however, these elements were changing, especially during the decades of the 20s and the 30s. Consequently, the time setting in which the movement for local health centers emerged and became institutionalized is important for understanding its further development.

The cessation of immigration during the war years and the restrictive legislation of 1921 and 1924 were undoubtedly important factors in changing the circumstances of the foreign-born. As the flow of new immigrants was cut down to a trickle, the foreign-born and even more so their children adapted to American life under the influence of economic and educational factors.[57] As they moved up the economic ladder, there was an increasing tendency to move out of the areas of initial settlement and toward the periphery of the community. Between 1920 and 1930 there appeared to be a growing trend toward less clustering of the foreign-born in ethnic neighborhoods. Movements within the cities and towards suburbs scattered members of these groups in areas that were mixed. Many of those involved in this process were younger persons of the second generation, largely native-born, with a greater earning capacity than their parents or older families with few children below working age. Hand-in-hand with these changes went higher levels of schooling among the children of the foreign-born and a wider use of English by their parents, changes clearly reflected in the foreign language press of the period.

As this potential clientele for local health centers changed its character, it turned more and more to the use of private health care. This tendency was reinforced by the limited nature of the services provided in most local health centers. Thus, there was practically no integration of preventive and curative services. As Michael Davis saw in 1921, "curative work furnishes the best approach to preventive" service. "In the field of preventive medical and health work," he said, "there is particular need for emphasizing . . . that the study of people must run parallel to the study of technique. As a corollary to this, curative work must be connected with preventive work, so that the service which the people seek of their own initiative can be supplemented by the service which we believe the larger interests of all require."[58] Therapeutic services were provided only to a limited degree, for the most part to patients with tuberculosis and venereal disease. At the same time medical practice was changing. Immunization, antepartum care and well child care were incorporated into the work of the private practitioner, and this was to happen later with the treatment of tuberculosis and venereal disease when the antibiotics became available.

The Depression of the 1930s retarded these tendencies, but they were reinforced indirectly as the attention of many concerned with the provision of medical care and its costs turned to the problem of organizing the financing of such care on a compulsory or voluntary basis. The improvement of economic conditions toward the end of the decade coincident with the outbreak of World War II made it financially possible for more people to seek private medical care, especially when labor-management negotiations provided varying forms of health insurance. Thus, the local health centers tended to lose one part of the rationale for their creation.

The same period also saw the erosion of another part of the theoretical underpinning of the health center movement. Need for coordination of health and welfare services had been adduced as a reason for bringing them together under one roof or at least in close contiguity. However, the role of social agencies changed greatly during the Depression as government, particularly on the federal level, assumed a larger and more active part in welfare, specifically in its financial aspects. At the same time social work was beginning to move away from an interest in social problems and reform. Case work became the dominant facet of social work, and in turn social work focused on the individual, on his personal strengths and weaknesses, and on individual psychological mechanisms, with psychoanalysis providing a theoretical rationale for this orientation.[59] Along this line of development, social agencies withdrew from health centers to other locations where they could centralize their therapeutic services and utilize them more efficiently.

In addition to the factors discussed above, there were a number of others that hindered the development of health centers and led to the decline of the movement. Thus, despite the often expressed aim of involving the local population in the neighborhood health program, this goal was hardly realized and remained more of a pious intention. Although Bellevue-Yorkville in New York City may have been envisaged as an experiment to crystallize community consciousness around health as a center, the demonstration was actually run by a group of voluntary health and welfare agencies, financed by a foundation in collaboration with the municipal health department.[60] In the New Haven Health Center Demonstration (1920–1923), efforts to develop active participation by local people were admittedly unsuccessful, mainly because the necessary rapport was not established with the largely Italian population.[61]

Another negative factor was the resistance by political forces in the broadest sense. The ability of government (municipal or state) to hinder or to facilitate the creation and development of health center programs is evident from the examples of Milwaukee, Cincinnati, and New York. Antagonism of professional groups such as physicians or welfare agencies were significant in some cases. Administrative infighting within the municipal health department was a factor in weakening the New York City health center program, and such a factor may have been operative elsewhere. Finally, one should note that the health center movement participated in the general pattern of development of public health during this period. In the late 1930s public health was beginning to approach the end of a period of development that had begun around the first decade of the century. World War II was an interlude in this transition which is still in process. By that time, however, the health center movement had run out of steam.

QUESTIONS?

Analysis of the earlier health center movement raises certain questions about the current neighborhood health centers. These too have come into being to provide for the needs of the urban poor, of people who have migrated to the city and who live under circumstances highly adverse to health. These centers clearly fill an immediate need, and no doubt fulfill their purpose better than did the earlier centers.[62] Today they are located in impoverished areas. But what should happen if and when the economic status of the population changes? One aim of the centers is job training, which implies a change in economic condition. Is it not possible that improved economic circumstances may lead to a shift of population, and thus to a loss of health center clientele? Or is there an unexpressed assumption that the poor will always be with us and a separate system is needed for them? Furthermore, should neighborhood centers remain purely local, or should they become part of a larger system of health care toward which we appear to be moving? Should they become part of a national health insurance system and of a larger health-care delivery system? Obviously, such questions have no immediate answer, but they do arise from a consideration of the earlier local health center movement.

NOTES

On April 14, 1971, this paper was presented to the John Shaw Billings History of Medicine Society, Indiana University School of Medicine, Indianapolis, Indiana. This paper is also based in part on the author's experience as a clinic diagnostician in the Bureau of Tuberculosis, as a district health officer and Borough health officer in the Office of District Health Administration, and as the director of the Bureau of Health Education in the New York City Department of Health (1940–1943, 1946–1950)

1 Sar A. Levitan, *The Great Society's Poor Law. A New Approach to Poverty* (Baltimore: Johns Hopkins Press, 1969), pp. 191–197.

2 Lisbeth Bamberger, "Health care and poverty: what are the dimensions of the problem from the community's point of view?" *Bull. N.Y. Acad. Med.*, 1966, *42*: 1140.

3 U.S. Bureau of the Census, *Historical Statistics of the United States: Colonial Times to 1957* (Washington, D.C.: Government Printing Office, 1960).

4 For the following see Moses Rischin, *The Promised City: New York's Jews, 1870–1914* (Cambridge, Mass.: Harvard Univ. Press, 1962); Hutchins Hapgood, *The Spirit of the Ghetto* (Cambridge, Mass.: Belknap-Harvard Univ. Press, 1967); Giuseppe Prezzolini, *I Trappiantati* (Milan: Longanesi, 1963), pp. 401–430; Phyllis H. Williams, *South Italian Folkways in Europe and America* (New Haven: Yale Univ. Press, 1938); Robert E. Park and Herbert A. Miller, *Old World Traits Transplanted* (New York: Harper & Bros., 1921). The literature on this theme is large and the above references are simply illustrative.

5 Henry George, *Social Problems* (New York, 1886), pp. 40–46, 161–162.

6 Barbara M. Solomon, *Ancestors and Immigrants. A Changing New England Tradition* (Cambridge, Mass.: Harvard Univ. Press, 1956). Quotation is from the edition published by John Wiley & Sons, 1965, pp. 140–141.

7 John Higham, *Strangers in the Land. Patterns of American Nativism, 1860–1925* (1955) (New York: Atheneum, 1963), pp. 88–94.

8 Richard C. Cabot, *Social Service and the Art of Healing* (1909) (New York: Dodd, Mead & Co., 1931), pp. 4–7.

9 R. L. Duffus, *Lillian Wald: Neighbor and Crusader* (New York, 1939), p. 147.

10 Jane Addams, "Hull House: an effort toward social democracy," *Forum*, 1892, *14*: 226; Jane Addams et al., *Philanthropy and Social Progress: Seven Essays* (New York, 1893), pp. 2–3, 15–16, 35–38; Lillian D. Wald, *The House on Henry Street* (New York: Henry Holt & Co., 1915), pp. 66, 184, 290, 310; Frank J. Bruno, *Trends in Social Work . . . 1874–1946* (New York, 1948).

11 Edward Thomas Devine (1867–1948) was General Secretary of the Charity Organization Society in New York City, 1896–1912, and Secretary until 1917; Director of the New York School of Philanthropy, 1904–1907, 1912–1917, and from 1905 to 1919 Professor of Social Economy at Columbia University.

12 Edward Thomas Devine, *Misery and Its Causes* (New York: Macmillan Company, 1910), p. 55. See the section on ill health in this book, pp. 53–112.

13 Wald, *The House on Henry Street*; Lillian D. Wald, *Windows on Henry Street* (Boston: Little, Brown & Co., 1934).

14 *Hull House Maps and Papers. A Presentation of Nationalities and Wages in a Congested District of Chicago, together with Comments and Essays on Problems Growing Out of the Social Conditions by Residents of Hull House* (New York and Boston: Thomas Y. Crowell, 1895), p. 228; Jane Addams, *Twenty Years at Hull House* (New York: Macmillan, 1910), pp. 342–358.

15 Kate H. Claghorn, "The foreign immigrant in New York City." In *United States Industrial Commission: Reports on Immigration* (Washington, D.C., 1901), XV, 449 ff.; see also *Harper's Weekly*, Jan. 12, 1895, pp. 42, 60–62, and June 22, 1895, pp. 586–587.
16 George Rosen, *A History of Public Health* (New York: MD Publications, 1958), pp. 344–349.
17 *Ibid.*, pp. 319–343.
18 "Health and national efficiency," *Modern Med.*, 1919, *1*: 2–3; H. W. Hill, "The new public health," *Ibid.*, 1919, *1*: 57–58.
19 Michael M. Davis, *Immigrant Health and the Community* (New York: Harper & Brothers, 1921), pp. 406–407.
20 *Annual Report of the Department of Health of the City of New York for the Calendar Year 1914* (New York, 1915), p. 25. *The House that Health Built. A Report of the First Three Years' Work of the East Harlem Health Center Demonstration, prepared under the Direction of Kenneth D. Widdemer* (New York, 1925), p. 4.
21 *The Health Units of Boston, 1924–1933* (City of Boston Printing Department, 1933), quoted in I. V. Hiscock, "The development of neighborhood health services in the United States," *Milbank Mem. Fund Quart. Bull.*, 1935, *13*: 30–51, p. 35.
22 Davis, *Immigrant Health*, p. 299.
23 *Ibid.*, p. 329.
24 *Ibid.*, p. 299.
25 Homer Folks, Preface, *House that Health Built*, p. 3.
26 Robert A. Woods, *The Neighborhood in Nation-Building* (Boston and New York: Houghton Mifflin Co., 1923), p. 279.
27 Wilbur C. Phillips, *Adventuring for Democracy* (New York: Social Unit Press, 1940). Unfortunately, Phillips rarely dates the events he describes so that the evolution of his activities and ideas has had to be reconstructed from other sources indicated below.
28 Charles E. North, "Milk and its relation to public health," in *A Half Century of Public Health*, ed. Mazyck P. Ravenel (New York: American Public Health Association, 1921), pp. 279–280; William H. Allen, "Health needs and civic action," in *The Public Health Movement* (Philadelphia: American Academy of Political and Social Science, 1911), pp. 3–12, see p. 7.
29 Rosen, *History of Public Health*, pp. 354–355.
30 Wilbur C. Phillips, "The achievements and future possibilities of the New York Milk Committee," *Proceedings of the Child Conference for Research and Welfare, 1909, Clark University, Worcester, Mass., July 6–10, 1909* (New York: G. E. Stechert & Co., 1910), pp. 189–192.
31 Wilbur C. Phillips, "The trend of medico-social effort in child welfare work," *Am. J. Public Hlth.*, 1912, *2*: 875–882, see pp. 881–882; Phillips, *Adventuring for Democracy*, pp. 46–47, 55–56, 63–114.
32 Phillips, *Adventuring for Democracy*, pp. 59–60.
33 A. C. Burnham, *The Community Health Problem* (New York: Macmillan Co., 1920), p. 108.
34 N. A. Nelson, "Neighborhood organization vs. tuberculosis," *Modern Med.*, 1919, *1*: 515–521; Courtenay Dinwiddie and A. G. Kreidler, "A community self-organized for preventive health work," *Modern Med.*, 1919, *1*: 26–31. Wilbur C. Phillips, "Democracy and the unit plan," *Proceedings of the National Conference of Social Work, Atlantic City, New Jersey, June 1–8, 1919* (National Conference of Social Work, 1920), p. 562.
35 William C. White, "The official responsibility of the state in the tuberculosis problem," *J.A.M.A.*, 1915, *65*: 512–514.
36 Davis, *Immigrant Health*, p. 381.
37 Shirley W. Wynne, "Neighborhood health development in the City of New York," *Milbank Mem. Fund Quart. Bull.*, 1931, *9*: 37–45.
38 *Annual Report of the Department of Health of the City of New York for the Calendar Year 1914* (New York, 1915), p. 25.
39 Davis, *Immigrant Health*, pp. 381–384. According to Herbert Kaufman, *The New York City Health Centers* (Inter-University Case Program #9) (Indianapolis: Bobbs-Merrill Co., 1959), the population was 35,000.
40 *Annual Report of the Department of Health of the City of New York for the Calendar Year 1916* (New York, 1917), pp. 23, 31; *Annual Report of the Department of Health of the City of New York for the Calendar Year 1917* (n.p., n.d.), pp. 12–13; Hiscock, "Development of neighborhood health services in the United States," pp. 38–39.
41 Charles F. Wilinsky, "The Blossom Street health unit," *Nation's Hlth.*, 1924, *6*: 397–398; Charles F. Wilinsky, "The health center," *Am. J. Public Hlth.*, 1927, *17*: 677–682.
42 Michael M. Davis, *Clinics, Hospitals and Health Centers* (New York: Harper & Brothers, 1927), pp. 354–355; Hiscock, "Development of neighborhood health services," p. 48.
43 [C.-E. A. Winslow], "The health center movement," *Modern Med.*, 1919, *1*: 327.
44 Burnham, *Community Health Problem*, pp. 99–100; E. A. Peterson and W. H. Brown, "The American Red Cross and health," *Nation's Hlth.*, 1921, *3*: 73–80.
45 James A. Tobey, "The health center movement in the United States," *Modern Hosp.*, 1920, *14*: 212–214.
46 Peterson and Brown, "American Red Cross," p. 79.

47 E. A. Peterson, "What is a health center?" *Nation's Hlth.*, 1921, *3*: 272–274.

48 Michael M. Davis, "Goal-post and yardsticks in health center work," *Am. J. Public Hlth.*, 1927, *17*: 433–440, p. 434.

49 *Ibid.*, p. 439.

50 *House that Health Built*, p. 4; *A Decade of District Health Center Pioneering, A Report of Ten Years Work of the East Harlem Center* (New York City, 1932), p. 23; George R. Bedinger, "Cooperative Health Plan in New York County," *Nation's Hlth.*, 1921, *3*: 486–489.

51 C.-E. A. Winslow and Savel Zimand, *Health Under the "El"* (New York & London: Harper & Brothers, 1937).

52 The exact number seems uncertain, but was probably close to 70. According to Hiscock there were 85, according to Kaufman about 65.

53 J. L. Pomeroy, "County health administration in Los Angeles," *Am. J. Public Hlth.*, 1921, *11*: 796–800; J. L. Pomeroy, "Health center development in Los Angeles County," *J.A.M.A.*, 1929, *93*: 1546–1550.

54 George Rosen, The impact of the hospital on the patient, the physician and the community," *Hosp. Admin.*, 1964, *9*: 15–33.

55 Milton Terris, "Hermann Biggs' contribution to the modern concept of health centers," *Bull. Hist. Med.*, 1946, *20*: 387–412; B. R. Rickards, "What New York State has done in health centers," *Am. J. Public Hlth.*, 1921, *11*: 214–216.

56 John B. Grant, "Health care for the community," *Selected Papers*, ed. Conrad Seipp (Baltimore: Johns Hopkins Press, 1963), pp. 5–6, 21–24, and *passim*.

57 *Recent Social Trends in the United States. Report of the President's Research Committee on Social Trends* (New York: McGraw-Hill, 1933), pp. 469, 560, 563–564, 582; John C. Gebhart, *The Health of a Neighborhood. A Social Study of the Mulberry District* (New York Association for Improving the Condition of the Poor, 1924), pp. 5–7.

58 Davis, *Immigrant Health*, p. 419.

59 George Rosen, *Madness in Society. Chapters in the Historical Sociology of Mental Illness* (Chicago: Univ. of Chicago Press, 1968), pp. 310–312.

60 Winslow and Zimand, *Health Under the "El,"* pp. 11–13, 38–48.

61 Philip S. Platt, *Report on New Haven Health Center Demonstration July 1920–June 1923* (n.p., n.d.), pp. 21–23, 98.

62 Gerald Sparer, "Evaluation of OEO neighborhood health centers," *Am. J. Public Hlth.*, 1971, *61*: 931–942.

Allied Professions

Although physicians have traditionally stood at the head of the healing arts, they have, for at least a century or so, shared many health care responsibilities with others: dentists, midwives, nurses, optometrists, podiatrists, pharmacists, psychologists, and various therapists and technicians. The division of labor among these diverse occupational groups seems at times to defy logic. Why, for example, did the treatment of most of the body evolve into medical specialties controlled by physicians, while the care of the teeth and feet fell to practitioners outside the medical profession? History provides some clues.

During the second quarter of the 19th century a handful of physician-dentists sought to turn their field into a medical specialty, like surgery or ophthalmology. But their suggestion that dentistry be included in the medical curriculum met with the response that it was too mechanical. After all, dentists filled and extracted teeth; they did not heal them. Rebuffed by their erstwhile colleagues, these dentists about 1840 founded their own society, started their own journal, and opened their own school, the Baltimore College of Dental Surgery. Within a few decades American dentistry was preeminent in the world, far surpassing American medicine in international repute.

Podiatry, also known as chiropody, developed from a similar quasi-medical background. When doctors specializing in the care and treatment of the feet urged medical schools at the turn of the 20th century to assume responsibility for training in this area, deans turned them away with the comment that corns and bunions were too trivial to warrant such attention. So with the medical profession's blessing, podiatrists, like dentists a half-century earlier, set up their own institutions.

Optometry and pharmacy trace their roots not primarily to medicine but to the business of drug selling and "spec" peddling. Over the years both professions worked out reasonably harmonious divisions of labor with physicians, distinctions ultimately sanctioned by law. Pharmacists prepared and dispensed drugs, but left the prescribing to physicians. Optometrists tested for corrective lenses, but referred all treatment of the eyes to ophthalmologists.

Midwifery offers a contrast to these four professions. As Francis E. Kobrin demonstrates in her study of the midwife controversy, the medical fraternity did not take too kindly to nonmembers competing for the same business. And it was not as easy for midwives and obstetricians to divide their work as it had been for optometrists and ophthalmologists. On the basis of these few examples, it seems that the medical profession welcomed, or at least tolerated, only those independent activities that physicians did not want, like dentistry and podiatry, or that did not encroach substantially on their preserve, like optometry and pharmacy.

These examples may also illustrate a reluctance on the part of male physicians to admit women into the healing arts — except, in the case of nurses, as clearly defined subordinates. (It is interesting that only members of largely male professions such as dentistry, optometry, and podiatry are allowed to use the title "doctor.") Although physicians encouraged the professionalization of nursing, they always insisted on being captains of the team.

15

Nursing Emerges as a Profession: The American Experience

RICHARD HARRISON SHRYOCK

In the midst of anxiety about hospital personnel in the United States, more than one writer has claimed that lack of nurses threatens even the survival of patients. If this is true, we still face dangers as serious as those recognized more than two centuries ago. Thus, an article in the famous *Encyclopédie* declared (1765) that "the lives of patients may depend" on the selection of their attendants; that is if well-qualified nurses were not at hand, the sick might not pull through.[1] Yet how can it be that, despite all the progress made since that "dark age of hospitals," we still confront this same, stark alternative?

The question is by no means trite: it is pertinent and pressing for all concerned. And it may help, in seeking answers, if we reconsider the evolution of secular nursing services. If, for example, one reason for the exploitation of nurses after 1875 was simply the fact that most of them were women, the cumulative results of this experience may have bearing even on current tensions. Or, again, when nursing — for better or for worse — was differentiated on several levels of training, this could hardly have been avoided after scientific progress led to similar distinctions within medicine. For when American physicians improved their schools, tightened licensing requirements, and moved into specialties, nurses were naturally propelled in the same direction. Or so it seems, to a hopefully objective historian.

As long as secular hospital nurses were little more than servants and provided only custodial care, their role changed very slowly — if at all. There was little which historians could say about them, and that little was rarely told because servants were taken for granted and few pertinent records of their work survived.[2] The recent era, however, finally brought changes which initiated new trends and inspired new vistas.

Many persons, of course, had always valued custodial care within families. One must recall, also, that there were no hospitals in the modern sense in the English-American colonies for more than a century after settlements were first established. And as long as nearly all patients were tended at home, relatives or friends looked after them as a matter of course. Or they employed neighborhood women who likewise served on a personal basis. Appreciation of care of this sort was often expressed during the 18th century, and some statements linked good nursing with effective treatments as a combination devoutly to be wished.

Thus Mrs. Henry Drinker of Philadelphia, writing in 1793 of her son's illness, recorded that:[3]

> — the particular care of our good Doctors Bard and Jones, *with good nurseing* and the kindness of the family we were with — brought William so forward as to attempt a journey homewards —.

At other times, appreciation was expressed in principle rather than in personal references, and it was noted that efficient nursing was preferable to poor "doctoring." In 1738, for example, a writer declared that if a medical man could not pass licensing examinations, patients would be:[4]

> safer without him; and its more prudent trusting to the care of Providence *and a good nurse . . .*

Richard Harrison Shryock (1893–1972) was William H. Welch Professor of the History of Medicine Emeritus, The Johns Hopkins University, and Professor of History Emeritus, University of Pennsylvania.

Reprinted with permission from *Clio Medica*, 1968, *3*: 131–147.

Obviously, those termed "good," and who in this context rated next to godliness, were viewed with some respect.

Nursing within voluntary hospitals, caring chiefly for the poor, was another matter. The first American institutions of this type (1751, 1791) were quite respectable, and their matrons and stewards were occasionally honored for faithful service. But even in this setting, nurses were trained only as apprentices ("on the job")—chiefly for housekeeping chores and bedside routine. Such work was tedious, involved certain risks, and offered little incentive. Matters were worse in early almshouses or city hospitals, where convalescents were used as attendants and where standards of good behavior were not always maintained. But these "nurses," men and women, were themselves given little consideration. Not until more was expected of them, could motives arise for improving their work and reputation. Meantime, it was probably unfortunate, for American hospital services, that no highly motivated Catholic or Protestant nursing orders were available until after 1840.[5]

Expectations for secular nursing did rise during the later 1700s, as a result of both social and medical developments. As far as social factors were concerned, one recalls that the 18th and 19th centuries were an era of humanitarian reform. Ameliorative efforts emerged from religious backgrounds but were beginning to take on secular forms. There were such strivings as the antislavery drive, the women's rights movement, the temperance upheaval, and so on. The demand for trained nurses is not usually viewed as one of these crusades, yet it was inspired in part by the growing sensitivity to suffering which characterized the age. Humanitarianism assured a response to reformers which earlier centuries would not have provided.

Humane feeling could be diffuse, however, and had to be related to specific need to be made effective. The first step in this direction, with respect to nursing, was the realization by physicians that this service could at times make all the difference. Laymen, as noted, had long recognized this in their homes — presumably because a good nurse provided moral support as well as physical comfort. But more promising was the recognition by doctors that such values were part of medical care as a whole, for these men envisaged nursing in hospitals as well as in homes.

Among the first who took hospital nursing seriously from a medical viewpoint were certain German authorities. Brief manuals of instruction had been prepared for the guild as early as the 16th and 17th centuries; but it was not until the later 18th century that attempts were made to provide some formal education. Thus, Dr. Franz May of Mannheim became convinced by 1780 that poor nursing caused hospital deaths, and he therefore urged probationers to attend lectures and to practice under supervision. In some cases, those already working in wards were brought into classes. Dr. May condemned the "slavery" in which nurses were held, hoping that he could attract intelligent women and then provide them with certification. Similar efforts were made in other German cities, and in some respects these plans anticipated the Nightingale reforms which came more than a half-century later.[6]

There were, however, serious weaknesses in the early programs. First, it was difficult to overcome social distinctions: well-qualified persons rarely could be lured into semi-domestic labor. Second, there was a built-in obstacle to any improvement of status: nursing as yet rarely called for knowledge beyond that which could be learned on the job. One can see, looking back, just the beginning of such a demand. Dr. May, for example, called attention to the need for well-informed attention to diet and to bleedings; and even earlier, an English manual had given nurses some guidance on aiding surgeons and obstetricians.[7] In the United States by the 1790s, Dr. Valentine Seaman of the New York Hospital, and perhaps a few other physicians, gave some instruction in obstetrical nursing. But the effectiveness of most nurses continued to depend simply on kindness, common sense, and experience.

Consequently, it is not until Florence Nightingale's era that we usually date the advent of "trained nurses." She was, at first, inspired by German Protestant traditions and by the humane heritage of certain Catholic orders. But she also had advantages — in addition to her own dedication and influence — which had been denied earlier reformers. Times were changing by the 1850s. Class distinctions had become less rigid and humanitarianism was more widespread. Miss Nightingale, moreover, was able to combine this sentiment with the nationalistic enthusiasm of her day. Had she not served Britain well in the Crimean War? In consequence, a patriotic people raised an endowment for her pioneer school and women of good background responded to her call.

The possession of its own funds provided this school with a degree of autonomy, although it operated within a hospital. And autonomy, in turn, protected students against exploitation as attendants. So also did Miss Nightingale's insistence that superintendents be women. Hence, although the founder demanded discipline, her program was at first in harmony with the feminist movement. It was more than coincidence that women began to receive training in nursing during the same era (1850–1875) when they were first admitted to medical schools.

After that period, both church-controlled and secular hospitals largely ceased to use men as nurses. The tendency to employ only women may have been encouraged by feminist views, but in any case reflected an old belief that they made more humane nurses than did men. (A serious scandal was caused by the brutality of male nurses in New York City mental wards in 1900, after which women were more generally employed.) Another factor, in secular institutions, was presumably women's willingness or compulsion to work for lower pay. Analogies may be found here with the earlier experience of elementary school teachers in the United States.

The Nightingale movement also benefited from a new outlook within medicine. Socially minded physicians of the mid-19th century, like social scientists in the 20th, emphasized environmental influences rather than biologic factors in causation. This meant, in medicine, a declining interest in contagious animalculae or in "viruses" (poisons), and greater concern with sanitary reform. Such reform had implications for institutions as well as for cities as a whole. Thus, Miss Nightingale sought the same order and cleanliness in hospital wards that health reformers desired in street cleaning, water supplies, and the like. Nurses therefore must be informed about both personal and public hygiene. Here was the first real impact of scientific concepts on nursing education. Although simple in technical content, the impact was a prophetic one.

Meanwhile, in the United States, social and medical trends similar to those in Britain — combined with experience gained during the Civil War — made the development of nursing schools almost inevitable. The Nightingale movement probably hastened this outcome and provided a model. Just which American programs were "firsts" is of no great moment: one can so designate the plan established at the New York Infirmary for Women and Children in 1859, that of the Woman's Hospital in Philadelphia in 1861, and that of the New England Hospital for Women and Children in Boston in 1862. Or priority can be claimed for the first schools established on the "Nightingale Plan"; namely, those set up in 1873 in New York, in New Haven, and in Boston.[8]

If attempts to follow the Nightingale model had entirely succeeded, educational objectives would have been emphasized. But no American program shared the patriotic appeal inspired in Britain by military nursing. A number of women had become famous as Civil War nurses, but none of them attempted to found schools; and there was no appeal to the nation to aid such an effort. Under these circumstances, it is not surprising that no one endowed a nursing school — particularly in a day when even medical colleges were expected to pay their own way. Means for the support of nursing education were found only when hospital authorities discovered (1) that improved nursing lessened mortality, and (2) that student nurses could provide much bedside care just for "board and keep." Meantime, nursing appealed to young women partly on humanitarian and partly on economic grounds: there were still few employment opportunities for their sex. Hence, during the 1880s and 1890s, the number of hospital schools and of trained nurses increased rapidly. Whereas in 1880 only 15 schools existed with 157 graduates, in 1900 there were 432 schools which produced 3,456 graduates. By 1920, these numbers had increased respectively to about 1,700 and nearly 15,000.[9]

One can understand the motives which led hospitals to organize schools and then to staff their wards as cheaply as possible. Population was expanding, and reports of medical progress aroused for the first time some public desire for hospitalization. But institutions rarely had adequate funds to meet this demand, even if private patients were charged on a sliding scale. Hospital boards were therefore tempted to use unpaid students in the wards, where they were offered little more than the old, apprenticeship type of training.

Hence, although nursing schools varied widely in quality, many were mediocre at best. Students were not only exploited during a 12-hour day (as were other workers), but even "trained nurses" had not yet acquired much status or been accorded much freedom. Although some American superintendents relaxed the discipline desired by Florence Nightingale, Miss Dock of the Hopkins School could still write in the 1890s that:

> The Nurse is a soldier. Absolute and unquestioning obedience is the fundamental idea of the military system . . . Strictness and exactness produce better nurses.

For better or for worse, a hospital environment of this sort encouraged among nurses an awe of authority, a devotion to exact routine, and a lack of initiative even in small things — attitudes from which, according to some critics, the vocation still suffers to this day.[10]

By the 1890s, the situation in American nursing must have been confusing. There were some able nurses with superior education, but at the other extreme were women with little or no training — including those who had drifted into the vocation before schools were available. Most of the first group cherished humane ideals, while the untrained element doubtless included those who needed a job. The majority, however, represented various points between the two extremes; and since no national standards had been set up, families and even hospitals must have found it difficult to make distinctions.

It was progress in science which finally brought some order into the picture. This was a matter of direct influence when bacteriology and other fields — reviving a biologic approach and so advancing beyond empirical sanitation — pressured schools into giving additional training. But the indirect influence of medical progress may have been even greater. The quarter-century when trained nursing was taking form, 1875–1900, was also the era when the American medical profession was at last raising *its* standards in response to the new science.

In the 1870s the country had endured many weak medical schools, and was served by large numbers of poorly trained "doctors." The situation was not unlike that in nursing, with no widely enforced standards. Some real physicians, however, had enjoyed the advantages of arts-college background, of two or three years in good medical schools, and of advanced training abroad — chiefly, by that time, in the German-speaking universities. Such men responded more promptly to the new science than could nursing personnel. By the 1890s they were urging a reform of medical education, with emphasis on research and on the development of specialties. When philanthropists provided funds to support this appeal, modern-type schools at last appeared — beginning with The Johns Hopkins in 1893. Meantime, state legislatures were persuaded to reintroduce the examining boards and licensing which had been abandoned a half century earlier.[11] By 1905 a reform of medical education and of the medical profession was under way.

Well-trained doctors, devoted to specialties, gradually took charge of services in the better hospitals — particularly in those connected with medical schools. And as therapy now required new techniques and equipment, physicians encouraged patients to enter hospitals which could provide these advantages. Doctors, moreover, found it more convenient to see patients in hospitals, and felt that they could best control treatments there — provided efficient nurses were available. The drift of patients into institutions was most obvious in the case of surgery, which was occasionally practised in homes as late as 1900–1905 but moved almost entirely into hospitals thereafter.[12]

Better-informed doctors naturally desired the aid of better-informed nurses. Whether the influence of leading physicians on nursing was greater in Europe than in the United Kingdom and the United States, is a question outside the province of this article. But it is suggestive that whereas the classic English works in this field were written by Florence Nightingale, the outstanding German text by 1880 was that of the great surgeon Billroth. My impression is that this Austrian publication revealed the implications of scientific advances more promptly than did contemporary works by English nurses or humanitarians. It may be that American medical leaders were influenced, in their expectations of nurses, by what they observed in Germany or Austria as well as by knowledge of the Nightingale plan.[13]

Whatever the sources of inspiration, when superior women became superintendents of nursing schools in university hospitals they were soon disturbed by confusion in their vocation. They were dedicated persons but realized that kindness was no longer enough; knowledge and skill were also essential. Both these motivations can be traced thereafter in the activities of American nurses, though economic and scientific interests gained ground throughout the ensuing era.

Continuing idealism was exhibited by individual hospital leaders, but was also manifested in the emergence of public health nurses whose activities transcended medical institutions. Social reform movements of the first three-quarters of the 19th century had reflected prevailing romanticism, but thereafter less dramatic, more realistic efforts were made to aid the poor and underprivileged. Nurses moved out into slum areas surrounding hospitals, where they founded "settlement houses" and became in effect the first medical "social workers." They also advocated medical services in public schools, and even displayed interest in early appeals — encouraged by German and British models — to establish compulsory health insurance. They apparently maintained this concern thereafter, for as late as 1961 nursing organizations supported bills in Congress which were precursors of the present "Medicare" law noted below.

Nurses were likewise attracted to such programs, led by physicians, as had immediate welfare implications; for example, some sought experience as "tuberculosis nurses" at a time when many of the guild shared the public fear of this plague. In due time, local authorities came to appreciate the services of such women and provided for the first "visiting nurses." The personification of social idealism among them can be observed in the career of Lillian D. Wald of New York City. Miss Wald, founder of the Henry Street Settlement House, also pioneered in securing school nurses and proposed the Federal Children's Bureau as established in 1908.[14]

Meantime, however, hard experience was forcing heads of schools to consider the needs of their own guild as well as those of society at large. Gradually they became convinced that — in the public interest, as well as their own — nurses should receive improved training and be granted better working conditions, salaries, and general status. Was this not the only way to attract high-grade personnel? Was it not, moreover, the nurses themselves who must initiate such efforts? By giving an affirmative answer to each of these questions, an often disregarded "calling" took the first, tentative steps toward professionalization.

American nurses had been preceded, in aspiring to a professional role, by the British Nurses Association founded in 1886. This body, granted a charter in 1893, had set up a General Register for those nurses whom it approved. The association still followed Miss Nightingale's leadership in some respects, as in supporting only women as directors of nursing schools, but questioned her discipline as lending itself to exploitation. Miss Nightingale, conversely, opposed the secular trend on the ground that ". . . nurses cannot be registered and examined any more than mothers," and also because she feared that a professional body would exhibit "a mercantile spirit" — as in "forcing up wages."[15] But British nurses, even as the American, were turning away from these semi-enclosed ideals and accepting rather the scientific model afforded by the medical profession. This shift in attitudes had both merits and limitations.

The first steps taken to organize American nurses are well known. In 1893 at the Chicago World's Fair, Miss Isabel Hampton — superintendent of The Johns Hopkins School — arranged a meeting of 20 women holding similar posts. This group formed, within a year, the body which later adopted as its name the "National League of Nursing Education." Then, in 1896, a society open to all "graduate nurses" in the United States and Canada was organized among the alumnae of some twenty of the better-known schools; and this group assumed in 1911 the title of the American Nurses' Association. Proposals for an official publication took form when the A.N.A. founded, in 1900, the *American Journal of Nursing*.

Other national societies, differentiated in one way or another, soon appeared — notably the public health ("visiting") nurses' organization, the association for practical nursing education, and a society of colored graduate nurses. (Although the latter were usually well regarded, the need for their separate body, founded in 1908, persisted for some years — reflecting old racial prejudices within American society.) When the American Hospital Association looked into the national situation in 1913, it found no less than nine types of nursing personnel. Most of these indicated training on different levels or the beginnings of specialization.

The American Nurses' Association evolved into the largest and most representative body, and set up a federal organization something like that adopted by the American Medical Association in 1901. (By the early 1960s, it had about 180,000 members.) The A.N.A. did not immediately imitate physicians in promoting state-board examinations, but it did adopt a procedure usually followed by groups desiring professional status. This was to seek laws to distinguish between those who had graduated from schools and those who had not.

In 1903 a "nurse practice act" was adopted in North Carolina, and by 1914 some forty states had passed similar laws. (Since the United States Constitution left education in the hands of states, there was no national legislation — except for Federal services — on the qualifications of either doctors or nurses.) In most cases these laws set up state nursing boards which defined educational standards, and which approved those schools whose graduates could be listed in official registers — hence the title "registered nurse" (R.N.) gradually replaced the terms "trained" or "graduate" nurse. Later, some states required individual examinations, just as was done for physicians and for other types of medical personnel.

During the Spanish American War, the army declined the proffered services of the A.N.A. and instead requested the Daughters of the American Revolution — an hereditary, patriotic society — to recruit nurses. No doubt this action reflected, among other things, the fact that national nursing bodies were young and not yet widely recognized. They gained ground, however, between 1900 and 1914; as when, in 1901, Mrs. Robb of the Hopkins school persuaded Columbia University to introduce an advanced course on teaching and administration in nursing — work taken over by her former pupil, M. Adelaide Nutting, when she became the first American professor of nursing in 1907.

During this period, moreover, nurses received some encouragement from the medical profession regarding professional goals. Thus, about 1908, the secretary of the American Medical Association stated that the newly organized A.M.A. "Hospital Section" (Council) was determined "to accept the trained nurse as a member of a learned profession, and contradistinct from a labour union. . . ." He emphasized, however, the "high calling" of the guild, and expressed the desire of his council "to help elevate" its ideals.[16] There were, it may be added, instances in which hospital directors opposed educational standards desired by nursing organizations.

During World War I the American Red Cross recruited army nurses, in cooperation with nursing organizations; and the record of these women increased respect for the guild as a whole.[17] Soon after the war the number of students declined sharply, however, and some observers urged that the length of training be shortened from three years to two. The surgeon Charles H. Mayo even headed an article: "Wanted, 100,000 Girls for Sub-Nurses" — who could be trained in a hurry. This disturbed A.N.A. leaders, who were by this time convinced that a three-year curriculum was needed. But Dr. Mayo implied that when schools provided courses in anatomy, physiology, and other medical subjects, their students were qualified to offer more than custodial care.[18] Hence, it seemed sensible to turn routine over in part to practical nurses.

Recruitment brought student enrollments up again in the 1920s, and "the White Cap Famine" was temporarily forgotten. Moreover, by that time, nursing schools had been set up within church hospitals, and some members of nursing orders became R.N.'s and members of the A.N.A. There was even an oversupply of nurses during the Depression of the 1930s, as a result of which small training schools closed and students were replaced in some hospitals by graduates. Partly in order to employ more nurses, hours were reduced — although this raised costs. "Nurses' homes" became more comfortable, discipline less rigid, and average weekly hours declined to about 45. But by the 1940s, new employment opportunities diverted many women into other fields and once again demand for nurses exceeded supply. The salaries of R.N.'s, nevertheless, lagged behind rising living costs, and this at a time when their duties became more technical.

Greater responsibilities now confronted nurses as a result of further advancements in diagnosis and therapy. As medical care became more complex and a shortage of doctors developed, functions once performed only by that guild — such as giving inoculations or transfusions — were turned over to nurses or to technicians.[19] Moreover, as many physicians moved into specialties, such as surgery, obstetrics, and psychiatry, they desired the aid of — respectively — surgical, obstetrical, and psychiatric nurses. Hence, in all such fields as well as in teaching and administration, there was a demand for more highly trained personnel.

In order to meet this need, certain schools made arrangements with universities whereby student nurses would combine general and professional education and take an arts degree. (As early as World War I, a program to encourage college graduates to qualify as nurses had been arranged at Vassar College under private auspices.) In other cases, universities organized — in cooperation with their hospitals — colleges of nursing which possessed their own faculties and budgets. A five-year program was usually involved, but this relieved an ambitious nurse from the struggle of securing a degree *after* going into practice.

The situation was similar to that once faced by school teachers, who had long worked for degrees after graduating from normal schools but who later completed "undergraduate work" before teaching. In addition to intrinsic merit, degrees had status values for teachers and nurses when "college education" came to be expected in the professions. In teaching, however, degree-holders became the rule; whereas, in nursing, their numbers remained relatively small and most of them became specialists, professors, or administrators. The contrast reflected the fact that states supported low-cost teachers' colleges, but provided little direct aid to nurses' colleges. Private foundations, which gave large grants to medical schools after 1910, likewise did little for nursing schools in particular.

While a small number of women were obtaining bachelors' degrees in nursing, the supply of traditional R.N.'s gradually declined. This trend continued despite the fact that the latter, like patients, were moving from homes into hospitals. The immediate cause of the decline was a renewed closing of hospital schools — despite in these years, a shortage of graduates. The total number of schools shrank, between 1926 and 1946, from about 2,150 to 1,300.[20] Some were weeded out as standards rose, much as low-grade medical schools had been eliminated a generation before. But institutions also closed because of dwindling registration. In order to provide enough bedside care in hospitals, efforts were then made by schools and also by vocational agencies to train more practical nurses. The latter, although taking shorter courses, had to meet requirements of state boards in order to be certified.

World War II brought a sudden call for nurses from the army and the navy, and the R.N.'s who responded — excepting a small number who were men — were given commissions. Hospitals also had to compete with a growing demand for nurses in industry, in "nursing homes" (for non-intensive care), and in visiting-nurse programs. Meantime, economic opportunities for women continued to expand in society at large. The net result of these trends was a second "white-cap famine" after 1940, which has become ever more serious since that time.

One effort to meet this situation was undertaken by the U.S. Public Health Service during the war. This was the organization of a Cadet Nursing Corps, out of which grew arrangements for nursing education within "junior" or "community" colleges. (Like the old normal schools for teachers, these were two-year institutions which rounded off — in sequence with high schools — a rough equivalent of secondary education in Europe.) After work in both arts and in nursing, students received an "associate degree" in the latter field; and were then permitted by some state boards to take examinations for nurses.

In this way there emerged a third level of R.N.'s; the other two being the graduates of hospital (diploma) schools, and those holding a bachelor's degree. This division of a field was not peculiar to nursing. There were, for example, various levels in teaching, in engineering, and in medicine itself. Certified specialists and general practitioners, to say nothing of sectarians, represented two types of physicians; and if "assistant doctors" also appear, these will comprise a third level even within the "regular" profession. Since some nursing specialists already served in effect as doctors' assistants, it was suggested that such women (with additional training) might move into this proposed rank of "assistant doctors." If the idea proved feasible, it would reduce the gap between nurses and physicians.[21] In other words, it would raise the medical guild ceiling under which even the better-trained R.N.'s operated and so afford them more leeway in achieving formal professional standing.

Whatever the outcome of this proposal, community college and baccalaureate programs meantime had brought nursing into "the main stream of American education." Hospital schools, on the other hand, still stood apart from arts colleges and universities. Their faculties served under hospital boards, and the status of graduates was probably not helped by the appearance of R.N.'s holding a degree. Yet diploma nurses made up most of those expected to give general care. And even when their absolute number did not decline, the relative supply fell. This resulted not only from circumstances already mentioned but also from further growth of population, and because annual admission rates to hospitals mounted — between 1935 and 1965 — from 56 to 132 per 1,000 persons.[22]

As the number of R.N.'s became inadequate, bedside care fell more and more into the hands of licensed practical nurses (L.P.N.) and/or of aids trained on the job. As Dr. Mayo had foreseen in 1920, this trend was desirable as far as routine was concerned.[23] (It was analogous to the tendency, among doctors, to assign what became medical routine to nurses or technicians.) But when half the posts for R.N.'s became vacant in some hospitals, and when one R.N. might find herself responsible for the care of an entire floor — with the assistance of only three or four aids or practical nurses — the difficulties confronted were obvious. In extreme cases, almost incredible conditions arose. In November 1967, officials of the Kings County Psychiatric Hospital (New York City) reported that "on some shifts there is only one nurse in the entire building" — although the budget called "for a total of 138 staff nurses." There is no need to labor the critical nature of this situation.

A sense of crisis pervaded public discussion of nursing by the 1960s. Concern about the quantity of nursing service was most obvious; but since the term "nurse" was often used to connote an R.N., anxiety about the quality of care was also implied. Typical of newspaper headlines were such statements as:[24]

> Nurse Shortage Plagues Hospitals and Shows Signs of Getting Worse

or:

> Nurses' Paradox: Hospitals Close Nursing Schools Despite Shortage.

To some degree, anxiety about nurses was but one phase of a concern about medical care as a whole. During the past five years, most news magazines and journals of opinion as well as many newspapers carried articles on the ominous lack of adequate services.[25] These articles, which repeated views expressed three decades earlier by liberal physicians and other critics,[26] emphasized such matters as rising hospital costs and the shortage of doctors and of nurses. Statements on the social and psychological aspects of medical care also began to appear in the sociological literature, as interest grew in "applied behavioral science." It is difficult to prove, but one suspects that old-fashioned family doctors and family nurses — however limited their technical knowledge — had done more to encourage patients than did either doctors or nurses whose motivation was largely a scientific one. In any case, the familiarity of home was often more reassuring to an invalid than was the strange, impersonal, and even threatening environment of the hospital. Sociologists surveyed and analysed, 1950–1965, the inter-personal relations of doctors, nurses, and patients; and, in the process, implied that all types of medical personnel could do more for the morale of the sick than was usually accomplished. Nurses were perhaps in the best position to do this, as some of their leaders had long noted, but only if they were present in adequate numbers. And this point brings one back to the ubiquitous problem of supply and demand in this field.

In order to understand the closing of nursing schools despite shortages, one must again recall the desire of nurses to improve their own status. As early as 1937, the National League of Nursing Education had provided a curriculum guide, and by 1941 its Grading Committee had begun to list accredited schools.[27] In these matters, nurses had again followed the example set by physicians under A.M.A. leadership some 30 years before. Although nurses had long lacked a unified body analogous to the A.M.A., an important step toward unity was taken in 1952 when several societies merged into the National League for Nursing (N.L.N.). Thereafter, this body and the A.N.A. cooperated in speaking for nursing as a whole.

The drive to improve status, 1930–1965, had naturally emphasized educational standards, and by 1966, baccalaureate and associate-degree programs finally became about as numerous (400) as the diploma schools.[28] Indeed, a recent "position paper" of the A.N.A. recommended college education for all future R.N.'s. But in advocating degrees and specialization, nursing leaders seemed to be diverting young women from hospital schools and from what might be termed general practice. Hence, some superintendents and physicians held nursing bodies responsible for the growing shortage of R.N.'s in hospitals. It was said, for example, that:

> The trouble with nurses is that they have just educated themselves out of nursing.

Or that:

> Any girl able to take a five-year training for a nursing degree, might as well go on and become a doctor.

What seems an extreme instance of such criticism was a statement, by a physician, that the N.L.N. had encouraged "the withdrawal of the student nurse from the bedside" and had "down-graded and even ridiculed the service ideal."[29]

One notes in passing the advantage which American physicians had had (1900–1925) in raising educational standards, in comparison with the difficulties faced by nurses during their own efforts after 1940. When the proportion of doctors to population had been reduced by raising school and licensing standards, there had long been an excess of practitioners — hence few persons were at first disturbed by a lack of medical men. And by the 1940s when worry finally arose about a doctor shortage, "medical reform" was firmly established.[30] But when educational programs seemed to reduce the number of *nurses*, such personnel was already in short supply and there was immediate criticism.

No doubt the basic causes of the shortage of nurses in recent years were economic in nature. Closely related to economic factors, however, was a growing concern about uncertainty of status and mounting obligations. The plain facts were that bedside nursing, for any type of R.N., was hard and responsible work, often done under difficult conditions and for relatively low pay. The salary of many R.N.'s, as recently as 1965, was not more than $4,500 to $5,000; and this at a time when the average income of physicians was over $20,000. Most nurses, moreover, "lived out"; that is, received no board and keep from hospitals. It is true that even a salary of $5,000 involved daily payments which were very high for patients who wished full-time, "private duty" nursing; but this often had to be viewed — however desirable — as a luxury service.

The attitude of doctors toward nurses became more liberal over recent decades, but there were still some who regarded R.N.'s as subordinates who merely carried out orders and were subject to reprimands. Meanwhile, hospital authorities, worried by rising expenses, were often unwilling or unable to augment costs by increasing nurses' salaries. Hence, the American Hospital Association was accused at times of blocking improvements in their economic position, and some resentment was aroused in consequence.[31] One cannot say how serious resentment was; but to the degree that it did exist, recruitment in the guild was probably discouraged. And this occurred just when there was need to make careers more rather than less attractive. For in an increasingly secular culture, many nurses — as well as other professional personnel — decided that dedication and hard work appealed less than did tangible rewards. Meanwhile, those probationers who still cherished ideals were in danger of disillusionment. One physician, concerned about this situation, exclaimed in 1967:[32]

> Who in the hell wants to be a nurse today? In nursing you take young, highly motivated people and clobber them.

It was no longer effective, under these circumstances, to assure nurses that their services were "above price." For many young women, nursing became just one type of work which looked less promising than did some others. Sensing all this, leaders of the guild realized that it must be made more attractive by improvements in income. Organized R.N.'s therefore began to move, even as Miss Nightingale had feared, toward "forcing up wages." In 1966, the A.N.A. House of Delegates approved a salary of $6,500 for R.N.'s as an official goal.

The urgency of this proposal was made clear by a continued decline of registration in nursing schools. Not only did many schools close, but hospitals shut down some beds because of the lack of nurses to attend them. And this occurred at about the time (1966) when the long-delayed adoption of Medicare and Medicaid programs[33] increased demand for these facilities.

A further complication arose when some R.N.'s became so unhappy about salaries that they began to consider "direct action." Affiliation with labor unions, or at least a following of union tactics, had proved successful for many school teachers and so appealed to other groups of government employees — including nurses in public hospitals. Matters came to a head in 1966 at 21 municipal hospitals of New York City, which possessed only 3,260 R.N.'s to fill 8,000 posts. The nurses demonstrated at City Hall in protest against low salaries and shortages, and were joined in this by some staff doctors. About 200 R.N.'s took other jobs, and 300 left the city system. There was no open strike, perhaps because of state laws on municipal employees, but some 1,400 resignations were submitted. The city finally met the issue by offering salary increases. Annual payments to staff nurses were raised from the 1966 level of about $6,000–$7,500 to $6,400–$8,200 for 1967. (New York City salaries were relatively high in most vocations.) There were similar difficulties that year in other cities, as in San Francisco.[34] Thus, at least in municipal systems, it appeared that direct action by nurses might "pay off" after *professional* protest had failed.

Obviously, at present, American nursing is in a transitional stage. There is still confusion within the vocation because of the different types of personnel involved. Indeed, it has been held that the term "nurse" is so ambiguous that it should be applied to only one of these types. But as noted, similar ambiguity is displayed by such titles as "doctor" and "engineer," yet these words have value as indicating all persons devoted to certain common, general fields of service. Subdivisions within these large areas can be expected to exhibit various levels of education, functions, and income, and nursing is no exception to the rule.

Over the past half-century, nursing has been transformed from a "calling" well endowed with ideals but otherwise neglected, into a professional or semi-professional guild. This transformation had been initiated by social trends and scientific advances, but nurses themselves had — like physicians before them — formed the organizations and defined the standards desired under these circumstances. "The nursing vocation," wrote one of its leaders in 1967, "need no longer operate on a survival basis. In fact, to do so is to promote mediocrity. We are arriving as a profession and should adopt open systems models so that we can ride with the rapid transitions taking place in society."[35]

More adequate salaries for R.N.'s appear essential and it may be hoped that these can be secured without resort to strikes or other drastic measures. But this economic problem is not peculiar to diploma nurses or even to R.N.'s in general. What *is* a special problem is whether to maintain and revive the hospital schools. In the case of reforms in medical education, 1910–1930, it is possible that too many schools were closed too quickly;[36] and this outcome is more likely and equally dangerous in the case of nursing.

One step toward strengthening diploma schools would be to provide their faculties with more autonomy within hospitals — a return to the Nightingale tradition. It is not inconceivable — though it would complicate matters — that hospital authorities could view nursing schools as coordinated entities rather than simply as subsidiary enterprises. (In certain cases, nurses have already been appointed members of the boards in municipal hospitals.[37]) Another possibility would be to make arrangements with adjacent colleges which would improve the status of graduates. And this group could be encouraged, by better salaries and other advantages, to continue bedside care — much as many teachers, holding degrees, still serve general educational functions.

The feasibility of strengthening diploma schools has been maintained by some of their graduates.[38] It has also been recognized by many hospital authorities, who were doubtless impressed by the three factors already mentioned: (1) the shortage of R.N.'s giving bedside care, (2) the desire of diploma nurses for improved status, and (3) the stronger bargaining position in which many nurses now find themselves. Administrators, while deploring attempts to move most training into colleges, stated that hospital schools must attain standards which would command "recognition in academic circles." This goal was envisaged by the American Hospital Association, which declared that the *education* of students in these schools was of prime importance, and that hospital boards should provide their faculties with "the autonomy and academic freedom appropriate" to educational objectives. The Association also stated, jointly with the National League for Nursing, that hospital schools "belong in the general system of education," that a "growing partnership" between them and other educational institutions is indicated, and that — whenever possible — such schools should be approved by the voluntary accrediting agencies.[39]

Although diploma programs raised the most obvious questions about recruitment, other means of increasing the number of R.N.'s also received attention. One way to do this was to enlarge the pool from which they could be drawn. Young Negro women, for example, had been admitted to nursing schools in the northern states as early as about 1880, and this practice had been continued on a small scale thereafter. Meantime, untrained Negro nurses had often been praised in the South, as by the distinguished surgeon Rudolph Matas of New Orleans, and separate schools were eventually set up for them in that section. The chief difficulty in recruiting more Negroes, over recent decades, was inability to meet academic standards. To the extent that educational opportunities for the race are improved, one may expect this source to be utilized more effectively.

Another pool for recruitment existed because, in this one instance, nurses reversed the policies of physicians. While the latter had remained a predominantly masculine guild, women had almost completely taken over nursing. The outcome today is that, while recruitment of more women is indicated in medicine, an enrollment of more men is called for in nursing. The national nursing societies approve the latter policy, and there has been some increase in the number of male students in certain schools.

One of the most promising means for securing more R.N.'s rapidly was to bring back into service nurses who had retired — usually as a result of marriage. Hospitals, schools, and nursing organizations began during World War II to recruit inactive R.N.'s, and offered refresher courses and part-time schedules to those who responded. Federal funds for this purpose became available in 1967, in those cases in which a responsible state body — the health department, a state nursing association, or a hospital council — contracted with the federal government to provide a program. Both on-the-job and classroom instruction were provided, and also allowances for some of the trainees. Oversight of the whole plan, which it was hoped would enroll some 30,000 additional R.N.'s, was placed in the hands of the U.S. Public Health Service.[40]

So much for both direct and indirect efforts to overcome the nursing shortage. One concludes that, at least during the present emergency, all the chief programs in nursing education merit further support. The difficulties in such a course are obvious — some arising from the need to adjust traditions, some from the mounting costs of nursing education and services. Here are encountered problems which involve colleges as well as hospitals, doctors as well as nurses, patients as well as the State.

A half century ago, the United States, in contrast to European nations, still left such matters largely to private initiative. But since that time, the State, operating on all levels, has gradually extended its influence into many aspects of medical care in America. One recalls, for example, the revival of licensing standards; regulations adopted concerning food and drugs; and provision of the costs of medical care for much of the population. At present, the American scene exhibits a balance of power between voluntary and governmental bodies — an arrangement reflecting the general structure and attitudes of American society.

Nursing has necessarily been involved in these developments. Whether or not the trend toward State control continues, there will be further efforts to increase the number of nurses and to improve their quality. It can hardly be otherwise, since their services constitute a major aspect of the whole complex of medical care. And this is a field of ever increasing concern, not only in terms of unmet needs but also because the very concept of "need" expands with growing confidence in medical science. Although this confidence can be exaggerated, the basic attitude is unlikely to change in the near future.

NOTES

In preparing this paper, I have been indebted to Miss Anne L. Austin, formerly Professor of Nursing, Western Reserve University, for helpful suggestions; and to Dr. Edwin L. Crosby, Director, American Hospital Association, for current statements by that body.

1 "Infirmier," *Encyclopédie* . . . , VII (Neufchâtel, 1765), 707. Similar views were doubtless held in the United States; see, e.g., L. K. Eaton, *New England Hospitals, 1790–1833* (Ann Arbor: Univ. of Michigan Press, 1957), p. 46.

2 The archives of the Pennsylvania Hospital, oldest in this country, reveal little about the selection or status of nurses prior to *c.* 1870.

3 *Not So Long Ago* . . . , ed. Cecil Drinker, (New York: Oxford Univ. Press, 1937), pp. 70 f., italics inserted.

4 *Boston Weekly News Letter*, Jan. 5, 1737/38. Italics inserted.

5 See, e.g., S. Lillian Clayton, "School of Nursing," in *History of Blockley*, ed. J. W. Croskey (Philadelphia: F. A. Davis, 1929), p. 146. Similar conditions obtained in many European hospitals; see A. Fischer, *Geschichte des deutschen Gesundheitswesens*, II, (Berlin: Herbig, 1933), 89; F. Bauer, *Geschichte der Krankenpflege: Handbuch* . . . (Kulmbach: Baumann, 1965), p. 159, etc. John Howard's accounts of inferior hospitals and poor nursing in Europe are well known; but it is often overlooked that he also reported good services in some Catholic and some Lutheran hospitals. No attempt is made here to trace the history of religious orders in nursing in the United States.

6 See F. May, *Unterricht für Krankenwärter* . . . Mannheim: Schwan, 1784), pp. 5 ff.; G. Pfähler, *Unterricht für Personen, welche Kranke warten* (Riga, 1793), *passim*; A. Fischer, *Geschichte des deutschen Gesundheitswesens*, II, 89–404 ff.; Bauer, *Geschichte der krankenpflege*, pp. 262–263.

7 Robert W. Johnson, *Friendly Cautions to the Heads of Families* . . . (1st ed., London, 1778; American ed. from 3rd London ed., Philadelphia: J. Humphreys, 1804).

8 Cf. E. H. L. Corwin, *The American Hospital* (New York, 1946), p. 122; and Agnes Gelinas, *Nursing and Nursing Education* (New York, 1945), p. 4—both published by the Commonwealth Fund for the N.Y. Academy of Medicine. On the scandal over male nurses in New York City, an episode called to my attention by Mr. Martin Kaufman of Tulane University, see the *New York Times*, issues from Dec. 16, 1900, to Jan. 12, 1901.

9 Corwin, *The American Hospital*, p. 123; Gelinas, *Nursing*, p. 5.

10 Quotation is from Ethel Johns and Blanche Pfefferkorn, *The Johns Hopkins Hospital School of Nursing, 1889–1949* (Baltimore: Johns Hopkins Press, 1954), p. 76. See also, L. B. Christman, "Nursing leadership — . . . ," *Am. J. Nursing*, October, 1967, *67*: 2093. The standard work in English on the *History of Nursing* is that of M. Adelaide Nutting and L. L. Dock, 4 vols. (New York: Putnam & Sons, 1907–1912). This gives a detailed factual account of American developments down to the years noted. (The later volumes were collaborative, and edited by Miss Dock alone.)

11 R. H. Shryock, *Medical Licensing in America: 1650–1965* (Baltimore: Johns Hopkins Press, 1967), ch. 2.

12 Early issues of the *American Journal of Nursing*, founded 1900, contained notes on "surgery in the home."

13 See [C. A.] Th. Billroth, *Die Krankenpflege im Hause u. im Hospitale* (Vienna: Gerold's Sohn, 1881), ch. 3–7, inclusive; and the comment thereon in Erna Lesky, *Die Wiener Medizinische Schule im 19. Jahrhundert* (Graz-Köln: H. Böhlaus Nachf., 1965), p. 445. T. N. Bonner, however, makes no reference to nurses in his standard *American Doctors and German Universities* (1963).

14 L. L. Dock, R. N., *A History of Nursing*, III (New York: Putnam & Sons, 1912), 215–234; Richard Harris, "Annals of legislation": III, *The New Yorker*, July 16, 1966, p. 46.

15 Sir Edward Cook, *Florence Nightingale*, II (New York: Macmillan, 1942), 359; R. H. Shryock, *The History of Nursing* (Philadelphia: Saunders, 1959), pp. 281–283.

16 Quoted in Dock, *History of Nursing*, p. 236. (Miss Dock did not give the exact year or the names involved.) A biography of Miss Nutting is being prepared by Professor Helen Marshall of Illinois State University. [Editors' note: Since the original publication of this article, the biography has been published: Helen E. Marshall, *Mary Adelaide Nutting: Pioneer of Modern Nursing* (Baltimore: Johns Hopkins University Press, 1972).]

17 Dock, *History of Nursing*, pp. 302–310.

18 See, e.g., D. C. Kimber and Carolyn E. Grey, *Textbook of Anatomy and Physiology* (New York; issued by Macmillan in many revisions beginning 1894, in conformity with a curriculum recommended by the National League of Nursing Education).

19 Note comment on the extent of this transfer by the 1940s, in Esther L. Brown, *Nursing for the Future* (New York: Russell Sage Foundation, 1948), p. 80; see also Corwin, *The American Hospital*, p. 123, *re* supply and demand for nurses.

20 Gelinas, *Nursing*, p. 9.

21 Joseph Stokes, III, "Physicians' assistants," *Am. J. Nursing*, July 1967, *67*: 1441 f. See also Patricia D. Horgan, "Nursing is not a profession," quoting Dr. Eli Ginzberg, in *RN Magazine*, January 1960, reprinted in B. and V. Bulloch, *Issues in Nursing* (New York: Springer, 1966), p. 58; and the *Wall St. Journal*, Jan. 17, 26, 1967.

22 Dr. John Parks, President-elect of the Association of American Medical Colleges, quoted in *U.S. News and World Report*, Jan. 23, 1967, p. 62.

23 Note, e.g., Brown, *Nursing for the Future*, pp. 56–72.

24 Philadelphia, *Evening Bulletin*, July 17, 1966; the *Wall St. Journal*, March 24, 1967. On the situation in the Kings County Hospital noted, see the *New York Times*, Nov. 25, p. 42C.

25 Among the most careful analyses were those published in *Harper's Magazine* and in *The New Yorker*.

26 See, e.g., *Henry E. Sigerist on the Sociology of Medicine*, ed. M. I. Roemer, M.D. (New York: M.D. Publications, 1960), for articles published *c.* 1940.

27 On the efforts of nurses themselves to upgrade education during the 1940s and 1950s, see Stella Goostray, "Challenge and change," a paper read at the annual N.L.N. convention, May 11, 1967, in New York City.

28 *Ibid.*

29 Thomas Hale, M.D., "A doctor's opinion," *Saturday Rev.*, Feb. 4, 1967, p. 62.

30 Shryock, *Medical Licensing*, ch. 2.

31 Barbara Carter, "Medicine's forgotten women", *The Reporter*, March 1, 1962, reprinted in B. and V. Bullough, *Issues in Nursing*, pp. 171–177. See also Evelyn B. Moses, "The continuing economic difficulties of nurses," *Am. J. Nursing*, January 1965, reprinted *ibid.*, pp. 178–185.

32 Baltimore *Evening Sun*, Jan. 12, 1967.

33 "Medicare": a federal program meeting most hospital charges, and offering voluntary low-cost insurance against doctors' bills for all over age 65. "Medicaid": a federal program for aiding states which support free medical services to low-income citizens.

34 *RN Magazine*, July 1966, p. 67; *New York Times*, July 3, 12, 1966. Cf. *ibid.*, Jan. 5, 1968.

35 Christman, "Nursing leadership—. . . ," p. 2093. See also D. D. Rutstein, *The Coming Revolution in Medicine* (Cambridge, Mass.: MIT Press, 1967), pp. 135 f.

36 Shryock, *Medical Licensing*, ch. 3.

37 See the *New York Times*, Aug. 2, 1966.

38 E.g., Ruth Sleeper, R.N., "A reaffirmation of belief in the diploma school of nursing," *Nursing Outlook*, 1958, *6*: 616–618.

39 See, e.g., Edwin L. Crosby, in *Medical World News*, June 16, 1967, p. 16; also "Role and responsibilities of the Board . . . conducting a diploma school of nursing," approved by the A.H.A., Nov. 17–19, 1965; and "Statement on hospital schools of nursing," approved by the N.L.N. and the A.H.A., May 8–10, 1967.

40 The program, whose funds are provided under the Manpower Development and Training Act, is described in the May, June, July, and September issues of the *Am. J. Nursing*.

16

The American Midwife Controversy: A Crisis of Professionalization

FRANCES E. KOBRIN

Although medicine itself has long been an established profession, many of the specialties within medicine have a much shorter history. This diversification is a result not simply of developments within the field itself but has also depended upon the attitude of potential patients — their feeling of a need for such specialization and their ability to take advantage of it. The role of this external factor, however, has varied considerably in the historical development of the several specialties. Surgery became differentiated as soon as the techniques developed enabling it to be practiced safely, whereas other specialties, such as dermatology, plastic surgery, or orthodontics, had to wait until a public attitude evolved which considered ills far less serious than malaria (itself once thought a natural state) as unnatural conditions which require treatment.

Such a specialty was obstetrics, which dealt with what many still consider to be the "natural process" *par excellence*. In the obstetricians' struggle for universal acceptance they faced both medical and nonmedical competition and an almost insuperable economic problem; the level of even the best obstetrical work was almost more of a hindrance than a help. The decade from about 1908 began the contest between the increasingly self-conscious obstetrical specialist and his adversaries, the midwife and her advocates. That such a debate could be carried on with great virulence is itself indicative of the importance of considerations other than the strictly medical. The result, the complete defeat of the United States' variety of midwife and the essential triumph of a "single standard of obstetrics," was not simply a function of the maturity of the obstetric profession.

In the United States in 1910, about 50 percent of all births were reported by midwives,[1] and the percentage for large cities was often higher. At the same time, and continuing well beyond this peak period, the maternal death rate in the United States was the third highest of countries which kept such records.[2] Midwives were employed primarily by Negroes and by the foreign-born and their children, and the midwives themselves usually shared race, nationality, and language with their customers.[3] Because this was a period of unrestricted and heavy immigration (one-third of the population was foreign-born or Negro),[4] the midwife population was swollen considerably.

At this time also, various local medical units in the nation began to assess the situation in their areas, and this resulted in a flood of articles and addresses on "the midwife problem in ——." The big eastern cities, most affected by the heavy immigration, were the most diligent in this regard and produced the bulk of the available data. In 1906, New York commissioned a study which revealed that the New York midwife was essentially medieval, very different from European midwives, for these did not emigrate as rapidly as those who expected such service. According to this report, fully 90 percent were "hopelessly dirty, ignorant, and incompetent."[5] These revelations resulted in the tightening up of existing legislation, and the creation of new, for the licensing and supervision of midwives and eventually in the establishment of the Bellevue School for Midwives, an institution which lasted for 30 years. Other areas reported similar conditions.

The major failing of the midwife, which this

Frances E. Kobrin is Assistant Professor of Sociology, Brown University, Providence, Rhode Island.

Reprinted with permission from the *Bulletin of the History of Medicine*, 1966, *40*: 350–363.

legislation was to correct, was responsibility for maternal deaths from puerperal sepsis and for neonatal ophthalmia, both preventable with the knowledge available at the time. But it became clear during the controversy that occurred over how to deal with this problem that the midwife was by no means the sole offender in these matters. A survey of professors of obstetrics reached the conclusion that general practitioners were at least as negligent as midwives, as well as being equally responsible for preventable deformities.[6] The overall picture of the obstetrical possibilities open to a prospective patient was not very good. Hospitalization was impossible for all but the very rich or the charity cases in the wards, obstetricians were few, and general practitioners unreliable. Use of a midwife involved many hazards, despite the fact that she was usually a sympathetic woman who would wait and work with the natural labor process (often, of course, for too long) and would also in many cases be in regular attendance for more than a week afterwards, not only caring for mother and infant, but also assuming such duties as were necessary to keep the household functioning normally.

The most obvious cause of this medically unsatisfactory situation was the general opinion that the midwife was an adequate birth attendant. Her success was due to the fact that the rigors of childbirth were still considered normal and risks in the process unavoidable. The general attitude was that nature really controlled the process so that there was little constructive assistance that could be given. This feeling was clearly dominant among the public, although there were signs of change; it was also an important attitude within the medical profession as a whole. One observer, in assessing the lack of interest in obstetrics generally, noted that the word "obstetrics" comes from a Latin word meaning "to stand before" and added, "or as a sneering colleague once said, 'to stand around.'"[7]

The best evidence that this was the judgment of the medical profession was the status of the teaching of obstetrics in United States medical schools. Dr. J. Whitridge Williams, Professor of Obstetrics at Johns Hopkins University, made a comprehensive report on obstetrics as it was studied in United States medical schools in 1912; he found that although medical schools had been improving rapidly, obstetrics was by far the weakest area.[8] He sent a questionnaire to professors of obstetrics of 61 schools rated by the American Medical Association as acceptable (they required entrants to have at least a high school degree) and to 59 nonacceptable schools, receiving 32 and 11 replies respectively. Among his results were the following: Of the 43 professors of obstetrics, only five limited their outside practice to obstetrics, 21 to obstetrics and gynecology, and 17 were in general practice. Only ten had served in lying-in hospitals for more than six months. Only nine had seen more than 1,000 cases of labor as preparation for their post, 13 had seen fewer than 500, five fewer than 100, and one had never seen a woman deliver. Six schools had no connection whatsoever with a lying-in hospital for teaching purposes, and only nine had as many as 500 cases a year for teaching material. The average medical student witnessed but one delivery, and the average for the best 20 medical schools was still only four. Half the schools required a period of service of less than a year in training assistants for their own staff, a level, according to Williams, at which a student is still unable to recognize, much less cope with, a serious emergency. Several of the professors admitted that they themselves were incapable of performing a Caesarean section. Williams concluded that there was only one medical school in the country properly equipped for teaching obstetrics, and he regretted that it was not Johns Hopkins. The result of this neglect of obstetrics, he saw clearly, was that poor schools with poor facilities and poor professors were turning out incompetent products who lost more patients from improper practices than midwives did from infection.[9]

But the obstetricians themselves were fighting this conception of the insignificance of their field. They argued again and again that normal pregnancy and parturition are exceptions and that to consider them to be normal physiologic conditions was a fallacy.[10] It was this view which contributed to much of the unnecessary operative interference that occurred in this period. Amused critics pointed out that women often delivered themselves while their doctors were scrubbing up for a Caesarean,[11] but other results, such as the use of high forceps previous to sufficient dilation, were less fortunate for the health of mother or child.

It was these two fundamentally different approaches to the process of childbirth, based on opposite views of its naturalness, which were responsible for many of the arguments which appeared during this period about the future of the midwife. At one extreme were those who advocated outright abolition of midwives, with legal prosecution of those who continued to practice. This was the official attitude of the state of Massachusetts and also that of most eminent obstetricians.[12] Less adamant was a second group, led by Dr. W. R. Nicholson of the Pennsylvania Bureau of Medical Education and Licensure, which favored eventual abolition, with the existing midwives closely regulated until substitutes could be furnished. A third group was pessimistic about ever abolishing the midwife and thus felt that regulation plus education would elevate the midwife to the relatively safe status she had achieved in England and on the continent. This attitude was reported from Newark, New York State generally, and New York City and Buffalo particularly. Finally, there were those, especially in the South, who felt that if, somehow, midwives could be made to wash their hands and use silver nitrate for the babies' eyes, that would, because of a host of economic and cultural reasons, be the most that could be expected.[13]

Since all but those who held the first position believed that at present there really was no substitute for the midwife, and thus she had at least temporarily to be endured, their views can be conveniently called the public health approach. Their concern was for the immediate future. The first group based its arguments on the necessity of developing obstetrics for the long-term good of American mothers, and so can be identified with the professional approach. An early analyst of this division in medical opinion described it as a conflict between the practical and the ideal,[14] but the actual arguments involved a great deal more than that.

The public health exponents did, in fact, always claim to be realistic, and they accused the professionals of "criminal negligence."[15] The aspects of the situation which they were in a position to consider were certainly important. Since midwives were registering 50 percent of all births, it did not seem likely that the medical profession could expand sufficiently to take care of all. Some public health officials were not even sure that such expansion was desirable. Arguments against it included the record of the medical profession as a whole, the economic problem of supporting the higher prices charged by doctors, and the attitude of the women themselves. There was also a subterranean problem of status: doctors were often considered less manageable than the more easily supervised midwife.[16]

With regard to the question whether the medical profession ever could absorb all the obstetric cases, Dr. Florence E. Kraker of the Children's Bureau in Washington felt that the midwife problem would actually grow as the preference for hospitals and laboratories among doctors increased, causing them to desert rural areas.[17] Even if sufficient expansion were possible, it would still be necessary, according to New York City Public Health official Dr. S. Josephine Baker, to keep midwives and make them safe, because immigrant women, and particularly their husbands, would allow no male attendants. They expected the simple nursing care and household help that a doctor would not provide, and for this they expected to pay the customary small fee. Providing only doctors for these groups would force them either to pay a higher fee or to use clinics with their implication of charity. Above all, they rejected hospital delivery, which would badly upset the home situation.[18]

What encouraged the proponents of the public health view most was the actual progress which had been made through legal recognition, education, and supervision of midwives. England was the chief source of inspiration, since Parliament had, as recently as 1902, established a Central Midwives Board "to secure the better training of midwives and to regulate their practice." Following this change, infant mortality, which had been 151 per 1,000 in 1901, dropped to 106, in 1910, with a commensurate decrease in maternal mortality.[19] A committee of the Russell Sage Foundation, after studying the results, was entirely in favor of the change. In particular, they found that rather than replacing obstetrical practice with trained midwives, it had "increased, improved, and upheld the work of the obstetrician."[20] Germany was also much admired by those of public health persuasion, since the midwife there was a scrupulously regulated institution, trained in government clinics and working in a set district in a defined relationship with a government doctor.[21] The level of obstetric training received by German midwives was recognized as superior to that of most United States doctors.[22]

Major progress had also been made in the United States itself. Newark, after adopting a program of "conference, lectures and personal visits," reported a drop in the three years, 1914–1916, in maternal mortality from 5.3 to 2.2 per 1,000 for the city as a whole, and a level of 1.7 per 1,000 among mothers who "received prenatal supervision from the Child Hygiene Division and were delivered by midwives." This was aggressively compared with the rate of 6.5 for Boston, where midwives were banned. For 1916, again, Newark's infant mortality rate below one month was 8.5 for the special category, as opposed to a city rate of 36.4. The reporting of births was greatly improved, silver nitrate was in universal use, and Board of Health Officer Levy was highly pleased with his results.[23] In Philadelphia a similar program, which emphasized in addition control through registration, gave its director "hope to show statistics unequaled in the history of the world."[24] Midwives, more secure in their licensed status, were calling doctors earlier and oftener, neonatal ophthalmia had vanished, and all at relatively little cost.

Besides pragmatically recognizing the midwife's possibilities, many of her promoters felt a strong sympathy for her and her deficiencies. Ira S. Wile defended her on the grounds that it was "unfair to criticize the lack of an educational standard which has never been established." He felt that abolition was no more the answer than it had been for nurses of the "Sairy Gamp type," 18th-century doctors, or present-day obstetricians, all of whom, by absolute standards, were very bad indeed.[25] Midwives also gained sympathy from their adherents because of the rudeness with which the "arrogant," "unrealistic" obstetricians treated them. Those most in favor of the midwife seemed bent on elevating her to a professional status well above that of a nurse. Recognition was to build self-respect and pride; caste and dignity would bring a more intelligent type of woman into the profession.[26]

It was with these general attitudes that the public health exponents faced the task of elevating the American midwife. The consensus which developed was that midwives should have training for at least six months to a year, including instruction on pregnancy, asepsis, care of labor, and of mother and child after confinement, and, above all, recognition of conditions that indicate when a doctor is needed. These requirements, coupled with legal proscriptions against vaginal examinations, drugs other than laxatives, douches, and the use of instruments, would, they felt, render the midwife a useful member of the community. The further elaboration of linking the midwife to a clinic and to a physician who would make examinations and be available for emergencies was advocated by some, but the problem of maintaining doctors in government employ presented such difficulties that many public health officials were forced to ignore the possibility that a doctor might not be available when needed.[27]

What is important in the plans discussed and occasionally established by public health officials is that in general these men were not simply embracing a distasteful necessity that would otherwise have been avoided. There were some, of course, who felt this way: the official who established the Philadelphia system was well aware of "the incongruity of allowing or actively sanctioning by license, the doing of distinctly medical work by non-medical persons. We cannot adduce a single argument in its favor except . . . *necessity*."[28] But the others were expressing an ideal of obstetric service whereby the ubiquitous process of childbirth could be carried on cheaply and easily, respecting modesty and the integrity of the household, and in a more natural and personal way than if rendered by doctors.

The solution offered by the obstetric profession, on the other hand, was not merely an ideal of obstetric care, but also a very realistic solution for the obstetricians' difficulties. Until this last great wave of immigration, graduating obstetricians had always found sufficient numbers of patients. J. L. Huntington, a Boston obstetrician who was partly responsible for Massachusetts' unique position and was the most vocally concerned of the professionals, observed that the midwife was not — yet — a native product of America. She comes with the immigrant, "but as soon as the immigrant is assimilated, . . . then the midwife is no longer a factor in his home."[29] It was this latest influx of immigrants from southern Europe which had given the midwife problem such dimensions, and, if left alone, her numbers would again dwindle with the slowing of immigration. But if she were given official recognition so that immigrants' sons and grandsons expected such service for their wives, the obstetric profession would, he felt, face grave difficulties. Huntington believed, therefore, that the greatest danger in recognizing the midwife lay in the effect of such recognition on the general public. If the midwife was sufficient, then calling a G.P. would be the height of caution, and there would be no need felt for obstetricians.[30] He and other obstetricians believed recognition of midwives would set the progress of obstetrics back tremendously. The 50 percent of all cases handled by midwives were useless for advancing obstetrical knowledge. Elevating the midwife and training her would decrease the number of cases in which the stethoscope, pelvimeter, and other newly developed or newly applied techniques could be used to increase obstetrical knowledge. The need for strengthening obstetrics courses in medical schools would diminish, and practicing doctors would think themselves so superior to the strengthened corps of midwives that they would feel no need for improvement.[31] Lowering the standard of adequacy would lower all standards.

Because they believed this situation existed, the obstetricians had very different perspectives from the public health exponents. Some physicians felt the arrangement in Germany was far from ideal, so that even if such a system could be transplanted to the United States the resulting standard of obstetrics would be inadequate. Although German midwives learned obstetrics of high quality in their six-month course, that time was considered insufficient to instill an "aseptic conscience." Further, even in Germany their relationship with the physician was not one of "perfect harmony." According to Huntington's analysis, since it was profitable for a midwife to deliver each case herself, she might postpone calling a physician in time of danger; the physician, as well, might also be insufficiently cautious if he were called in, since the responsibility for complications remained with the midwife. Huntington argued further that in the United States such a plan would be impossible because (stating clearly the issue which so troubled some public health officials) the American medical profession could never be forced by law to respond to the call of the midwife in trouble.[32]

From the professional standpoint, the solution in England was also a bad one. In fact, the more midwives there were, and the more successful they were, the worse the situation would be for the community at large, according to Huntington, because this would aggravate a "double standard of obstetrics." The 30,000 English midwives had not only taken cases that would have been better cared for by doctors but had also taken enough practice away from physicians to obtain a livelihood.[33] Dr. Charles Ziegler, who was later to become cynical about the whole debate, also complained of the estimated five million dollars collected annually in the United States by midwives "which should be paid to physicians and nurses for doing the work properly."[34] The relationship between the ideal of a "single standard" and the issue of economic competition came up clearly again when obstetricians saw the midwife to be in league with "outside" influences — optometrists, osteopaths, neuropaths, Christian Scientists, and chiropractors — who were all invading the legitimate field of medicine.[35] Massachusetts had just licensed optometrists; "if the midwives are now to be recognized we may fairly ask, where is it going to end?"[36]

The professional ideal, of course, was that all women be delivered by an obstetrician, privately, or, if they could not afford such care, in a hospital-medical school complex. Thus, at a stroke, the midwife would be eliminated and the basis established for enormous advances in obstetrics, since students would then get ample training. In suggesting such a system for New York City, Dr. J. Van D. Young felt that even if it were inaugurated at state expense, "the ultimate good to the profession and to the people would be enormous" and rapidly repaid, and, also, that it would attract serious obstetrical students to New York.[37]

The professionals saw only one way by which their goals could be reached and those of the public health approach thwarted. There had to develop a demand from the public for a higher standard of obstetrics. "We can teach the expectant mother what she deserves, and when she demands it she will get it."[38] They urged accordingly that every mother has a right to such care as shall preserve her and hers in life and health, the care which, they said, the midwife cannot provide since the necessary skills are difficult to teach. Combating the "fallacy" of normal pregnancy and delivery was necessary not only to enhance the value of obstetric skills but also to make the American mother not merely respect, but fear, possible danger and so consider no precaution excessive.

Behind both these perspectives on the midwife problem was a complicating factor with which neither side dealt adequately. The economic realities of the situation and the costs of the various programs should have been given far more consideration. Since these economic aspects were working against the obstetricians in particular, they were the most guilty in this respect. In general, the public health approach overstated the economic obstacles to the realization of the obstetricians' ideal, whereas the obstetricians tended to ignore such obstacles, with one significant exception. The problem was that the training of an obstetrician was expensive, and his practice had to be sufficiently lucrative to draw able men into the field. In addition, the expansion of hospital and laboratory facilities to train new men and for their use in practice was expensive. Public health officers, who always have many places to spend every appropriation, are not in a position to weigh these facts and their possible consequences; the chief attraction of the midwife for them was that she was cheap. Levy, who established the Newark system, considered as only rhetorical the question whether those who can only afford midwives "should be delivered in finely appointed hospitals at public expense."[39] Others presented the obstetric ideal as a sort of *reductio ad absurdum*. The obstetricians, on the other hand, ignored this difficulty altogether because of their hope of changing what was then a very annoying fact: the same family will pay easily for surgery but expect to pay meagerly for attendance during pregnancy and confinement.[40] All that would be needed was propaganda to solve what they felt was not really an economic problem.

Huntington felt he had another answer to the "economic necessity for the midwife." Boston Lying-in Hospital ran an Out-Patient Department to provide obstetric training for medical students, and the patients, contributing an average of $1.28 each, in 1910 paid "all the expense" of the department, with a surplus of $807.82.[41] But his conclusion that the finest hospital care was itself inexpensive can be seriously questioned. The Boston medical school complex attracted prospective obstetricians from all over the country. Cases used for teaching amounted to nearly 20 percent of the total number of births in Boston in 1913.[42] Huntington thus claims an amazing percentage, and few other areas could hope to rival it, considering the scarcity of obstetricians at that time; yet it still left 80 percent of the births unaccounted for. It can perhaps be safely inferred that the costs of giving the rest similar treatment would rise rapidly, once deliveries had to be accomplished without the help of unpaid medical students. Yet even if the costs were indeed relatively low for caring for everyone on such a basis, the necessary expenditures on facilities to make room for all would be beyond the economic horizon of public officials forced to account closely for their use of public funds.

Only two writers proposed a solution which would make ideal obstetric care possible for all, given all the existing conditions. A. K. Paine, Huntington's only apparent critic in his home state, said that our method of government was not suited to the rigid requirements which the properly regulated midwife demands, but that the "obstetric poor" could be handled on a community basis, if the community would assume the responsibility.[43] Because of the stress Paine gave community responsibility, his argument clearly implied public institutions staffed by government employees and run with tax funds on some level or another.

Charles Ziegler, who earlier had complained of the money wasted on midwives, was a Pittsburgh obstetrician who was concerned with the midwife problem. What happened to him when he attempted to approximate ideal obstetric care for all puts an interesting light on the importance of the "ideal" elements in the original professional argument. Ziegler's experiment also involved inexpensive delivery of the poor and, although he got his funds privately, he had even then the idea that what was essentially obstetric charity should not be borne solely by obstetricians, but should be subsidized by the community.[44] Although he had no access to public funds, he evidently could generate other sources of aid by his enthusiasm for his project. Ziegler wanted to establish a dispensary which could give the best care to those who usually did not get such care, i.e., those not in either of the extreme income categories. The aim was to demonstrate how much mortality statistics could be improved, in the hope, of course, that the result would provide encouragement for others to try to achieve the same result. Six years after opening the dispensary in 1912, $80,000 in contributions had been spent caring for 3,384 confinements on both an in- and an outpatient basis. Fifty-six percent of the cases were foreign-born and 16 percent were Negroes. There were two sets of results. First, maternal mortality was 17 per 10,000 as opposed to a national average of 88.5.[45] This was a remarkable result for the time and clientele. The other result was that the Alleghany County Medical Society found Ziegler guilty of breaches of professional ethics by "solicitation and attendance on cases in families able to pay for a physician [and] . . . solicitation and attendance on cases where a physician had previously been engaged."[46]

Ziegler himself was suspended from the society, and, in 1918, his hospital was commandeered for government service, finishing his experiment.[47] Ziegler concluded after all this that, given the existence of such patients, the cost of caring for them properly (about 20 times Huntington's figure of $1.28), and the strength of the enemies made in the process, the only solution would be municipal, state, and federal aid, not as charity, "but as a matter of wise public policy and of justice to those to whom we look for the perpetuation of our family and national life."[48] He saw the whole obstetric problem as an economic one in which many people could not pay for the services they deserved; an institutional redistribution of such services was therefore necessary.

He believed that his solution would bring opposition from the medical profession, "as they are opposed to any plan which includes municipal or state aid looking toward the solution of the problem on a public-health or public-welfare basis."[49] For although Ziegler's solution ostensibly fulfills the obstetric ideal by granting every American mother her "right," by his method the natural elevation in status of obstetricians which would otherwise have occurred might be jeopardized.

Today the prospective American mother theoretically has access to high quality obstetric care. If she is from a relatively urban environment, this is available through clinics, or through a private obstetrician, for whom a group insurance plan might help pay. If she is from a rural area, a general practitioner graduated from a medical school, whose quality, both overall and in obstetrics, has greatly improved, is likely to be available. Obstetrics, both as a branch of medicine and in professional status, has advanced significantly. Can this result somehow be attributed to the developing superiority of obstetrics as performed by obstetricians, or could the forces arrayed against them have been exaggerated by the obstetricians, making the whole issue just a paper debate?

It appears that despite the potential obstetric superiority of obstetricians over midwives, the triumph of the former was probably due most to the fact that the circumstances debated in this period changed radically. It is certain that the relevant health conditions were not improving in those areas where the midwife was first being superseded. Although in Washington the percentage of births reported by midwives shrank from the 1903 high of 50 percent to 15 percent in 1912, infant mortality in the first day, the first week, and the first month of life had all increased in this period. Also, New York's dwindling corps of midwives achieved significant superiority over New York's doctors in the prevention of both stillbirths and puerperal sepsis.[50] Rather, the obstetricians triumphed because, before the public health programs became firmly established in the public mind, the obstetrician gained tremendous advantages from other sources. Immigration decreased significantly during the war and was afterwards reduced legally to a small fraction of the numbers experienced just before the war. This put time entirely on the side of the physicians, a considerable advantage in itself, while concurrently the economic problem *per se* was greatly reduced. This did not occur simply because of the "prosperity" of the 1920s, which may have had no impact at all; rather, the secular trend towards limitation of family size accelerated to include nearly the entire population. In 1919 in New York City there were 1,700 midwives who were responsible for 40,000 births, or 30 percent of the total. In 1929, though there were still 1,200 midwives, they delivered but 12,000, 12 percent of the total.[51] Not only did the average deliveries per midwife shrink decidedly from 23 to 10 births a year, but also total births decreased by 25 percent. With the limitation of births, it is possible that pregnancy and anticipated delivery seemed sufficiently rare to be generally equated with major operations and worthy of greater expense.

The other secular shift in attitudes from which the obstetricians benefitted was a new, general demand for improved obstetrics, the change for which they had been most devoutly hoping. The midwife controversy itself was in some ways a reflection of this change. It was not merely the benevolent concern of public health officials about their vital statistics which was instrumental in effecting all the legislation regulating the midwife. Also responsible was a growing public demand from women, who were becoming increasingly self-conscious about their own welfare, and who were still infected with the reforming zeal of the Progressive Era which was to lead to their enfranchisement. These were, after all, the women who shortly afterward were to deluge their congressmen and senators with pleas for the passage of the Sheppard-Towner Bill. This bill, which Ziegler worked for, provided federal money to the states for the "protection of maternity." With "womanhood" no longer rooted in the domestic, "natural" environment, or perhaps reflecting the struggle for release from such roots, the "natural" way of doing things was losing its appeal for the many emerging American women, and the obstetrician was increasingly there to reap the results of a growing anxiety about childbirth.

In summary, then, the professionalization process was very sensitive to external conditions and attitudes. If conditions had not changed so propitiously, if an economic problem and a conflict of attitudes had continued to exist, the obstetrician might well have found himself in the position of the present-day psychoanalyst with the public realizing that his skills solve but a small part of a complicated problem.

NOTES

1 Thomas Darlington, "The present status of the midwife," *Am. J. Obst. & Gynec.*, 1911, *63*: 870.

2 E. R. Hardin, "The midwife problem," *Southern Med. J.*, 1925, *18*: 347.

3 See nearly any discussion of the subject at this period, e.g., Darlington, "Present status of the midwife"; J. Clifton Edgar, "The remedy for the midwife problem," *Am. J. Obst. & Gynec.*, 1911, *63*: 882.

4 Darlington, "Present status of the midwife."

5 Edgar, "The remedy for the midwife problem."

6 J. Whitridge Williams, "Medical education and the midwife problem in the United States," *J.A.M.A.*, 1912, *58*: 1–7.

7 C. E. Ziegler, "How can we best solve the midwifery problem," *Am. J. Public Hlth.*, 1922, *12*: 409.

8 Abraham Flexner came to much the same conclusion in his discussion of the clinical years in American medical schools. *Medical Education in the United States and Canada: A Report to the Carnegie Foundation for the Advancement of Teaching*. Bulletin No. 4 (New York, 1910), p. 117.

9 Williams, "Medical education."

10 See, for example, J. F. Moran, "The endowment of motherhood," *J.A.M.A.*, 1915, *64*: 126; J. L. Huntington, "The midwife in Massachusetts: her anomalous position," *Boston Med. & Surg. J.*, 1913, *168*: 419.

11 "Discussion — midwife problem," *N.Y. St. J. Med.*, 1915, *15*: 300.

12 For an impressive list, see Huntington, "The midwife in Massachusetts," p. 420.

13 W. A. Plecker, "The midwife problem in Virginia," *Virginia Medical Semi-Monthly*, 1914–1915, *19*: 457–458; Helmina Jeidell and Willa M. Fricke, "The midwives of Anne Arundel County, Maryland," *Johns Hopkins Hosp. Bull.*, 1912, *23*: 279–281.

14 A. K. Paine, "The midwife problem," *Boston Med. & Surg. J.*, 1915, *173*: 760.

15 Clara D. Noyes, "The training of midwives in relation to the prevention of infant mortality," *Am. J. Obst. & Gynec.*, 1912, *66*: 1053.

16 "Discussion — midwife problem."

17 Hardin, "The midwife problem," p. 349.

18 Josephine Baker, "The function of the midwife," *Woman's Med. J.*, 1913, *23*: 197.

19 Noyes, "The training of midwives," p. 1054.

20 *Ibid.*, p. 1052.

21 A. B. Emmons and J. L. Huntington, "The midwife: her future in the United States," *Am. J. Obst. & Gynec.*, 1912, *65*: 395–396.

22 Hardin, "The midwife problem," p. 347; Emmons and Huntington, "The midwife," p. 395.

23 Julius Levy, "The maternal and infant mortality in midwifery practice in Newark, N.J.," *Am. J. Obst. & Gynec.*, 1918, *77*: 42.

24 W. R. Nicholson, "The midwife situation . . . ," *Tr. Am. Gynec. Soc.*, 1917, *42*: 632.

25 "Schools for midwives," *Med. Rec.*, 1912, *81*: 517.

26 *Ibid.*, p. 518.

27 See, among others, Hardin, "The midwife problem," p. 349; Plecker, "The midwife problem in Virginia," p. 457; J. A. Foote, "Legislative measures

against maternal and infant mortality," *Am. J. Obst. & Gynec.*, 1919, *80*: 550; Edgar, "The remedy for the midwife problem," p. 883.

28 Nicholson, "The midwife situation . . . ," p. 626.

29 Emmons and Huntington, "The midwife," p. 399.

30 Huntington, "The midwife in Massachusetts," p. 419.

31 *Ibid.*

32 Emmons and Huntington, "The midwife," pp. 397–400.

33 *Ibid.*, p. 394.

34 Charles E. Ziegler, "The elimination of the midwife," *J.A.M.A.*, 1913, *60*: 34.

35 "Discussion — midwife problem," p. 299.

36 Huntington, "The midwife in Massachusetts," p. 419.

37 J. Van D. Young, "The midwife problem in the State of New York," *N.Y. St. J. Med.*, 1915, *15*: 295.

38 George C. Marlette, "Discussion," in Hardin, "The midwife problem," p. 350.

39 Levy, "Maternal and infant mortality," p. 41.

40 Paine, "The midwife problem," p. 761.

41 Huntington, "The midwife in Massachusetts," p. 421.

42 Paine, "The midwife problem," p. 762.

43 *Ibid.*, pp. 763–764.

44 Ziegler, "The elimination of the midwife," p. 34.

45 Ziegler, "How can we best solve the midwifery problem," pp. 407–408.

46 *The Weekly Bulletin. Official Journal of the Allegheny County Medical Society*, *5*, No. 7 (Feb. 12, 1916), 5.

47 Ziegler, "How can we best solve the midwifery problem," pp. 412–413.

48 *Ibid.*, p. 407.

49 *Ibid.*, p. 413.

50 Baker, "The function of the midwife," p. 196.

51 Hattie Hemschemeyer, "Midwifery in the United States," *Am. J. Nursing*, 1939, *39*: 1182.

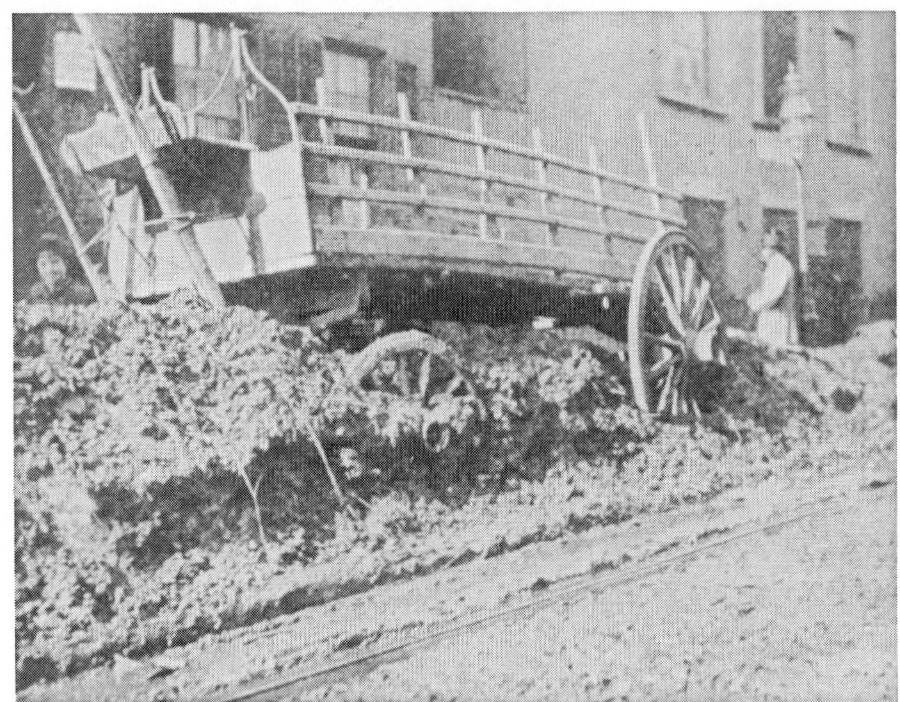

Harper's Weekly, 1895, *39:* 586 (State Historical Society of Wisconsin)

These photographs, taken by the muckraking journalist Jacob Riis, illustrate the transformation brought about by New York City Street Commissioner George Waring after he took office in 1895. Both pictures show the same paved block in front of 212 Sullivan Street. The top photo, taken in March, 1893, depicts a scene typical of American cities in the late 19th century.

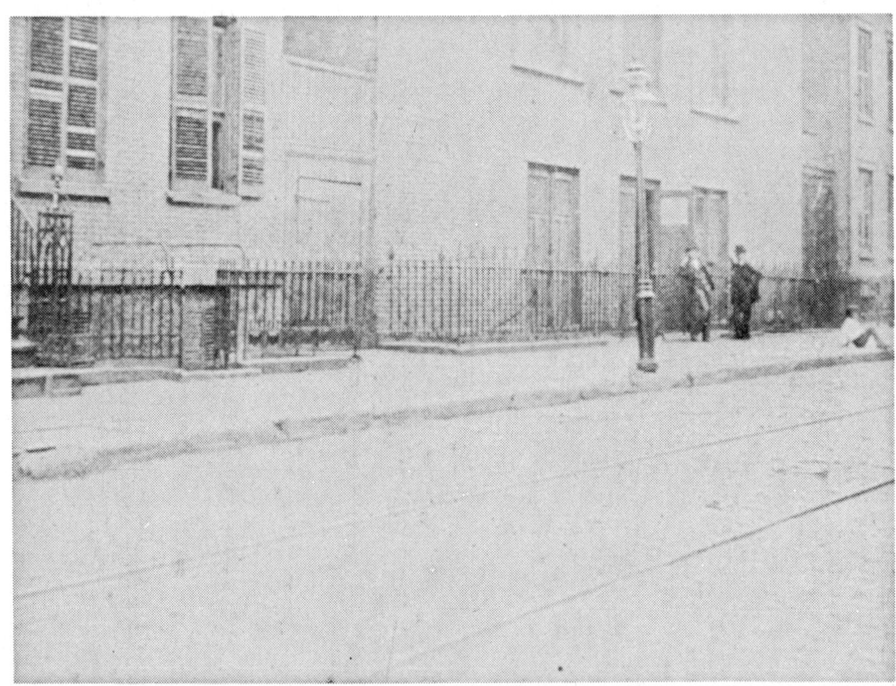

Harper's Weekly, 1895, *39:* 586 (State Historical Society of Wisconsin)

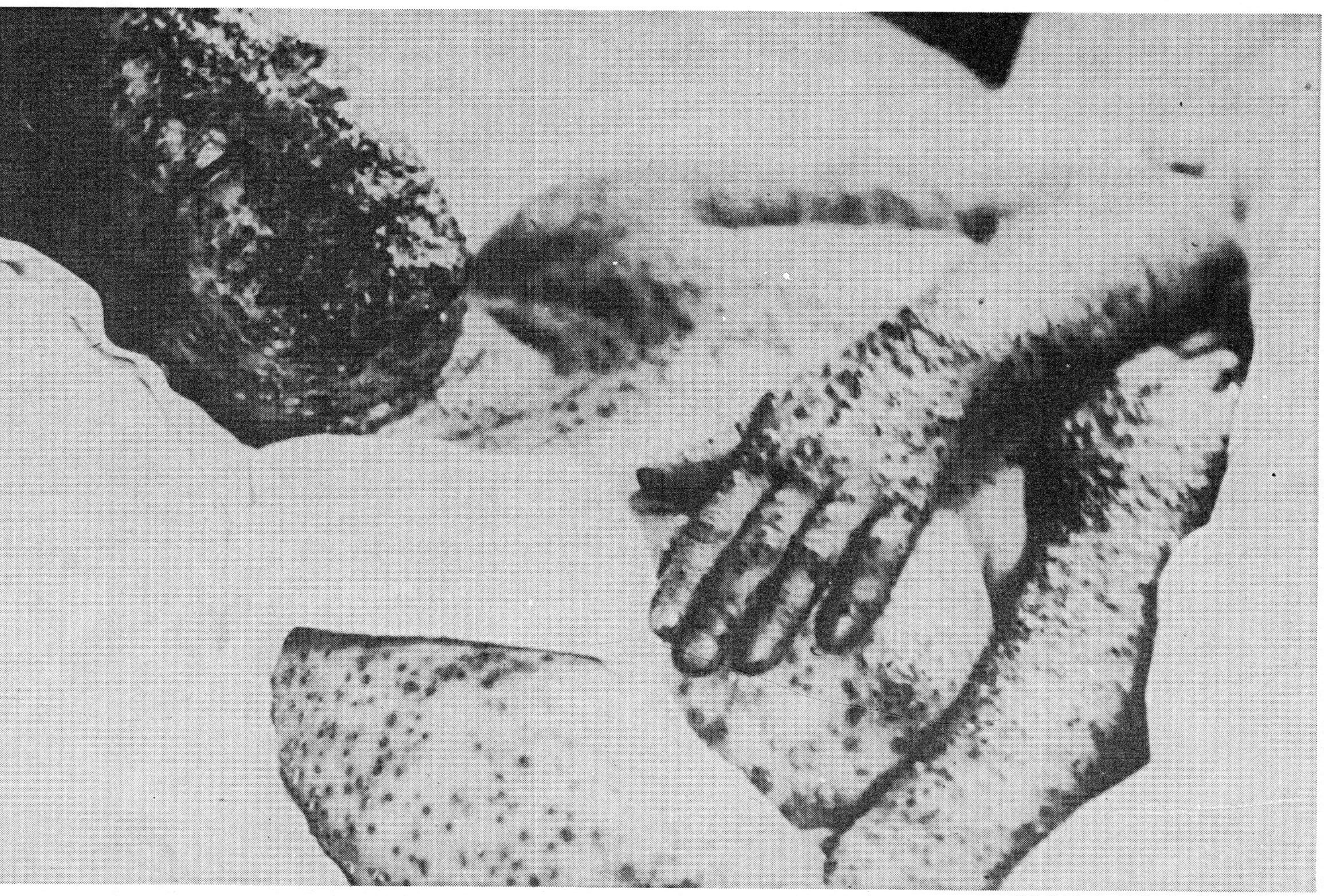

U.S. Public Health Service, National Archives

Of all 19th-century threats to health, epidemic diseases aroused the greatest concern. Besides taking many lives, the loathsome smallpox left many of its victims permanently disfigured.

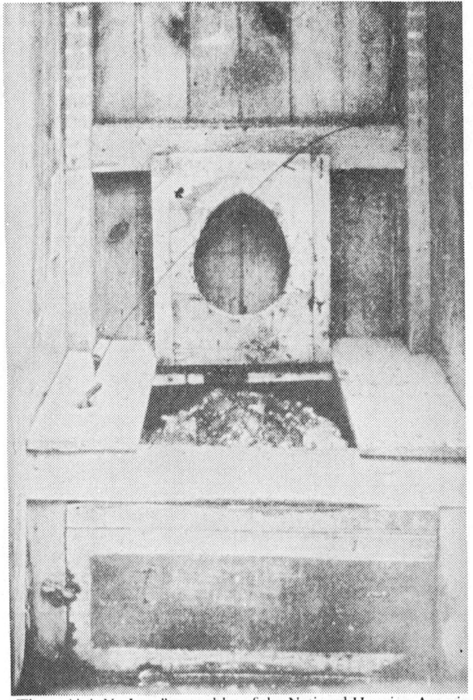

"There Ain't No Law," pamphlet of the National Housing Association (New York, 1913). Courtesy of Clay McShane

Contaminated milk and overflowing privies contributed to the poor health of American city dwellers. The 1858 drawing (below) illustrates one dairy's attempt to obtain the last drop of milk from an obviously sick and dying cow. The 1913 photograph of a privy in Yonkers, New York, graphically portrays the unsanitary condition of one American community in the early 20th century.

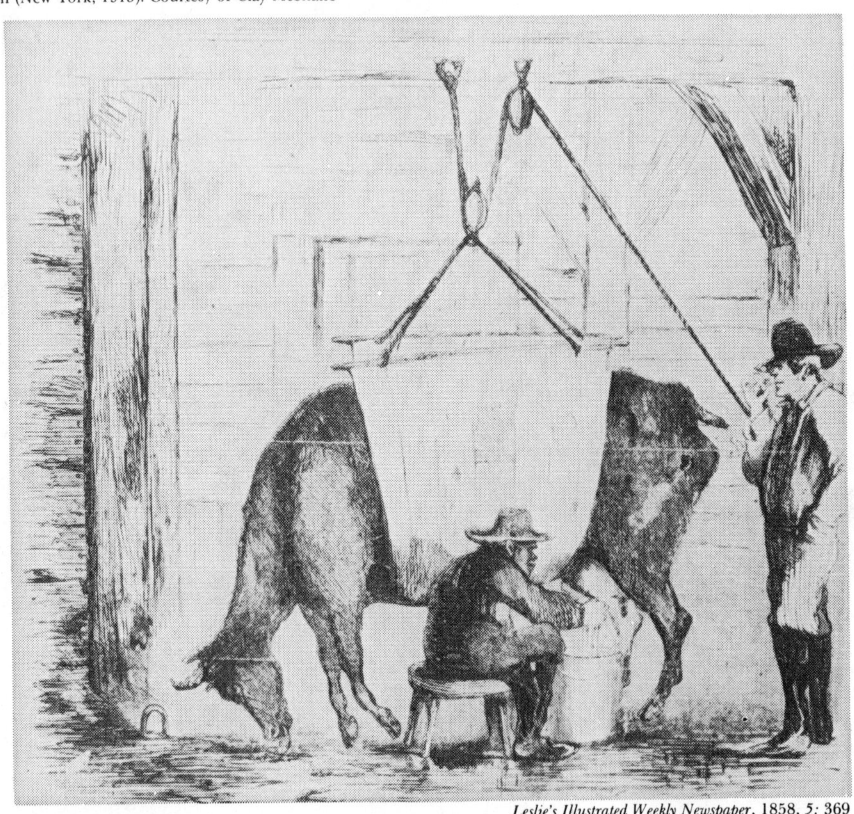

Leslie's Illustrated Weekly Newspaper, 1858, *5:* 369

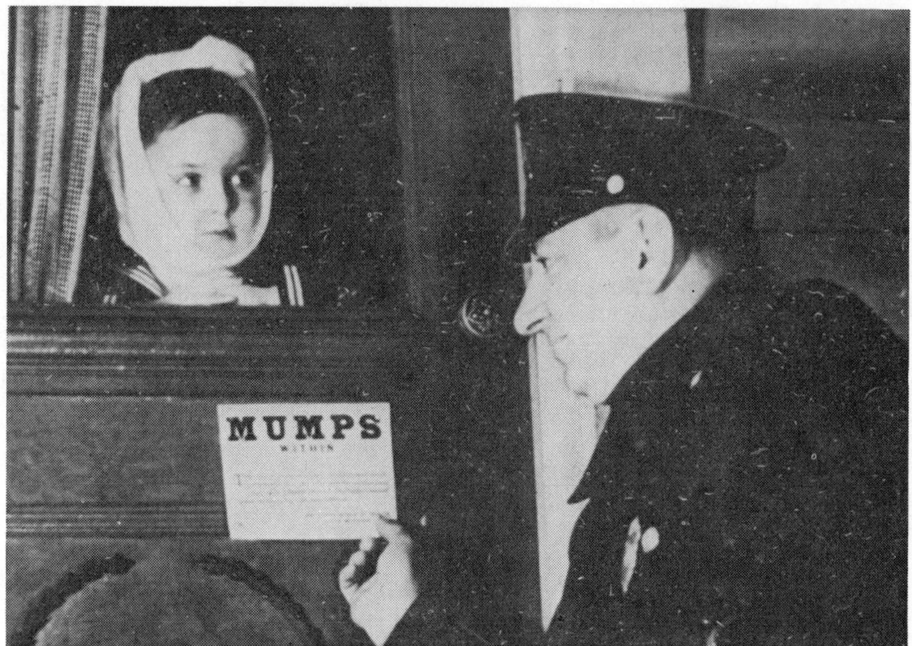

City of Milwaukee Health Department

Quarantines and school medical inspections were two of the measures urban health departments employed to reduce sickness among children. These photographs show a Milwaukee health inspector placarding the home of a little boy suffering from mumps and a New York City public health nurse examining the cleanliness of school children.

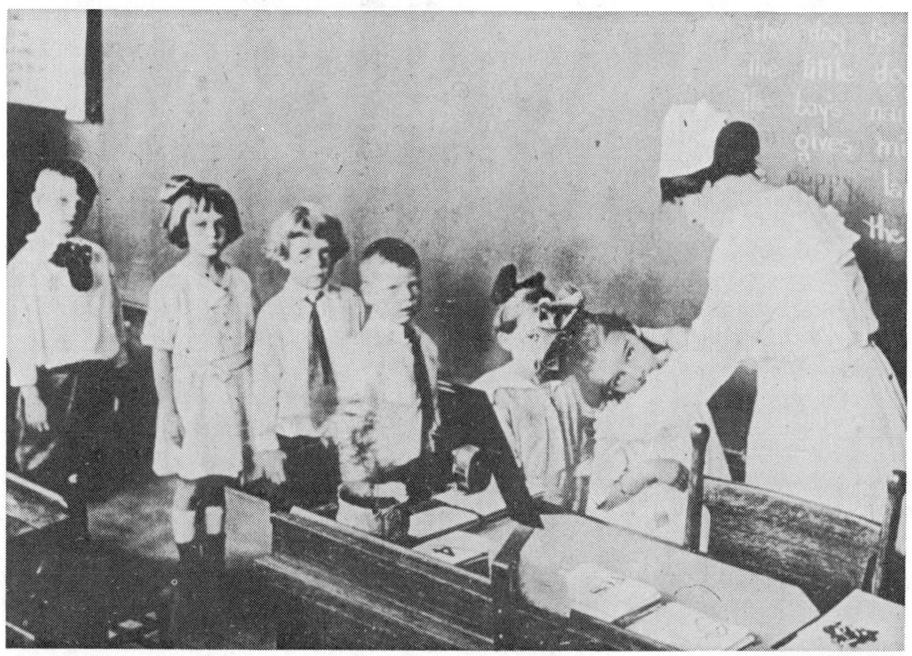

National Library of Medicine

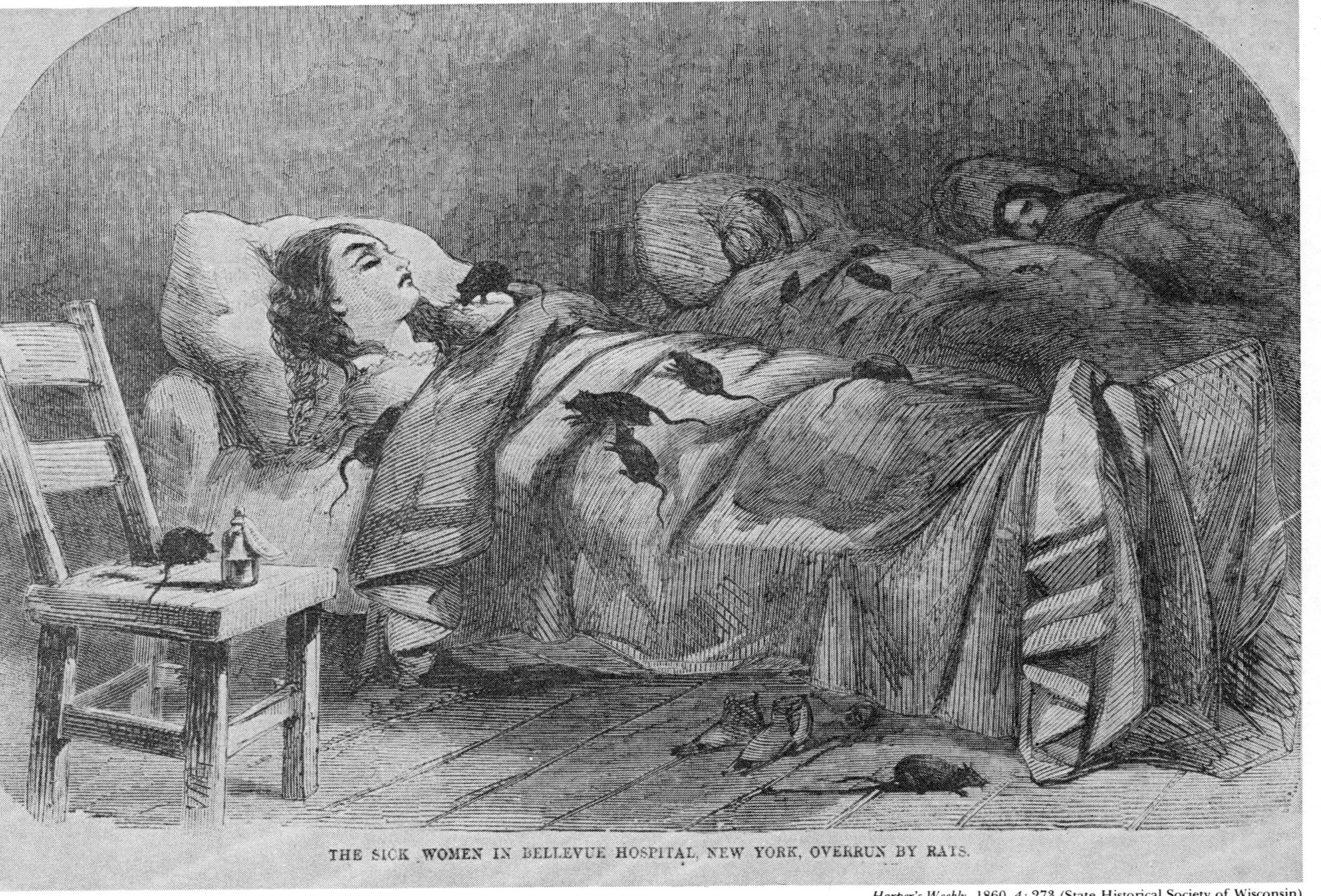

THE SICK WOMEN IN BELLEVUE HOSPITAL, NEW YORK, OVERRUN BY RATS.

Harper's Weekly, 1860, *4:* 273 (State Historical Society of Wisconsin)

Nineteenth-century hospitals sheltered the suffering poor, but their filthy and understaffed facilities sometimes did more harm than good. In 1860 a woman in New York City's Bellevue Hospital actually lost her newborn baby to the institution's rats.

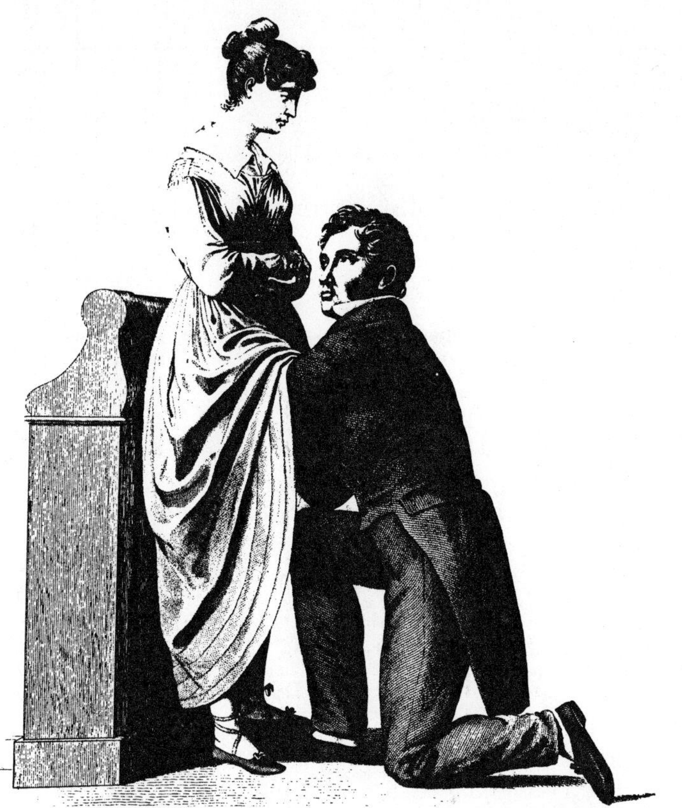

J. P. Maygrier, *Midwifery Illustrated* (New York: Harper Bros., 1834), p. 90

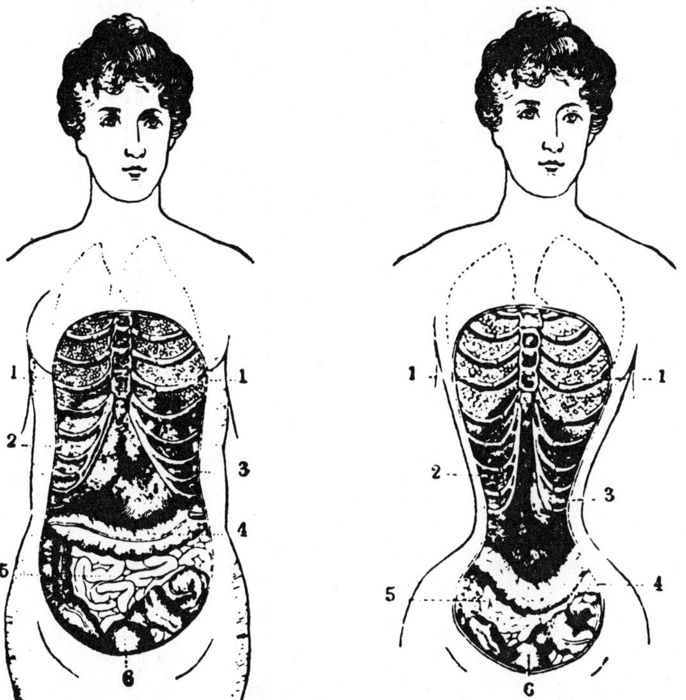

From *The Unfashionable Human Body* by Bernard Rudofsky. Copyright © 1971 by Bernard Rudofsky. Used by permission of Doubleday and Company, Inc.

Modesty frequently inhibited women from seeking assistance for sensitive ailments and sometimes affected the treatment they received, as this pelvic examination illustrates. Several health problems resulted from the fashionable 19th-century custom of wearing waist-restricting corsets.

FEE-BILL,

Adopted by the Western Medical Society of the State of Wisconsin, December, 1849.

Ordinary office prescription,	$ 0 50
Venesection, or extracting tooth at office.	50
Opening abscess,	50 *to* 5 00
Dresing wound,	50 " 5 00
Vaccination,	" 1 00
Dividing Fraenum,	50 " 2 00
Cupping,	1 00 " 2 00
Introducing Seton or Issue	1 00 " 2 00
Scarifying Eye,	1 00 " 5 00
Verbal advice,	1 00
Written advice,	2 00 " 5 00
Ordinary visit in Town,	1 00
Visit after 10 o'clock P. M.,	2 00
Additional patients, same family, (each)	50
Consultation visit,	3 00 " 5 00
Malignant Contagious diseases, (first)	3 00 " 5 00
Subsequent visits, each,	2 00
Natural Parturition, (ten hours.)	6 00 " 10 00
Extra Detention, (pr hour.)	50
Unnecessary Detention, (pr hour.)	1 00
Twin cases,	10 00 " 15 00
Instrumental Labor, or Turning,	15 00 " 25 00
Removing Placenta,	6 00 " 10 00
Visits after two days, charged as ordinary.	
Visit in country under two miles,	2 00
Do. over two miles, pr mile,	50 " 1 00
Visit, same neighborhood half price.	
Gonorrhœa, (in advance.)	5 00 " 20 00
Syphilis, (Do.)	10 00 " 25 00
Introducing Catheter, (first time.)	2 00
Do. Subsequently,	1 00
Paracentesis,	5 00 " 20 00
Excision Tonsils,	5 00 " 10 00
Operation for Hydrocele,	5 00 " 25 00
Do. Phimosis, Paraphimosis,	5 00 " 10 00
Do. Fistula Lachrymalis,	10 00 " 30 00
Do. " in Ano,	10 00 " 35 00

Operation for Imperforate Anus.	$ 5 00 *to* 25 00
Do. Vagina.	10 00 " 50 00
Do. Hare-Lip,	10 00 " 30 00
Do. Hernia.	25 *to* 100 00
Do. Cataract,	50 " 100 00
Do. Strabismus,	10 " 25 00
Do. Club-Foot,	25 " 100 00
Do. Stone.	100 " 200 00
Ligating Arteries,	10 " 200 00
Extirpating Eye,	50 " 100 00
Do. Testicle,	25 " 100 00
Do. Tumors,	5 " 100 00
Trephining.	25 " 100 00
Reducing Hernia,	5 " 15 00
Do. Prolapsus Ani.	2 " 10 00
Do. Fracture of Thigh,	25 " 50 00
Do. " Leg,	10 " 30 00
Do. " Clavicle,	10 " 25 00
Do. " Arm, Forearm,	10 " 25 00
Do. " Fingers, Toes,	3 " 10 00
Dislocation Hip-Joint,	25 " 100 00
Do. Shoulder-Joint,	15 " 35 00
Do. Elbow, Wrist, Ankle,	10 " 25 00
Do. Finger, Toe,	3 " 10 00
Amputation Thigh,	50 " 100 00
Do. Leg, Foot,	25 " 100 00
Do. Finger, Toe,	5 " 15 00
Do. Arm, Forearm, Wrist,	25 " 75 00
Do. Hip, or Shoulder Joint,	100 " 200 00
Do. Breast,	25 " 100 00
Do. Penis,	10 " 50 00
Inducing Premature Labor,	50 " 100 00

In all Surgical cases, the charge for subsequent attendance, to be according to time occupied and trouble incurred.

Visits in the country after dark to be considered as night visits, and charged double.

Resolved, That the moral, professional and pecuniary interests of this Society, require of its members a uniformity in charges.

Resolved, That we, the undersigned, members of the Western Medical Society of the State of Wisconsin, mutually pledge ourselves faithfully to adhere to the foregoing rates of charges.

(SIGNED,)

J. W. Clark,	H. Van Dusen,	Azel P. Ladd,	A. Sampson,
J. S. Russell,	Geo. D. Wilber,	Wm. Stoddart,	C. A. Mills,
Edward Cronin,	David Ross,	Geo. W. Phillips,	T. R Kibbe.

Attest, GEO. D. WILBER, *Secretary*. J. W. CLARK, *President*

History of Medicine Department, University of Wisconsin-Madison

Local medical societies attempted to regulate the costs of medical care and stabilize the income of physicians by publishing schedules of fees like this one for the Western Medical Society of the State of Wisconsin in 1849. Such documents can often tell us as much about the practice of medicine as about medical economics.

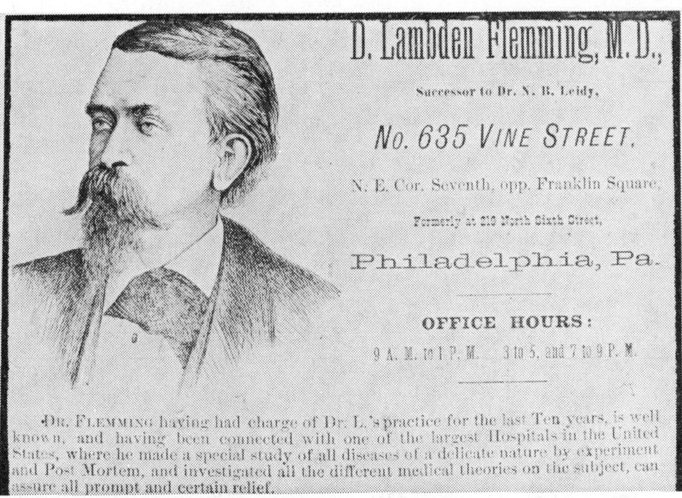
D. Lambden Flemming, M.D.,
Successor to Dr. N. B. Leidy,
No. 635 Vine Street,
N. E. Cor. Seventh, opp. Franklin Square,
Philadelphia, Pa.
OFFICE HOURS:
9 A. M. to 1 P. M. 3 to 5, and 7 to 9 P. M.
Dr. Flemming having had charge of Dr. L.'s practice for the last Ten years, is well known, and having been connected with one of the largest Hospitals in the United States, where he made a special study of all diseases of a delicate nature by experiment and Post Mortem, and investigated all the different medical theories on the subject, can assure all prompt and certain relief.

Picture Collection, New York Public Library

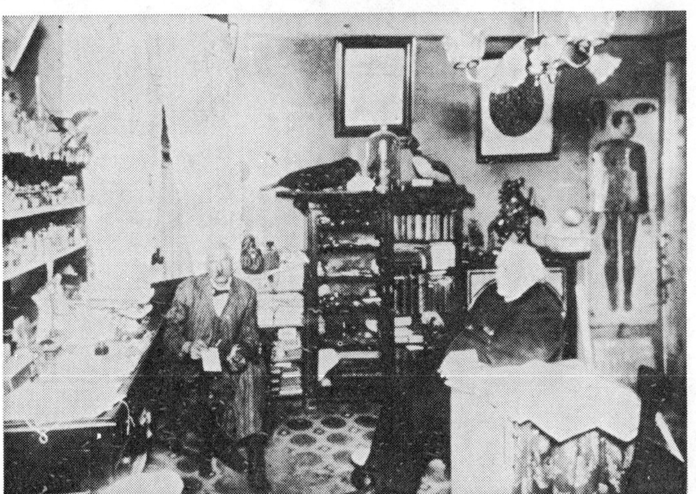

State Historical Society of Colorado

These illustrations suggest changes in the image of the American doctor: the businessman-physician of the 19th century, the family practitioner of the early 20th century, and the striking house staff of a major New York hospital in the 1970s.

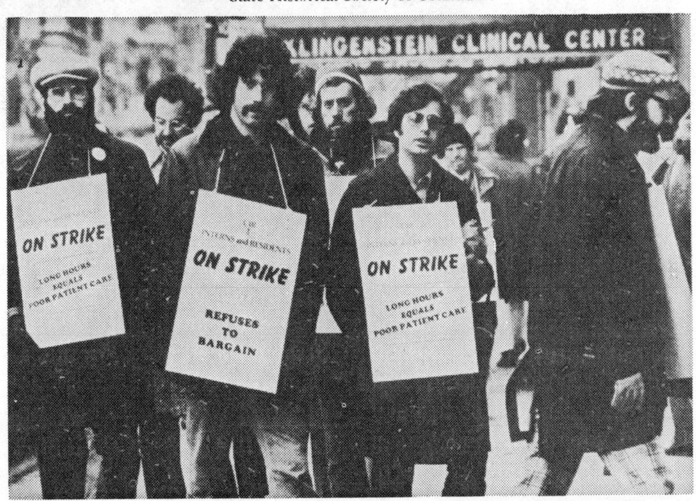

Medical Dimensions, June, 1975, p. 14

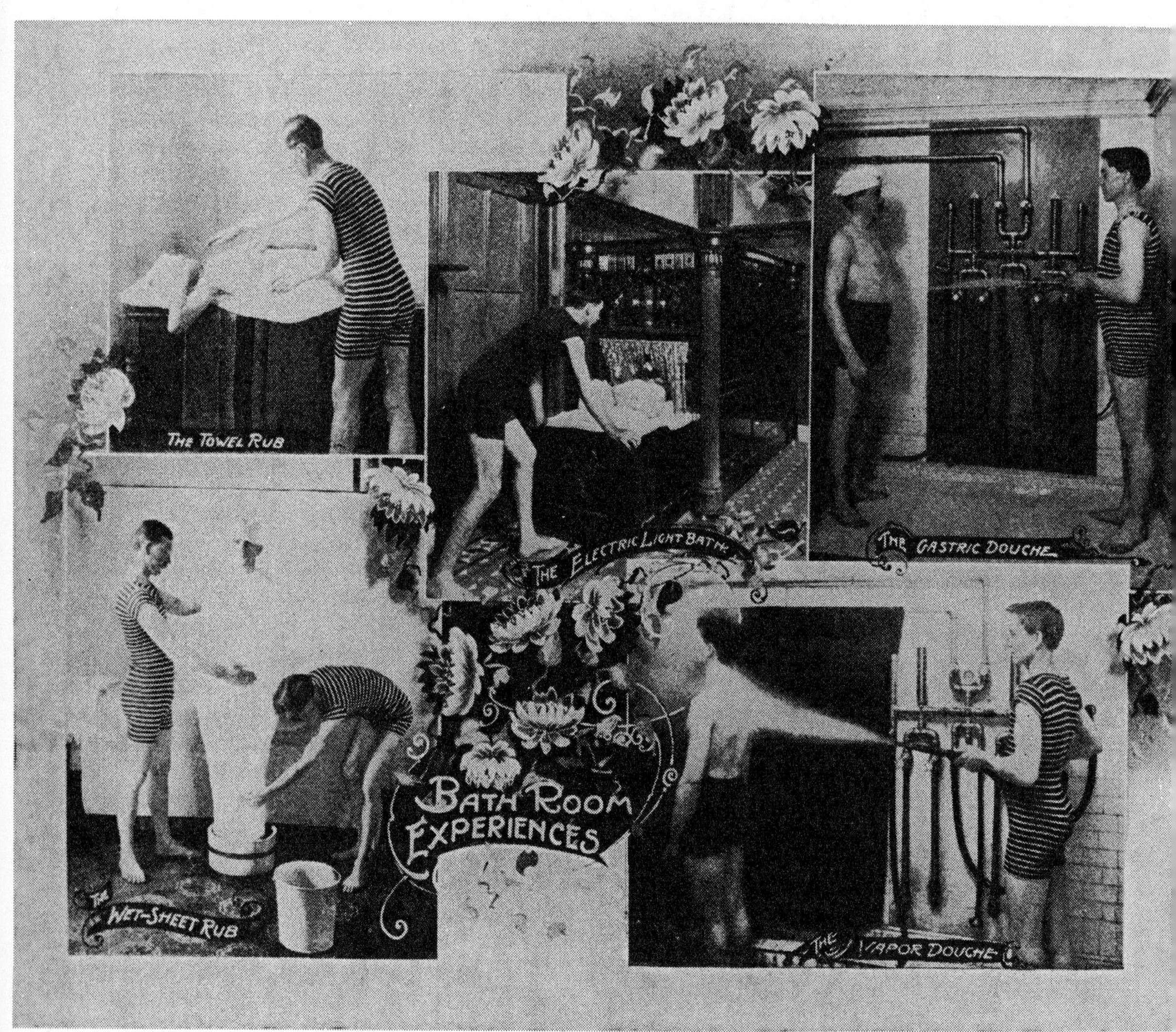

Smithsonian Ins

Hydropathy was only one of several medical sects that flourished in 19th-century America. These photographs show the va treatments available at Dr. John Harvey Kellogg's Battle Creek Sanitarium, which prospered well into the 20th century.

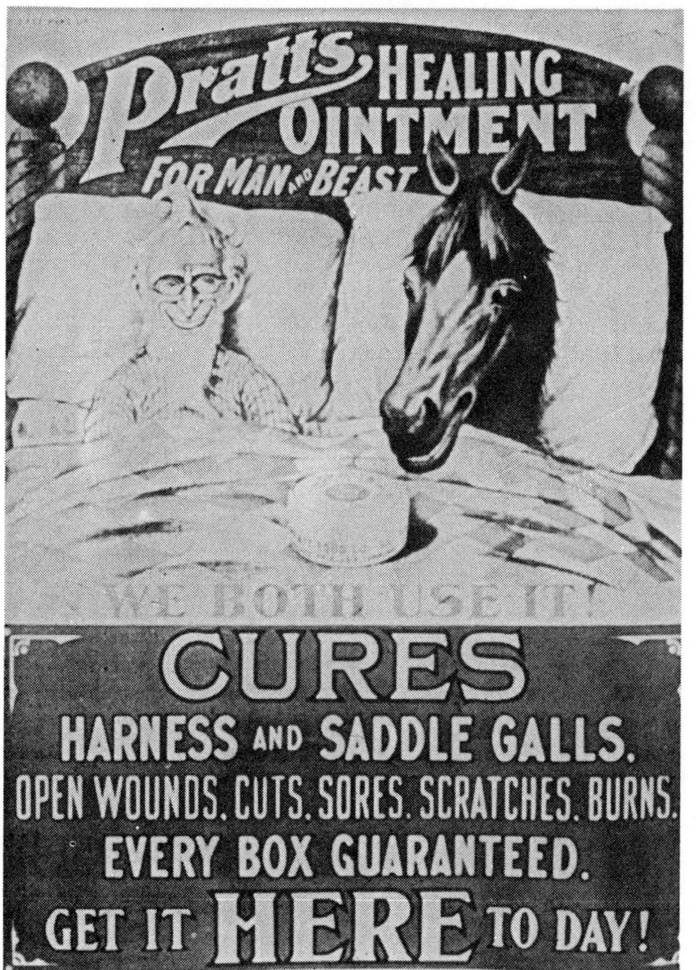

School of Pharmacy, University of Wisconsin

In addition to its regular and sectarian physicians, America offered its sick an almost infinite variety of quacks and cures, from ubiquitous patent remedies like Pratt's Healing Ointment to more elaborate and costly devices like the worthless Electric Couch and Dry Bath.

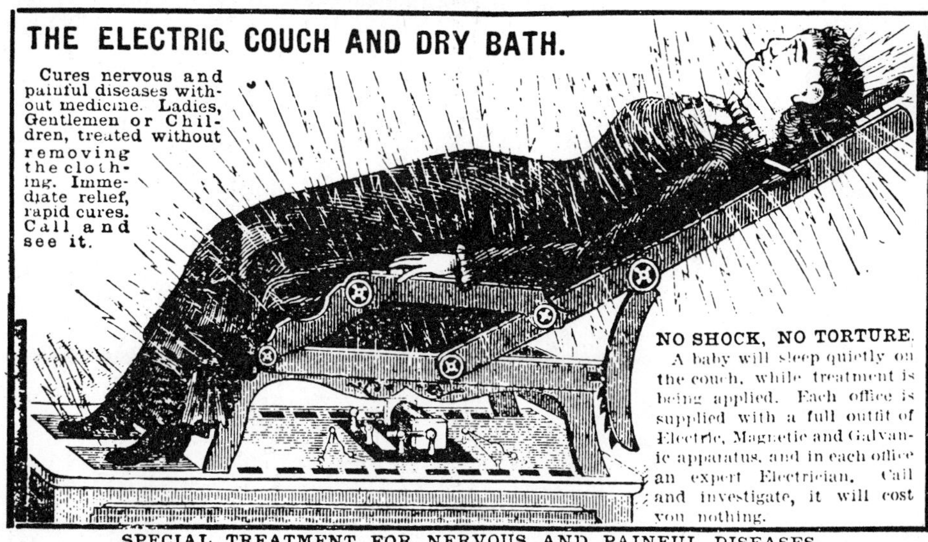

Smithsonian Institution

Bellevue Hospital Medical College.

CITY OF NEW YORK.

SESSION 1874–'75.

.... *is entitled*

To all the Privileges of the Department of

PRACTICAL ANATOMY,

Until March 1, 1875.

A. Flint Jr M. D., Sec'y of the Faculty.

☞ This Ticket is not an evidence that the holder of it has actually dissected, unless certified by the Professor of Practical Anatomy. [OVER.]

Bellevue Hospital Medical College.

CITY OF NEW YORK.

SESSION 1874–'75.

Admit..

LECTURES

ON

Physiology and Physiological Anatomy.

A. Flint Jr *M. D., Professor.*

Bellevue Hospital Medical College.

SESSION 1874–'75.

LECTURES ON SURGERY.

Admit..

Frank H. Hamilton *M. D.,*

Prof. of Practice of Surgery with Operations.

Lewis A. Sayre *M, D.,*

Prof. of Orthopedic Surgery.

Alex. B. Mott *M. D.,*

Prof. of Clinical and Operative Surgery.

Wm. Van Buren *M. D.,*

Prof. of the Principles of Surgery with Diseases of the Genito-Urinary System.

Bellevue Hospital Medical College.

CITY OF NEW YORK.

SESSION 1874–'75.

Admit..

LECTURES

ON

THE PRINCIPLES AND PRACTICE OF MEDICINE.

Austin Flint. *M. D., Professor.*

Richard W. Schwarz Collection

Until late into the 19th century medical students paid for their tuition by purchasing tickets from each professor whose lectures they wanted to attend.

PART II

Public Health and Personal Hygiene

Epidemics

Although epidemics seldom took more lives than endemic diseases, they have always attracted the most attention. Sweeping inexorably through town after town, these unpredictable plagues aroused more fear and anxiety than the more deadly but common everyday killers like pneumonia and tuberculosis. Even today the threat of an epidemic that might cost a few thousand lives excites more concern than automobile accidents, for example, which annually take tens of thousands of lives. Of all epidemics, the most feared were smallpox, yellow fever, and cholera.

Smallpox, a physically repulsive and often disfiguring disease, arrived in the New World with the European settlers. It decimated many Amerindian groups and took the lives of numerous immigrants. When smallpox struck, colonials typically quarantined the affected area and isolated the sick, either at home or in a pesthouse. In 1721 Cotton Mather attempted to introduce another means of stopping this loathsome disease. John B. Blake tells about the controversy in Boston that the introduction of inoculation (or variolation) ignited. Although this preventive measure seemed to lower mortality from smallpox, it was not without its risks, as opponents vigorously pointed out. A second debate over smallpox immunization developed in the 19th century, after Benjamin Waterhouse brought William Jenner's method of vaccination with cowpox virus to America. Even with this safer technique, resistance — political as well as medical — continued until the 20th century.

Yellow fever, a distinctive disease characterized by yellowish skin, black vomit, and high death rates, likewise stirred political and medical passions, as Martin S. Pernick shows in his study of the Philadelphia epidemic of 1793. That epidemic served as a terrifying model of yellow fever's destructive abilities for the next hundred years. Although yellow fever disappeared from the northern states after the early 19th century, it remained a threat in the South until 1900, when Walter Reed and his associates discovered the role of the mosquito in transmitting the infection.

Cholera visited the United States only four times — in 1832, 1849, 1866, and 1873 — but the mere thought of this viciously dehydrating disease struck fear in the heart of virtually every American throughout the 19th century. Charles E. Rosenberg traces the evolving medical and lay interpretations of its cause and cure. The contagionist-anticontagionist controversy he describes represented a major medical dilemma of the 19th century and applied to many other diseases besides cholera.

With the exception of the 1918–19 influenza epidemic, which killed more Americans than World War I, the United States has been remarkably free of major epidemics during the 20th century. But as the swine flu scare of 1976 illustrated, we still live in fear of an attack by a mysterious new killer.

17

The Inoculation Controversy in Boston: 1721–1722

JOHN B. BLAKE

Of all the diseases affecting colonial America, none caused more consternation than smallpox. Highly contagious, once it gained a foothold, it spread rapidly and with fearful mortality. Recognizing these facts, the authorities of Massachusetts developed certain techniques designed to keep this scourge under control. They required incoming vessels with smallpox aboard to perform quarantine at Spectacle Island in Boston harbor, and when cases appeared in town, the selectmen removed the patients to a pesthouse or placed guards about the infected dwellings. Although these precautions often proved successful, they were unable entirely to prevent periodic epidemics. During one of these outbreaks, in 1721, inoculation of the smallpox was first tried in the colonies. It enraged the town and called forth a bitter newspaper and pamphlet war, but it was the earliest important experiment in preventive medicine in America.

The practice was not new in 1721. People in certain parts of Africa, India, and China had been using inoculation for centuries. Even in Europe there was some reference to it in a verse production of the School of Salerno in the 10th or 11th century. The first authentic reports were published in Leipzig between 1670 and 1705. In other parts of Europe it was employed as a part of folk-medicine.[1] Late in the 17th century, accounts of the Asiatic practice began arriving in England, and in February 1699/1700, Dr. Clopton Havers called it to the attention of the Royal Society. Certainly by this time many Englishmen had heard of the art.[2]

In the following two decades, after inoculation had become popular in Turkey, it was more fully studied, reported, and recommended in the western world. During a smallpox epidemic in 1713 it agian came up for discussion in the Royal Society. In May 1714, Dr. John Woodward, Professor of Physic at Gresham College, communicated to this scientific organization an enthusiastic endorsement from Dr. Emanuel Timonius of Constantinople.[3] Other correspondents also reported on the practice, and two years later the society published another favorable account by Jacobus Pylarinus.[4] Not until April 1721, however, did the first recorded inoculation take place in England, on the daughter of Lady Mary Wortley Montagu. Another child received the treatment in May. Princess Caroline became interested, and in August six felons offered themselves for experiment. After other trials the two royal daughters were successfully inoculated in April 1722.[5]

In Massachusetts, meanwhile, some of Cotton Mather's parishioners gave him a Negro slave in 1706. No doubt Mather asked him if he had had the smallpox, and received then his first confused intimation of the practice of inoculation as some of the African natives carried it out. Further questioning of several other Negroes and some Guinea slave traders confirmed the tale. Sometime before July 1716, Mather also received a copy of Timonius's communication in the *Philosophical Transactions*. In a letter to Dr. Woodward of July 12, 1716, he corroborated this account with what he had heard and inquired why the practice was not tried in England. "For my own part," he wrote, "if I should live to see the *Small-Pox* again enter into our City, I would immediately procure a Consult of our Physicians, to Introduce a Practice, which may be of so very happy a Tendency."[6] At least five years in advance, therefore, Mather had

---

JOHN B. BLAKE is Chief of the History of Medicine Division, National Library of Medicine, Bethesda, Maryland.

Reprinted with permission from the *New England Quarterly*, 1952, *25*: 489–506.

seriously considered the policy he was later to follow.[7]

On April 22, 1721, among several ships arriving from the West Indies was H.M.S. *Seahorse*, which brought the smallpox. Not until May 8, however, did the selectmen learn that a Negro who came on the naval vessel was in town with the disease. When they heard of another case at Captain Wentworth Paxton's house, they ordered two men to stand guard there and let no one in or out without their permission. A few days later, at the request of the town, the governor and council ordered the *Seahorse* down to Bird Island to prevent further infection from this source, but not until after several other sick members of the company had come ashore. As late as May 20 the selectmen could find no more cases, but two days later the town nevertheless instructed its representatives to seek further legislation to enable the selectmen to prevent the spread of infectious sickness. On the twenty-fourth the selectmen set 26 free Negroes to work cleaning the streets as a preventive measure, but without avail. On May 27 there were eight known cases, and by the middle of June the disease was in so many houses that the selectmen abandoned the system of guards.[8]

By this time Cotton Mather had decided to carry out his previous plan. Considering it his Christian duty — and worrying about his own children — on June 6 he circulated a letter about inoculation among the physicians of Boston, along with an abstract of the accounts by Timonius and Pylarinus. "*Gentlemen*," he wrote, "My *request* is, that you would *meet for a Consultation* upon this Occasion, and to *deliberate* upon it, that whoever first begins this practise, (*if you approve that it should be begun at all*) may have the concurrence of his *worthy Brethren* to fortify him in it."[9] Whatever their reasons, they made no reply. On June 24, after the guards had been taken off the houses, he wrote another letter strongly recommending the technique to Dr. Zabdiel Boylston.[10] This may have convinced the physician, for two days later he inoculated his six-year-old son Thomas and two of his Negroes. After several anxious days the experiment proved successful, and on July 12 he inoculated Joshua Cheever. Two days later John Helyer and another Negro underwent the operation. On the seventeenth Boylston treated his son John, and on the nineteenth three more people, bringing the total to ten.[11]

The populace was quickly aroused. The idea had caused talk soon after Mather brought it up; within four days after Boylston's first experiment it "raised an horrid Clamour. . . ."[12] In an advertisement in the *Boston Gazette* on July 17 the physician justified his action on the grounds of the reports of Timonius and Pylarinus and his own successful experiments, but when he indicated his intention to continue by the announcement that "*in a few Weeks more, I hope to give you some further proof of their just and reasonable Account*," he no doubt increased the people's wrath. Cotton Mather, convinced of the value of the practice, thought the Devil had "taken a strange Possession of the People," and noted sadly in his diary that not only Boylston but he himself was also "an Object of their Fury; their furious Obloquies and Invectives."[13]

Soon the selectmen felt they must act. On July 21 they and some justices of the peace met with several members of the medical profession. Disregarding Boylston's invitation to see some of his patients,[14] they accepted instead Dr. Lawrence Dalhonde's statement that inoculation in Italy, Spain, and Flanders had led to horrible sequelae, and pronounced that it "has proved the Death of many Persons," that it "Tends to spread and continue the Infection," and that its continuance "is likely to prove of most dangerous consequence."[15] On this basis the selectmen and justices severely reprimanded Boylston and forbade him to continue the practice.[16]

Three days later Dr. William Douglass, who led the professional opposition, tried a new attack in a communication to the *News-Letter*. He credited Mather with "a Pious & Charitable design of doing good," but attacked Boylston for "*His mischievous propagating the Infection* in the most Publick Trading Place of the Town. . . ." He called on the ministers to determine "how the trusting more the extra groundless *Machinations of Men* than to our Preserver in the ordinary course of Nature, may be consistent with that Devotion and Subjection we owe to the *all-wise Providence* of GOD Almighty." Of the lawyers he inquired "how it may be construed a *Propagating of Infection and Criminal*."[17] On the thirty-first the ministers' reply appeared in the

Gazette, signed by Increase and Cotton Mather, Benjamin Colman, Thomas Prince, John Webb, and William Cooper. After upholding Boylston's professional skill, they declared that if, as they believed, inoculation could save lives, they accepted it "with all thankfulness and joy as the gracious Discovery of a *Kind Providence* to Mankind. . . ." Use of this operation, they said, like that of any other medical treatment, depended on God's blessing and was fully consistent with "*a humble Trust . . . and a due Subjection*" to the Lord. When James Franklin's new paper, the *New-England Courant*, appeared on August 7, the anti-inoculators had their medium, and a furious newspaper and pamphlet war ensued.

Boylston, meanwhile, backed by the six ministers, disregarded the selectmen's orders and on August 5 resumed inoculating. During that month he performed the operation on 17 people, in September on 31, and the next month on 18. Among the last were three men from Roxbury who, after their recovery, returned to recommend it there. November was his busiest month, with 104 inoculations. Several ministers and other prominent men encouraged the practice by their example. On September 23 the Honorable Thomas Fitch, Esq., tried the new technique. Others included the Reverend Thomas Walter on October 31, and in November, the Reverend Ebenezer Pierpont, Anthony Stoddard, Esq., John White, Esq., the Honorable Judge Quincy's son Edmund, Edward Wigglesworth, and William Welsteed, professor and fellow respectively at Harvard, Justice Samuel Sewall's grandson Samuel Hirst, the Honorable Jonathan Belcher's son Andrew, and the Reverend Nehemiah Walter. On December 8, even a doctor, Elijah Danforth of Roxbury, submitted to the test.[18]

Whatever the clergymen and esquires may have thought of inoculation, the people as a whole continued to oppose it violently. They were urged on by most of the local physicians, one of whom went so far as to assert that it would breed in Boston bubonic plague, which was then devastating southern France.[19] One man vented his feelings about three in the morning of November 14 by throwing a lighted grenade into Cotton Mather's house.[20] Ten days previously, shortly after Boylston began receiving patients from Roxbury and Charlestown, the town had expressed its official attitude by voting that anyone who came into Boston to be inoculated should be forthwith sent to the pesthouse unless he returned home, "Least by alowing this practis the Town be made an Hospital for that which may prove worse then the Smal pox, which has already put So many into mourning. . . ."[21] The selectmen thereupon requested the justices for warrants to remove such persons.[22] When several ministers were accused of encouraging country people to come into Boston to be inoculated despite the town's vote, the selectmen called them to a meeting, but "after some hot Discourse on both sides" they denied it.[23]

Meanwhile the epidemic also raged. Soon after it began, trade was disrupted, and many people fled. One person died in May, 8 in June, 11 in July, and 26 in August.[24] That month the General Court, which was sitting at the George Tavern on the Neck, appointed three men to stand guard at the door of the House of Representatives to prevent anyone from Boston entering without special license.[25] In September, when the deaths jumped to 101, the selectmen severely limited the length of time funeral bells could toll.[26] When the sloopmen who normally supplied the town with wood refused to bring it in, the selectmen made special arrangements to allay their fear and avert a fuel shortage, perhaps on the suggestion of Cotton Mather.[27] When the General Court met again on November 7, in Cambridge, the members were "very solicitous of Returning to their Homes as soon as may be,"[28] for by then the smallpox was in the college town. The session lasted only ten days, most of the time being taken up with the Indian war in Maine and quarrels with the governor. The legislators did find time, however, to tighten up the law against peddlers, who were charged with spreading the disease.[29] More helpful was the thousand pounds voted from the public treasury for the selectmen and overseers of the poor to distribute among the many people "reduced to Very Great Strieghts & Necessitous Circumstances," who could otherwise have supported their families comfortably.[30] Along with the contributions from other towns, it was no doubt gratefully received.[31]

By then the epidemic was beginning to decline. October had been the worst month, with 411 deaths. In November the total dropped to 249, and by mid-December, according to the selectmen, the mortality was not much higher than in time of health.[32] During January and February Boylston inoculated only 12 people, none in Boston.[33] On February 26 the selectmen issued an official statement that there were no more known cases in the town. Altogether, since April, 5,889 people, of whom 844 died, had had the smallpox. This one disease caused more than three-fourths of all the deaths in Boston during the year of the epidemic.[34] During the same period Boylston inoculated 242 persons, with 6 deaths.[35] Except for a few recurrences in April and May the epidemic was over in the capital.[36]

Then, on May 11, 1722, Boylston inoculated Samuel Sewall, a Boston merchant and nephew of the diarist, his wife, three boys in his household, and Joanna Alford, the first he had done since February 24, and the first in Boston since December.[37] The people were incensed. The selectmen quickly removed these new cases to Spectacle Island to keep them from communicating the infection to anyone else,[38] and called Boylston before the town meeting, where he "did solemnly promise to Inoculate no more without the knowledge & approbation of the Authority of the Town."[39] Douglass gloated:

> Last January *Inoculation* made a Sort of *Exit*, like the Infatuation Thirty Years ago, after several had fallen Victims to the mistaken Notions of Dr. *M–r* and other learned Clerks concerning Witchcraft. But finding Inoculation in this Town, like the Serpents in Summer, beginning to crawl abroad again the last Week, it was in time, and effectually crushed in the Bud, by the *Justices, Select-Men*, and the *unanimous Vote* of a general Town-Meeting.[40]

The voters also instructed their representatives to seek legislation regulating inoculation and prohibiting it in any town without the selectmen's permission. Since some question had arisen over the interpretation of the act relating to contagious diseases, the people wanted their officials "Clothed with full power to obtain the great End & Designe of that Law, which is for the Preservation, Health, and Safty, of the Inhabitants."[41]

The House had already passed a "Bill to prevent the Spreading of the Infection of the Small-Pox by the practice of Inoculation" in March 1721/1722, but the council had turned it down.[42] Perhaps for this reason the representatives made no further attempt to pass a general law. Their attitude, however, was unchanged. When the Boston assemblymen brought up the subject of Samuel Sewall and the others sent to Spectacle Island, the General Court resolved on June 2, 1722, that they should not come to Boston as long as the legislature was in session. As late as July 3 the House denied a petition passed by the council to rescind this order.[43]

An analysis of the whole controversy shows that several factors were involved. One source of opposition to inoculation was the religious scruples of earnest and devout people. Some maintained that it was a sin for a healthy person to bring the sickness upon himself, especially since he might otherwise escape it altogether, and that he should in submission to God's will leave it to Him to determine whether or not he would suffer the disease. Another argument was that since the epidemic was sent by God, the only proper recourse was repentance and reformation; inoculation only increased the guilt because it was a rebellious attempt to take God's work out of His hands and showed distrust in His promises:[44]

> It is impossible that any *Humane Means*, or *preventive Physick* should defend us from, or Over-rule a *Judicial National Sickness*; for were it so, Wicked and Atheistical Men would have the same terms and conditions of *Security* in a *Physical Respect*, with the most Holy and Religious. And *National Judgments* would not have the Designed Ends for which they were sent *National Amendment*.[45]

Some of Boston's leading ministers, however, easily answered these arguments. It was not unlawful to make oneself sick in this manner, they declared; rather it was a duty because it was a protection against a worse sickness. In the same way, they pointed out, other preventive medicines such as purges and vomits were used, and no one considered that sinful. William Cooper provided the most complete rebuttal. It was not faith, he said, but presumption for anyone to think that God would preserve him when walking in an infected atmosphere. One must, of course, rely primarily on the Lord, he said, but this did not preclude the use of the best human help afforded by His providence. Recourse to inoculation did not take God's work from His hands, for both inoculated and natural smallpox were secondary causes and therefore under Him the First Cause. While agreeing that the epidemic was God's judgment for the sins of the community, he believed that the people should be thankful for His mercy in sending the means to escape the extremity of destruction. Inoculation, he said, might be God's chosen instrument to preserve life as long as He had predestined it; no one, he pointed out, relied on predestination to keep himself from starving. Admittedly there was no guarantee that an inoculated person would not die. But after serious consideration of this, the knottiest problem of all, Cooper believed that if a person died under this operation, he died in the use of the most likely means he knew to save his life in time of peril, and, therefore, in the way of duty and so in God's way.[46]

The religious question, though significant, should not be overemphasized. While much of the argument was couched in religious terms, the real dividing point was medical. The Sixth Commandment was frequently mentioned, but whether for or against depended on what the medical results of inoculation were alleged to be. None of the opponents was content to rest his case on the necessity of trusting in God's providence; however they phrased it, they all thought the practice harmful to the health and lives of their fellow-citizens.

In the passion of the fight both sides exaggerated either the ease and safety of the practice on the one hand, or its horrors and dangers on the other. The proponents' fundamental argument, however, was that it gave the patient a mild case of smallpox which protected him from the natural one. They cited the reports of Timonius and Pylarinus, and Boylston published Mather's abstracts.[47] They pointed out that in Africa the Negroes had long carried on this practice to great advantage. They ridiculed the assertions that it would cause plague or debilitate the constitution. In particular they called to witness the results of Boylston's own trials. Old and young, weak and strong, had been inoculated, they said, with success beyond expectation. After making excuses for the sole death at the time he wrote, Increase Mather declared:

> It is then a wonderful Providence of GOD, that all that were *Inoculated* should have their Lives preserved; so that the Safety and Usefulness of this Experiment is confirmed to us by Ocular Demonstration: I confess I am afraid, that the Discouraging of this Practice, may cause many a Life to be lost, which for my own part, I should be loth to have any hand in, *because of the Sixth Commandment.*[48]

When we see how easily it enables people to pass through smallpox, said Benjamin Colman, we should praise the Lord for His mercy in providing it.[49] "*In fine*;" added Cotton Mather, "*Experience has declared, that there never was a more* unfailing Remedy *employed among the Children of Men.*"[50]

Although some objections were fantastic and some picayune, anti-inoculators also had sound arguments. They emphasized the known deaths among the inoculated — which the Mathers tried to explain away — and hinted of others. They said, rightly, that the technique endangered the individual who submitted to it. Their chief contention was that inoculation as performed by Boylston spread the epidemic. John Williams maintained that anyone who voluntarily took the smallpox violated the moral law of God — "Therefore all things whatsoever ye would that Men should do to you, do ye even so to them" — by bringing the disease to his neighbor.[51]

The anonymous author of *A Letter from One in the Country, to His Friend in the City* expressed this viewpoint ably. As he saw it, Boylston introduced the practice without the consent of the other physicians soon after the guards had been removed from stricken houses, when there was still a possibility that the epidemic would not spread. Is it not an offense against the government, he asked, to infect one's own family with the smallpox despite the cries of civil authority, professional brethren, and neighbors? "If a man should wilfully throw a Bomb into a Town. . . . ought he not to die? so if a man should wilfully bring Infection from a person sick of a deadly and contagious Disease, into a place of Health; is not the mischief as great?"[52] The author was willing to allow those who favored inoculation to practice it, but only where they would not threaten the rest of the community. He felt sure, and he was right, that the people who urged the new technique never thought of regulating it, "which ought to have been the very first step in a matter of such concernment to a people."[53] He hoped the General Court would act:

> That if they allow it, there may be proper Pest Houses in solitary places, to receive those that have a mind thus voluntarily to infect themselves, with severe penalties on those that shall dare to do otherwise, to the endangering the lives of their honest Neighbours. . . .[54]

This was a sound suggestion. Unfortunately it was not carried out for many years.

Religious and medical divisions were not the only causes of the heat of the controversy. In part they were due to the personalities involved, particularly those of Cotton Mather and William Douglass. The former, pedantic, tactless, egotistical, convinced that those who opposed him were possessed of the Devil, yet rejoicing in the prospect of martyrdom at the hands of Satan's minions (the town), asserted that raving and railing against "*the* Ministers, *and other serious* Christians, *who favour this Practice, is a very crying Iniquity; and to call it a* Work of the Devil . . . *is a shocking* Blasphemy. . . ."[55] He or one of his cohorts accused the anti-inoculation physicians of being another "Hell-Fire Club," a current, notorious group of blasphemers in England.[56] Douglass, on the other hand, accused Mather of credulity, whim, and vanity, of omissions and errors in his abstracts of Timonius and Pylarinus, and of misrepresentation; and he called Boylston an illiterate quack.[57] Douglass, apparently, thought he should be the leader of whatever was happening in local medical affairs and was prone to disparage any who were not his sycophants. Nine years later he declared that Mather had "surreptitiously" set Boylston to work, "that he might have the honour of a New-fangled notion."[58] One suspects that some of his bitterness resulted from his own failure to take the lead. Eventually he came to favor the practice, but he never forgave his two opponents.[59]

The clash between Mather and Douglass stemmed from more than their personalities, for they also stood for two different principles. The minister was in effect maintaining the right of his profession to interfere with and control the life of the community. This is why he and his father — the ordained leaders in all things — became so incensed when others defied them. We say that inoculation is good and lawful, they seemed to assert; therefore all men must believe it. The wise and judicious people of Massachusetts approved it, wrote Increase Mather, referring to the magistrates and ministers, himself and his son. Those who opposed were of a different breed:

> Furthermore, I have made some Enquiry, Whether there are many Persons of a Prophane Life and Conversation, that do Approve and Defend *Inoculation*, and I have been answered, that they know but of very few such. This is to me a weighty Consideration. But on the other hand, tho' there are some Worthy Persons, that are not clear about it; nevertheless, it cannot be denied, but that the known Children of the Wicked one, are generally fierce Enemies to Inoculation.[60]

To those with a troubled conscience, Mather suggested that they seek guidance from their religious advisers. But as for Douglass, no one could "in rational Charity" think that he had

> the least spark of Grace in his heart . . . ; for in his Pamphlet there are many impudent and malicious Lies, and the whole design of it is to jeer and abuse the faithful Messengers of GOD, which is far from a sign of Piety. 2 Chron. 36. 16.[61]

Douglass, on the other hand, was defending the integrity of the medical profession against the interference of those whom he considered to be credulous laymen. He pointed out that no one should accept all the quaint things published in the *Philosophical Transactions*, that Mather's sources of information — accounts from the Levant and from untutored Negroes — were at best questionable.[62] His principal complaint was that despite the opposition of the town, the selectmen, and the medical profession, "*Six Gentlemen of Piety and Learning, profoundly ignorant of the Matter*," rashly advocated a new and doubtful procedure in "a Disease one of the most intricate practical Cases in Physick. . . ."[63] By January 1721/1722, Douglass was willing to admit that inoculated smallpox was frequently more favorable than natural and that the practice was at least a temporary, palliative preventive.

Though pessimistic, he thought that it might with improvement become a specific smallpox preventive. But, he declared, it must be allowed by an act of the legislature and carried out by "abler hands, than *Greek old Women, Madmen and Fools.*" He wanted a period of cautious experimentation. "For my own Part," he said, "*till after a few Years, I shall pass no positive Judgment of this bold Practice.*"[64]

Douglass' attitude toward the clergy brought him allies who opposed them chiefly for political reasons. Among them was John Williams. Much of his stuff was nonsense, some of it mildly amusing, but a large part was devoted to comprehensive attacks on the ministers. Claiming that inoculation was "a Delusion of the Devil," he compared it to "the Time of the Witchcraft at Salem, when so many innocent Persons lost their Lives. . . ."[65] He blasted the ministers for going outside their calling by trying to control such public affairs as inoculation and paper money. "Now the People are afraid," he declared, "the Ministers do affect a Rule over them in Temporals, as the Pope of *Rome* does temporally as well as spiritually, rule and determine things."[66]

James Franklin also seized this opportunity to belabor the clergy. "I pray Sir," asked "Layman" in a debate with "Clergyman" printed in Franklin's *Courant*:

> who have been Instruments of Mischief and Trouble both in Church and State, from the Witchcraft to Inoculation? who is it that takes the Liberty to Villify a whole Town, in Words too black to be repeated? Who is it that in common Conversation makes no Bones of calling the Town a MOB?[67]

Another *Friendly Debate* which he published just before the annual meeting for choosing town officers used the controversy to introduce an attack on the ministers, particularly Cotton Mather, for electioneering against the incumbent selectmen, for attempting to run the town, and for scorning the "Leather Apron Men."[68]

Boston's religious leaders were not the sort to turn the other cheek. One of their supporters damned "this Impious and Abominable Courant" as a weekly libel sheet whose "main intention" was to "Vilify and Abuse the best Men we have, and especially the Principal Ministers of Religion in the Country."[69] Increase Mather added his condemnation and his lamentations for the degeneracy of his native land. "I can well remember," he declared, "when the Civil Government could have taken an effectual Course to suppress such a *Cursed Libel*!"[70] The most thorough rebuttal was a pamphlet inspired by Cotton Mather,[71] the *Vindication of the Ministers of Boston.* The anonymous author lauded the clergy as worthy men seeking the best for their people and gave the pro-Mather version of the beginning of the whole controversy. He was chiefly concerned, however, with maintaining the ministers' leadership in all things:

> If this *impious* & Satanic Custom [of attacking the clergy] prevail, we shall involve our selves into a thousand pernicious *Evils.* . . . Our *Reprovers* and *Prophets* being Silenced, *Iniquity* and every *Abomination* will break in among us, and bear down like an irresistible Torrent, all *Virtue*, and *Religion* before it. And what is mostly to be deprecated, all manner of *Spiritual Plagues* will follow this our degeneracy; and the *Town* grow ripe for a *Wrath unto the Uttermost.*[72]

Inoculation had become a bitter party cause.

Reviewing the controversy, we must credit Cotton Mather and Boylston for their courage in experimenting with and continuing what seemed on fairly good evidence to be a means of saving life. But they cannot escape censure for their neglect of the rights of the community by their failure to take any steps to prevent those who were inoculated from transmitting the disease to others. Moreover, though Mather was not as credulous in this case as Douglass thought, it is difficult to escape the conclusion that he and Boylston were lucky that the experiment worked so well. On the other hand, Douglass' cautious approach toward an obviously dangerous medical innovation was a sane one. Unfortunately the vehemence of his opposition and his credulity in accepting Dalhonde's report becloud the positive values of his attitude. Furthermore, despite his expressed preference for cautious experiments, he himself would probably never have undertaken them.

NOTES

1 Arnold C. Klebs, "The historic evolution of variolation," *Johns Hopkins Hosp. Bull.*, 1913, *24*: 70; Charles G. Cumston, "Historical notes on smallpox and inoculation," *Ann. Med. Hist.*, 1924, *6*: 469.

2 Raymond P. Stearns and George Pasti, Jr., "Remarks upon the introduction of inoculation for smallpox in England," *Bull. Hist. Med.*, 1950, *24*: 106–108.

3 Emanuel Timonius, "An account, or history, of the procuring the small pox by incision, or inoculation; as it has for some time been practised at Constantinople," Royal Society of London, *Philosophical Transactions*, No. 339, April-May-June 1714, *29*: 72–82.

4 Jacobus Pylarinus, "Nova & tuta variolas excitandi per transplantationem methodus, nuper inventa & in usum tracta," Royal Society of London, *Philosophical Transactions*, No. 347, January-February-March 1716, *29*: 393–399.

5 Stearns and Pasti, "Introduction of inoculation in England," pp. 109–114; Klebs, "Evolution of variolation," pp. 71–72.

6 George L. Kittredge, "Introduction," Increase Mather, *Several Reasons Proving That Inoculating or Transplanting the Small Pox, Is a Lawful Practice, and That It Has Been Blessed by God for the Saving of Many a Life* (Cleveland, 1921), p. 5.

7 *Ibid.*, pp. 2–6; George L. Kittredge, "Some lost works of Cotton Mather," Massachusetts Historical Society, *Proceedings*, 1911–1912, *65*: 420–427.

8 Boston Record Commissioners, *Report* (Boston, 1876–1898), VIII, 154–155; XIII, 81–83; Massachusetts General Court, *The Acts and Resolves, Public and Private, of the Province of the Massachusetts Bay* (Boston, 1869–1922), X, 105; *Boston News-Letter*, May 22, 29, 1721; William Douglass to Cadwallader Colden, May 1, 1722, New-York Historical Society, *Collections*, 1917, *50*: 141–142.

9 *A Vindication of the Ministers of Boston, from the Abuses & Scandals, Lately Cast upon Them, in Diverse Printed Papers* (Boston, 1722), p. 8; Cotton Mather, *Diary* (Massachusetts Historical Society, *Collections*, 7th series, VII–VIII, 1911–1912), II, 620–622.

10 Reginald H. Fitz, *Zabdiel Boylston, Inoculator, and the Epidemic of Smallpox in Boston in 1721* (n.p., [1911], reprinted from *Johns Hopkins Hosp., Bull.*, 1911, *22*: 315–327), p. 10.

11 Zabdiel Boylston, *An Historical Account of the Small-Pox Inoculated in New England, upon All Sorts of Persons, Whites, Blacks, and of All Ages and Constitutions . . .* 2nd ed. (London, 1726; reprinted at Boston, 1730), pp. 2–7.

12 C. Mather, *Diary*, II, 628.

13 *Ibid.*, p. 632.

14 Boylston, *Historical Account*, pp. 3–4; *Boston Gazette*, July 31, 1721.

15 *News-Letter*, July 24, 1721.

16 [Cotton Mather], *An Account of the Method and Success of Inoculating the Small-Pox, in Boston in New-England* (London, 1722), p. 11; *New-England Courant*, Aug. 7, 1721.

17 *News-Letter*, July 24, 1721. As was his wont, Douglass added several gratuitous insults to Boylston.

18 Boylston, *Historical Account*, pp. 7–31, 50; *News-Letter*, March 5, 1729/30.

19 *Courant*, Aug. 14, 1721.

20 C. Mather, *Diary*, II, 657–658; *News-Letter*, Nov. 20, 1721.

21 Boston Record Commissioners, *Report*, VIII, 159.

22 Boston Record Commissioners, *Report*, XIII, 90–91.

23 *Courant*, Nov. 20, 1721. Yet as late as Jan. 13, 1721/22, Cotton Mather recorded in his *Diary* (II, 670): "Make an offer to a Minister at *Marble-head*, likely to be murdered by an abominable People, that will not lett him save his Life, from the Small-Pox, in the Way of Inoculation. Offer to receive and cover him."

24 *News-Letter*, Feb. 26, 1721/22.

25 Mass. *Acts and Resolves*, X, 105.

26 Boston Record Commissioners, *Report*, XIII, 87.

27 *Ibid.*, pp. 88–89; *News-Letter*, Sept. 25, 1721; C. Mather, *Diary*, II, 646.

28 Massachusetts General Court, House of Representatives, *Journals* (Boston, 1919—), III, 146.

29 1721–1722, ch. 6, Mass. *Acts and Resolves*, II, 232.

30 Mass. *Acts and Resolves*, X, 123.

31 Boston Record Commissioners, *Report*, VIII, 159; *Courant*, Jan. 1, 1721/22.

32 *News-Letter*, Feb. 26, 1721/22; Boston Record Commissioners, *Report*, XIII, 92.

33 Boylston, *Historical Account*, pp. 32-duplicate 31.

34 *News-Letter*, Feb. 26, Mar. 12, 1721/22.

35 Boylston, *Historical Account*, p. 50; *News-Letter*, March 5, 1729/30.

36 Boston Record Commissioners, *Report*, XIII, 96; *News-Letter*, April 16, 1722; *Gazette*, May 21, 1722.

37 Boylston, *Historical Account*, pp. duplicate 31-duplicate 32; Frederick G. Kilgour, "Thomas Robie (1689–1729), colonial scientist and physician," *Isis*, 1939, *30*: 486–487.

38 Boston Record Commissioners, *Report*, VIII, 165; XIII, 97–98; *Gazette*, May 21, 1722.

39 *Gazette*, May 21, 1722.

40 *Courant*, May 21, 1722.

41 Boston Record Commissioners, *Report*, VIII, 166–167.

42 House *Journals*, III, 178, 181, 184–185; Thomas Hutchinson, *The History of the Colony and Province of Massachusetts-Bay*, ed. Lawrence S. Mayo (Cambridge, Mass., 1936), II, 208.
43 Mass. *Acts and Resolves*, X, 161; House *Journals*, IV, 66.
44 *The Imposition of Inoculation as a Duty Religiously Considered in a Letter to a Gentleman in the Country Inclin'd to Admit It* (Boston, 1721), pp. 4–15; *Courant*, Aug. 28, 1721.
45 *Imposition of Inoculation Religiously Considered*, p. 9.
46 [William Cooper], *A Letter to a Friend in the Country, Attempting a Solution of the Scruples & Objections of a Conscientious or Religious Nature, Commonly Made against the New Way of Receiving the Small-Pox* (Boston, 1721), pp. 3–11.
47 Zabdiel Boylston, publisher, *Some Account of What Is Said of Inoculating or Transplanting the Small Pox* (Boston, 1721).
48 I. Mather, *Several Reasons*, p. 72.
49 Benjamin Colman, *Some Observations on the New Method of Receiving the Small-Pox by Ingrafting or Inoculating* (Boston, 1721), pp. 1–5.
50 Cotton Mather, *Sentiments on the Small Pox Inoculated* (with I. Mather, *Several Reasons*, Cleveland, 1921), p. 76.
51 John Williams, *Several Arguments, Proving that Inoculating the Small Pox Is Not Contained in the Law of Physick, Either Natural or Divine, and Therefore Unlawful*, 2nd ed. (Boston, 1721), pp. 3–4.
52 *A Letter from One in the Country, to His Friend in the City: in Relation to Their Distresses Occasioned by the Doubtful and Prevailing Practice of the Inocculation of the Small-Pox* (Boston, 1721), pp. 3–4.
53 *Ibid.*, p. 7.
54 *Ibid.*, p. 8.
55 C. Mather, *Sentiments on the Small Pox Inoculated*, pp. 78–79; Mather's *Diary* for the period (II, 620–674) is full of such opinions.
56 *News-Letter*, Aug. 28, 1721.
57 [William Douglass], *The Abuses and Scandals of Some Late Pamphlets in Favour of Inoculation of the Small Pox, Modestly Obviated, and Inoculation Further Consider'd in a Letter to A—— S—— M. D. & F. R. S. in London* (Boston, 1722), pp. 6–7; [William Douglass], *Inoculation of the Small Pox as Practised in Boston, Consider'd in a Letter to A—— S—— M. D. & F. R. S.* (Boston, 1722), pp. 1–13; *News-Letter*, July 24, 1721.
58 [William Douglass], *A Dissertation Concerning Inoculation of the Small-Pox* (Boston, 1730), p. 2.
59 William Douglass, *A Summary, Historical and Political, of the First Planting, Progressive Improvements, and Present State of the British Settlements in North-America* (London, 1755), II, 409.
60 I. Mather, *Several Reasons*, p. 73.
61 Increase Mather, *Some Further Account from London, of the Small-Pox Inoculated*, 2nd ed. (Boston, 1721), p. 5.
62 [Douglass], *Inoculation as Practised in Boston*, pp. 1–9; [Douglass], *Abuses and Scandals*, pp. 6–10.
63 *Courant*, Aug. 7, 1721.
64 [Douglass], *Inoculation as Practised in Boston*, p. 20.
65 John Williams, *An Answer to a Late Pamphlet, Intitled, a Letter to a Friend in the Country* (Boston, 1722), p. 4.
66 *Ibid.*, p. 11.
67 *Courant*, Jan. 22, 1721/22.
68 *A Friendly Debate; or, a Dialogue between Rusticus and Academicus about the Late Performance of Cademicus* (Boston, 1722).
69 *Gazette*, Jan. 15, 1721/22.
70 *Gazette*, Jan. 29, 1721/22.
71 Kittredge, "Introduction," I. Mather, *Several Reasons*, pp. 39–41.
72 *Vindication of Ministers*, p. 12.

18

Politics, Parties, and Pestilence: Epidemic Yellow Fever in Philadelphia and the Rise of the First Party System

MARTIN S. PERNICK

The omens were not auspicious for Philadelphia in the summer of 1793. Unusually large flocks of migrating pigeons filled the daytime sky. By night a comet streaked the heavens. Increased numbers of cats were dying, their bodies putrefying in the streets and sinkholes, as the rains that usually washed them away were replaced by prolonged drought. Most ominously, the swarms of flies seemingly indigenous to the city had been driven off by a dense mass of "moschetoes" that hung over the city like a cloud.[1] Warned by these signs and portents, the learned Philadelphia medical community had prepared itself for the appearance of a somewhat more virulent strain of "autumnal fever" than was usual. By early August, though, the doctors were puzzling over isolated cases of a new disease involving yellowing of the skin and vomiting of an unknown black substance. On August 19, Dr. Benjamin Rush, signer of the Declaration of Independence and dean of Philadelphia medicine, proclaimed that yellow fever had returned to the city for the first time since 1762.

Initial disbelief turned rapidly to panic as the death toll mounted. By the end of the month between 140 and 325 Philadelphians had died of the fever. On one October day, 119 dead were buried. Between August 19 and November 15, 10 to 15 percent of the estimated 45,000 Philadelphians perished, while another 20,000, including most government officials, simply fled.[2] An extralegal committee of citizen volunteers, called upon by the mayor following the hasty departure of the regular municipal officers, gradually brought the panic under control. Growing slowly from a nucleus of ten men who answered Mayor Matthew Clarkson's September 10 call, the committee commandeered the vacant Bush Hill estate for use as a hospital, set up an orphanage, distributed food, firewood, clothes, and medicine to the poor, buried the abandoned corpses, and undertook a complete cleanup of the city.[3]

Good intentions and hard work were not enough; the hospital could do little when no cure was known. Sanitary efforts were random at best when no one understood the cause of the sickness. The city of Philadelphia needed immediate resolution of three crucial medical questions: what caused the fever and how might its spread and recurrence be averted? how should the sick be treated? and should the people evacuate or stay?

Philadelphia was the medical capital of the United States. Franklin's Pennsylvania Hospital, the prestigious College of Physicians, and the American Philosophical Society combined to attract to the city the best of the new nation's scientific and medical talent. But the medical problems posed by yellow fever were simply not soluble by even the best 18th-century physicians — or, more accurately, medical science alone provided no definitive way of choosing from among the scores of conflicting causes, preventives, and cures, each presented as gospel by its learned advocates. This uncertainty provided the opening by which influences initially quite removed from medical science entered the medical debate.[4]

The yellow fever epidemic of 1793 provides an early example of the complex links between health and politics in American society. In addition, the epidemic reveals the respective roles of local and national events in the creation of America's first two-party system.

MARTIN S. PERNICK teaches in the Department of Humanities, College of Medicine, Pennsylvania State University, Hershey, Pennsylvania.

Revised by author and reprinted with permission from the *William and Mary Quarterly*, 1972, *29*: 559–586.

Philadelphia in 1793 was not only the medical center of America but the political capital of a new republic as well. And in politics as in medicine, the presence of a large body of experts did little to expedite agreement. In fact, 1793 found the political leadership of the nation more divided than at any time in its short past. The year began amid an increasingly bitter verbal duel between Treasury Secretary Alexander Hamilton, writing in John Fenno's *Gazette of the United States*, and Secretary of State Thomas Jefferson, whose views appeared in Philip Freneau's *National Gazette*. The battle, begun over fiscal policy, took on added significance with the news at mid-spring that Revolutionary France had executed America's benefactor, Louis XVI, and had declared war on England. Jefferson and his followers feared English "monarchism" as much as Hamilton and his supporters detested French "anarchy." The arrival of Citizen Genêt, the new French Republican Minister to the United States, inspired sympathetic popular demonstrations in Philadelphia and elsewhere, events organized in part by the newly formed Pennsylvania Democratic Society. The exact purposes of this organization may well have been as unclear to the founders as they are to modern historians, but everyone agreed that it was pro-French and pro-Republican.[5]

In spite of such signs of pro-French sympathy, Jefferson's political standing underwent a marked decline in the summer of 1793. Hamilton gained increased influence over foreign policy within the administration following the April Neutrality Proclamation, while Genêt's rapid success in alienating almost everyone in America further discouraged Jefferson. On July 31, Jefferson notified Washington of his intention to resign by year's end.

Local Philadelphia politics grew more involved following the arrival in early August of over two thousand French refugees from the black revolution in Haiti. Unlike the earlier royalist refugees, the new arrivals included many white radicals and moderates, ousted when the slaves seized control of the revolutionary movement.[6]

Both Hamilton and Jefferson feared dividing the young Republic, but their debate provided the core around which local and congressional factions crystalized to form the first institutional American party system. As Jeffersonians became Democratic-Republicans and Hamiltonians became Federalists, both sought to arouse public interest by taking sides in a variety of local or nonpolitical disputes. Local factions likewise often tried to identify their cause with a national party for ideological, rhetorical, political, or moral support against their local rivals. In either case local antagonisms were deepened and prolonged while the national party gained new grass roots significance.[7] Not surprisingly, the national parties first found themselves embroiled in local issues in the capital city of Philadelphia. The medical controversies generated by the 1793 epidemic over the cause of the disease, its proper treatment, and the conduct of those caught in the crisis, thereby became an integral chapter in the history of the first party system.

DIRTY STREETS OR DIRTY FOREIGNERS?: THE CAUSE

Since it was not until 1901 that Walter Reed demonstrated the process by which the *Aëdes aegypti* mosquito transmits yellow fever from an infected person to a healthy one, Philadelphia physicians of 1793 divided bitterly over the cause of the epidemic. Doctors who saw the roots of the disease in domestic causes — the poor sanitation, unhealthy location, or climatic conditions of Philadelphia itself — disputed those who placed the blame on the unhealthy state of the still disembarking refugees and their ships. In fact, both sides were right, since a yellow fever epidemic requires both locally bred mosquitoes and an initial pool of infected persons, such as the exiled Haitians. In 1793, however, there was simply no known medical theory to resolve the dispute.[8] The etiological debate revealed, moreover, a medical community split along partisan political lines. In general, Republican physicians, including the refugee doctors, believed the fever to be local. The "importationists" were almost all nonpartisans or Federalists.

Dr. Michael Leib, a founder of all three branches of the Philadelphia Democratic Society and a member of the key correspondence committee of the "mother society," argued the domestic origin case before the College of Physicians. Joining him was his old professor, Dr. Rush, an outspoken opponent of Hamilton. Rush, a founding fellow of the College, leader of the medical school faculty, and probably the best known physician in Philadelphia, insisted that "miasmata" from local swamps and "effluvia" from unsanitary docks bred the fever. A second member of the Democrats' correspondence committee, Dr. James Hutchinson, who as Secretary of the College and Physician of the Port was responsible for deciding to admit or bar the refugee ships, reported to Pennsylvania Governor Thomas Mifflin on August 26, "It does not seem to be an imported disease; for I have learned of no foreigners or sailors that have hitherto been infected." Dr. Jean Devèze, himself a refugee, attributed importationism to ignorance and party influence.[9]

The advocates of importation included Philadelphia's lone confessed Federalist physician, Dr. Edward Stevens, a future diplomat and close boyhood friend of Hamilton. The other leading importationists were Drs. Adam Kuhn, Isaac Cathrall, and William Currie. Although prominent in the profession, they took no part in party politics in 1793. On November 26, after Hutchinson's death in the epidemic enabled Kuhn and his supporters to gain a majority, the College of Physicians passed a resolution firmly asserting, "No instance has ever occurred of the disease called the *yellow fever*, having been generated in this city, or in any other parts of the United States . . . but there have been frequent instances of its having been imported." The resolution was the work of Drs. Thomas Parke, John Carson, and Samuel P. Griffitts, none of whom was politically active in 1793.[10] Benjamin Rush had resigned from the College a few days earlier. Benjamin Smith Barton was the only Republican physician in Philadelphia to support importationism in this epidemic.[11] (See Table 1.)

Politics entered the issue by different doors with different doctors. As a topic for medical debate "The Origin of Pestilential Fevers" was an old favorite, and several physicians were committed to one side or the other before 1793. One such was Benjamin Rush. His 1789 comments belittling both importationism and its advocates created hostilities which may help explain why few importationists would join Rush in the Jeffersonian councils.[12]

For most physicians, though, the whole issue remained a somewhat remote subject for scholarly speculation until the crisis of 1793 suddenly forced each practitioner to choose a course of immediate action. Many turned for guidance to trusted colleagues — teachers and friends whose opinions on medical, political, and other matters they had shared in the past.[13] In addition, Republican doctors were the most likely to have come in contact with the localist doctrines which dominated French medicine. In the case of Dr. Hutchinson, politics may have influenced medical decisions more directly. An importationist prior to the epidemic, the Republican port physician apparently switched to localism to avoid closing the city to the French refugees.[14]

Table 1
1793 Party Affiliations of Physicians Who Expressed an Opinion on the Cause of Yellow Fever

	Republicans	Federalists	Uncommitted
Importationists — 10	1	1	8
Domestic origin — 14	6	0	8

Note: Twenty-four Philadelphia physicians, the most prominent third of the practicing healers in town, left evidence of their opinions on the cause of the fever. One-third of this medical elite was actively involved in the earliest stages of party building. The prominence of this elite gave their views social significance despite their lack of statistical significance.

Like the physicians, the political leaders of Philadelphia split by party over the cause of the fever. Although Republican editor Freneau vehemently condemned the disputes of the medical men, declaring that "no circumstance has added more to the present calamity," he actually strongly supported a local origin. He made his viewpoint clear in the following poem:

Doctors raving and disputing,
Death's pale army still recruiting —
What a pother
One with t'other!
Some a-writing, some a-shooting.

Nature's poisons here collected,
Water, earth, and air infected —
O, what pity
Such a City,
Was in such a place erected![15]

On September 23, the *National Gazette* published a discussion of more than a dozen theories of the origin of the disease without once mentioning the possibility of its being imported.[16] In medicine as in politics only one's opposition was seen as the "divisive faction." Local Republican civic leaders like editor Andrew Brown and merchants John Swanwick and Stephen Girard supported Dr. Devèze's explanation that burying the dead inside the city had produced the disease. Jefferson explained to Madison that the fever was "generated in the filth of Water street."[17]

On the other hand, Philadelphia Federalists John Fenno, Oliver Wolcott, Thomas Willing, Benjamin Chew, Levi Hollingsworth, J. B. Bordley, Ebenezer Hazard, Bishop William White, and printer Benjamin Johnson led their party in publicly proclaiming yellow fever a foreign disease.[18] In his days as a Federalist after 1794, William "Peter Porcupine" Cobbett, the Anglo-American pamphleteer, penned a series of libelous attacks on Rush's theories. But in 1793, as a supplicant of the patronage of Secretary Jefferson and a tutor to the refugees, Cobbett spoke of the yellow fever as a typical product of the unhealthy American climate.[19]

More than one-third of the most prominent national and local political leaders in Philadelphia took a public position on the cause of the epidemic. With few exceptions the Republicans backed a domestic source of the fever, while Federalists largely blamed importation. Governor Mifflin, who endorsed importation theories, has been called a Republican although he usually appeared as the nonpartisan "Father of his State." Benjamin Franklin Bache, editor of the Republican *General Advertiser*, believed the disease imported but blamed the *British* West Indies, later calling the fever "a present from the English." The least typical was Republican printer Mathew Carey, who included his native Ireland as well as the French islands among the possible sources of the fever.[20] Timothy Pickering, an intimate friend of Dr. Rush, was probably the only Federalist leader in Philadelphia to claim the yellow fever as a domestic disease.[21]

The party leaders, moreover, moved rapidly to exploit the many political implications they discovered in the medical controversy. Federalists used the importation doctrine to back demands for the quarantine or exclusion of the radical French, and for limitations on trade with the French islands, while Republican merchants saw importationism as a cover for plans to wreck their lucrative trade with the West Indies. Girard and Dr. Devèze denounced the proposed quarantine as "disastrous to commerce." In June 1798, during the "Quasi-War" with France, the newly drafted quarantine laws were in fact successfully invoked to block the immigration of suspected Haitian subversives.[22]

A novel twist was provided by Dr. Currie's theory that the disease originated on board the French privateer *Sans Culotte*, which brought a prize to Philadelphia in July. Accusing both the French and Port Physician Hutchinson, the Federalists charged that sickness on the ship had been covered up to protect the Republican political and financial stake in her activities. Benjamin Johnson blamed the epidemic on the French "licensed plunderers of the Ocean," adding that "if particular men had done their duty; and had not betrayed more indulgence to French cruizers, than genuine friendship for this city," the disease would have been averted.[23] Federalist charges fed a growing Francophobia. "AMOR PATRIAE" warned Philadelphians not to trust the city's benevolent French physicians. Persistent rumors that the wells had been contaminated preparatory to a French invasion led to threats of mob violence against the hapless refugees.[24]

Although the Federalists talked of closing all trade with the French islands, they seemed far more anxious to arouse public suspicion of the French and the Republicans than to create any precedent for a government embargo on commerce. Indeed, the Federalist merchants feared that localism was part of a Republican conspiracy to discredit Philadelphia and all large commercial centers and to force relocation of the capital in a rural setting. Richard Peters warned Timothy Pickering against Rush's doctrine on October 22: "His Assertion that the Philadelphia Hot beds produced this deadly Plant is . . . a mischievous Opinion . . . and will be eagerly caught at by the Anti-Philadelphians. Stifle this Brat if you can."[25] Rush noted the result by October 28: "A new clamor has been excited against me in which many citizens take a part. I have asserted that the yellow fever was generated in our city. This assertion they say will destroy the character of Philadelphia for healthiness, and drive Congress from it."[26] John Beale Bordley wrote an importationist pamphlet for the admitted purpose of convincing Congress to remain in Philadelphia. Federalist editor John Fenno worried that the domestic origin theory would "not only render multitudes uneasy and interrupt the usual course of business, but injure the interest and reputation of the city in several-respects."[27]

Such political fears could easily distort medical objectivity. "Is there a city in the world," asked Levi Hollingsworth, "kept cleaner than Philadelphia?" The College of Physicians answered flatly, "No possible improvement with respect to water or ventilation can make our situation more eligible" — this at a time when Philadelphia had no sewage system, no fresh water supply, and no provision for regular garbage disposal![28]

Republicans did attack large cities as unhealthy, and Jefferson later expressed confidence that the "yellow fever will discourage the growth of great cities in our nation."[29] Yet most Republicans protested that they wanted not to destroy commercial cities but to preserve them through sanitary reform.[30] Federalist fears of a plot to move the capital also proved groundless. In the debates over whether or not Congress could legally meet elsewhere to avoid the fever, the Republicans, for strict constructionist reasons, favored convening in Philadelphia.[31]

The Federalist endorsement of importation proved to be a very effective and popular position as the idea of a native American plague irritated a highly sensitive patriotic nerve. Rush noted that "Loathsome and dangerous diseases have been considered by all nations as of foreign extraction."[32] Importationists made much of the widely held feeling that independent America was the New Eden. Reaching the farthest extreme of this argument, one importationist asserted in 1799 that the doctrine of domestic fevers was "treason," perhaps hoping that the Alien and Sedition Acts gave the Federalists the power to deport foreign diseases along with foreign agitators.[33]

The people of Philadelphia urged their officials to agree on specific actions to prevent the return of yellow fever, but the political implications of the issue made adoption of any single course of action unacceptable. Thus, immediately following the 1793 epidemic, Pennsylvania and other threatened states undertook *both* quarantine and sanitary reform projects. Simple political compromise provided a way around the bitter medical deadlock.[34] Considering the state of medical knowledge in 1793, the imposition of a political settlement may well have been the best result that could have been expected.

In 1793, the division between medicine and theology was still young. Not everyone in Philadelphia believed the cause of the plague was strictly medical; rather, the wrath of the Deity appeared to many as manifest in the fever, and before the debate over the epidemic had ended, theology, like medicine, had become enmeshed in political developments. The devout saw most early American diseases, such as cholera and typhoid, as punishment for the individual sins of vicious immigrants and slothful poor. Unlike these diseases, though, yellow fever was spread not by poor individual hygiene but by infected mosquitoes which could and did bite high and low with complete republican egalitarianism. Some physicians even declared that blacks and the West Indian immigrants were more immune than respectable white Philadelphians, a costly error. At any rate, the pious saw the yellow fever as a communal punishment rather than as retribution against individual sinners.[35]

The issue that remained, of course, was to identify and root out those communal transgressions which had provoked the pestilence. With no shortage of suggestions as to where the country was going astray, the Republicans first gave political content to the religious debate. At the very height of the plague, Freneau devoted front page coverage to a series of articles and letters which pointed to the pride and vanity of the communal leaders as the major transgression. Mathew Carey joined in the attack. And Benjamin Rush, the Enlightenment man of science, commented in retrospect, "I agree with you in deriving our physical calamities from moral causes. . . . We ascribe all the attributes of the Deity to the name of General Washington. It is considered by our citizens as the bulwark of our nation. God would cease to be what He is, if he did not visit us for these things."[36]

Federalists too put the religious issue in political harness. An official thanksgiving-fast sermon by the Reverend William Smith linked the pestilence with French immorality and with the "wild principles and restless conduct of their partisans here, impatient of all rule and authority."[37] Connecticut

Senator Chauncey Goodrich saw the divine anger resulting from Republican adoration of Genêt, while Alexander Graydon recalled the "state of parties in the summer of 1793, when the metropolis of Pennsylvania, then resounding with unhallowed orgies at the dismal butcheries in France, was visited with a calamity which had much the appearance which heaven sometimes sends to purify the heart."[38]

A peculiar coincidence gave added depth to these speculations, for the fever had miraculously appeared just as Philadelphia completed construction of what one Republican termed its "Synagogue for Satan" — the city's new Chestnut Street Theater. Many in Revolutionary America saw the theater as an extremely complex negative symbol, part bordello and part palace. The new theater, with fluted marble columns and pure golden ornaments, was indeed palatial.[39] While a few Republicans like Swanwick owned stock in the theater company, the major backers were prominent Federalists.[40] They in turn tried to portray opposition to the theater as a Republican scheme to subvert private property. One Francophobe detected the same "rigourous enthusiasm" which spawned the French Revolution motivating the foes of the drama. Opponents of the stage did appeal to Anglophobic, antimonarchical, and Republican imagery to justify their cause, although not all Republicans were antitheater.[41]

Philadelphia's embattled defenders of public virtue had all but given up when the epidemic provided the ammunition for yet another crusade. Sixteen of the city's leading clergymen joined with the Quakers in petitioning the state to shut the new theater. "We conceive that the solemn intimations of Divine Providence in the late distressing calamity which has been experienced in this city, urge upon us in the most forcible manner the duty of reforming every thing which may be offensive to the Supreme Governor of the Universe." Devout Republicans found it significant that "the actors and retainers of the stage, who actually arrived here at the time when the fever raged with the utmost violence," were Englishmen.[42] The opponents of stage plays eventually lost their struggle, even with the arguments gained from the epidemic. The issue, however, helped strengthen the growing bond between Quakers and Republicans in Philadelphia.[43]

BLEEDING VS. BARK: THE CURE

Medical science today can do little more to cure a case of yellow fever than it could in 1793, a sobering fact that helps explain the continued controversy over the treatment of the disease long after the question of etiology had been shelved. The number of treatments attempted in the sheer desperation of the Philadelphia epidemic was astounding, yet the medical community rapidly split into two main schools. One favored the use of "stimulants" — quinine bark, wine, and cold baths — a method long used in both British and French West Indies. Opposing these "bark and wine murderers," a second group advocated the "new treatment" concocted by Dr. Rush, who believed it advisable to draw an amount of blood which we know today to be in excess of the quantity possessed by most people, and whose doses of mercury caused severe disfiguration of the teeth and skin. But by 18th-century standards his "experimental" approach appeared more advanced than the "traditional" bark cure.[44]

Many factors helped determine which doctors adopted what cure, not the least of which was chance. Rush himself tried the bark and wine method before his "discovery" but lost three of four patients. Another variable was the infamous, tangled infighting among Philadelphia physicians. Almost any medical opinion rendered by Benjamin Rush eventually drew the ridicule of Dr. William Shippen, the man Rush had hauled before a court-martial over their disagreements in the Revolution.[45] Partisan differences were at first unimportant in a doctor's choice of a cure. True, Rush counted among his followers many ardent Republicans such as Dr. Leib, Dr. George Logan, the Quaker pacifist, Dr. Benjamin Say, and most of his former students. However, a large body of Republican "bark and wine doctors" included Hutchinson, Dr. Benjamin Smith Barton, and the French-trained Bush Hill staff under Devèze and Girard. Republican bark doctors did learn the cure from the French refugees, while the Federalist Dr. Stevens and other non-Republican physicians adopted the procedure from the British or Dutch islands, but their actual methods of treating patients were almost identical. Although it was inaccurate, many Philadelphians persisted in the conviction that there was a "Republican cure" and a "Federalist cure."[46]

The man initially responsible for politically polarizing this nonpartisan jumble was Alexander Hamilton. Seeing an opportunity to do a favor for an old friend, Hamilton published a glowing personal tribute to Dr. Stevens, attributing his own recovery to the bark and wine cure. In so doing, Hamilton could not resist a sneer at his old critic, Dr. Rush. Hamilton's tool, Secretary of War Henry Knox, followed, airing his thoughts on Rush a few days later. The local and national Federalist press took the cue and began a barrage of political-sounding attacks on Rush's cure, terminated only by the 1799 libel judgment against Cobbett. Fenno's unkind attempt to derive Rush's bloodletting from that of the French terror resulted in a libel action against him as well, but the case was never tried.[47]

By simply declaring long enough and loud enough that bark and wine was the Federalist cure, these editors were able to make a considerable political issue out of a basically nonpartisan dispute. Their appeal was meant to gain political support among the many users of the mild wine and quinine therapy while personally discrediting Rush. The political element in the attack on bleeding seemed obvious to Rush. "I think it probable that if the new remedies had been introduced by any other person than a decided Democrat and a friend of Madison and Jefferson, they would have met with less opposition from Colonel Hamilton," Rush complained. "Many of us," he later told General Horatio Gates, "have been forced to expiate our sacrifices in the cause of liberty by suffering every species of slander and persecution. I ascribe the opposition to my remedies in the epidemic which desolated our city in 1793 chiefly to an unkind and resentful association of my political principles with my medical character."[48] Rush did not deny the Federalist charge that his cures were associated with his politics. Attacked as a democrat, he replied as a democrat, hoping to rally Republican political support for his medical views. Rush declared his cure the only truly egalitarian form of medicine in that it was easy to master and could be practiced by anyone with little formal training. Putting his beliefs into practice, he trained a group of free blacks as itinerant bleeders during the epidemic and published "do-it-yourself" directions in the newspapers, actions which did not endear him to the guardians of the professional mysteries any more than to the Federalists. Rush declared it unnecessary "to send men educated in colleges . . . to cure . . . pestilential disease," assuring his followers that "men and even women may be employed for that purpose, who have not perverted their reason by a servile attachment to any system of medicine." "All that is necessary," he added, "might be taught to a boy or girl twelve years old in a few hours."[49]

Rush also adopted the Federalists' derogatory identification of his cures with the French Revolution, affirming "I am in the situation of The French Republic surrounded and invaded by new as well as old enemies, without any other allies." He went so far as to imply that the true treatment, no less than the true politics, could be derived in good democratic fashion: "The people rule here in medicine as well as government." The best cure could be decided by the will of the majority. On October 2, Rush wrote to Elias Boudinot that "Colonel Hamilton's remedies are now as unpopular in our city as his funding system is in Virginia or North Carolina."[50]

Public support of bark and wine by several prominent Federalists gave credence to its reputation as the "Federalist cure." Rush, however, failed in his attempt to rally the Republican leadership behind his "egalitarian" medicine. Prominent Republican leaders largely ignored the issue on which Republican physicians were themselves divided.

No clear political division over the issue of therapy actually existed, despite the highly publicized attempts of Hamilton and Rush to create such a polarization. Republican "bark and wine" physicians denied that bleeding was the Republican cure, but they could not compete for public attention with the colorful and prolific Dr. Benjamin Rush. Many Republican "bark doctors" were refugees, barred from political office and lacking public influence, and Hutchinson's death deprived them of their most prominent and articulate spokesman. The failure of "bark and wine" Republicans to counter the publicity attracted by Hamilton and Rush made the cure of yellow fever seem a clear-cut party issue.[51] Moreover, the injection of politics into this medical debate probably had some adverse side effects. The partisan taint of arguments against mercury and bleeding delayed rejection of the Rush cure long after the medical evidence pointed to its inefficacy and danger.

TO FLEE OR NOT TO FLEE: THE CREDIT

The first days of the epidemic produced a mad scramble to escape town. Benjamin Rush warned all who could to leave the city; even his bitter rivals Drs. Shippen and Kuhn took his advice this time and quickly departed. The panic was so great that "many people thrust their parents into the streets, as soon as they complained of a headache."[52] Exceptions to the general exodus soon appeared, however. Most of the physicians stuck to their posts. Rush, following his discovery of a "cure," publicly advised everyone to remain in town. The French, familiar with the disease and trained to believe it noncontagious, did not flee. Many shopkeepers and middle-class merchants with no one to look after their affairs, and the poor with no place else to go, stayed as well. A handful of true philanthropists remained. As the epidemic wore on, observers noted that the leaders of each of these groups were often Republicans.[53]

Several Federalists did play major roles in the heroic relief work. Mayor Clarkson organized the citizens' committee while Samuel Coates and John Oldden headed a merchants' distribution organization which handled supplies for the mayor. Coates, an intimate of Rush and Girard, was nonetheless a Federalist and was often criticized by Girard for his Francophobia.[54] Levi Hollingsworth and Caspar W. Morris joined the merchants' group. Clement Humphreys, son of the shipbuilder, remained at his post as a guardian of the poor. Three Federalist clergymen, William Smith, William White, and Robert Blackwell, also remained to comfort the ill. Although these nine men were the only identifiable Federalists at all involved in the organized relief work, an additional five, Jacob Hiltzheimer, Postmaster Timothy Pickering, ex-Postmaster Ebenezer Hazard, Congressman Thomas FitzSimmons, and John Stillé, chose not to join the organized effort but rendered important aid to their families and neighbors individually.[55]

Active Republicans, however, performed the greatest share of the work. Of the 18 men cited in the minutes as the leaders of the citizens' committee, nine were definitely Republicans, one was the brother of an ardent Republican, and seven could not be identified with either party. The mayor was the only Federalist. The Republican leaders of the committee were Vice-chairman Samuel Wetherill, Secretary Caleb Lownes, Stephen Girard of Bush Hill, Israel Israel (orphans), Mathew Carey (printing), Jonathan Dickinson Sergeant (counsel), James Sharswood (accounts), James Kerr (orphans), and John Connelly (accounts). Treasurer Thomas Wistar was the brother of Republican Dr. Caspar Wistar.[56] The other committeemen were Andrew Adgate (at large), Peter Helm of Bush Hill, Daniel Offley (at large), Joseph Inskeep (at large), John Letchworth (orphans), Samuel Benge (burials), and Henry Deforest (supplies).

Three of the four members of the key correspondence committee which ran the Democratic Society were leaders in fighting the fever. Two, Hutchinson and Jonathan Dickinson Sergeant, lost their lives while caring for the sick. The third was Dr. Leib, who had charge of Bush Hill in the first chaotic days of its existence. Alexander B. Dallas, the fourth member, claimed with some justification that his state office required him to follow the state government to its exile in Germantown.[57] At least 17 men listed as active in the Democratic Society played major roles in aiding the sick. Israel Israel directed the relief and orphanage work of the committee. Well-known in Philadelphia for his Revolutionary War exploits and for his antifederalism, Israel was treasurer of the Democratic Society. The president of the society, David Rittenhouse, went on call with his nephew Dr. Barton, arranging for free treatment of the poor. After the death of his son-in-law Sergeant, Rittenhouse left town briefly, but returned before the end of the epidemic to resume his work.[58]

The Quaker Dr. George Logan was an ardent Democrat who had left both medicine and Philadelphia in 1781. Returning now from his retirement at Stenton near Germantown, he served as the committee's inspector at Bush Hill, from where he reported to the world the incredible efforts of the managers, "Citizens Girard and Helm." The one-eyed merchant Girard, who almost alone turned Bush Hill from a pesthouse to a hospital, was also active in the Democratic organization.[59] The labors of Dr. Rush, who formally joined the society in early 1794, were comparable to those of Girard. Visiting hundreds of patients while ill himself, Rush stuck to his post even after the death of his sister. Also members of the Democratic group were John Connelly and James Kerr of the citizens' committee; George Forepaugh, Jeremiah Paul, William Robinson, Sr., James

Swaine, and William Watkins of the merchants' committee; volunteer John Barker; and John Swanwick, owner of the committee's orphanage. Others of Republican persuasion cited for their roles were aldermen Hilary Baker and John Barclay, and merchants' committeeman Caspar Snyder.[60]

Among Philadelphia newspapers, only Republican Andrew Brown's *Federal Gazette* appeared throughout the epidemic, keeping the remaining citizens in touch with the relief workers.[61] Freneau, who vowed to publish for as long as possible, held on longer than any editor except Brown. The *National Gazette* last appeared on October 16, a victim of financial losses rather than of editorial dereliction. His work ended, Freneau did not flee the city but remained until mid-December.[62]

The list of Republican heroes also included Frenchmen. In addition to Devèze, all four physicians' aides and most of the staff at Bush Hill were French. The French specialist in tropical medicine, Citizen Robert, hearing of the epidemic while en route to France, rushed to Philadelphia from Boston in what one writer termed a "confirmation of the sincere attachment of the French patriots, to the truly republican Americans!" The largest individual contribution to the relief fund came from Citizen Genêt. Even "THE REPUBLICAN SEAMEN OF FRANCE" got involved, forming Philadelphia's only intact fire company during the epidemic. Freneau credited them with saving the city from the fate of London.[63]

While Republicans dominated the relief work, Federalists often joined the ranks of the refugees, not necessarily from cowardice, as Republicans charged, but rather because of their belief in importation and contagion. No prominent importationist leaders of either party stayed in Philadelphia. The one anticontagionist Federalist official remained; the one importationist Republican fled. Illustrative of the disappearance of Federalists was the case of the Dutch Minister, Francis Van Berkle, who believed himself ill. Since Dr. Stevens had left for New York, Hamilton (from his refuge in Albany) suggested that the minister consult Oliver Wolcott on the use of bark and wine. The minister soon discovered that Wolcott too was gone. Tired of looking for someone to instruct him in the "Federalist cure," Van Berkle was treated by Rush and recovered.[64]

It appeared that the Republicans would receive high praise for their efforts. Benjamin Rush "is become the darling of the common people and his humane fortitude and exertions will render him deservedly dear," noted one observer.[65] Bravery and leadership make popular American campaign fare, and the Republicans were not slow to present their political bill for services rendered. Among the first to make an issue of bravery was Jefferson, whose Revolutionary War record had recently come under unkind Federalist scrutiny. His scornful cut at Hamilton as the Treasury Secretary prepared to flee is considered by Dumas Malone to have been Jefferson's most vicious political remark. "His family think him in danger," wrote Jefferson, "and he puts himself so by his excessive alarm. He has been miserable several days before from a firm persuasion he should catch it. A man as timid as he is on the water, as timid on horseback, as timid in sickness, would be a phenomenon if his courage of which he has the reputation in military occasions were genuine. His friends, who have not seen him, suspect it is only an autumnal fever he has." Jefferson also attacked Henry Knox, who had already fled, but after waiting to make sure Hamilton had really gone first, Jefferson himself left town over a week ahead of his planned departure.[66]

Freneau took over the task of castigating the "deserters." His poem, "Orlando's Flight," ridiculed the fugitives:

> On prancing steed, with spunge at nose,
> From town behold Orlando fly;
> Camphor and Tar where'er he goes
> Th' infected shafts of death defy —
>   Safe in an atmosphere of stink,
>   No doctor gets Orlando's chink.

Freneau also implied it was greed that made the fugitives so anxious to preserve themselves. Speaking of the afterworld, he concluded:

> Monarchs are there of little note,
> And Caesar wears a ragged coat.
> . . . .
> Blame not Orlando if he fled, —
> *So little's got by being dead.*[67]

The last evacuees had not yet returned when a special election brought the heroism issue to the fore. State Senator Samuel Powel, Philadelphia's beloved Revolutionary War mayor, had died of the fever. On December 12, a Republican meeting put forth the name of Israel Israel for Powel's seat. Israel's platform was simple and direct. He was "a gentleman whose philanthropy on a late melancholy occasion is well known, and whose firm and steady attachment to the people will, it is hoped, bring forth the united suffrages of the citizens in his favour."[68] The Federalist response came swiftly. The day after the Israel nomination, Fenno revealed a move to draft Mayor Clarkson as the Federalist choice. In an attempt to outdo the Republicans, Clarkson's backers asserted that "gratitude demands a particular tribute of acknowledgement to him for his assiduity, and perseverance in relieving the distresses of our fellow citizens during the calamity from which we have just emerged."[69] Clarkson, however, was content to be mayor, and the nomination went instead to William Bingham, the extremely wealthy associate of the powerful Willing-Morris partnership. Bingham had followed the progress of the fever from his New Jersey shore retreat. The actual management of his campaign, however, was placed in the hands of relief workers John Oldden and John Stillé. Their efforts apparently countered the appeal of Israel's candidacy, and Bingham won the December 19 contest by a three to two margin.[70]

The return of the "deserters" further complicated Republican use of the heroism issue. While many of the Federalists had fled the fever, most of the evacuees were not Federalists. One-third of all Philadelphians had left, and the majority of the rest remained hidden behind locked doors, venturing out only for necessities. Their initial gratitude toward the members of the committee was mingled with a good deal of shame, guilt, and envy. As one perceptive reviewer noted in commenting on Mathew Carey's account of the epidemic, "To panegyrize our contemporaries, without attracting censure on ourselves, requires a very delicate hand."[71] The Republicans realized that a campaign based solely on praising their own heroics while damning the opposition's defections was politically unwise. They usually attempted to temper their attacks by expressing sympathy with the difficulties encountered by the fugitives, many of whom had been brutally repulsed by the panicked citizens of neighboring cities.[72]

The returnees meanwhile countered criticism with charges of their own, terming the epidemic a "doctors' harvest." The citizens' committee was attacked as too expensive and as growing insolent with power. "Unless the Committee feel *tickled* with their employment," wrote one critic, "they ought to surrender it to the Guardians of the poor, who are competent to the service, and who will perform it at a *much less expence* and *with far less state*." Rush's black bleeders were easy targets for Federalist charges of profiteering. Actually, the committee and most physicians offered free medical service to the poor, while Rush even distributed free mercury. Yet the boast of Rush's student, Dr. Mease, that the fever had made his fortune for life, and the activities of Samuel Wetherill, whose drug business took precedence over his committee duties, gave the charges just enough credibility to undermine the Republican appeal to public gratitude.[73] A common complaint charged the committeemen with usurping powers reserved for the traditional political elite. "The bulk of them," wrote one resentful critic, "are scarcely known beyond the smoke of their own chimnies."[74] Further, many Philadelphians simply wished to forget the entire painful scene as quickly as possible. The heroes of the epidemic were living reminders of the horror and the suffering. "If the disease has disappeared as it no doubt has, every memento of its existence should disappear with it, that the citizens may once more enjoy repose."[75]

Despite the strenuous efforts of the party organization, Republican heroism was a complete flop as a political issue. A 1797 election in which Israel Israel had defeated Federalist Benjamin Morgan was invalidated when Morgan claimed his backers had been disenfranchised by holding the election while the Federalists were "driven from their homes" by the epidemic of that year. With the fleeing Federalists safely home again, the hapless Israel lost the second election despite heavy contributions from Girard and Sharswood.[76]

CONCLUSION: HEALTH AS A POLITICAL ISSUE

The yellow fever struck a Federalist Philadelphia in 1793 and left both local and national Federalist rule considerably strengthened. For one thing, the epidemic seriously weakened the national Republican organization. The deaths of Hutchinson and Sergeant eliminated two of the four men responsible for creating and directing new Democratic Society branches. Years later, John Adams declared that these two deaths alone saved the nation from an imminent revolution.[77] The collapse of the *National Gazette* under the financial strain of the epidemic created another void which Bache's *Aurora* could not immediately fill. Even the little-noted death of Citizen Dupont, the French consul, had its political effect, leaving France's critical relations with the United States in the hands of a vice-consul for months until the arrival of a replacement for Genêt.

In issues as well as institutions the Federalists gained, at least in the short run. The Republicans were unable to convert their heavy organizational losses into an effective sympathy vote. By denying any local source of the pestilence, the Federalists won much national chauvinist and local booster support, while their espousal of importationism heightened American Francophobia. In addition, the Federalists managed to identify their opponents with Benjamin Rush's advocacy of a dangerous and controversial remedy. Although Philadelphia Republicans found some additional Quaker support in the theater issue, the national party gained at best a minor new point against large cities.[78]

More important, the epidemic served to introduce new issues and attract new supporters to the two developing parties, thereby extending and broadening the base of the new party system. This development was sometimes local in its origins, as in the debate over the cause of the fever, where the already politically polarized local controversy introduced issues that the national politicians adopted and used. In other issues, such as the bleeding *v.* bark debate, a nonpolarized initial conflict had political meaning imposed from the outside by the intervention of national leaders. Furthermore, the process of giving political significance to social issues was highly selective. The issue which seemed logically closest to politics was that of courage and leadership, but despite the efforts of the local antagonists and the party organization, human feelings of gratitude proved too flimsy a foundation on which to build a political platform.

Neither the risks of disease nor the costs of fighting it are evenly distributed in American society. This inequality, resulting from both biological and social conditions, creates the potential for political division over almost all aspects of public health. But not every health issue actually produces a political conflict. Interest groups overlap in complex ways. Consider, for example, the dilemma facing Federalist merchants, who would gain from a quarantine of the French islands, but simultaneously would suffer from any increase in the rigor of quarantines in general.

Political influence in late 18th-century medicine did not always signify irresponsible meddling. Political compromise permitted concerted public action to fight future epidemics at a time when medical opinion seemed hopelessly deadlocked, although the political significance of the potentially lethal Rush "cure" helped assure its continued use, needlessly endangering the lives of patients.

Finally, not everyone was willing to be drawn into partisan debate over a medical question. Expressing the hope that the next epidemic might be met by the united efforts of "all parties" in the City of Brotherly Love, an anonymous satirist poked fun at both the Federalist and Republican views of the fever:

> Be patient ye vivid sons of mercury with the medical baptisms of your *cold bath brethren.* For had that therapeutic process been tried under the cataract of Niagara, no body can tell the wonders which might have been produced by it . . .
>
> Cease ye yellow fever heroes to censure, those of your brethren whose delicacy of nerves and previous engagements called them suddenly crochet and forceps a la main to Nootka Sound, to catch Otters and Beavers. Be assured, important discoveries have been made by the Jaunt.
>
> Lend a kind ear to the graduates of Montpelier, who inform you that the late disease arose from the burying grounds in the heart of your city, since in France they never bury the dead under Churches, but in balloons high up in the air.[79]

> Ye learned and long robed sons of Esculapius, pity and pardon poor Absolam Jones and Richard Allen,[80] two sable Ethiopians, who being ignorant of the Greek and Latin languages, were under the necessity of curing their patients *in English*.[81]

But neither the political nor the medical debates would be silenced so simply.

NOTES

I would like to thank Eric L. McKitrick for his guidance and encouragement at every stage of this project.

1 J. H. Powell, *Bring Out Your Dead: The Great Plague of Yellow Fever in Philadelphia in 1793* (Philadelphia, 1949), pp. 1–64; Charles E. A. Winslow, *The Conquest of Epidemic Disease: A Chapter in the History of Ideas* (Princeton, 1943), p. 198.

2 Powell, *Bring Out Your Dead*, pp. 8–12, 219, 232. The exact number of deaths is unknown. The figure 4,040, derived from burial lists, includes deaths from all causes in the city but does not include the many fever victims buried elsewhere. The burial lists are appended to Mathew Carey, *A Short Account of the Malignant Fever*, . . . 4th ed. (Philadelphia, 1794). See also Richard H. Shryock, *Medicine and Society in America, 1660–1860* (New York, 1960), pp. 82, 108.

3 Powell, *Bring Out Your Dead*, pp. 143, 242–243.

4 Erwin H. Ackerknecht, "Anticontagionism between 1821 and 1867," *Bull. Hist. Med.*, 1948, *26*: 562–593. An opposing view is J. B. Blake, "Yellow fever in eighteenth century America," *Bull. N.Y. Acad. Med.*, 1968, *64*: 681.

5 Eugene P. Link, *Democratic-Republican Societies, 1790–1800* (New York, 1942); Harry M. Tinkcom, *The Republicans and Federalists in Pennsylvania, 1790–1801: A Study in National Stimulus and Local Response* (Harrisburg, 1950).

6 Frances S. Childs, *French Refugee Life in the United States, 1790–1800: An American Chapter of the French Revolution* (Baltimore, 1940), pp. 22, 103, 142–143, 159.

7 A general picture of the events and mechanisms of party development may be found in Joseph Charles, *The Origins of the American Party System* (New York, 1956); Noble E. Cunningham, Jr., *The Jeffersonian Republicans: The Formation of Party Organization, 1789–1801* (Chapel Hill, 1957); Richard Hofstadter, *The Idea of a Party System: The Rise of Legitimate Opposition in the United States, 1780–1840* (Berkeley and Los Angeles, 1969); and Richard P. McCormick, *The Second American Party System: Party Formation in the Jacksonian Era* (Chapel Hill, 1966).

8 Winslow, *Epidemic Disease*, pp. 195, 200, 231. Related to, but distinct from, the etiology question was the problem of contagion. Almost all importationists believed the fever contagious, but advocates of a local origin differed over whether it could become contagious after appearing. For examples, see David Nassy, *Observations on the Cause, Nature, and Treatment of the Epidemic Disorder Prevalent in Philadelphia* (Philadelphia, 1793), p. 13; Benjamin Rush, *An Enquiry Into the Origin of the Late Epidemic Fever in Philadelphia* (Philadelphia, 1793), p. 14; Benjamin S. Barton, "On yellow fever," n.d. [1806?], Benjamin Smith Barton Papers, Delafield Collection, American Philosophical Society, Philadelphia.

9 Powell, *Bring Out Your Dead*, pp. 43–44; Carey, *Short Account*, p. 12; Benjamin Rush, *An Account of the Bilious Remitting Yellow Fever . . .* (Philadelphia, 1794); *Dictionary of American Biography*, s.v. "Hutchinson, James"; Jean Devèze, *An Enquiry into, and Observations upon; the Causes and Effects of the Epidemic Disease* (Philadelphia, 1794), p. 16; Powell, *Bring Out Your Dead*, pp. 36–44. On the importance of the correspondence committee, see Edward Ford, *David Rittenhouse: Astronomer-Patriot, 1732–1796* (Philadelphia, 1946), p. 190.

10 Records of the College of Physicians, I (1787–1812), 175, Nov. 19, 1793, College of Physicians of Philadelphia; Rush, *Account*, p. 146; Adam Kuhn, Yellow Fever Manuscripts (1794), p. 6, College of Physicians of Philadelphia, Philadelphia; Stacey B. Day, ed., *Edward Stevens: Gastric Physiologist, Physician and American Statesman* (Montreal, 1969); William Currie, *A Treatise on the Synochus Icteroides, Or Yellow Fever . . .* (Philadelphia, 1794), pp. 1, 67, 84; Currie, *An Impartial Review of that Part of Dr. Rush's Late Publication . . . In Which His Opinion is Shewn to be Erroneous; the Importation of the Disease Established; and the Wholesomeness of the City Vindicated* (Philadelphia, 1794), pp. 6–14.

11 Rush, *Account*, p. 146; *Independent Gazetteer* (Philadelphia), Jan. 22, 1794; Benjamin S. Barton to Thomas Pennant, April 11, 1794, Barton Papers. Later epidemics in 1797 and 1798 introduced some blurring of party lines. By 1797, Republican Dr. Caspar Wistar had definitely joined the importationists. See College of Physicians of Philadelphia, *Facts and Observations Relative to the Nature and Origin of the Pestilential Fever . . .* (Philadelphia, 1798), pp. 43, 52; Samuel D. Gross, ed., *Lives of Eminent American Physicians and Surgeons of the Nineteenth Century* (Philadelphia, 1861), pp. 134–135; College of

Physicians Records, I, 216, 225, 250. The political allegiance of Dr. William Shippen, Jr., is uncertain. An importationist, he chaired a largely Republican town meeting in 1795 but also appeared in the rolls of the Federalist marching society. See *Independent Gazetteer*, Nov. 30, 1793, July 25, 1795; and General Roll of McPherson's Blues, Hollingsworth Manuscripts, Business Papers Miscellaneous, undated, Historical Society of Pennsylvania, Philadelphia. An unlikely suggestion was made that Shippen did not know who was behind the 1795 meeting, "thus committing himself as a puppet to be moved at the pleasure of very bungling artists." *Gazette of the United States* (Philadelphia), July 25, 1795. Dr. Charles Caldwell continued to champion localism even after his 1796 conversion to Federalism, but in 1793 he was loyal to both the politics and the medicine of Benjamin Rush. See Charles Caldwell, *Autobiography* (Philadelphia, 1855), pp. 174, 182, 254, 267, 278; Caldwell to James Hutchinson, Aug. 1, 1793, Hutchinson Papers, American Philosophical Society.

12 Benjamin Rush, *Medical Inquiries and Observations* (Philadelphia, 1789); Carl Binger, *Revolutionary Doctor: Benjamin Rush, 1746–1813* (New York, 1966), p. 228.

13 Rush, for one, expected just such deference from former students. See *Letters of Benjamin Rush*, ed. L. H. Butterfield, II (Princeton, 1951), 681.

14 Powell feels Hutchinson was "obviously confused." *Bring Out Your Dead*, p. 43. See also n. 23 below.

15 "Pestilence," quoted *ibid.*

16 *National Gazette* (Philadelphia), Sept. 23, 1793.

17 Thomas Jefferson to James Madison, Sept. 1, 1793, in *The Writings of Thomas Jefferson*, ed. Andrew A. Lipscomb and Albert E. Bergh (Washington, D.C., 1903), IX, 214–215; *Federal Gazette* (Philadelphia), Dec. 17, 21, 28, 1793; *Gazette of the United States*, Dec. 18, 1793. Democratic Society leader Israel Israel requested the city to dig sewers following the epidemic. Israel to Clarkson, Jan. 29, 1794, Philadelphia Streets and Alleys Manuscripts, Historical Society of Pennsylvania.

18 For Fenno, see Nathan Goodman, *Benjamin Rush: Physician and Citizen, 1746–1813* (Philadelphia, 1934), p. 198; for Wolcott, see Charles Francis Jenkins, *Washington in Germantown . . .* (Philadelphia, 1905), p. 76; for Willing and Chew, see College of Physicians of Philadelphia, *Additional Facts and Observations Relative to the Nature and Origin of the Pestilential Fever* (Philadelphia, 1806), pp. 10, 11; for Hollingsworth, see "An Old Resident" [Hollingsworth] to David Claypoole, Hollingsworth MSS; for Bordley, see J. B. Bordley, *Yellow Fever* (Philadelphia, 1794); for Hazard, see "Hazard letters," Massachusetts Historical Society, *Collections*, 5th series, III (1877), 338, and Powell, *Bring Out Your Dead*, p. 86; for White, see Bird Wilson, *Memoir of the Life of the Right Reverend William White, D.D., . . .* (Philadelphia, 1839), pp. 158, 288; for Johnson, see Benjamin Johnson, *Account of the Rise, Progress, and Termination of the Malignant Fever* (Philadelphia, 1793), p. 5.

19 Lewis Saul Benjamin [Lewis Melville], *The Life and Letters of William Cobbett in England & America, Based Upon Hitherto Unpublished Family Papers* (New York, 1913), pp. 85–87.

20 For Mifflin, see Powell, *Bring Out Your Dead*, pp. 52–53, Samuel Hazard et al., eds., *Pennsylvania Archives*, 4th series, IV (Harrisburg, 1900), 264–269, and Tinkcom, *Republicans and Federalists*, pp. 72, 112, 219–220; for Bache, see Donald H. Stewart, *The Opposition Press of the Federalist Period* (Albany, 1969), p. 137; for Carey, see Mathew Carey, *Observations on Dr. Rush's Enquiry into the Origin of the Late Epidemic Fever in Philadelphia* (Philadelphia, 1793), and Carey, *Short Account*, p. 67.

21 Charles W. Upham, *The Life of Timothy Pickering*, III (Boston, 1873), 56, 62. Some Federalists from rival cities, such as Harrisburg's Alexander Graydon, encouraged the idea that Philadelphia was an unhealthy place. Alexander Graydon, *Memoirs of a Life* (Harrisburg, 1811), pp. 336–338. However, most Federalist merchants in New York, Baltimore, and Trenton remained importationists, leading the local efforts to cut off the trade of their stricken rival. See *General Advertiser* (Philadelphia), Sept. 18, 20, 23, 1793; and James Weston Livingood, *The Philadelphia-Baltimore Trade Rivalry 1780–1860* (Harrisburg, 1947). Even anticontagionist New York Federalist Noah Webster believed this Philadelphia epidemic contagious. Noah Webster, *A Collection of Papers on the Subject of Bilious Fevers* (New York, 1796), p. 233.

22 Harry Emerson Wildes, *Lonely Midas: The Story of Stephen Girard* (New York, 1943), pp. 121, 126; Albert J. Gares, "Stephen Girard's West Indian trade, 1789–1812," *Penn. Mag. Hist. & Biography*, 1948, *72*: 316; J. Thomas Scharf and Thompson Westcott, *History of Philadelphia, 1609–1884* (Philadelphia, 1884), I, 493.

23 Johnson, *Account*, pp. 5, 9; *Dunlap's American Daily Advertiser* (Philadelphia), Dec. 20, 1793; Rush, *Account*, p. 147. Leib and others defended Hutchinson against the charges raised by the College. *General Advertiser*, Nov. 30, Dec. 10, 1793.

24 *Independent Gazetteer*, Dec. 14, 1793; Henry D. Biddle, ed., *Extracts from the Journal of Elizabeth Drinker* (Philadelphia, 1889), p. 193.

25 Richard Peters to Timothy Pickering, Oct. 22, 1793,

Timothy Pickering Papers, Massachusetts Historical Society, Boston, quoted in *Rush Letters*, ed. Butterfield, II, 729–730. Pickering may have shown the letter to Rush. Fearing government restrictions on trade, one Federalist importationist appealed to the benevolence of the merchants and ship captains to impose a voluntary quarantine. "A Philadelphian," in *Occasional Essays on the Yellow Fever . . .* (Philadelphia, 1800), pp. 8–11, 13.

26 Benjamin Rush to Julia Rush, Oct. 28, 1793, in *Rush Letters*, ed. Butterfield, II, 729.

27 Goodman, *Benjamin Rush*, p. 198; Bordley, *Yellow Fever*, p. 1; Blake, "Yellow fever," p. 682.

28 "An Old Resident" to Claypoole, Hollingsworth MSS; College of Physicians, *Facts and Observations*, p. 24.

29 Jefferson to Rush, Sept. 23, 1800, in *Writings of Jefferson*, 10, ed. Lipscomb and Bergh, quoted in Charles N. Glaab, *The American City: A Documentary History* (Homewood, Ill., 1963), p. 52.

30 For example, *Federal Gazette*, Dec. 6, 21, 1793; John Redman Coxe Letters on the Yellow Fever [1794], p. 139, College of Physicians of Philadelphia; Joseph McFarland, "The epidemic of yellow fever in 1793 and its influence upon Dr. Benjamin Rush," *Med. Life*, 1929, *36*: 468. Both sides in the medical split claimed to be the true friends of commerce. Blake, "Yellow fever," p. 681.

31 Powell, *Bring Out Your Dead*, pp. 260–263. Constitutional principles did not limit the state's power to move its own capital out of Philadelphia in 1799 as a result of the yellow fever. Scharf and Westcott, *Philadelphia*, I, 501.

32 Rush, *Account*, p. 147.

33 College of Physicians, *Facts and Observations*, pp. 15–16; *Rush Letters*, ed. Butterfield, II, 798; Hazard et al., eds., *Pennsylvania Archives*, 4th series, IV, 269.

34 Blake, "Yellow fever," p. 681.

35 For a discussion of the theological perception of cholera, 1832–1866, see Charles E. Rosenberg, *The Cholera Years: The United States in 1832, 1849, and 1866* (Chicago, 1962). See also Shryock, *Medicine and Society*, p. 94; *Rush Letters*, ed. Butterfield, II, 659; Horace W. Smith, *Life and Correspondence of the Rev. William Smith, D.D., . . .* I (Philadelphia, 1880), 395; *General Advertiser*, Jan. 8, 1794.

36 Rush to William Marshall, Sept. 15, 1798, in *Rush Letters*, ed. Butterfield, II, 807. Rush also blamed party spirit in general. See also *National Gazette*, Oct. 9, 12, 16, 1793; Carey, *Short Account*, p. 10.

37 Smith, *Life of William Smith*, I, p. 392.

38 Graydon, *Memoirs*, p. 335; Stephen G. Kurtz, *The Presidency of John Adams: The Collapse of Federalism, 1795–1800* (Philadelphia, 1957), p. 190; Charles D. Hazen, *Contemporary American Opinion of the French Revolution*, Johns Hopkins University Studies in Historical and Political Science, XVI (Baltimore, 1897), pp. 185–186.

39 *National Gazette*, Oct. 16, 1793; Scharf and Westcott, *Philadelphia*, II, 966–967.

40 Scharf and Westcott, *Philadelphia*, II, 966–967.

41 *Gazette of the United States*, Dec. 19, 28, 1793; *General Advertiser*, Jan. 6, 1794; Arthur Hornblow, *History of the Theatre in America*, I (Philadelphia, 1919), 174–175; *National Gazette*, Oct. 16, 1793.

42 *Gazette of the United States*, Dec. 14, 26, 1793, Feb. 8, 1794; René La Roche, *Yellow Fever . . .* (Philadelphia, 1855), p. 73; William Priest, *Travels in the United States of America . . .* (London, 1802), p. 13; [John Purdon], *A Leisure Hour; or a Series of Poetical Letters, Mostly Written During the Prevalence of the Yellow Fever* (Philadelphia, 1804), p. 27.

43 Several leading Republican literary figures remained aloof from this alliance. Bache, whose son-in-law was an actor, was accused of misrepresenting rank-and-file Republican sentiment on the theater for family reasons. Roger Griswold, *The Republican Court; or, American Society in the Days of Washington* (Philadelphia, 1854), p. 316; *General Advertiser*, Jan. 10, 1794. On January 8, though, Bache attributed his stand to anticlericalism. See also Mathew Carey, *Autobiography* (New York, 1942 [reprint of 1837 ed.]), p. 29.

44 W. H. Hargreaves and R. J. G. Morrison, *The Practice of Tropical Medicine* (London, 1965), pp. 183–185; Powell, *Bring Out Your Dead*, pp. 64, 125, 292. Wine is generally not a stimulant although it was believed to be one. Chris Holmes, "Benjamin Rush and the yellow fever," *Bull. Hist. Med.*, 1966, *60*: 246–262, believes Rush's cures were not lethal, but does not fully distinguish patients like Hazard, who left Rush after one or two treatments, from those who stayed for the full course of bloodletting.

45 David Freeman Hawke, *Benjamin Rush, Revolutionary Gadfly* (Indianapolis, 1971), pp. 208–223, 236–240; Powell, *Bring Out Your Dead*, p. 78; Goodman, *Benjamin Rush*, pp. 90–116.

46 Powell, *Bring Out Your Dead*, pp. 82, 153, 203; George Logan to "Citizen Bache," in *General Advertiser*, Sept. 18, 1793; *The Papers of Alexander Hamilton*, ed. Harold Syrett and Jacob E. Cooke, XV (New York, 1969), 325 n. 1. Say's party affiliation is derived from Tinkcom, *Republicans and Federalists*, p. 240.

47 *Dunlap's American Daily Advertiser*, Sept. 13, 1793; *Hamilton Papers*, ed. Syrett and Cooke, XV, 331–332; Powell, *Bring Out Your Dead*, p. 135; Goodman, *Benjamin Rush*, p. 215; Jenkins, *Washington in Germantown*, p. 25.

48 B. Rush to J. Rush, Oct. 3, 1793, to Horatio Gates,

Dec. 26, 1795, to John Dickinson, Oct. 11, 1797, in *Rush Letters*, ed. Butterfield, II, 701, 767, 793; Goodman, *Benjamin Rush*, pp. 203, 209.

49 McFarland, "Yellow fever and Dr. Rush," pp. 486–487; John E. Lane, "Jean Devèze," *Ann. Med. Hist.*, n.s., 1936, *8*: 220; Margaret Woodbury, *Public Opinion in Philadelphia, 1789–1801*, Smith College Studies in History, V (Northampton, Mass., 1920), p. 16; Goodman, *Benjamin Rush*, p. 208. Some Republican bark physicians agreed that Rush's cures were egalitarian but denied that political Republicanism required opposition to medical elitism. See letter of "Citizen Robert, M.D.," *General Advertiser*, Dec. 6, 1793, whose combination of titles reflects his attempt to combine egalitarianism and professional distinctions.

50 Powell, *Bring Out Your Dead*, p. 201; *Rush Letters*, ed. Butterfield, II, 692.

51 McFarland, "Yellow fever and Dr. Rush," p. 462.

52 Goodman, *Benjamin Rush*, p. 183.

53 Stephen Girard to Pierre Changeur & Co., Sept. 11, 1793, Girard Papers, Am. Phil. Soc.; Powell, *Bring Out Your Dead*, pp. 175, 179–180.

54 Powell, *Bring Out Your Dead*, pp. 179, 242. Samuel Coates is not to be confused with William Coates, a founder of the Democratic Society. Henry Simpson, *The Lives of Eminent Philadelphians, Now Deceased* (Philadelphia, 1859), p. 218; *Gazette of the United States*, Dec. 14, 1793.

55 Carey, *Short Account*, pp. 27, 28. Carey seems to slight Federalists in his stories of heroism. For their side, see also *Extracts from the Diary of Jacob Hiltzheimer, of Philadelphia*, ed. Jacob Cox Parsons (Philadelphia, 1893), pp. 195–197; Smith, *Life of William Smith*, I, 379; Upham, *Life of Pickering*, III, 62; "Hazard letters," p. 334; Powell, *Bring Out Your Dead*, p. 138; and Simpson, *Eminent Philadelphians*, pp. 908–922. For party affiliations of Morris (as of 1798), see letter of Nov. 19, 1798, Hollingsworth MSS; of Humphreys, see Scharf and Westcott, *Philadelphia*, I, 490; of Hollingsworth, see David Hackett Fischer, *The Revolution of American Conservatism: The Federalist Party in the Era of Jeffersonian Democracy* (New York, 1965), p. 339; of Hiltzheimer and FitzSimmons, see Tinkcom, *Republicans and Federalists*, pp. 138, 152. In addition, Samuel Pancoast of the merchants' committee was listed as a Federalist by 1817. Scharf and Westcott, *Philadelphia*, I, 588.

56 For Wetherill, see Simpson, *Eminent Philadelphians*, p. 940, and Tinkcom, *Republicans and Federalists*, p. 252; for Lownes, see Scharf and Westcott, *Philadelphia*, I, 477; for Girard, see Link, *Democratic Societies*, pp. 75–76; for Israel, see Powell, *Bring Out Your Dead*, p. 178; for Carey, see Carey, *Autobiography*; for Sergeant, see *Dictionary of American Biography*, s.v. "Sergeant, Jonathan Dickinson"; for Sharswood, see Simpson, *Eminent Philadelphians*, p. 885; for Kerr and Connelly, see Minute Book of the Democratic Society, pp. 29, 47, Historical Society of Pennsylvania, and Scharf and Westcott, *Philadelphia*, I, 507, 588; for Wistar, see Powell, *Bring Out Your Dead*, p. 179. The list of leaders of the committee was compiled from names most frequently cited in *Minutes of the Proceedings of the Committee Appointed on the 14th September, 1793* (Philadelphia, 1848); and Carey, *Short Account*, p. 95.

57 Powell, *Bring Out Your Dead*, pp. 72, 87, 179; Ford, *David Rittenhouse*, p. 190; Kenneth R. Rossman, *Thomas Mifflin and the Politics of the American Revolution* (Chapel Hill, 1952), p. 225.

58 Powell, *Bring Out Your Dead*, p. 177; Ford, *David Rittenhouse*, pp. 190–192.

59 Helm was Girard's assistant in charge of "external affairs." He was a second generation German-American but little else is known of him. The chronology of Bush Hill is as follows: Aug. 31 — Mayor authorizes seizure of estate, hospital set up under Leib and others; Sept. 16 — Girard and Helm volunteer to manage and administer the hospital for the committee; Sept. 18 — Girard appoints Devèze to assist Leib and the medical staff; Sept. 21 — Leib resigns in dispute over the proper cure. Powell, *Bring Out Your Dead*, pp. 140–172.

60 Democratic Society Minute Book, pp. 29, 39, 42, 47, 48, 52, 95; Link, *Democratic Societies*, pp. 77, 90; Carey, *Short Account*, pp. 20, 27, 30, 37; Tinkcom, *Republicans and Federalists*, pp. 57, 84, 283. Snyder is identified as of 1799 in Scharf and Westcott, *Philadelphia*, I, 507, 588. There were two John Barclays; this one was president of the Republican Bank of Pennsylvania. Duplication of names makes it impossible to say whether merchants' committeeman William Clifton was the Federalist poet or one of two shopkeepers of that name. Likewise, William Sansom, Guardian of the Poor, may have been either the Federalist or the Republican of that name. Simpson, *Eminent Philadelphians*, p. 210; General Roll of McPherson's Blues, Hollingsworth MSS; J. Hardie, *The Philadelphia Directory and Register . . .* (Philadelphia, 1793), p. 182 and *passim*.

61 Powell, *Bring Out Your Dead*, pp. 85–86. To avoid confusion over the new implications of its old name, the *Federal Gazette* became the *Philadelphia Gazette* on Jan. 1, 1794. Clarence S. Brigham, *History and Bibliography of American Newspapers, 1690–1820*, II (Worcester, Mass., 1947), 91.

62 Lewis Leary, *That Rascal Freneau: A Study in Literary Failure* (New Brunswick, N.J., 1941), pp. 240–246; Dumas Malone, *Jefferson and the Ordeal of Liberty*, Vol. III of *Jefferson and His Time* (Boston, 1962), p. 142.

63 *National Gazette*, Sept. 11, Oct. 9, 1793; Scharf and Westcott, *Philadelphia*, II, 1606; *Minutes of the Committee*, p. 232.

64 Powell's account, *Bring Out Your Dead*, p. 135, differs from Rush's version of the Van Berkle business, B. Rush to J. Rush, Oct. 3, 1793, in *Rush Letters*, ed. Butterfield, II, 701. Wolcott fled with Knox in early September. Jenkins, *Washington in Germantown*, p. 22.

65 Powell, *Bring Out Your Dead*, p. 123.

66 Jefferson to Madison, Sept. 8, 1793, in *The Writings of Thomas Jefferson*, ed. Paul Leicester Ford, VI (New York, 1895), 419; Malone, *Jefferson and the Ordeal of Liberty*, pp. 140–142.

67 *National Gazette*, Sept. 4, 1793. The version in Powell, *Bring Out Your Dead*, p. 240, is not the original 1793 poem but a printed edition of 1795. The original attacks all deserters; the later one absolves all but the fleeing physicians. Condemnation of the fugitives often stressed their wealth. *Gazette of the United States*, letter of Feb. 20, 1794.

68 *Dunlap's American Daily Advertiser*, Dec. 14, 1793; Nathaniel Burt, *The Perennial Philadelphians: The Anatomy of an American Aristocracy* (Boston, 1963), pp. 156–157. "Nomination," "platform," etc. are all useful metaphors in spite of the anachronism.

69 *Gazette of the United States*, Dec. 13, 1793.

70 *Ibid.*, Dec. 14, 20, 1793; Robert C. Alberts, *The Golden Voyage: The Life and Times of William Bingham, 1752–1804* (Boston, 1969), p. 246. Out of 14,000 eligible, only 1,282 Philadelphians came out to vote. *Independent Gazetteer*, Dec. 21, 1793.

71 *Dunlap's American Daily Advertiser*, Dec. 14, 1793.

72 *Hamilton Papers*, ed. Syrett and Cooke, XV, 332 n; Carey, *Short Account*, p. 93; Powell, *Bring Out Your Dead*, pp. 216–232.

73 *General Advertiser*, Dec. 2, 1793; *Rush Letters*, ed. Butterfield, II, 736; Johnson, *Account*, p. 28; Powell, *Bring Out Your Dead*, pp. 87, 178. Carey printed rumors of black profiteering similar to Johnson's but he hastily withdrew them. Richard Allen, *Life Experiences and Gospel Labors . . .* (Philadelphia, 1933), pp. 34–35.

74 *General Advertiser*, Dec. 2, 3, 1793; *Federal Gazette*, Dec. 9, 14, 1793.

75 "HOWARD," in *General Advertiser*, Jan. 8, 1794; see also Nov. 27, 1793.

76 Tinkcom, *Republicans and Federalists*, pp. 176–179; John Bach McMaster, *The Life and Times of Stephen Girard, Mariner and Merchant*, I (Philadelphia, 1918), 352. The career of Israel Israel and his role in Philadelphia class politics is traced in John K. Alexander, "The City of Brotherly Fear: the poor in late eighteenth century Philadelphia," in Kenneth T. Jackson and Stanley K. Schultz, comps., *Cities in American History* (New York, 1972), pp. 86–90.

77 *The Works of John Adams, . . .* , ed. Charles Francis Adams, X (Boston, 1856), 47. Jefferson declared the death of Hutchinson to be as great a setback as the Genêt fiasco. Merrill D. Peterson, *Thomas Jefferson and the New Nation: A Biography* (New York, 1970), p. 508.

78 Tinkcom, *Republicans and Federalists*, p. 173.

79 Jean Pierre Blanchard had recently introduced the city to the French hot air balloon.

80 Two of Rush's black apprentices.

81 *Gazette of the United States*, Dec. 23, 1793.

19

The Cause of Cholera: Aspects of Etiological Thought in 19th-Century America

CHARLES E. ROSENBERG

Cholera was a new and unavoidable challenge to the medical world of the 19th century. At its first appearance in the West, it represented as much a mystery as had the plague five centuries earlier, for the theoretical resources of the average physician in 1832 were not greatly different from those of his medieval predecessor. Yet, by 1866, only 34 years after their first experience with cholera, even provincial Americans were familiar with the names of Snow and Pettenkofer, Liebig and Berzelius. Traditional concepts had been changed, infiltrated and supplanted by new ideas.

In 1832, when cholera first appeared in this country, American medical men were convinced that it was not contagious. Its cause lay in the atmosphere.[1] Experience with vaccination and smallpox, the one new and extremely pervasive element in etiological thought, served only to reinforce the dominant anticontagionism. Unable to abandon older ideas, medical thinkers failed to generalize from their experience with vaccination and to assume that a similar, though as yet undiscovered, process might take place in other diseases. Any disease not conforming to the rigid and arbitrary "laws" assigned smallpox could not be contagious.

Nor was it difficult to show by analogy that cholera was not contagious. Even if transmitted from place to place, cholera was certainly not passed "from one body to another, or through the medium of those morbid secretions of the human system which preserve and multiply the sources of infection in contagious diseases." Cholera could be contracted more than once, while a contagious disease — defined in terms of smallpox — could not. Moreover, smallpox was not influenced by atmospheric variations as were cholera and other "epidemic" diseases. Regardless of atmospheric conditions, all exposed to its poison would inevitably fall victim unless they had been vaccinated or had recovered from an attack. This was manifestly not the case in cholera. The poison secreted by a person suffering with a contagious disease was specific in character and always caused precisely the same disease. For this to happen, wrote the irascible Charles Caldwell, only part of the time, or only in certain circumstances, would be a change as drastic as the transformation of a rattlesnake into a blacksnake, or aconite to asparagus.[2]

Physicians naturally assumed that smallpox was a specific disease. Unlike other ills, it had a specific and "known" cause, one that could be placed in a glass vial and carried to a distant city, there infallibly to produce the same disease. But in this, smallpox was unique. At this time, indeed, the very concept of disease specificity was more than a little suspect. Following Broussais, many American physicians disclaimed belief in what they termed "ontology." ("That is, in the idea that disease is an *entity* — a being — a something added to the system."[3]) Disease was a protean and dynamic condition. Psychic and somatic ills were not rigidly demarcated. The etiology and symptoms of disease were constantly affected by climatic, hygienic, mental, and moral factors.

Even before they had seen the "oriental scourge," some American physicians wrote soothingly that cholera was but another form of "sinking typhus," others that it was a variety of bilious fever or a "Lymphatic Hemorrhage." In the midst of fighting a cholera epidemic, a Philadelphia physician found time to note that he was treating a

---

Charles E. Rosenberg is Professor of History, University of Pennsylvania, Philadelphia, Pennsylvania.

Reprinted with permission from the *Bulletin of the History of Medicine*, 1960, *34*: 331–354.

"malignant congestive fever." A rural New York physician cited Rush to lend authority to his classification of cholera as a "suffocated fever."[4]

Most common was the opinion that Asiatic cholera was only an aggravated form of common cholera — a flexible term used to describe ailments as diverse as dysentery and diarrhea. Comforting in its familiarity, this nomenclature also played another role, implying a local origin for the disease, and hence nonimportation and noncontagion. In the words of Daniel Drake, cholera bore "to cholera morbus, a relation similar to that of the influenza to a common cold." It differed only in virulence. One physician reported finding three or four different degrees of cholera in the same family, ranging from the mild common cholera to the malignant. "The common Cholera heightened by panic" seemed less threatening than a completely new and spectacularly fatal ailment.[5]

With "disease" so flexible a concept, it was only natural that mental and moral factors should be presumed to play a role in its causation. Those succumbing to the ubiquitous "epidemic influence" had somehow predisposed themselves, had overeaten, been intemperate, or had capitulated to panic. Despite the obvious moralism[6] of such injunctions, medical thinkers did not regard the disease as a direct imposition of the Lord. Its onset was an inevitable result of the debilitating physical effect of transgressing His physical and moral laws. An active exercise of faith in God and His justice would protect one from fear and thus from cholera, but, however, "preeminently by the physical influence of that faith." For fear has

> a more specific operation upon the human body, than any other passion; it spasmodically contracts the mouths of thousands of our perspiring or exhaling vessels, flings the acrid perspirable matter upon the insides of our digestive organs, which it stimulates, and causes by abstracting much of the watery part of our blood, a looseness and congestion in our bowels, the very proximate cause of the Epidemic Cholera.

Indeed, the entire epidemic might be explained as a mass psychological phenomenon, akin to the "jerks" at a camp meeting. William Beaumont was only expressing a truism of his time, when he wrote that "the Greater proportional number of deaths in the cholera epidemics are, in my opinion, caused more by fright and presentiment of death than from the fatal tendency of the disease."[7] Even more directly than fear, sexual excess, gluttony, or an improper diet would weaken the "system" and predispose it to cholera.

This doctrine of predisposing causes, however, played more than a monitory role. It reinforced one of the weak spots in the atmospheric theory by explaining how some were stricken while others remained exempt, though all breathed the same atmosphere. Concentrations of cholera cases in circumscribed slum areas might be charged — and were — either to the moral qualities of the victims or to the presence of crowded tenements, decaying filth, resident pigs — anything which might produce miasmata or somehow vitiate the air needed to maintain normal respiration. Only those so weakened would then be attacked by the latent cholera poison in the atmosphere. In another variation of this theory, the cholera poison in the atmosphere did not become virulent unless it combined with locally produced miasmata. Only when "local" and "general" causes acted in concert did cholera break out. Thus was avoided a repetition of the local origin versus importation controversies which had raged so bitterly during yellow fever epidemics.

The sudden and widely scattered outbreak of cholera cases in many areas also implied that cholera was an atmospheric and not a contagious disease. Dr. Kane of Plattsburg, appointed by his community to observe the disease in Montreal, became convinced that it was not contagious, for it had descended in many parts of the city simultaneously, "like a shower of hail." An American physician, observing the disease in Vienna, concluded that its cause must be some alteration of the atmosphere — the only thing which could have affected so many people at the same time. A similar conclusion was reached by Daniel Drake, after observing the disease in Cincinnati.[8]

There were but few to question.[9] The atmospheric theory was too convenient. Flexible and amorphous enough to explain the varied phenomena of the disease, it served also as an effective weapon against the "antisocial" and "antiquated" doctrine of contagion. The more precise attributed the disease either to some change in the normal constituents of the atmosphere, or the addition to it of some deleterious substance of terrestrial origin. A greater number found such intellectual refinement unnecessary, content to intone such phrases as "epidemic influence," "choleraic distemperature," or "uncontrollable atmospheric peculiarity."

Although they might disagree as to the nature of this epidemic influence, all physicians could testify to having observed occurrences that only an atmospheric disease could have produced. Outbreaks of cholera were foreshadowed by a "universal tendency toward bowel complaints." When the epidemic began, it "drove out all other diseases" or made them "assume its livery."[10] A St. Louis newspaper noted during a cholera epidemic that there was "scarcely any other disease in the city — all others determining in cholera." An observer in New York reported that there were few cases of any other disease, though all the inhabitants were afflicted with some of the symptoms, which "in proper subjects amount to actual cholera." Even the lower animals were said to succumb to this pervasive atmospheric contamination.[11]

Though the "common people" might regard all diseases as contagious, many of the educated shared the physician's belief that the cause of cholera lay in the atmosphere. Joel Munsell protested to his diary that it was fruitless to burn pitch in an attempt to purify "a boundless element of the noxious particles floating in it." Though not contracting the disease, many laymen noted that their health was affected adversely by exposure to a "cholera atmosphere." Public-spirited newspaper editors, wishing to scotch the antisocial idea of contagion, filled their columns with expositions of the atmospheric theory, "made clear to the meanest capacity." Stories were circulated, telling of a piece of "fresh, wholesome beef," placed on the Cathedral spire in Montreal, "and taken down after an hour and twenty minutes in a tainted and corrupt state."[12]

Perhaps the most compelling reason for the dominance of the atmospheric theory was the absence of alternatives. The animalcular theory — subject of so much historical interest — was, in effect, a variation of standard atmospheric ideas, differing in that the cholera causing substance in the air was specified as being a "small winged insect not visible to the naked eye." Daniel Drake, the only physician to hold this view in a sample of over one hundred, conceived of the animalculae as "poisonous, invisible, aerial insects, of the same or similar habits with the gnat." This theory which did recognize a need for assuming some specific material cause for disease and which did suggest that it might be organic, found few converts. It was a notion with "but few enlightened advocates," though it was more popular outside of medical circles. Finding few scientific backers, "the little, infernal, greedy, choleric *critters*," became easy prey for the wit of journalistic sophisticates.[13]

Other variants of the atmospheric theory attracted even less interest. At least one physician suggested that some deficiency in atmospheric electricity might be the cause of the disease, but this idea was not treated seriously. Nor was the belief that the disease might be due to some lack of oxygen in the air. The hoary view that epidemics might be caused by the vagaries of extraterrestrial bodies was held by at least two physicians. (Samuel Cartwright felt that the cause of the disease was a "moving non-electric meteor," while another physician suggested that "the approach of comets to the earth is a great link in the chain of their causation.") Yet even this early in the century, such ideas, "so utterly repugnant to the established principles of physical science," were generally scouted.[14]

Contagionism, though handicapped by being defined in terms of smallpox, seemed the only serious alternative to the atmospheric theory. Lacking the physician's theoretical knowledge, many intelligent and articulate lay observers, in common with ordinary folk, were impressed by evidences of contagion. Charles Francis Adams noted in his diary that the disease followed the tracks of commerce, which "would seem to sustain the doctrine of contagion." To canny old Deborah Logan, "contagion was too apparent to be doubted." In nine cases out of ten, the outbreak of cholera in a community could be traced to immigrants or to communication with an infected city. To some physicians, the opinion that contagion "under certain circumstances, belongs properly to every malignant disease," was not an extreme one.[15] Nevertheless, only one physician in my sample could be considered a consistent and thoroughgoing contagionist.

Bernard Byrne, in a short treatise on cholera

published in 1833, argued that cholera, like smallpox, was caused by an "animal poison" and was always contagious. Other diseases, "accidental" and not "specific," were caused not by a poison, but by anything else which might disturb the "system." This theoretical argument was reinforced by an intelligent analysis of the peregrinations of the disease. Whenever, he noted, we see a disease leave its place of origin, we have *prima facie* evidence of its contagiousness; "for in the present state of our knowledge, there is no other mode, than that of human intercourse, by which progress of any disease can be accounted for." If there was such a thing as an epidemic constitution of the atmosphere, how could we account for cholera and yellow fever having prevailed at the same time? Which was the "epidemic"? Was it not a strong coincidence that a disease of local origin should originate in a place where immigration was greater than any other, "and that too at the critical moment when an infected vessel arrived there?"[16]

Byrne, almost alone in his belief, could be ignored. The more numerous contingent contagionists had to be answered. On the face of it, they were admonished, belief in a second cause, when one was sufficient, was "unphilosophical" and reeked of "empiricism." Dr. S. H. Pennington, for example, reporting on a group of cholera cases at Whippany, New Jersey, stated that though he could not explain them on any basis other than contagion, he could not consider cholera contagious, for he had seen instances where it had not spread by contagion, and it was "unphilosophical" to suppose that there were more causes responsible for a given effect than are absolutely necessary.[17]

American physicians were still thinking in scholastic terms, hoping by elaborate chains of reasoning to discover the true philosophy of a disease. (Thus high value was placed upon the word "philosophical" and a correspondingly low evaluation given the word "empirical.") Certainly this kind of reasoning, formal in its rhetoric, based perhaps on a random observation, recalled the 18th century rather than prefigured the second half of the 19th.[18]

When, 17 years after its first appearance on this continent, cholera next returned, the etiological thinking of most American physicians had not greatly changed. A significant minority,[19] however, were becoming aware that to provide a name for a thing was not to understand it. Chemistry and biology had, moreover, provided new alternatives to older ideas. The work of Bassi, Ehrenberg, Schönlein, Cagniard-Latour, Berzelius, and especially Liebig, was known, even if in an attenuated form.

Advances in clinical medicine and pathology had also begun to exert an important influence, making respectable the idea of disease specificity.[20] The Americans who had studied in the Paris clinics in the 1830s were the teachers of a new generation of medical students. In addition, personal experience with so striking a disease as cholera had convinced many of its specificity during the first cholera pandemic. In the words of Sir Thomas Watson: "The malady was too striking, to be overlooked, or ever forgotten, by any who had once seen it." John W. Francis had written in the midst of the cholera epidemic of 1832 in New York City, that "nosology [could] not classify a more distinctive disease."[21] By 1849, most physicians agreed that cholera was a specific disease caused by a specific poison.

Certainly, those who had abandoned or attempted to give precision to the atmospheric theory, found it entirely natural to assume that cholera was a specific disease. A specific cause would produce a specific effect — a vague "epidemic influence" would produce effects equally amorphous. For example, a medical man who considered disease to be caused by a fungus would naturally argue that measles always produces measles and smallpox always produces smallpox, "as wheat produces wheat, and rye produces rye; each after its kind."[22]

Still, ideas of specificity were hardly rigid: to many, the variability of disease remained an article of faith. It was difficult to believe that disease could remain the same, while social, even geological and climatic, conditions were changing: "Constitutions, and habits of life, and modes of living are constantly changing; hence new diseases are making their appearance from time to time, while others have vanished from the world." When threatened by cholera, doctors were still urged to study "the antecedents to its approach, its aspect on first manifesting itself, its associations with other forms of disease, its absorption into itself of its Typhoid predecessors, and its final immersion into Dysentery and an Asthenic form of Fever." Many observers noted influenza and intestinal disorders heralding its arrival. Where it raged, cholera was charged with having postponed births. And, as President Polk was warned by a physician, "all diseases of the bowels had a tendency to run into cholera when that disease prevailed." Particularly bad environmental conditions might, of themselves, give rise to "sporadic cholera." Though sporadic cases might arise in such places as the holds of emigrant ships, they would not spread as an epidemic unless the peculiar "epidemic influence" was also present. This belief was extremely pervasive, reflecting a growing concern with environmental sanitation.[23]

Naturally, the socially useful doctrine of predisposing causes was still preached. Journalists, ministers, and others of the public spirited, as well as physicians, published long catalogues of the disreputable actions which might lead to cholera. Newspaper readers were urged to "have peace with God, through the Lord Jesus Christ," for "your peace will be of essential service in enabling you to throw off the malady." The doctrine of predisposing causes was completely unquestioned by the medical profession. Even the moderate report of the American Medical Association's Committee on Practical Medicine and Epidemics reasoned that cholera could not be contagious, for a debauch or a drinking bout had never caused a *contagious* disease.[24]

The great majority of physicians still believed that the cause of cholera lay in the atmosphere. But now the mere profession of this belief seemed inadequate. Believers had to be more precise: they could no longer rely exclusively on affirmation and intonation, but must attempt to define whatever it was in the atmosphere that caused the disease. The number of physicians content to assign the disease to an "epidemic influence," or an "imponderable atmospheric peculiarity," decreased markedly. Now, one blamed the disease upon electricity, or ozone, or carbonic acid, or at least a "specific aeriform poison." Local exciting causes continued, however, to play a prominent role in etiological thinking. To a generation increasingly conscious of the relation between disease and environment, local filth and lack of ventilation and pure water were the obvious reasons for the concentration of cholera cases among the poor and in circumscribed slum areas.

Other, older patterns of thought endured as well. Few questioned the assumption that an epidemic disease drove out other diseases or made them "wear its livery." (Epidemics "seem ever to exercise upon the atmosphere a controlling power, as exemplified in the fact that the ordinary diseases of the country partake in some measure, of the character of the prevailing epidemic.") When cholera was epidemic, ran a popular saying, all other diseases disappeared. One newspaper editor encouraged his readers by noting that rather than increasing during a cholera epidemic, the bills of mortality were less crowded than usual.[25]

As was not the case in 1832, however, a few critics appeared. The Philadelphia Board of Health proved, by comparing mortality statistics for the years 1846 through 1849, that cholera had not driven out other diseases, but that these had on the contrary, increased during the cholera year. Observers in New Orleans and Brooklyn also noted that cholera did not swallow up other diseases or force them to wear its livery.[26] Moreover, fundamental criticisms of the atmospheric theory itself became more frequent.

Alexander Stevens, president of the New York State Medical Association in 1849 and a believer in the atmospheric origin of cholera in 1832, could now call that theory only an excuse for thought: "It is improperly called an explanation. It is only a confession of ignorance; and just as strong proof might be adduced that diseases were induced by witchcraft, or the influence of comets and fiery dragons in the heavens; . . . it should be discarded from science; it belongs in the middle ages." John Evans, editor of the *Northwestern Medical and Surgical Journal*, charged the atmosphere with being "made the scape-goat to bear off the sins of our ignorance." What evidence, he continued, had ever been presented for this theory other than the fact that everyone contracts cholera while breathing? One might as well blame the stars or the moon for having caused the disease.[27]

The rhetoric of progress could cut two ways, however, and the anticontagionists were the ones who employed it most frequently in their attacks on quarantine regulations. The quarantines implied by a belief in contagionism were regarded with some ambivalence even by contagionists, while their opponents labelled them inhuman "relicts of superstition and barbarism." It seemed a mystery indeed, "that this absurd system [was] still maintained, in spite of all sense, science and experience." The abolition of quarantines marked triumphs "of truth over error, not only for the honor of the human mind, but for the benefits of commerce; and above all for the good of humanity."[28]

Some modifications did appear in the arguments which had been so effective in fighting contagionism two decades earlier. Contingent-contagionism could no longer be dismissed as "unphilosophical." Arguments based on analogies with smallpox did not cease, but were vigorously criticized and less frequently utilized. Jonathan Knight, professor at Yale Medical School, held that such arguments by analogy were responsible for "more errors in reasoning" than had arisen from all other sources.[29]

> It is because we continually try to study one disease by looking at another, that we so often run astray. One specific disease can furnish us no data from which to judge of the nature of another. It is because cholera is a specific disease, and differs from any other, that it needs to be studied by actual observation, not by comparisons . . .

By 1849, the idea that cholera was "portable," though not contagious, seemed a moderate one, consistent with the great bulk of evidence. Even decided anticontagionists had to account for this portability. (As early as 1836, Sir Thomas Watson had concluded that the disease must be portable and could be transported from place to place by persons "who were themselves proof against its effects.") Especially in rural and isolated communities in the United States, the circumstances surrounding cholera outbreaks pointed unmistakably to its having been imported from infected areas.[30]

Nevertheless, there were anomalies in the spread of this "portable" disease not easily explained by believers in either the contagionist or atmospheric theories. Fortunately, the natural sciences had provided new alternatives. One, stemming from microscopy and biology, visualized a microorganism, either plant or animal, as causing the disease. The second, originating in the work of chemists on catalysis and fermentation, conceived of the epidemic as a kind of delayed chemical reaction, taking place either in the atmosphere or the patient's body and caused by the introduction of a small portion of cholera ferment or catalyst.

The idea that microscopic organisms might be the cause of disease was a novel, but not entirely new, one to American medical thinkers in 1849. As early as 1836, John L. Riddell, Adjunct Professor of Chemistry at the Cincinnati Medical College,[31] had outlined at some length a theory in which diseases were caused by "corpuscles," "transmicroscopic" in size, and holding "nearly the same grade in respect to animate and sentient beings which the more simple and minute of the *Fungi* and *Algae* do to the more perfect tribe of vegetables." The cause of cholera must, he reasoned, be organic, for only in living organisms is found the ability to reproduce indefinitely. Chemical reactions are self-limiting, and take place in definite proportions. The unpleasant ulcer caused by the application of caustic potash to the skin could not possibly be communicated to another person.

In the fall of 1849, readers of the Philadelphia *Medical Examiner*[32] would have come across an editorial marshalling the evidence for the idea that a microorganism was the cause of cholera. Reference was made to the work of Bassi and Balsamo, Schönlein and Henle, and even to Boehm, who as early as 1832 had found microscopic fungi in the dejecta of cholera patients. The editorial concluded with a notice of the recent writings of Dr. William Budd. The English physician had, it seemed, adopted the fungoid theory and urged that all cholera evacuations be placed in a chemical fluid known to be fatal to the "fungous tribe." Water should be supplied from uninfected districts, he also counselled, for it was "the principal channel through which this poison finds its way into the human body."

The fungous or cryptogamous theory was, in the United States, identified with the name of John Kearsley Mitchell. A professor at Jefferson Medical College, Mitchell concluded that cholera and other diseases were, in all probability, caused by a fungus, the spores of which could be wafted from place to place in the atmosphere.[33] Others, willing to make the assumption that the cause of the disease was organic and capable of reproduction by "germs," could not, like Mitchell, assume these "germs" to be fungi. Some considered "infusoria" or "animalculae" the cause, while others were willing to admit anything other than that the cause was "specific, reproductive, and infectious."

A growing interest in microscopy, followed by the discovery of animalculae and fungi in cholera evacuations, naturally suggested that they might be the cause of the disease. Interest was shown in this work by a number of American physicians. Some, like Waldo Burnett and D. H. Storer of Boston, did not regard the "vibriones" they saw as being peculiar to cholera, while at least one Cincinnati microscopist, W. H. Mussey, felt that he had seen the organisms responsible for cholera. This work, incomplete and fragmentary though it was, promised much for the future. The significance of a general acceptance of a "germ theory" was not lost on all physicians. In the prophetic words of one: "If such a theory should eventually be proved to be founded on facts, the hypothetical etiology of medical philosophers will be discarded, and medicine be rescued from much of the obloquy which now attaches to it."[34]

The most prominent and consistent of believers in this proto-germ theory was Samuel Henry Dickson, Professor of the Practice of Medicine at New York University. A firm believer in the contagiousness of cholera since 1832,[35] Dickson had, in the interim, been supplied with the theoretical arguments to bolster his position. He had become convinced that the cause of the disease, though "ultra-microscopic," must be living matter: "Whether simply cellular or of complicated structure, whether a fungous sporule or an animalcule, its capacity of self-multiplication, of infinite reproduction, necessarily implies its vitality." Though not certain of their exact nature, Dickson confidently suggested a procedure by which microorganisms could be proven to cause disease.[36] "A *contagious cell*," was one found only in the animal body when a particular disease was present and which then regularly produced the disease when introduced into the body of another person. Though none of the causative organisms of the great epidemic diseases had as yet been found, Dickson was positive that their nidus was the human body. In a public lecture in New York, Dickson urged rigid quarantines. Their very laxity in the past, he argued, was reason enough for their failure. Moreover, he continued, it was senseless to argue that contagionism was antisocial. It was much less likely to produce a panic than the vague idea of some mysterious epidemic influence pervading the atmosphere.[37]

However, even those firm in the belief that cholera was caused by a microorganism could not free themselves completely from the complex of ideas which had dominated epidemiological thought for so many centuries. For example, with the conflict over spontaneous generation as yet unsettled, there was no real necessity to assume that a disease could not originate *de novo* as a result of peculiar local conditions. Even S. H. Dickson assumed that many diseases originated spontaneously. Certainly typhus, "which none will doubt to be generated by filth and want of air, and low living," was one. Other physicians who might agree with Dickson in his supposition that the cause of cholera was organic and microscopic, could not agree that its nidus was the human body, could not forsake completely the older atmospheric and local origin theories. Most physicians who believed that a fungus was the cause of the disease, still maintained a belief in these traditional concepts by assuming that the seeds of the disease were spread through the atmosphere, "germinating" only in those places where conditions were appropriate.[38]

Most members of the medical profession, however, still regarded the fungoid and animalcular theories as unproven, if not bizarre. Austin Flint lamented J. K. Mitchell's treatise on the fungoid origin of the disease, for the "author had identified himself with a fanciful hypothesis, which would only serve as a fresh occasion for sarcasm for those who search the annals of medical literature for subjects of ridicule or reproach." The very idea of looking "for an ague in a mushroom, and for a pestilence in a crop of cryptogamous plants" was absurd. Joseph Leidy, the eminent botanist, ridiculed the idea that there could be spores or animalcula in the atmosphere too small to be detected. "It is," he said, "only saying in other words that such spores and animalcula are liquid and dissolved in the air, or in a condition of chemical solution."[39]

An "animalcular" theory was also popular with the public, which failed, however, to distinguish these newer ideas from traditional ones. Animalcula were still minute insects, just a bit too small to be seen by the naked eye. Xavier Chabert, one of the most spectacular and successful of quacks, and certainly conscious of what people were prepared to believe, wrote that the "aerial cholera poison" was a "small green insect, invisible to the naked eye, but easily to be seen under the action of a powerful microscope." Many physicians, as well, were unable to make a clear distinction. Witness an army surgeon, who supported a belief in the "cryptogamous theory" by mentioning that during the prevalence of cholera in San Antonio, the atmosphere some miles distant, "was filled with *grasshoppers*, visible to the naked eye."[40]

Far more pervasive than the fungoid or animalcular theories, was the idea that cholera was caused by a "ferment."[41] Accepted wholeheartedly by only a minority of physicians, this theory nevertheless found a place in the ideas of many others. On what other basis, besides that of personal contagion, could the portability of the disease be explained? (One need only assume that a minute quantity of the "cholera ferment" had been somehow introduced into a receptive environment.) The atmospheric theory need not be discarded, for it seemed probable that this "fermentation" process took place in the atmosphere.[42] The same theory might also explain how local nuisances fostered cholera. A deadly miasma might well be produced by fermentation in the filth, offal, and confined air of the slums. Not inherently inconsistent with older ideas, it served to clothe them with the scientific garb necessary in a more critical generation. Nor was the fermentation theory inconsistent with the idea that cholera was caused by a microorganism. It was logical to suppose that the ferment might be organic in nature. Only a "nucleated cell" with its indefinite powers of reproduction could "leaven" whole continents.[43]

New and promising elements were clearly apparent in American etiological thought in 1866, as the United States faced an epidemic of Asiatic cholera for the first time in a dozen years. "Exact methods of investigation," used during the epidemics of 1849 and 1854, had shown that the poison responsible for the disease was propagated "in the diarrhoeal and vomited fluids of infected persons."[44] These ideas, associated with the names of Snow and Pettenkofer, and current in medical circles for a dozen years, were widely accepted by American physicians. In the spring of 1866, the New York Academy of Medicine resolved *unanimously*:[45]

> . . . that in the judgment of the Academy the medical profession throughout this country should, for all practical purposes, act and advise in accordance with the hypothesis (or the fact) that the cholera diarrhoea and "rice-water discharges" of cholera patients, are capable, in connection with well-known localizing conditions, of propagating the cholera poison; and that rigidly enforced precautions should be taken in every case of cholera to permanently disinfect or destroy those ejected fluids . . .

A few physicians rushed forward with claims that they had been teaching this doctrine for over a dozen years — a conclusive symptom of intellectual fashionability. By 1866, there were few intelligent physicians who doubted that cholera was portable and transmissible: many considered the evacuations of cholera patients the most likely channel for this spread. Even the most cautious could agree that "if cholera is communicable, it is probably so through the stools."[46]

The rapid assimilation of these new ideas should not be surprising. Many American physicians were readers of European medical journals. A greater number kept abreast through the "eclectic" sections of the better American medical journals.[47] (These consisted of summaries of the more important articles in the major French, English, and, by the time of the Civil War, German medical journals.) The ideas of Snow, Budd, Pettenkofer, and Griesinger were no more distant than the nearest post-office. So rapid, indeed, was the assimilation of Snow's work in the eastern United States, that as early as the summer of 1855, his principles were being applied in the administration of the New York State quarantine hospital on Staten Island.[48] Immigrant physicians provided another source of knowledge. In Cincinnati, St. Louis, and New York, such men were leaders in advocating contagionism. By settling in these opinion-forming urban centers, a few emigrees might exert an influence far out of proportion to their numbers.

But opponents were still numerous in 1866. Cholera might be portable, but it certainly did not seem to be contagious. There were still physicians who could deny that cholera was contagious, "rather in the interest of humanity than on the side of mere theory." Older men, like John H. Griscom,

Edwin Snow, and Henry G. Clark, who had spent decades in fighting for sanitation and against filth, could not easily accept a doctrine which promised to destroy the rationale of their work. Commercial interests also found these new ideas — and the rigid quarantines they implied — unpalatable. When William Read, Resident Physician of Boston, announced his conversion to the ideas of Snow, he was quickly reprimanded for espousing doctrines "detrimental to the health, happiness and pecuniary interests of the citizens at large."[49]

But now the anomalies which had confounded contagionists in past epidemics could be explained. Knowing that cholera might be spread through a water supply or carried by seemingly healthy persons, the followers of Snow and Pettenkofer were able to display in the progress of the epidemic irrefutable evidence for their convictions. Its transmission by human intercourse seemed too apparent to admit of doubt. In Chicago, the outbreak of the disease was traced to a Mormon immigrant. In Pittsburgh, a few seemingly spontaneous cases on the outskirts were all eventually traced to contacts inside the city. New York, however, was the scene of the most striking demonstration of the validity of the "Snow-Pettenkofer" theory. The Metropolitan Board of Health, created in the early spring of 1866 to fight the epidemic, succeeded, by using prophylactic methods based on these theories, in limiting the epidemic in New York City itself to a few hundred cases.[50]

The common people, of course, continued in their unchanging belief that cholera was contagious. Mobs were still one of the normal operating hazards of cholera hospitals. But now, the theories of Snow and Pettenkofer, rather than ozone and electricity as in 1849, were urged upon their readers by newspapers and magazines. Contagionism had become respectable. In Chicago, for example, a correspondent noted that the general opinion "was that the foecal matter from the cholera patient spreads the disease. Whether it becomes contagious to the attendant or filters from cess-pool into well, it is sure to carry cholera."[51]

Naturally, most physicians, as well as laymen, confused the concepts of Snow and Pettenkofer with each other, as well as with other ideas, older and more accustomed. Belief in predisposing causes continued, regardless of any other ideas a medical man might entertain. Many physicians able to espouse these newer ideas continued to assign a role to the atmosphere in the spread of the disease. One Yankee physician, who quoted Griesinger and cited Pettenkofer, Snow, and Budd, could also marshal an imposing catalogue of predisposing causes, among them "lewdness," and remark that after an epidemic had broken out, an "infection pervaded the air." Other physicians believed that the cholera evacuations had an "infective" or "zymotic" quality only in an atmosphere contaminated with exhalations from decomposing organic matter. (Or perhaps, as many felt, a contaminated atmosphere — as in a slum — must weaken the "system" and predispose it to cholera.[52])

Many doctors who accepted the notion that human excreta had something to do with the spread of the disease, failed to understand that these evacuations could spread cholera only if they contained a specific organism or poison. "It has been supposed," wrote one California physician, "that fecal discharges, under some circumstances, favor the production of cholera — especially those from patients suffering with the disease." A New Orleans doctor agreed with the general opinion that the cholera poison was spread through the excrements, "but not to the extent that many represent. It has to be concentrated and confined."[53] The idea that some interval or "fermentation" period was necessary before the feces could become infectious was quite common, though Pettenkofer's elaborate theory justifying this was unknown or misunderstood.

It is unnecessary to outline the many ways in which older ideas survived: unnecessary, because they differed in most cases only in detail from those held in 1832 and 1849. Almost half of the physicians sampled in 1866, for example, continued to believe that the atmosphere was a primary medium for the spread of the disease. The vagaries of the epidemic were still explained in terms of "local exciting causes." But new habits of thought, perhaps less conspicuous, betokened the future.

Arguments based on formalistic philosophical assumptions almost ceased. Statistics and careful observation replaced tortured and abstract reasoning. (The imperfections which marred this work do not invalidate the importance of a newly felt need to perform it.) Perhaps most striking was an almost unquestioned assumption of the specificity of the disease. One heard almost nothing of "universal bowel complaints," of diarrhea "shading into cholera," of cholera transforming itself into typhus.

One might admit the specificity and portability of cholera and still find fault with the theories of Snow and Pettenkofer. Pettenkofer especially was the object of much criticism. To some, his *Grundwasser* theory was nothing more than an "irreconcilable absurdity." Cholera had spread in the frozen snows of Russia and in the deserts of Arabia. It had made its appearance in places where there could not have been the slightest trace of sub-soil filtration. It had prevailed in a citadel perched on the top of one thousand feet of solid rock, while the city at the foot of the mountain escaped. Many other critics emphasized the inability of Snow or Pettenkofer to explain the "isolated cases" which had occurred.[54]

The assumption that cholera might be caused by microorganisms met with a mixed, though promising, reception in the United States. Twenty years of scientific advance had made this idea seem less bizarre than it had in 1849. The popular furor, for example, over the "trichina disease" was at its height in the spring of 1866.[55] Even those who opposed the idea that "mere worms" could cause such a serious illness, frequently were led to argue that such parasites were normal inhabitants of the body and hence harmless. Moreover, the work of Pasteur and other scientists on fermentation and spontaneous generation was, at the same time, becoming known to the general public.[56]

Let us not distort our understanding through hindsight. Physicians believing in some sort of "germ-theory" were still in a small minority — roughly one in seven — while their ideas were often crude and inconsistent. But they were listened to and could no longer be dismissed with a few words of casual ridicule. The painstaking studies of Snow and Pettenkofer had provided the epidemiological underpinning for the rapid and natural acceptance in the United States of Koch's discovery of the cholera *vibrio* (1883). As early as 1869, even a firm believer in miasmas had to concede that he was "very fond of the cell theory," and predict that there was "more truth to be developed from that idea than from any other view before the professional mind."[57]

The most compelling of arguments for the organic causation of the disease rested on the assumption that only living things had the power of indefinite reproduction, while epidemiological evidence indicated that the cause of cholera was some specific and indefinitely reproducible poison. Though no chemical or microscopic analysis had as yet discovered such subtle organisms, "yet their existence cannot be denied, or we must admit that these diseases can exist without a cause." The very rapid transmission of the poison and the lethal effect which could be produced by the ingestion of a very small quantity also implied that it had the power of reproduction and was hence organic.[58]

The ferment theory, even more pervasive than it had been in 1849, did not clash with the ideas of Snow and Pettenkofer, or with the conviction that cholera might be caused by living organisms. (The morbid fermentations within the body — which constituted the disease — might well be caused by a microorganism, as were the fermentations which produced beer and wine.) Almost all those who held that cholera evacuations were not immediately infectious, believed that it was some "fermentation" process which transformed the once harmless excreta. The ideas of Snow could be easily assimilated as well.

> The researches of the late Dr. Snow render it highly probable that the disease often arises from drinking water, impregnated with the *fermenting* excreta of persons suffering from the disease.[59]

When, in 1873, cholera again attacked the United States, few physicians clung to traditional anticontagionist theories. Their inadequacy had become more apparent with each succeeding cholera epidemic. Dozens of communities, large and small, now utilized the prophylactic methods which had protected New York in 1866. The success of these procedures provided conclusive evidence for the theories upon which they were based.

American medical thought had passed seemingly through centuries rather than decades in the years since cholera had first appeared on this continent. New ideas, new assumptions, and new habits of thought had supplanted those dominant 40 years before. American physicians readily accepted the discovery of the cholera *vibrio* in 1883. Many had expected it, for they had been brought, step-by-step, to an intellectual position which could easily assimilate it.

NOTES

This investigation was carried out during the tenure of a Predoctoral Fellowship from the National Institute of Mental Health, United States Public Health Service.

1 A sample of the opinions expressed by 109 American physicians during the years 1832–1834 shows that 90 did not consider the disease to be at all contagious, while only 5 considered it to be primarily contagious. The other 14 considered the disease to be primarily noncontagious but admitted that under some circumstances it might be communicable (contingent-contagionism). Of the 87 physicians who clearly expressed their opinion as to the actual cause of the disease, 48 considered it to be due to some substance added to the atmosphere or some change in its constituents. Others, expressing only their opinion tnat the disease was an "epidemic," may also be presumed to have believed in its atmospheric transmission, since an "epidemic" disease was usually defined as one spread through the atmosphere. Ten physicians regarded the disease as being caused by some substance of "terrene" origin in the atmosphere. These opinions have been gathered from books, pamphlets, medical journals, newspapers, diaries, letters, and journals. A similar procedure has been followed for the 1849–1854 and 1866 epidemics.

2 Patrick Macauley, *How is the Cholera Propagated?* . . . (London: Miller, 1831), p. 6; N.Y.C. Board of Health, *Reports of Hospital Physicians and other Documents* . . . ed. Dudley Atkins (New York, 1832), p. 140; *Boston Recorder*, June 27, 1832; Joseph M. Smith, *Discourse on the Epidemic Cholera* . . . (New York: Seymour, 1831), pp. 24–25; Charles Caldwell, *Maryland Med. Recorder*, 1831, *2*: 574.

3 "On the contrary," he continues, disease "is virtually disorder, an alteration of the natural state or actions of the tissues of organs of the economy," Hugh L. Hodge, "On the pathology and therapeutics of cholera maligna," *Am. J. Med. Sci.*, 1833, *12*: 388. Hodge cites Broussais and Bichat and, like most American physicians, seems not to have assimilated the work of those opposed to Broussais.

4 John Esten Cooke, "Remarks on spasmodic cholera," *Transylvania J. Med.*, 1832, *5*: 481–500; Thomas Miner, *Boston Med. & Surg. J.*, 1832, *6*: 397; William Darrach, Diary, MS, Historical Society of Pennsylvania, Aug. 19, 1832; E. Cutbush, *Western Med. Gaz.*, 1833, *1*: 63.

5 Daniel Drake, *Western J. Med. & Phys. Sci.*, 1832, *6*: 79; "Diocles," Washington *National Intelligencer*, Sept. 4, 1832; James McNaughton, *Letter on the Epidemic Cholera of Albany* . . . (Albany, 1832); Ossining, N.Y., *Westchester Herald*, July 10, 1832.

6 This is discussed at greater length by the author in "The cholera epidemic of 1832 in New York City," *Bull. Hist. Med.*, 1959, *33*: 40–45.

7 "Progress of the Indian cholera," *Methodist Magazine*, 1832, *3*: 468–469; C. L. Seeger, *A Lecture on the Epidemic Cholera* . . . (Boston: Wright, 1832), p. 25; Sylvester Graham, *A Lecture on Epidemic Diseases Generally and Particularly the Spasmodic Cholera* . . . new ed. (Boston: Cambell, 1838), p. 29; Jesse S. Meyer, *Life and Letters of Dr. William Beaumont* (St. Louis: Mosby, 1912), pp. 142–143. Local newspapers, seemingly without exception, printed admonitions warning of the effects of fear and panic.

8 New York *Evangelist*, June 30, 1832; Charles T. Jackson, "Cholera in Vienna," *Boston Med. Magazine*, 1832–33, *1*: 214; Cincinnati *Chronicle*, Oct. 13, 1832. Compare the typical shift of the Albany Board of Health from cautious support of quarantine to violent anticontagionism after the quarantine had proved unavailing, and the disease had broken out in Albany. Albany *Argus*, June 19, July 10, 1832.

9 It was hard to admit that "we are still wandering in a mazy labyrinth; blind and without a leader," and to criticize the "stale resort of reference to the occult, unknown, and unascertained qualities of the atmosphere. This last, this dernier resort, although it has the authority of Sydenham, is in truth, and in fact nothing more than a confession of ignorance, total ignorance!" Joseph Comstock, "Remarks on the cause of epidemics," *Boston Med. & Surg. J.*, 1832, *6*: 149–159. In a sample of over a hundred physicians, however, only one other physician criticized the atmospheric theory as such. Henry Bronson, "The chlorides and chlorine . . . Preventives of cholera," *ibid.*, 1832, *7*: 85–94.

10 In other words, the epidemic influence so dominated the atmosphere that the symptoms of other ills were altered so as to resemble those of cholera.

11 St. Louis *Missouri Republican*, July 12, 1833; Dr. Isaac Hartshorne, New Haven *Palladium*, July 21, 1832;

J. Mauran, S. H. Tobey, and T. H. Webb, *Remarks on the Cholera, embracing Facts and Observations Collected at New York* . . . (Providence: Marshall, 1832), pp. 26–27.

12 Joel Munsell, Diary, MS, New-York Historical Society, July 10, 1832; Charles G. Finney, *Memoirs* (New York: Barnes, 1876), p. 320; J. G. Birney, Huntsville, to Ralph S. Gurley, Washington, June 29, 1833, in *Letters of James Gillespie Birney* . . . , 2 vols. (New York: D. Appleton-Century, 1938), I, 77; William Lyon MacKenzie, *Sketches of Canada and the United States* (London: Wilson, 1833), p. 235.

13 St. Clairsville, Ohio, *National Historian*, June 30, 1832; Daniel Drake, *A Practical Treatise on the History, Prevention, and Treatment of Epidemic Cholera* (Cincinnati: Corey and Fairbank, 1832), p. 44; Benjamin Lundy, *Life, Travels, and Opinions* . . . (Philadelphia: Parrish, 1847), pp. 32–33; New York *Constellation*, Aug. 11, 1832.

14 Samuel Cartwright, *Some Account of the Asiatic Cholera* . . . (Natchez, 1832), p. 8; J. A. Allen, "Remarks on the etiology and character of epidemics," *Boston Med. & Surg. J.*, 1832, 7: 55; "A. C." offers this criticism in the Boston *Christian Watchman*, Oct. 12, 1832, a Baptist paper.

15 Charles Francis Adams, Diary, Adams Papers, Microfilm, Reel 61, June 24, 1832; Deborah Norris Logan, Diary, MS, Pennsylvania Historical Society, Aug. 4, 1832; Thomas Miner, "Case of malignant cholera," *Boston Med. Magazine*, 1832–3, *1*: 161.

16 Bernard M. Byrne, *An Essay to Prove the Contagious Character of Malignant Cholera* . . . (Baltimore: Carey, Hart, 1833), pp. 3–4, 7, 9, 59, and *passim*. A representative review termed this treatise "specious" but "interesting." *Boston Med. Magazine*, 1833–34, *2*: 393–395.

17 S. H. Pennington, "Report for the eastern district," *Tr. Med. Soc. St. N.J.*, 1833, p. 308. Dr. Pennington, who could not believe the evidence of his own senses, is only an extreme example of this very common view.

18 Social status was also bound up with education and the formal reasoning which was its symbol. For some of the very few criticisms of this kind of reasoning, see *Boston Med. & Surg. J.*, 1832, *6*: 338; Alfred Woodward, *Information for the People on Cholera* (Philadelphia: Griggs & Dickinson, 1832), p. 12; Richard Sexton, "Remarks on malignant cholera," *North Am. Arch. Med. & Soc. Sci.*, 1835, *2*: 325.

19 One hundred and three out of 146 medical men whose opinions were sampled considered the disease to be noncontagious. Twenty-three considered it to be primarily contagious, while 20 were contingent-contagionists. A representative position was that taken by the St. Louis Medical Society, when it voted 26 to 10 against contagionism. Prairie du Chien *Patriot*, Aug. 13, 1851, cited in Peter T. Harstad, "Sickness and disease on the Wisconsin frontier," (Master's thesis, Univ. of Wisconsin, 1959), p. 55.

Of the 146 opinions tabulated, 33 were unclassifiable. Thirty-five favored some atmospheric influence, while 16 held a miasma responsible for causing the disease. Seven favored a deficiency — or excess — of electricity in the atmosphere. Four physicians considered a lack of oxygen — or an excess of nitrogen — to be the cause. Five held fungi or animalculi responsible, while three attributed it to a "specific animal poison." Four doctors considered microscopic "germs" to be the cause of the disease. Other theories attributed cholera to an excess of carbonic acid or limestone, to an "Act of God," or to an improper diet. Both in England and in France, anticontagionism continued to be dominant.

20 Specificity in therapy still bore the stigma of quackery, however. For an excellent survey of advances in clinical medicine in this period, see Knud Faber, *Nosography*, 2nd ed. rev. (New York: Hoeber, 1930).

21 Sir Thomas Watson, *Lectures on the Principles and Practice of Physic* (Philadelphia: Lea and Blanchard, 1844), p. 718; J. W. Francis, *Letter on the Cholera* . . . (New York: P. G. Scott & Co., 1832), p. 32; Robert W. Haxhall, Richmond, Va., *Constitutional Whig*, July 31, 1832.

22 W. C. Wallace, "Practical and theoretical reasons for the necessity of cleanliness . . . ," *N.Y. Med. Gaz. & J. Hlth.*, 1854, *5*: 389.

23 W. Taylor, "Changeability of disease," Medical Association of the State of Alabama, *Proceedings*, 1852, pp. 68–71; Z. Pitcher, "The cholera of 1854 in Detroit," *Peninsular J. Med. & Collateral Sci.*, 1854, *2*: 145; New York *Day-Book*, Dec. 5, 1848; George Mendenhall, "An account of cholera as it appeared in Cincinnati during the year 1850," *Tr. A.M.A.*, 1851, *4*: 191; Washington *National Era*, Dec. 14, 1848; *The Diary of James K. Polk* . . . ed. Milo M. Quaife, 4 vols. (Chicago: McClurg, 1910), IV, 142.

24 New York *Evangelist*, June 14, 1849; "Report of the Committee on Practical Medicine and Epidemics," *Tr. A.M.A.*, 1850, *3*: 127–129. The report is signed by J. K. Mitchell, R. La Roche, and Francis West.

25 Frank A. Ramsey, *Cholera* (Knoxville: Helms, 1849), p. 2; W. H. Scoby, "Remarks on the influence of cholera on other diseases," *Western Lancet*, 1850, *11*: 91–93; John Butterfield, *Ohio Med. & Surg. J.*, 1849, *1*: 576; A. G. Lawton: "On the epidemic cholera," *Am. Med. Monthly*, 1855, *3*: 182; Philadelphia *American Model Courier*, June 16, 1849; Boston *Christian Register*, Aug. 11, 1849. In the East, and in large cities, such ideas were no longer entertained with

such assurance by physicians. For example, the four medical men cited above hail, respectively, from Knoxville, Tennessee, Rossville, Ohio, Columbus, Ohio, and La Salle, Illinois.

26 Philadelphia, Board of Health, *Statistics of Cholera* . . . (Philadelphia, 1849), p. 47; The use of statistics, typical of such reports in 1849, was almost unknown in 1832. Lunsford P. Yandell, *Western J. Med.*, 1849, *3*: 143; Joseph C. Hutchinson, "History and observations of Asiatic cholera in Brooklyn, N.Y., in 1854," *N.Y. J. Med.*, 1855, 2nd series, *14*: 52–53.

27 Alexander Stevens, "On the communicability of Asiatic cholera," *Tr. Med. Soc. St. N.Y.*, 1850, p. 33; *North-Western Med. & Surg. J.*, 1849, *2*: 278.

28 *St. Louis Med. & Surg. J.*, 1851, *9*: 418; New Orleans *Bulletin*, June 16, 1849; New Orleans *Daily Picayune*, Nov. 15, 1848; Henry G. Clark, *Superiority of Sanitary Measures over Quarantines* . . . (Boston: Thurston, Torry and Emerson, 1852), pp. 25–26. Professor E. H. Ackerknecht has connected this anticontagionism and hostility to quarantine with the growing political and scientific liberalism of the first half of the century. "Anticontagionism between 1821 and 1867," *Bull. Hist. Med.*, 1948, *22*: 567. Cf. also Ackerknecht, *Rudolf Virchow* (Madison: Univ. of Wisconsin Press, 1953), and J. M. D. Olmsted, *François Magendie* . . . (New York: Schuman's, 1944). Much of the feeling against quarantine in the United States can also be charged directly to the influence of the merchants. Cf. Charleston *Courier*, June 30, 1849.

29 Jonathan Knight, *An Introductory Lecture to the Course of 1849–50 . . . On the Propagation of Communicable Diseases* (New Haven: Hamlen, 1849), p. 11; *North-Western Med. & Surg. J.*, 1849, *2*: 278.

30 This was the position taken by the A.M.A. Committee on Practical Medicine and Epidemics. *Tr. A.M.A.*, 1850, *3*: 105–133. Both Samuel Smith Purple and Valentine Mott held similar views. Mott, *An Inaugural Address Delivered Before the New-York Academy of Medicine* . . . (New York: Ludwig, 1849); Purple, *N.Y. J. Med.*, 1849, 2nd series, *2*: 252–254; Watson, *Lectures*, p. 719; D. P. Holloway, Richmond, Indiana, to Caleb Smith, Washington, Aug. 4, 1849, Caleb B. Smith Papers, Library of Congress.

31 "Memoir on the nature of miasm and contagion," *Western J. Med. & Phys. Sci.*, 1835, *9*: 401–412, 526–532.

32 1849, *5*: 685–688.

33 *On the Cryptogamous Origin of Malarious and Epidemic Fevers* (Philadelphia: Lea and Blanchard, 1849). Mitchell states that he has taught such doctrines for years (p. iii). Though he cites Bassi and others for their work on fungous diseases, he remarks that his ignorance of German has prevented him "from knowing how far the authors of that country, Henle, Muller [*sic*], and others, have carried their ideas." (p. iv).

Theories similar to those of Mitchell, and based on microscopic observation of cholera stools, were advanced in England during the 1849 epidemic and created a furor both in England and the United States. These reports were finally discountenanced by a committee of the College of Physicians, which reported that the microscopic organisms discovered in the evacuations of cholera patients were not specific for the disease.

34 Robert Southgate, "Medical sketch of West Point, N.Y., during the summer of 1849," *N.Y. J. Med.*, 1850, 2nd series, *4*: 188.

35 Samuel Henry Dickson, "On the communicability of the cholera," *Am. J. Med. Sci.*, 1833, *13*: 359–366. He was convinced of the contagiosity of the disease after witnessing an outbreak at isolated Folly Island near Charleston, where the disease had, to him, obviously been brought by a beached emigrant ship on which the disease had been raging.

36 Samuel Henry Dickson, "On contagion," *Am. J. Med. Sci.*, 1849, *18*: 107–118. It is not clear from Dickson's writings whether he had read Henle. Experience with vaccination may have also been a source of his ideas.

37 The lecture was reported in the New York *Independent*, Dec. 28, 1848. Dickson was, of course, the recipient of much criticism for espousing so "antisocial" a doctrine. Cf. Charles B. Coventry, *Epidemic Cholera* . . . (Buffalo: Derby, 1849), p. 38.

38 Dickson, "On contagion," *Am. J. Med. Sci.*, p. 107; William Hort, "Remarks on cholera," *New Orleans Med. & Surg. J.*, 1849, *6*: 297; A. B. Palmer, *North-Western Med. & Surg. J.*, 1849, *2*: 362.

39 Austin Flint, *Buffalo Med. J. & Monthly Rev.*, 1849, *5*: 60; Theodore S. Bell, "Cholera," *Western J. Med. & Surg.*, 1849, *3*: 315; Joseph Leidy, "A flora and fauna within living animals," *Smithsonian Contributions to Knowledge* (Washington, D.C., 1853), V, 15; Columbus *Ohio State Journal*, June 15, 1849; Thomas D. Mitchell, *Lecture on the Epidemic Cholera* . . . (Philadelphia: Craig and Young, 1849), p. 4.

40 J. X. Chabert, *Observations on the Origin, Treatment and Cure of Asiatic Cholera* . . . (New York: Marks, 1852); J. B. Wright, "Report on the topography of San Antonio, and the epidemic cholera that prevailed there in the spring of 1849," *Southern Med. Rep.*, 1849, *1*: 431.

41 The works of Liebig were amazingly popular in the United States. By the middle of the 1840s, readers of even the most remote small town newspapers knew of his work. The interest of American medical men in the so-called ferment theory of disease

seems, however, to mirror the interest shown it in England.

42 William MacNeven, "Remarks on the mode by which cholera is propagated," *N.Y. J. Med.*, 1849, 2nd series, *2*: 194–195, 201; E. B. Haskins, "Some remarks on the febrile stage of cholera; with the suggestion of a new theory of the propagation and spread of cholera," *Western J. Med. & Surg.*, 1849, *3*: 384.

43 A. B. Palmer, "Observations on the cause, nature, and treatment of epidemic cholera," *Peninsular J. Med. & Collateral Sci.*, 1854, *1*: 339; Thomas White, *The True Cause of the Cholera Explained* . . . (Cincinnati: James, 1850), p. 3.

44 New York State, Metropolitan Board of Health, *Annual Report, 1866* (New York, 1867), p. 204 appendix. This portion of the report was signed by Elisha Harris, a prominent New York sanitarian. Elsewhere (*Tr. A.M.A.*, 1867, *18*: 431–437) Harris states that he has believed in this doctrine of the infection of cholera since 1854.

45 This resolution was printed in full in the *Med. & Surg. Reptr.*, 1866, *15*: 54. The clause referring to "well-known localizing conditions," was obviously necessary if a unanimous vote was to be recorded.

In a sampling of the opinions of 128 physicians — not including the above-mentioned vote — 55 were found to have taken a thoroughly contagionist stand: 21 were contingent-contagionists. Fifty-two remained anticontagionists. Forty-five accepted at least some of the conclusions of Snow and Pettenkofer, while 22 were believers in some variation of the germ-theory. The atmospheric theory found 29 believers, while a sprinkling of others believed in variations of it (electricity, miasma, aerial ferment). Thirteen who favorably cited the work of Snow or Pettenkofer also felt that the atmosphere played a role in the communication of the disease.

It should be noted that Pettenkofer was in the context of his time a contagionist, for he emphasized the role of human beings in the spread of cholera and stated, moreover, that it was probably caused by some microorganism.

46 From a circular prepared by a committee of the Buffalo Medical Society, *Buffalo Med. & Surg. J.*, 1866, *5*: 389. George Sutton ("A summary of observations on the cholera," *Med. & Surg. Reptr.*, 1866, *14*: 281–283) and Thomas Rochester ("A few remarks on cholera," *Buffalo Med. & Surg. J.*, 1866, *5*: 461–464; *6*: 1–9) both asserted that they had been teaching this doctrine for many years.

47 John Shaw Billings noted in 1876 of the *Am. J. Med. Sci.*, that so excellent were its, "abstracts and notices of foreign works, that from this file alone, were all other productions of the press for the last fifty years destroyed, it would be possible to reproduce the great majority of the real contributions of the world to medical science during that period." *A Century of American Medicine, 1776–1876* (Philadelphia: Lea, 1876), p. 333.

48 New York State, Metropolitan Board of Health, *Annual Report, 1866*, p. 217 Appendix.

49 William Read, *A Letter to the Consulting Physicians of Boston* . . . (Boston: Mudge, 1866), p. 5; John F. Geary, *Epidemic Cholera* . . . (San Francisco: Bancroft, 1866), p. 43; Edwin M. Snow, *A Report upon Sundry Documents Relating to Asiatic Cholera*, Providence City Document No. 5 (Providence: Knowles, Anthony, 1865), p. 9; for Griscom, see *Bull. N.Y. Acad. Med.*, 1866, *3*: 6 ff., and for Clark, see *Boston Med. & Surg. J.*, 1865, *73*: 225, and *Med. Rec.*, 1866, *1*: 437–439.

50 T. Bevan, "The recent epidemic of cholera at the County Hospital, Chicago, 1866," *Chicago Med. J.*, 1866, *23*: 450–459; Thomas J. Gallagher, "Report of the Allegheny County Medical Society," *Tr. Med. Soc. St. Penn.*, 1867, p. 202.

51 Letter from "Mosely," dated Chicago, Sept., 1866, New York *Evangelist*, Sept. 13, 1866. Cf. "Epidemics, past and present," *Catholic World*, 1866, *2*: 427; William H. Draper, "The march of the cholera," *Galaxy*, 1866, *1*: 107–115; Chicago *Daily Republican*, Aug. 13, 1866; Cincinnati *Volksfreund*, Aug. 10, 1866; *Brownlow's Knoxville Whig*, Aug. 22, 1866; Cincinnati *Daily Gazette*, Aug. 21, 1866; *New York Times*, Jan. 21, March 12, April 9, 1866; Chicago, *North-Western Presbyterian*, Oct. 20, 1866; Baltimore *Catholic Mirror*, May 5, 1866; Yorkville, S.C., *Enquirer*, Feb. 8, 1866.

52 Linus P. Brockett, *Asiatic Cholera* . . . (Hartford: Stebbins, 1866), pp. 62, 96, 99–103, 144–146, 175, 185. The International Sanitary Commission, for example, which met at Constantinople in 1866 and reported unanimously in favor of the transmissibility of the disease, endorsing unanimously the idea that the cause of the disease was reproduced in the body of the sufferer, also voted that "the principle of cholera . . . is volatile, and acts in this respect after the manner of miasma; that is to say, by infecting the atmosphere." International Sanitary Conference, *Report . . . of a Committee from that Body, on the Origin, Endemicity, Transmissibility and Propagation of Asiatic Cholera*, translated by Samuel Abbott (Boston: Mudge, 1867), pp. 24, 38, 40, 94–95.

53 H. Gibbons, "Hygiene of cholera," *Pacific Med. & Surg. J.*, 1865, *8*: 243; Warren Stone, "Cholera and its treatment," *New Orleans Med. & Surg. J.*, 1866, *19*: 17; J. H. P. Frost, "Report of the Committee on Cholera," *Tr. Homoeopathic Med. Soc. St. Penn.*, 1866–67, pp. 94–105.

54 Thomas Kennard, "Cholera — its history, causes, pathology, and treatment," *St. Louis Med. & Surg. J.*,

1867, n.s. *4*: 123; N. S. Davis, *Chicago Med. Exam.*, 1867, *8*: 656; A. P. Morrill, *Galveston Med. J.*, 1866, *1*: 143; William Elmer, *Tr. Med. Soc. St. N.J.*, 1867, p. 252, and J. S. B. Alleyne, *St. Louis Med. Reptr.*, 1866, *1*: 192, all argue that the erratic spread of the disease is not adequately explained by these new ideas.

55 For representative articles on the "trichina disease," see the Green Bay, Wis., *Advocate*, April 26, 1866; Chicago *Republican*, April 14, 1866; Boston *Christian Register*, March 31, 1866; New York *Journal of Commerce*, March 26, 1866; New York *Sunday Dispatch*, Feb. 11, 1866.

56 "W" in the Boston *Zion's Herald*. An unsigned article in the *New York Times*, March 12, 1866, significantly enough, calls the organisms which cause cholera — and upon which Pasteur has been working — insects.

57 Remarks of Dr. John O. Stone, at a meeting of the New York Academy of Medicine, Feb. 11, 1869. *Bull. N.Y. Acad. Med.*, 1869, *3*: 396 ff.

58 W. S. Haymond, "The collapsed stage of cholera," *Tr. Indiana St. Med. Soc.*, 1867, p. 101; William Schmoele, *An Essay on the Cause . . . of the Asiatic Cholera and other Epidemics* (Philadelphia: King and Baird, 1866), pp. 17–20; J. M. Toner and Charles A. Lee, "Facts and conclusions bearing upon the questions of the infectious character of Asiatic cholera," *Med. Rec.*, 1866, *1*: 201–205; Kennard, "Cholera," p. 133; Henry Hartshorne, *Cholera: Facts and Conclusions as to its Nature, Prevention, and Treatment* (Philadelphia: Lippincott, 1866), pp. 46–47.

59 "Epidemics, past and present," *Catholic World*, p. 427; significantly enough, the passage continues: ". . . and if this be so, from what we know of other diseases, it is not unreasonable to infer that, in certain conditions of the atmosphere, the poison of the cholera may be generated during the fermentation of the excreta of healthy persons." M. Herzog, "Our present knowledge of the causes of cholera," *Med. Rec.*, 1867, *2*: 193; L. Ch. Boisliniere, *St. Louis Med. & Surg. J.*, 1866, n.s. *3*: 489, suggests that "either Liebig's albumoid, or Pasteur's animalcular," theory may be adopted to account for the fermentation. Cf. Phillip Harvey, "Asiatic cholera," *Iowa Med. J.*, 1868, *5*: 55–56; John Ordronaux, *Prophylaxis*, an Anniversary Oration Delivered Before the New York Academy of Medicine . . . (New York: Ballière, 1867), pp. 48–57.

Sanitation

Most 19th-century physicians attributed rising mortality rates in American cities to the filthy urban environment. This "miasmatic" theory, linking dirt with disease, motivated much public health activity: street cleaning, garbage collection and disposal, water and sewer systems, and food regulation.

Control over milk supplies emerged as a serious problem in the 1840s and continued to plague cities until the widespread adoption of pasteurization in the 1920s. Norman Shaftel describes the long battle New Yorkers fought to obtain clean milk. Cities also attempted to regulate ice cream shops, bakeries, and slaughterhouses. But it was not until 1906 that most municipalities were able to put meat-packing under effective controls. With the establishment of health-department laboratories and the passage of the Pure Food and Drugs Act, food control became truly scientific.

Polluted water sources presented another public health problem. In 1801 Philadelphia opened its municipal water system, designed to bring fresh country water into the city. This action helped to save Philadelphia from devastation by cholera in 1832. New York and Boston, recognizing the benefits, followed suit, and other cities across the country copied the eastern model. Although located at the edge of Lake Michigan, an ample body of water, Chicago faced a peculiar problem. Louis P. Cain describes the lengths to which that city went to supply its inhabitants with water. The Chicago hero Chesbrough, like other engineers, achieved national prominence for his urban sanitation efforts.

Engineers, plumbers, and other nonmedical sanitarians were as important to the public health movement as physicians. The medical profession may have perceived the necessity of sanitation, but engineers provided the technical ability needed to execute the massive urban cleanups. James H. Cassedy explores the methods and influence of one filth-oriented sanitation expert during the early days of the bacteriologic era.

In the 20th century sanitation lost its dominant position in the public health movement. The germ theory changed the focus of health activity from cleaning the environment to tracking down specific bacteria, shifting disease control from the streets to the laboratory. Today, however, in a world beset with new environmental pollutants, sanitation is once again assuming a central role.

20

A History of the Purification of Milk in New York, or, "How Now, Brown Cow"

NORMAN SHAFTEL

It is now generally conceded that milk is one of our most important foods and therefore of outstanding importance in determining, in large measure, the health and welfare of the community. Because of the close relationship between milk and public health it is essential that milk be uncontaminated and wholesome. Although this is so today it was not always thus, and this paper is written to trace the evolutionary changes in the history of milk purification.

To attempt to portray the struggle for milk purification in each of these 48 states is far beyond both the compass of the author's knowledge and the space limitations of this paper. Therefore the following is limited to a history of the most significant developments in New York State. But as is so often the case with an historical process, the successive stages of milk purification in New York do represent rather accurately, in developmental if not strict chronologic order, the picture in the country as a whole.

Although the bibliography on milk is rather extensive there has been little or no attempt to present the complete history of those sequential developments which our fortunate position in time now permits. A detailed search of the literature of the last decade uncovers no attempt to fulfill this need, and the story is so unexpectedly fascinating that it compels recording.

To the naive and unitiated the unfolding may prove a shocking exposé as all the essential elements of drama crowd across the stage. Involved in this story are racketeering, politics, picturesque customs of bygone eras, American history, scientific achievement, and the often unpredictable peculiarities of man. The developments and advances in milk purification will be discovered to follow in causal relationship social, political, and scientific maturity. But these advances have been made in most instances only where the dangers have been previously exposed, emphasized, or outlined by reformers, public-spirited citizens, or the stark factuality of scientific achievement.

Ancillary factors such as transportation, refrigeration, and even distillation (of alcoholic beverages) will also be discovered to play important roles in the complete synthesis of the story. Behind all is man, who gives direction and propulsion whether in the social, political, or scientific sphere. This therefore will be a portrayal of man's humanity, and sometimes inhumanity to man, and as in the truly popular drama, of a righteousness born of knowledge, triumphant in the end.

COLONIAL TIMES

No milk problem existed in this country, much less in what was later to become New York State, when in 1609 Henry Hudson, searching for a northwest passage to India, explored the river which now bears his name. No milk problem existed because the American aborigines had no domesticated animals but dogs. When Hudson's favorable reports were confirmed by subsequent Dutch voyagers, trading settlements developed in New Netherlands by 1614. Among the privations of these earliest settlers was lack of food, and it is therefore completely understandable that they would import cattle as soon as feasible in order to rectify this defect. The first such shipment into New York occurred in 1625 with the arrival of 103

NORMAN SHAFTEL is Assistant Clinical Professor of Medicine at the State University of New York College of Medicine, Brooklyn, New York.

Reprinted with permission from *New York State Journal of Medicine*, 1958, *58*: 911–928.

animals. This livestock included cows and bulls thought to have come from the Isle of Trexel near the coast of Holland.[1] The cows are believed to have been the black and white variety (Friesians) common to that locale. The distinction of importing this country's first cattle, however, goes to the colony at Jamestown, Virginia, where cattle were landed on these shores in May 1611.

As the population of New York increased from 270 in 1629 to 1,000 by 1650 the need for cattle and milk also increased, and there continued to be importation of cattle into the settlement. The colonists were industrious and despite many handicaps successful, so that by 1656 a market place had been built. The colonists were then able to discontinue importing butter and cheese and indeed were even beginning to export these products. As the farmers realized profits they cleared additional land and increased their stock of cattle to produce greater surpluses for export. By such economic transistions frontiers were often pushed westward to supply the growing herds.

The consumption of milk by the colonists was undoubtedly small in comparison to what it is today, but we know that milk of both cows and sheep was being drunk. In 1670 a Dr. Wellman attributed the good health of the rural population to "sheep's milk and fresh air," and indeed he recommended milk for "scrophulous people," a very questionable procedure in light of what was subsequently to be learned about the transmission of this same disease through cow's milk.

During the colonial period and for the first two centuries following after the initial colonization of New York there was little or no concern with the problem of milk purification. This was due to justifiable ignorance, as Leeuwenhoek did not discover bacteria until 1687, plus the socioeconomic conditions of the times which required very little marketing of milk. A study of 1790[2] indicated that most families owned one or more cows and therefore consumed fresh milk, the short interval between milking and consumption preventing putrefaction. In addition the milk cows were highly regarded and treated with care and respect, particularly as their welfare in large measure determined the health of the children. The cattle of the villages were often pastured in a common field and cared for by a cowherd who would pass through the streets each morning while sounding his horn and the same evening would return the cows to their proper owners.

The price of milk sold in New York after December 23, 1763, was regulated by a resolution passed by the Common Council of New York City[3] and was set at the rate of "six coppers by the quart." For comparison, at the same time the price of beef was "four pence half penny by the pound weight . . . the price of veal for hind quarter at . . . the rate of sixpence by the pound weight."

AFTER 1800

More intense regulation by law governing the sale of milk began when the marketing of milk became an important business, but such status was not present until the earlier decades of the 19th century, when we witness the beginnings of a large-scale population increase in urban centers. In 1800, for example, only 4 percent of the total population lived in cities of more than 8,000. By 1850 this figure had grown to 12.5 percent, by 1900 it had jumped to 32 percent, and to 49.1 percent in 1930. By 1940 this figure had reached 77 percent! The rate of urban concentration is perhaps most dramatically emphasized by the figures for New York City. The population of New York in 1800 was 79,216; in 1850, 696,115; in 1900, 2,437,202; in 1930, 6,930,446; the census just completed shows us to be today a city of seven and a half million.

Up to the time of the Treaty of Paris in 1763 (ending the Indian wars) the settlers, in almost constant conflict with the Indians, had been confined to restricted areas. When the farmers were released from this geographically constricting influence there was a movement toward the better agricultural lands west of the Appalachian mountains. There pasture was richer, and after 1800 the development of farm machinery made it possible to cultivate large tracts of the newly settled land, increases in dairying following proportionately with each agricultural advance.

And yet in 1806 the area covered by individual milk deliveries was so small that milk was generally carried by hand. Since the farm was still within easy walking distance of the customer each man supervised his own milk purchases. The milk vendor of that day[4] was described as "sweating beneath a wood yoke of labour . . . instead of awkwardly traveling along, with a heavy bucket of milk in one hand only, they are thus accoutred. A piece of wood, about two feet long, is made to fit around the back of the neck, and rest upon the shoulders. To each end is affixed a chain, with a hook at the end. The chain is of such length as to enable them, the carriers, by stooping a little, to hook the handles of two milk vessels, made of tin, resembling a grocer's tea-canister; containing three or four gallons of milk. One of these is thus carried on each side to the house of their customers. A loud cry of 'Milk's come,' awakened me from a late nap this morning; and when I arose, and went to the window, saw a Dutchman thus yoked."

In 1800 when the population of New York City was approximately 80,000, little knowledge was available concerning the relationship of the health of dairy animals to the wholesomeness of their milk. Fortunately the animals were generally kept in small groups and therefore less likelihood of spread of infection existed than might have been expected. Nevertheless it has been adequately proved that impure milk was responsible for a shameful infant mortality during the colonial and revolutionary periods.

There was little popular awareness at the time of the relationship between the quality of the milk and the epidemics of diseases which were so devastating, particularly to the infant population. Such ignorance was not always world wide. As far back as 1599 the Senate of Venice provided the death penalty for anyone selling milk or milk products during an epidemic. And in the 18th century Johan Petrias Frank laid down such principles for a more sanitary milk supply as we were still struggling to have recognized and legislated more than one hundred years later. Frank[5] stated that "Those who sell milk should have clean, well-lighted, and healthful stables. They should give the cows fresh food or pasture them, which latter method gives the cows healthful exercise. Colostral nor watered milk should not be sold."

Milk-borne outbreaks were to continue into the modern era, although gradually reduced in numbers and severity by the application of sanitary principles with utilization of scientific discoveries.

In 1830 New York City was still a comparatively small town, but as the population grew the enclosed pasturage shrank to smaller and smaller proportions. When it seemed that milk production would disappear from the cities with the disappearance of pasturage, a solution to the problem was supplied by the city's distilleries.

It having been more or less accidentally discovered that cows could be induced after a period of enforced semi-starvation to eat the waste products or slop from the distilleries, and that at least for a time the cows fed on such distillery slop (brewer's grains in large proportion) would give larger amounts of milk, the marriage of the cowshed and the distillery was arranged by the interested parties. While the cows were being "debauched" on alcoholic dregs, their milk when boiled would smell "strongly of beer and would coagulate into a hard lump." Such milk was "likely to produce death in the infant fed upon it."[6] It was known that infant mortality increased from 32 percent in 1814 to 50 percent in 1841 and that these figures coincided with those of other cities where milk was similarly produced. By contrast, mortality in European cities where this condition did not exist decreased during this same period, indicating a probable causal relationship between the use of this poisonous brew and the rising infant mortality.

Despite this dangerous association the practice of feeding cows distillery slop persisted, because it was financially profitable (to the extent of one million dollars per year) to the parties concerned in this diabolic agreement. There were estimated in 1835 to be 18,000 cows in New York City and Brooklyn (which did not become a part of New York City until 1896) fed on distillery slop. The cow stalls were owned by the distillers and rented to different milk men for from four to five dollars per year per cow.

This rather alcoholic solution to the problem of feeding cows without an adequate pasturage brought forth upon the scene, uniting the man and the hour, a courageous eccentric who made the first real, fruitful protest against the conditions of milk production in New York. The man was Robert M. Hartley who, in a memorable book published in 1842, elaborately described in deservedly unflattering terms the disgusting conditions which existed and their consequent threat to the public health.[7] The publication of this book constituted the first serious effort to improve the purity of milk in New York State, and this represented the pioneer effort in milk sanitation in the State.

Robert Milham Hartley was born in Cockermouth, Cumberland County, England, on February 17, 1796. He came to New York when he was three years old and was nurtured on the Bible and the religious fervor of his parents. This boy, fanning his religious flames, constantly sought some "sign," and his patience was duly rewarded on the evening of July 22, 1814, when, after pouring his heart out in prayer, his diary tells us, ". . . There, in the stillness and darkness, I fervently supplicated the Lord for the pardon of my transgressions. . . . I became more and more rapt in ecstasies of devotion; and I was sensibly impressed they were spiritual visitations. . . . During the fervor of my feelings, I heard a fluttering sound, as if a bird was flying rapidly around me, and so near, that I felt the vibration of the air from the movement of the wings. The ecstasy, as it may be termed, gradually left me; but in fervor of my gratitude and love, I continued to praise Him for His wonderful mercy. On returning to my chambers, at my closet devotions, and after retiring to rest, the visitations were repeated."[8]

These wing beats of the ethereal dark beckoned Hartley to enlightened earthly endeavors, and for the succeeding 15 years he continued to pray, to plead, and to read his Bible while awaiting some worthy mission. When he was 33 years old he chose his particular mission and joined the Temperance Society. Four years later in 1833 he was elected corresponding secretary. Once established in an idealistic endeavor he lost no time in additional revery but deployed his activities in a prodigious outburst of journalism, speech, and investigation. In one year he is said to have distributed more than 30 million pages of literature. It is neither inconsistent nor should it have been unpredictable therefore that in this same year 9,986 people signed the "pledge."

In Hartley's investigation of distilleries he discovered that they sold mash (remaining after the whiskey was made) to dairy men. He hoarded this fact as a weapon to be used to destroy alcoholism and continued to investigate the conditions of the stables which flanked the distilleries. Discovering sanitary conditions which in the mildest language can only be described as unbelievably disgusting, he proceeded to acquaint the populace with his findings in a vigorous attempt to abolish distillery slop dairies. It would be difficult to improve on his colorful description of these slop dairies, so the author will simply and humbly quote Mr. Hartley: ". . . if the wind is in the right quarter, he will nose the dairy a mile off. . . . a high distillery, sending out its tartarean fumes, and blackened with age and smoke, casting a sombre air all around. Contiguous, (he will see) numerous low, flat pens, in which more than five hundred milch cows owned by different persons are closely huddled together amid confined air and the stench of their own excrements. He will also see various appendages and troughs to conduct and receive the slops, smoking hot from the still, with which to gorge animals so inhumanly condemned to subsist on this most unnatural and disgusting food; and all within an area of a few hundred yards. He will discern, moreover, numerous slush carts in waiting and in motion, for the supply of the distant dairies; empty milk-wagons returning and others with replenished cans, as constantly departing."[9]

A typical stall is described in Mr. Hartley's pamphlets as housing 2,000 cows in the winter. The slop would be supplied to the cows via large tanks and wooden troughs to the stalls. The cattle, head to tail, stood in rows about three feet wide which would permit the cows no movement, and none there was for the entire nine months, during which they would be milked while standing, weak and sickly, up to their bellies in filth and excrement. Each cow ate daily about 32 gallons of slop which cost nine cents per barrel, and the results of the digestion was a malodorous issue compounded by an equally stinking lack of ventilation.

Very few cows survived the year, the weak and diseased being sent to the butcher for the "coup de grace." When a cow died on the day she was milked, her contribution could be said to have been delivered posthumously.

Mr. Hartley claimed that the high infant mortality in New York was largely the result of the milk from these cows. When it is known that the ancillary equipment and the dairy men themselves were in no greater state of cleanliness than the conditions under which the milk was produced, this would seem to be a reasonable assumption.

Mr. Hartley, whose campaign was matched only by his naiveté, requested the distilleries to relinquish their association with dairying. This met with predictable and prodigious failure. Undaunted, in the best tradition of any courageous reformer, he appealed to the press in 1836 and 1837 but achieved no real support. He was instead physically attacked by hirelings of the slop dairy owners in the neatest and best of racketeering tradition.

In 1842 Mr. Hartley, shifting his *locus operandi*, became corresponding secretary and agent of the New York Association for Improving the Conditions of the Poor, but he continued his fight for a better milk supply. He modified his direction of attack, suggesting that country milk be sent into the city in competition with the swill milk. Thaddeus Selleck, only one year before in 1841, was the first man to ship milk to New York City by train.* As a result of Hartley's exhortations and suggestions several groups of farmers formed into combines and by 1844 were shipping milk into New York City in competition with local swill dairymen. During this competition the combines learned that in order to prevent the souring of milk, which often occurred in transit, cooling was necessary during shipment. In this way the necessity for refrigeration and the importance of transit time came under study. Ice had been available since 1825, although Dr. William Cullen had made an ice machine, using a vacuum pump, 50 years earlier in 1775. Jacob Perkins in 1834 made a vital contribution to the dairy industry with his discovery of the compression cycle. This was utilized many years later in the production of mechanical refrigerating machines, a marked improvement over ice refrigeration. Refrigerator cars (not mechanical) were not to appear until 1867 (between New York and Chicago), and artificial ice itself was not produced in appreciable quantities until 1878.

Despite early reverses due to inadequate train services on the Erie Railroad and resultant souring of milk in transit, the "importing" of country milk increased gradually, so that by 1853 one of the combines, the Orange County Milk Association, was distributing 7,000 quarts daily.[10] Despite this increase in milk sales by the milk associations, there was no corresponding decline in the sale of city swill milk. This anomaly is explicable on the basis of a concomitant and compensating increase in the population of the city during these years. But Mr. Hartley had achieved a signal success, and for the first time country milk was brought into New York.

In 1848 the New York Academy of Medicine, stimulated by Mr. Hartley's exposé, appointed a committee headed by Dr. Augustus K. Gardner to investigate swill milk. Their report stated that slop milk contained only one-half to one-third the amount of butter fat of Orange County milk and that children fed on slop milk were susceptible to such diseases as scrofula and cholera infantum as well as being increasingly susceptible to any epidemic disease existing at the time.[11]

In 1850 the defeat of a court action by a distillery dairyman to collect for the sale of what was testified to be unwholesome milk augured some hope for the future disappearance of slop milk, but a campaign against swill milk by the *Sunday Dispatch* in the same year, 1850, met with complete disregard and apathy. Although the handwriting was beginning to appear on the wall, swill milk continued to be sold in Brooklyn even into the present century.

---

*Note by editor of *New York State Journal of Medicine:* In 1841, the only railroad running into New York City was the Harlem River Railroad chartered in April 1831. It ran from Park Row to Williamsburg by September 1842, and was extended to White Plains in 1844. See *Westchester County Historical Bulletin*, Vol. 29, No. 4, October 1953, p. 90.

The Erie Railroad was chartered April 24, 1832. In 1841–1842 it was opened from Piermont-on-the-Hudson inland to Goshen, Orange County, a distance of 46 miles. Source: *Encyclopedia Americana*, copyrighted 1918.

In his *A History of New York Dairy Industry* (New York: Orange Judd Publishing Co., Inc., 1941), p. 2, Mr. John J. Dillon, editor of the *Rural New Yorker* says, "It was a tradition in Orange County sixty years ago that the first shipment of milk from that county to New York City was made in a churn in the year 1842. The milk was not popular. The consumers complained that a yellow scum gathered on the top of it when held for a time. Cows fed on brewery waste did not produce milk rich in butter fat." Dillon also says: "About the same time (1844) considerable quantities of milk were shipped into the city by farmers of the Harlem River Valley over the New York and Harlem Railroad."

Concerning Mr. Thaddeus Selleck, a personal communication from Miss Adele Hiester, Librarian of the New York State Department of Health says, "Spring of 1842 milk was shipped by Erie Railroad from Chester to Piermont, a distance of 41 miles and then by boat the remaining 21 miles to New York City. The regular milk train into New York City did not operate until five years later. Cold water was used to keep the milk cool.

Thaddeus Selleck was the contractor for shipping and collecting milk from farmers who were paid two cents a quart. This was a higher return than they received for butter, and the Orange County farmers were glad to furnish him with their product."

The example set by Mr. Hartley was soon to be followed, and the torch he lit was to be passed into other hands. In 1853 a volume entitled "The Milk Trade in New York and Vicinity" was published, and with this instrument John Mullaly, the author, and Dr. R. T. Trall, who wrote the introduction, launched a second creditable attack on unhealthy milk. The authors pointed out the morbid effects of unwholesome milk on children, and in describing the deplorable conditions under which milk was being produced by the remaining 400 slop milk dealers in the city, painted with graphic and sensational detail a picture of unbelievable filth and squalor. Mr. Mullaly, for purpose of contrast and comparison, made an inclusive examination of milk dairies outside New York and showed that Orange County alone could supply the entire city with fresh milk. In colorful prose Mr. Mullaly proceeded to lambaste adulteration and in doing so described among other things the milk concoction euphemistically known to the trade as "the cow with the iron tail." The formula for this adulterated product was: to a gallon of milk add one pint of water, then a dash of chalk and plaster of Paris. This would produce a product of sickly blue hue. On rare occasions a soupçon of egg would be added to increase the "body." To the whole, molasses was then added to produce a deceivingly rich yellow color. When this macabre mixture was allowed to stand overnight any number of exotic transformations might occur, depending on the exact ingredients of the adulteration. A supernatant yellowish slime would indicate the (rare) addition of the egg, the astral blue of the body of this watery mixture proclaimed the anemic qualities of what remained of the milk, while the more solid adulterants could be seen dumpily vibrating at the bottom in a thick slime. O yes, we forgot to add: mix and serve.

As a result of his survey Mr. Mullaly recommended an increase in the number of country milk associations, such as the Orange County, that milk wagons be licensed, and that there be power of permit revocation and fine for those selling injurious milk. Unfortunately these recommendations were sterile of immediate results, and many years were yet to lapse before adequate licensing in the milk industry would become a reality.

Nevertheless, agitation against slop milk increased, and by 1856 there were ordinances in several of the Brooklyn wards against keeping more than three cows on a city lot. On December 26, 1856, the Brooklyn Common Council passed a law providing that between May 1 and November 1 no person should keep more than four cows on a half acre, or more than six cows on an acre, and not more than 12 on any lot whatsoever. A fine of ten dollars for each cow over the legal number was to be levied.[12]

This enactment, which promised speedy relief from the evils of swill milk, was just as speedily emasculated by litigation. A Mr. S. L. Husted, the owner of a large distillery with adjoining stables, gathered his colleagues with similar nefarious interests, and by political manipulation succeeded in calling a special meeting of the Common Council. This meeting, being called so hurriedly, was sparsely attended, yet this minority modified the law to except owners of distilleries then in operation, including "milkmen employed in the milk business." This shoddy legality counteracted any possible gains that the original enactment might have secured.

In 1858 the "vast and filthy" stables of Mr. Husted became the target for the deservedly invidious assault of the crusading *Frank Leslie's Illustrated Weekly*. Where previous appeals to reason by such as Mr. Hartley and Mr. Mullaly had failed, the roisterous cartoons and journalistic sensationalism of the press succeeded. As a result of the pressure exerted by this weekly, the Common Council of Manhattan appointed a committee of aldermen to investigate distillery stables in that borough. While examining Mr. Husted's stables the aldermen were regaled with "generous spirit," and shamefully in the final analysis this factor prevailed. The committee subsequently voted three to one in favor of the swill dairies and their "generous" host, Mr. Husted. This political whitewash was no rarity in the history of milk control, but Frank Leslie's disgust at this decision could only be equated with a superceding glee at the prospect of prolonging his forceful attack.

The majority report of the committee of aldermen had been sent to the Board of Health for affirmation, and by a vote of 16 to 11 the board accepted the majority report. At the same time they requested the Academy of Medicine to appoint another committee to reinvestigate the same situation. Most of the work of this latter committee was done by Dr. Samuel R. Percy. Dr. Percy affected disguises[13] so that he could more accurately acquaint himself with the usual day-to-day conditions of the stables he investigated. Had his true identity been known he felt the stable owners would have adopted temporary improvements in honor of his official visits. Dr. Percy would use the personification of "a farmer eager to sell cows . . . a butcher wishing to buy savory beef; sometimes . . . a grocery man wanting to make arrangements for a steady supply of wholesome and pure milk; and frequently as an idler 'looking for Patrick McLaughlin.'"

Two other members of the committee made major gastronomic sacrifices and actually ate distillery slops. They were rewarded with diuretic and laxative outpourings far beyond their most sanguine fears or expectations.

Dr. Percy unearthed sickness in children which he attributed to milk and realistically described several examples. The report of his committee, which was delivered to the president of the New York Academy of Medicine in 1859, was to the effect that slop milk was not a proper food. The discontinuance of the entire slop milk traffic was then strongly recommended.

In 1861 Senator Francis M. Rotch of Otsego County introduced a bill to stop the sale of swill milk. The senate passed but the assembly rejected it, but in the following year (1862) the law was enacted. This law, intended to prevent adulteration of milk, was the first Milk Law to be passed in New York State. There had been an antecedent law prohibiting adulteration of milk passed in Massachusetts in 1856 and still another in Boston in 1859 against adulteration with water and the use of distillery slops for feeding cattle.[14] Such laws were not new to the European continent, however, for as far back as 1742 Paris had specifically forbidden the feeding of spoiled malt or poisonous food to any animals producing milk.

The legal victory of 1862 with the enactment of New York's first Milk Law was heartily enjoyed by the New York Academy, but the fruits of this victory were in no way commensurate with the aspirations of its sympathizers. The law itself made the sale of "any impure, adulterated, or unwholesome milk" a misdemeanor and as such punishable by a fine of 50 dollars or a jail sentence when in default of payment of the fine. The law further forbade both the feeding of cows on food which would produce unwholesome milk and crowded or unhealthy conditions of cows in the stables. It also provided that the correct source of milk be marked on the delivery carts. Unfortunately the legal technicalities of rigid adherence to the letter rather than the spirit of the law resulted in test cases. In decisions handed down in such trials[15] Justices Ingraham, Barnard, and Clark made a mockery of justice by ruling that simply adding water to milk did not constitute an adulteration under the terms of this statute. And so the academy appealed to the legislature to specifically forbid either swill feeding or adulteration with water. In 1864 their request was granted by an amendment which specifically defined "the addition of water or any substance other than a sufficient quantity of ice to preserve the whole milk while in transportation" to be an adulteration. The milk of cows fed on swill was also stated to be unwholesome and impure.

This enactment legally ended swill milk in Manhattan. In Brooklyn the swill milk trade was protected by the local amendment to the milk ordinance of 1856, which had excepted those distillers and farmers employed in the milk business and in operation at the time. These latter continued unmolested therefore into the early years of our present century. When Dr. Thomas Darlington became Health Commissioner in 1904 (to get ahead of the story), there were "over 6,000 cows still being fed on distillery slop in Brooklyn,"[16] but under his leadership this abomination was speedily thenceforth eliminated.

Between 1864 and 1900 control and improvement of milk was spasmodic and essentially ineffectual. The Health Department never had sufficient police forces to adequately patrol the milk supply. As the swill dairies decreased in number and their obvious filthiness became less evident, so did the public interest in milk sanitation wane. For want of a *casus belli*, no further campaign materialized during these years, and as the germ theory of disease, promulgated about 1880, had not yet gained general acceptance, people were unconcerned about what they could not understand.

The Department of Health, organized in 1866, took no action against skimming or adulteration until June 2, 1873, when "the keeping, selling, or sending to the city of watered or adulterated milk or milk known as swill milk"[17] was forbidden by the sanitary code. This encouraged action, and in the succeeding two years 37 convictions were brought in. Unfortunately the assessment of fines, which were inconsequential, did not abolish adulteration, which proved an infinitely more prosperous operation than the punishment a deterrent.

As the dairies moved (and were pushed) further and further from the cities, the milk producers found it increasingly difficult to handle both production and distribution and were forced therefore to choose between them. As the milk industry grew, the interests of the milk producers were often antagonistic to those of the distributors. So, in addition to the battle between the milkmen and the Health Department, there were price wars between the country producers and city retailers. Since most of these battles ended in stalemate, the net result was a bitter travesty. The milkman of that day was not the benign unnoticed servant we take for granted today. According to the *Tribune*,[18] the milkman was so brutal that his horse invariably died in harness and was left on the street where he fell, and his wagon was so noisy as to excite the envy of any producers of other nocturnal disturbances. The milkman and his wagon are then described as "plunging with a bloodthirsty whoop into the areas of defenseless customers on his route" and of disseminating "a saturated solution of assorted zymotic disease at twelve cents a quart in advance."

We learn from contemporary reports that racketeering was rife in these "Roaring Seventies" and that "each milkman owned his own route and assassinated every presumptuous trespasser." This frequently left the independent American consumer only with a choice of either buying the "mysterious fluid" dispensed by the milkman or of buying condensed milk.

During the 1880s and later it was not uncommon for unscrupulous dealers to remove the cream, substitute water, and with diabolical though unappropriate humor label their concoction "pure" or "Board of Health" milk.[19] The New York State Inspector reported the addition of 3 to 5 quarts of water and 10 of skimmed milk to every 25 quarts of this "pure milk" concoction.

As previously mentioned, the farmers and city milk retailers were constantly warring about the prices for the country milk. In what was supposed to be an attempt to adjudicate this dispute, the Milk Exchange Limited was organized under the laws of the State of New York in October 1882. But the Milk Exchange failed from the start to fulfill its purpose when it offered the milk producers a minority representation on the board of directors. This offer was declined and the exchange became a spokesman for the city retailers who were left with sole representation. The succeeding eventualities were then fairly predictable. The three cents a quart originally offered to the farmers was declared unfair by them and a livelier milk war ensued with strikes, strike breaking, sabotage, and accompanying violence. In the milk industry the "Roaring Seventies" had now extended into the "Uproarious Eighties." By 1886 the farmers were getting one-half cent less per quart than originally while the powerful Milk Exchange continued to dictate prices until January 1891. At that juncture a court action, which was to last for four years, was begun, and this finally dissolved the exchange as a combination to lessen the supply of milk and to control prices.

While this drama was being played out on one set the Health Department continued its inspection of adulterated milk on another. The overwhelming necessity for such vigilance can better be appreciated when it is known that one instance of kerosene in bottled milk was uncovered following the complaint of a woman living at Gramercy Park, and in another instance of the same chronological vintage, reported by Dr. Henry Dwight Chapin,[20] an examination of 500 quarts of milk "from one of the better dairy farms" dredged out almost a pint of amorphous material, including blood, hair, and detritus of various kinds. And so we leave this sketchily portrayed period of violence and racketeering (which despoils the 20th century of any claims of priority in this regard) to examine the beginnings of an era more fruitful of advances in milk sanitation and, scientifically speaking, more exciting.

THE GERM THEORY OF DISEASE

Progress occurs only when man has fashioned the appropriate tools. With the elaboration of the tools of discovery advances can then be swift, often in geometric progression. Up to the last decades of the 19th century all improvement in milk sanitation was directed toward the correction of gross adulteration and improvement in over-all sanitation. The empirical knowledge of milk-borne diseases awaited the elaboration of the germ theory before proper evaluation could be made. Once this causal relationship between bacteriologic organism and specific disease was established, appropriate countermeasures could then be taken to eliminate the last factors producing milk-borne disease. A clearer scientific perspective can perhaps be obtained if we look briefly at the antecedent scientific discoveries that constituted the bricks and mortar used so advantageously by those scientists who eventually promulgated the germ theory of disease.

Milk-borne diseases of man are either those due to the transmission of animal diseases to humans or, the more important and larger group, diseases transmitted through milk as a result of the intermediary of the cow and her product. Included in the former group are bovine tuberculosis, brucellosis, milk sickness (or trembles), anthrax, and "Q" fever. The latter group includes tuberculosis, typhoid fever, paratyphoid fever, scarlet fever, diphtheria, and dysentery to name the more important. Many of these diseases had been clinically described centuries ago. For example, diphtheria was described by Arataeus in the first century A.D. and typhoid by Willis in 1643, but it remained for later bacteriologists to isolate and prove the causal relationships between organisms and disease and place the struggle for milk purification on a scientific basis.

Although it is not directly pertinent to a proper portrayal of the history of milk purification, it is certainly historically correct and scientifically germane to trace, albeit sketchily, the background of the germ theory of disease so accurately propounded by Koch and Pasteur.

Leeuwenhoek, who first saw protozoa in 1675, was the first to see bacteria in 1687 with the use of his simple microscope. The typhoid bacillus was discovered by Carl Joseph Eberth in 1880,[21] seven years after William Budd insisted that typhoid fever was spread by contagion originating in human dejecta.[22] The Corynebacterium diphtheriae was discovered in 1883 by Klebs,[23] the Brucella abortus by Bernhard Bang[24] in 1897, and the paratyphoid bacillus by Emile Achard and Raoul Bensaude in 1896.[25] In 1884 Koch isolated the Vibrio cholerae and proved its transmission through drinking water and food.[26] In 1882 Koch made his greatest discovery,[27] the tubercle bacillus, and in the same paper in which this was announced there appeared his rules for the proof of the pathogenicity of any given organism, the Koch's postulates. In 1898 Theobald Smith distinguished bovine from human tuberculosis,[28] and in 1898 Kiyositi Shiga discovered the organism responsible for bacillary dysentery.[29]

Last the other great pioneer in bacteriology (along with Koch) and the pioneer in preventive inoculation was Louis Pasteur, whose contribution to milk purification is perhaps the "first" in terms of importance. From his original observation of the spoiling of wine by microorganisms (1863–1865) and his demonstration of its prevention by heat sterilization, followed by his demonstration of a similar relationship and correction (1876) in the case of beer,[30] it was then a simple and logical progression to apply this knowledge to the purification of milk by a process now universally known as pasteurization. Pasteur showed that partial heat sterilization could be accomplished by temperatures of 55° to 60°C. It is a pathetic commentary that the use of the principle was not obligatory in New York State until 1912.

Once the basic concept of the bacteriologic relationship of milk-borne disease was established and accepted on a firm foundation, the further necessary steps toward milk purification could be taken. Actually no mention of bacteria was made by the Health Department until 1896. And it was not until 1909 that the board enlarged its definition of adulterated milk to include that milk "which contains an excessive number of bacteria." That these "steps" were not to be too promptly taken by the infant milk industry was soon evident, but, the die having been cast, the results were inevitable.

THE STRUGGLE FOR PASTEURIZATION

In the 1890s there appeared on the scene two men who pioneered in the utilization of the newest scientific discoveries. These men were Nathan Straus and Dr. Henry Leber Coit, each of whom made a significant and lasting contribution to the establishment of a pure and wholesome milk supply.

Nathan Straus, a New York merchant, was one of the first and most formidable champions of pasteurized milk, and the story of his accomplishments will rightfully start the section of this paper outlining the stages of the struggle for pasteurization. Another important figure in the same regard is Dr. Henry Leber Coit, one of our great American pioneers in the broader field of public health and particularly respected for his great contribution to milk sanitation. Dr. Coit's great contribution was the concept and realization of a raw milk which could be "certified" to be pure and wholesome. In a splendid article by Dr. Fred Rogers[31] it is noted that Dr. Coit was stimulated to his interest as a result of a fruitless attempt to purchase wholesome milk (from a neighboring farm) with which he hoped to nourish his first child, dying of milk-borne diphtheria in 1888. After the death of this child Coit made a personal crusade of inspection of the neighboring farms and dairies, which work extended over a period of several years. Thus, he acquired a first-hand knowledge of the problems of milk sanitation which was so effectively utilized later.

In an attempt to improve the conditions under which milk was being produced and retailed, Coit first tried to obtain state legislation. This failing, he proceeded to get the backing of the Practitioners Club of Newark, New Jersey. In 1892 he outlined to this group his historic plan for supervision of milk by chemical, bacteriologic, and veterinary standards, to be policed by routine inspections. These standards represent in essence the sanitary code for purity of milk accepted today.

The Medical Milk Commission of Essex County, New Jersey, was established as a result of this work. This commission was headed by Coit and in 1893 became the first organization of its kind in the world. Thus was born the concept of a "certified milk," the assurance at long last of a perfectly pure and safe milk for infants, convalescents, and expectant mothers. With the establishment of this first Medical Milk Commission the first bottle of certified milk was appropriately delivered to Mrs. Coit by its producer, Mr. Stephen Francisco of the Fairfield Dairy (New Jersey), who with Dr. Coit copyrighted the name "Certified Milk."

Certified milk was to become for many years the only raw milk available and accredited by physicians. It is therefore reasonable to assume that this was a healthful product, and an examination of some of its major requirements will clearly indicate the reason for the correctness of this supposition. These requirements included: (1) preliminary tuberculosis test of all animals added to certified herds, (2) regular semiannual tuberculosis test (alternating intradermal with subcutaneous test), (3) regular monthly veterinary inspection of all cows, (4) thorough examination of all new employees, (5) regular weekly medical inspection of all employees on every farm by physicians in the employ of the Milk Commission, (6) monthly sanitary inspection of the farms and their equipment, and (7) weekly chemical and bacteriological examinations of every farm's milk and every distributor's milk.

Standards for quality included: milk must be in its natural state, not having been heated, and without the addition of coloring matter or preservatives; nothing may be added and nothing taken away from the milk; milk must contain an average of 4 percent butter fat; milk must contain not more than 10,000 bacteria per cc on an average when delivered to the consumer.

Some of the regular routine details carried out on certified farms were: (1) hands washed before and rinsed and dried after milking each cow, (2) cows' udders washed and dried before milking, (3) employees dressed in white during milking hours, (4) sterilization of bottles, apparatus, and tinware either by steam or dry heat, (5) testing of the foremilk of each cow before milking, (6) the immediate cooling of the milk to 45°F, and (7) bottling and sealing of milk on the farm where produced.[32]

At the turn of this century Dr. Abraham Jacobi stated that the production and distribution of certified milk represented the greatest advance in infant feeding of the time, and, although there was no overwhelming necessity for pasteurizing certified milk, as shown by its sanitary and bacteriologic balances and counter-balances, the discussion of this problem was to occupy the profession for many succeeding years.

The importance of certified milk, particularly for the feeding of infants, can best be understood by a quantitative analysis of the methods of infant feeding. In the first decades of the 20th century Holt estimated that 85 percent of the babies were breast fed. There were 48,000 babies born in Brooklyn, for example, in 1921. Of these, 7,200

(15 percent) were artificially fed. Actually about 85 to 90 percent of the certified milk sold went for infant feeding.

The danger of unwholesome cow's milk for infants was emphasized by a study in the late 1910s in New York City, which showed that, although more than 75 percent of the infants were breast fed, 78 percent of the infants that died of enteritis were fed on cow's milk or patent foods. Another study reported 6,000 deaths from diarrhea in children under five years of age in 1910, while in 1930, when most milk fed to children was either certified or pasteurized, the deaths were less than 900.[33] Another study of groups of infants fed different kinds of milk (in summer) yielded the following interesting comparison: Of 79 children drinking nonpasteurized store milk, 15 died and 20 did "badly."[34]

The subject is perhaps best summed up in a statement from the address of Clarence W. Barron before the convention of the American Association of Medical Milk Commissions and Certified Milk Producers Association of America at Harvard Medical School in June of 1921: "More babies have been slain in the United States with impure milk than in all the rest of the world put together. More than 250,000 babies die every year in the United States within one year of birth. At least 90 percent could be saved with prompt medical attention and pure or natural milk from cows certified by the supervision of a Medical Milk Commission."[35]

Although Dr. Coit originally worked out the 70 rules which every certified milk producer obligated himself to follow, these were later revised and came to constitute the Methods and Standards for the production of certified milk as adopted by the American Association of Medical Milk Commissions and as such accepted throughout the United States.

Although these last paragraphs have not really constituted a digression, it is now necessary to return to the earlier years of the certified milk era so that a clearer chronologic picture may be had. In 1896 the Board of Health of New York took a major step forward in the fight for pure milk when it included in its sanitary code the prohibition of the sale of milk except under a permit, the milk being subject to the regulations of this board. Powerful interests opposed this ruling, but the right of the Department of Health to prevent the sale of milk without a permit was finally upheld by the United States Supreme Court in 1905.[36]

The case began with the conviction of a milk dealer for not having a written permit from the Board of Health. This conviction had been upheld by the New York Court of Appeals but finally went to the Supreme Court of the United States, since the milk dealer claimed in his defense that the permit requirement constituted a violation of the due process of law guaranteed to him by the Fourteenth Amendment. The Supreme Court nevertheless upheld the conviction on the grounds that the Sanitary Code was a constitutional use of the authority of a city to safeguard the health of its citizens in a reasonable manner.

And so at last began the period of effectual control of city milk supplies in New York State. The tuberculin test was applied for the first time in 1896, simultaneously uncovering the infection of a large proportion of the cows with the tubercle bacillus. It is pertinent to note that only certified milk avoided the stigma of infection, since it came from tuberculosis tested cows, and in addition its production and marketing were accomplished with scrupulous cleanliness as detailed earlier in this paper.

In New York City the production of certified milk, which was under the aegis of the County Medical Society, was under the supervisory control of Dr. William H. Park at the Research Laboratory. It was Dr. Park's observations of a direct ratio between rises in temperature of milk and increases in its bacterial count that resulted in an additional amendment to the Sanitary Code (in 1896) defining as adulterated milk which showed a temperature of more than 50°F.

The Milk Commission of the Medical Society of the County of New York was formed in 1896, and in March 1902, the Kings County Pure Milk Commission, under Dr. E. H. Bartley, held its first meeting. In 1907 The American Association of Milk Commissions was organized to include the many separate commissions that had arisen by that time.

With an ever-increasing awareness of the relationship of impure milk to disease and an even more rapidly increasing consciousness of the bacterial role in milk adulteration, it was only a logical next step to pasteurization. This new chapter in our history may appropriately be begun by stating that Pasteur reported lactic fermentation as far back as 1857, although the isolation of the causative organism (the Streptococcus lactis, which causes milk to sour) by Lister did not occur until 1873.

When the varied sources of milk and the many factors determining its production and marketing are considered, it would appear logical to assume that without pasteurization milk could not be considered a wholesome product for general public consumption. The milk that finally comes to the consumer is produced from thousands of cows on hundreds of farms. Milkers, utensils, transportation, and the human element of inspection are all involved in its final chemical and bacteriological makeup. Negligence, cupidity, stupidity, or ignorance could conceivably act to produce a potentially dangerous product, and so, despite all other precautions, it was felt necessary to provide for the destruction of all pathogenic bacteria.

In Europe, near the end of the 19th century, Dr. Soxhlet achieved a comparable result by boiling milk, which rendered the product sterile but not particularly palatable to most people. In 1898 the pasteurization of all bottled milk had been made compulsory in Denmark.

Dr. Abraham Jacobi, the Nestor of American pediatrics, was one of the first to recognize the value of pasteurization in this country. However, it was a layman, Nathan Straus, who had interested himself in milk for infants, who actually spearheaded the movement for a scientifically pure supply of milk in New York through his advocacy of pasteurization. During the controversy of the last decade of the 19th century, which raged about the topic of the relative merits of raw versus pasteurized milk, Straus vigorously championed the latter cause. It has been acknowledged by the son of L. B. Halsey, the president of the original Sheffield Farms, that his father became interested in pasteurization as a result of Mr. Straus' work in 1892.[37] In this year milk was pasteurized for the first time at the Chicago World's Fair. In 1893 Mr. Straus established the first milk station in this country and began the first free distribution of boiled milk at his infant milk depot located on the East Third Street pier. This was done two years before the first pasteurizing machines were invented and 19 years before pasteurization finally became law in this state. When pasteurization appeared mechanically feasible, Mr. Straus erected a plant for this purpose on Randall's Island in 1898.

Even in an historical paper, an occasional scientific digression in the interest of clarity is permissible, and so a short discussion of the details of pasteurization would seem to be in order. Pasteurization and sterilization obviously differ. Sterilization concedes the complete destruction of all living matter, which in milk requires prolonged boiling at high temperatures under pressure. Such a process does not improve the taste of milk and is generally unnecessary. Pasteurization, involving lesser degrees of temperature, makes milk safe, relatively palatable, but not sterile. However it does destroy all pathogenic nonspore-producing bacteria, thereby eliminating all pathogens responsible for milk-borne diseases. The only exception is anthrax, which is practically nonexistent in this country. Pasteurization likewise destroys most bacteria but not the lactic acid-producing bacteria, the survival of which is desirable, since these prevent the development of proteolytic bacteria.

Pasteurization was originally introduced into this country by dairy owners who wished to prevent their milk from spoiling. Jacobi was one of the first, however, to recognize its public health aspects in 1875.[38] By 1898 the pasteurization of all bottled milk was compulsory in Denmark. In this country we imported pasteurizing machines from Denmark in 1895, and some of the earliest experiments in their use were performed at Bloomville, New York, about that time. There is no agreement about the very first pasteurizations in this country, but Henderson attributes this honor to Cincinnati, in 1897, and believes it was next used in New York a year later.

As pasteurization was originally an economic device designed solely to prolong the life of milk and thus to earn greater profits for the producer, it was used in secret and accordingly viewed with deep suspicion by the public. In 1906 the aspect of secrecy was prohibited in New York City when it was decreed that all pasteurized milk had to be labeled as such, and with the time and temperatures of pasteurization stated on the package.

There were two general methods of pasteurization, known as the "flash process" and the "holding method." The first machines, imported from

Denmark in 1895, were of the flash process variety. In this method the temperature of the milk is brought to about 160°F and maintained for 15 seconds. In 1902 certain physicians encouraged experiments in pasteurization by the holding method. In this method the temperature is raised to the range of 140 to 145°F but maintained for 20 to 30 minutes. These experiments were apparently successful, and the first pasteurizer of this type was installed and used commercially in New York in 1907. It had been proved that a temperature of 140°F maintained for 20 minutes would destroy all pathogenic bacteria and in addition destroy between 90 and 99 percent of the total microorganisms in milk. The general acceptance of this process was slow, so that in 1909 only 25 percent of the milk was so pasteurized, and by 1912 only 33 percent. In 1908 the New York City milk ordinance required a temperature of 142° to 145°F for 30 minutes, and these standards were gradually accepted over the entire country. When the importance of pasteurization in disease prevention became increasingly apparent, it was adopted more frequently, even in the smaller towns.

Although the holding method remained the more important up until 1948,[39] there was a gradual change in popularity in recent years to the high-temperature, short-time (HTST) variation, using 161°F and 15 seconds. The reasons for the change in popularity again were economic. Up to recent years the volume of cream, as noted by the cream line, was of prime importance in the sale of milk, and temperatures over 143°F were known to destroy this evidence by causing disappearance of the cream line. Therefore, in 1917, for example, when it was initially noted that a temperature of 145°F would destroy the cream line, the temperature was dropped, and eventually in 1928 stabilized at 143°F. When homogenization became popular in the past decade or so, the cream line no longer was a factor.

Another factor involved in the recent trend to the HTST method concerns the relationship of exact timing of very high temperatures and the quality of the milk and therefore its salability. In recent years mechanical devices of extreme accuracy in timing have been perfected which now make the HTST more efficient and the quality of the milk more palatable and predictable. As a result, although this method of pasteurization is optional, practically all our milk is thus treated today.[40]

Along with pasteurization came the grading of milk on the basis of purity. Under the administration of the New York Health Commissioner, Dr. Thomas Darlington, a systematic mechanism of inspection of country dairies was introduced and within a few years had spread to include effectively all dairies in the New York "milkshed." Thus, while bacterial counts had been reported in 1906 to be usually between 2 and 20 million, the figures for 1908 averaged only 45,000 bacteria per cc, a remarkable improvement. When public acceptance of the bacterial count as a criterion of milk purity was at last achieved, it was a simple matter to include this as an indication of adulteration. This was actually done by an amendment to the Sanitary Code in 1909.

Between 1910 and 1912 there was a series of typhoid outbreaks in New York, and in 1911 the Board of Health, under Commissioner Ernst J. Lederle, adopted a system of grading milk and of defining pasteurization in terms of a particular temperature (145°F at that time) and a definite time (30 minutes). Under this system there were three grades of milk differentiated from each other by different bacterial count standards both before and after pasteurization. Grade A was the purest and the only one of the three permitted to be sold either raw or pasteurized. Most of the milk to reach the ultimate consumer was grade B, and therefore the requirement of pasteurization proved to be of tremendous sanitary import. Unfortunately World War I intruded during this time, and enforcement of pasteurization was not complete. Eventually, by 1926, with the reorganization of the milk inspection service, the regulation for pasteurization of grade B milk was strictly enforced.

The sale of grade C milk was prohibited after May 1926, when only grades A and B milk were permitted to be sold in New York. At the same time the bacterial standards were gradually being raised. As the standards for milk purity became stricter, the quality of grade B milk improved to the point that, for all practical purposes, it was as healthful as grade A milk. Actually the grade B then satisfied most of the requisites formerly in effect for grade A milk. The upgrading of grade B milk narrowed the gap between the grades and presented a situation with an illogical economic differential. Therefore, around 1940 the New York City Board of Health discontinued the system of grading of milk and established a single grade in this area known as approved milk.

The first pasteurized certified milk was marketed in 1929, and in June 1935 the American Association of Medical Milk Commissions voted to include permissive pasteurization of certified milk in the Methods and Standards. This provided a final, inevitable seal of safety for a clean milk. By 1936 certified milk could be purchased in almost 50 cities and towns in New York State. In 1943 the Board of Health changed its attitude with respect to certified milk and required all such milk or milk of certifiable grade to be pasteurized unless the raw product was specifically prescribed by a physician.

PRESENT-DAY DEVELOPMENTS

Practically all the milk sold in the United States before 1900 was delivered as raw, loose milk. In the succeeding decade more and more of this milk sold in the larger cities underwent pasteurization but was still sold loose. The usual method was for the milk to reach the retailer in three-gallon cans and thence emptied into the buyer's milk can (or other receptacle) by means of a measure or dipper. Despite the fact that Thatcher had invented a milk bottle in 1886, milk continued to be carried in cans and ladled out to customers in this obviously unsanitary way.

Since 1928 the New York State Sanitary Code required the bottling of all milk sold, other than that sold on the premises, but this code was not effective in New York City, where loose milk continued to be sold into the 1930s.

The question of loose milk as a health hazard had been debated for many years, but not until the *New York World-Telegram* published the results of analyses of loose milk in 1931 did the danger become pinpointed. The generating force apparently was the unsubtly veiled implication that the poliomyelitis epidemic of 1931 was somehow associated with the sale of loose milk. Under Health Commissioner Shirley W. Wynne a board of eminent scientists, social workers, and public health experts was appointed to study the situation and to make appropriate recommendations to the Board of Health, the only body empowered to modify conditions under which milk is produced and sold. In 1931 the Milk Commission recommended, in view of the opinion that loose milk was a health hazard, that the sale of loose or dipped milk not consumed on the premises be prohibited, that milk be dispensed only in and from bottles filled and sealed at the milk plant, and that such restrictions be made effective before January 1933. It further recommended that the "continued sale of loose milk to hospitals . . . be permitted under regulations prescribed by the Board of Health" and that other loose milk permitted in cooking or for manufacturing purposes was likewise to be regulated by the Board of Health.[41]

Such excepted loose milk could only be sold from dispensing devices specifically approved. The supervision of these devices was so exacting that any necessary repairs to them had to be made under the seal of the Board of Health. This last regulation did not however become completely effective until 1936, largely due to the time required for the satisfactory engineering developments necessary for the perfection of these specifically designed milk dispensing machines. Loose milk, under the specific regulations noted, continues to be sold in restaurants today, but the machines are specially handled, filled, and sealed at the milk factories where any required servicing is likewise attended. Such control is excellent and effective and regulated by the Board of Health.

An acceptable and yet dramatic indication of the public benefit from improvements in milk sanitation can be obtained from an analysis of the decrease in the death rate from typhoid fever (and of course its incidence) over a period of years. Experience has adequately demonstrated the close relationship between typhoid and milk sanitation and the steady fall in morbidity and mortality with improvements in milk purification quite proves the equation. In New York City the death rate from typhoid fever fell from 40 per 100,000 in 1868 to 16 in 1896, to 12 in 1908. In 1919 the rate was two per 100,000 and after 1927 but one per 100,000 population.[42]

When the now practically extinct "summer diarrhea" or cholera infantum is considered, the proof is even more convincing. Where there were 71 deaths per 10,000 each summer in children under five years of age as late as 1910, by 1930 the rate had been reduced to six per 10,000 population.[43] The connection between cholera infantum and impure milk is too well authenticated, and the significance of the figures too obvious to belabor or reemphasize the point. The arduous and extensive struggles for milk purification represent an expensive effort, yet the tremendous savings of life and the accompanying prevention of illness more than justifies it.

Finally, on the subject of milk-borne epidemics, the last reported epidemic of this nature was in 1918–1920, but in these instances it was shown that they were due to milk allegedly but actually not pasteurized. Authorities at the New York Board of Health predict today that our herds of cows will probably be completely free of brucellosis (a heretofore common milk-borne disease) within two years.[44]

Certain trends in the milk industry may now be noted. There is first a distinct trend toward a smaller number of dairy farms supplying the New York area. These fewer farms subscribe to a policy of more intensive farming. Whereas in 1930 there were probably 60,000 dairy farms, today there are perhaps 45,000, yet the present smaller number produces a greater amount of milk. There is an accompanying, although not necessarily related decline in the number of country milk receiving stations, whose numbers have been halved from the 1930 total of 800. This is due to consolidation of operation and more efficient means of transporting milk by motor trucks over improved roads.

In New York City today there is a great concentration in the number of milk pasteurizing plants which now number only about 35. Although the number of dealers has increased, the number of these central plants has been steadily reduced. This makes for a simpler and therefore more efficient control.

In addition, there are major changes in transportation and refrigeration of the milk produced by our modern dairy farms. More than 95 percent of the dairy farms which supply the New York City area are equipped with mechanical refrigeration, there is increasing use of pipe line milking machines (eliminating the local transport via the bucket), and increasing use is being made of refrigerated bulk tank trucks for cooling milk in transit from the country. This also eliminates the well-known milk can. Approximately 25 percent of the delivery trucks are also equipped with mechanical refrigeration.

The use of paper containers was originally designed for metropolitan marketing, and today more than 57 percent of New York's milk is "in paper." The first milk plant to use paper bottles exclusively was one in Ozone Park, Long Island, in 1935.[45]

Hand in hand with the reduction of numbers of dairy farms and a greater total yield of milk is the definite long-term trend of the farmer to keep the animals which give milk of lower fat content and higher total yields. Translated into terms of cattle eugenics, this heralds the decline of the Jersey and Guernsey cows and the ascendancy of the Holstein type of breed. Fortunately for the industry, the consumer trend has also been to deemphasize the role of fat, although this has been of more recent vintage. The producer trend in this regard began to be evident first about 15 years ago, while the consumers' predeliction for lower fat has been noted mainly in the last four to five years, especially evidenced by their greater demand and use of skimmed milk. The recent warnings against animal fats and their role in atherosclerosis can only serve to heighten this perfect and harmonious blending of producer and consumer preferences.

In addition to the increased consumption of skimmed milk, there is also an increased tendency to use skimmed milk powders, and this tendency has been accelerated in the past two years by the production of more readily skimmed powders than were available before. One unusual aspect of the use of powdered milk is that it is not restricted as to its source and the original milk need not be inspected. It therefore cannot be affirmed that it is completely without risk, because the temperatures used in its manufacture may not be sufficient to destroy certain preformed toxins such as that of the staphylococcus. This toxin is heat labile and can withstand temperatures of 300°F or more, although the staphylococcus organism itself is destroyed at much lower temperature levels. There have been milk powders manufactured in this country which have been implicated in food-borne diseases after shipment to England and certain South American countries.

The New York State Federal Milk Marketing Order, which was formed in 1937 to determine the price the farmer receives for his milk, has dominated certain economic aspects of milk marketing in the past score of years. Although this committee was suspended for a short interval after its original formation, as a result of legal actions, it has been in force directly thereafter and uninterruptedly ever since. This organization derives its ultimate authority from the Secretary of Agriculture and (in New York) the Commissioner of Agriculture of New York State. The existence and action of this body has the salutary effect of providing an orderly marketing of milk and preventing strikes and the problems that lead to strikes and disruption.

In the past year a considerable journalistic literature has been building up with relation to the effects of antibiotics, DDT, and radioactive fallout on milk and the subsequent effects on the milk-consuming public. Although there is no unanimity of opinion in lay circles, the better and scientifically informed feel that, although the situations bear watching, there is no real cause for alarm. The recent DDT sprayings in New York have created a modest journalistic furor, and allegations have been made that dangerous quantities of the insecticide get into milk.[46] And yet the laboratory determinations upon which these statements are based are conducted with suspicious speed, in contrast to similar determinations by the Board of Health which are accurate enough to reflect a much longer period of appraisal by their trained technicians. Another factor of safety implicit in DDT spraying lies in the choice of wooded areas rather than pasture, so that only by misdirection or accident would the insecticide reach the cow and her milk.

Strontium 90, the dangerous element of radioactive fallout, is absorbed like calcium, and if a significant amount were to find its way into the milk supply, a serious health problem would result. A close examination of the reports of the Atomic Energy Commission, however, gives no cause for alarm. The testing program is being handled not only by the United States Public Health Service but also by the individual states involved. If the situation should ever become threatening, the public will be quickly advised.

A peculiar and unique situation exists with respect to antibiotics and milk. Mastitis in cows, not uncommon, is treated frequently with antibiotics, but there is no law that controls the distribution of antibiotics for animal use. Hence there is unsupervised dosing of cows with these drugs administered largely by farmers. These drugs are known to appear in the milk, and it is often impossible to keep such milk out of the general supply. It is therefore possible for some individuals who are allergic to the particular antibiotic "contaminant" to develop a reaction. The United States Food and Drug Administration has taken the position that this might be harmful only in "exquisitely sensitive people," and to date there have been reported no such cases in the New York area.

Antibiotics in milk are also concerned in possible inhibiting effects on some lactic organisms with resultant future regrowths of temporarily inhibited bacteria. It would thus appear worth while to have some regulation to bar the promiscuous and uninhibited use of antibiotics in animals or at least to have such use supervised by a veterinarian. Perhaps one day this too will be history.

A discussion of the role of allergens in milk would be incomplete without a word about goat's milk. Its present frequent use is a matter of general knowledge, but it was not approved for public consumption until 1938. Today goat's milk may be purchased both certified pasteurized or certified raw. There are in the New York milkshed five goat dairies under the supervision of the Board of Health, and the milk produced represents a lifeline to many infants who are extremely sensitive to cow's milk, a sensitivity which the infants fortunately often outgrow.

Today we are justifiably proud of the high standards and purity of milk in New York, which rank among the best in the world. To those who have made the hope the realization, we express our gratitude and thanks by this reconstruction in words of their activities.

NOTES

The author wishes to acknowledge his indebtedness to his wife, Sheila, for invaluable editorial assistance in the preparation of this manuscript.

1 T. R. Pirtle, *History of the Dairy Industry* (Chicago: Mojonnier Bros. Co., [c. 1926]), p. 17.

2 C. L. Roadhouse and J. L. Henderson, *The Market*

Milk Industry, 2nd ed. (New York: McGraw-Hill, 1950).

3 J. Flexner, "The battle for pure milk in New York City," in *Report of the Milk Commission: Is Loose Milk a Health Hazard?* (Milk Commission, Dept. Health, New York City, [c. 1931]), p. 162.

4 *Manual of Incorporation of the City of New York*, Jos. Shannon, Clerk of the Common Council (E. Jones, printer for the city, 1832), in *Report of the Milk Commission*, p. 163.

5 Roadhouse and Henderson, *Market Milk Industry*, p. 2.

6 J. E. Allen, "The milk supply in New York," report of a paper, *Arch. Pediat.*, 1893, *10*: 519.

7 R. M. Hartley, *An Historical, Scientific, and Practical Essay on Milk as an Article of Human Sustenance* (New York: J. Leavitt, 1842).

8 I. S. Hartley, *Memorial of Robert Milham Hartley, D.D.* (Utica: Curtiss and Childs, 1882).

9 Hartley, *Milk as an Article of Human Sustenance*.

10 J. Mullaly, *The Milk Trade in New York and Vicinity* (New York: Fowlers and Wells, 1853).

11 Proceedings of the Brooklyn Common Council, 1856, as quoted by Flexner, "Battle for pure milk," p. 168.

12 Mullaly, *The Milk Trade*.

13 S. R. Percy, "On the food of cities." Read before the Medical Society of the State of New York at its annual meeting, February 1865.

14 J. A. Tobey, *Legal Aspects of Milk Control* (Chicago: International Association of Milk Dealers, 1936), p. 1.

15 Flexner, "Battle for pure milk," pp. 182, 184.

16 *Ibid.*

17 Department of Health (New York) Sanitary Code, June 2, 1873.

18 *New York Tribune*, Dec. 28, 1876.

19 Allen, "Milk supply."

20 H. D. Chapin, in Report to the New York Academy of Medicine, Section on Pediatrics, May 11, 1893, *Arch. Pediat.*, 1893, *10*: 521.

21 C. J. Eberth, "Die Organismen in den Organen bei Typhus Abdominalis," *Arch. pathol. Anat.*, 1880, *81*: 58.

22 F. H. Garrison, *An Introduction to the History of Medicine*, 4th ed. (Philadelphia: W. B. Saunders Co., 1929), p. 781.

23 T. A. E. Klebs, "Über Diphtherie," *Verhand. d. Cong. inn. Med.* (Wiesbaden), 1883, *2*: 139.

24 B. L. F. Bang, "Die Aetiologie des Seuchenhaftens ("infectiösen") Verwerfens," *Ztschr. Tiermed.*, 1897, *1*: 241.

25 E. C. Achard and R. Bensaude, "Infections paratyphoidiques," *Bull. et mém. Soc. méd. hôp. Paris*, 1896, *13*: 820.

26 R. Koch, "Über die Cholerabakterien," *Deutsche med. Wchnschr.*, 1884, *10*: 725.

27 R. Koch, "Die Aetiologie der Tuberkulose," *Berl. klin. Wchnschr.*, 1882, *19*: 221.

28 T. Smith, "A comparative study of bovine tubercle bacilli and of human bacilli from sputum," *J. Exper. Med.*, 1898, *3*: 451.

29 K. Shiga, "Über den Dysenteriebacillus (Bacillus dysenteriae)," *Zentralbl. Bakt.*, 1898, *24*: 817, 870.

30 Garrison, *History of Medicine*, p. 576.

31 F. B. Rogers, "H. L. Coit, 1854–1917, pioneer in public health," *J. Med. Soc. N.J.*, 1955, *52*: 36.

32 H. Moak, "Raw milk in relation to nutrition, the work of the Milk Commission of the Medical Society of the County of Kings," *Long Island Med. J.*, 1922, *16*: 55.

33 C. F. Bolduan, "Milk regulation from 1900 to the present," in *Report of the Milk Commission*, p. 204.

34 Roadhouse and Henderson, *Market Milk Industry*.

35 C. W. Barron, *Boston Evening Transcript*, June 7, 1921.

36 Tobey, *Legal Aspects of Milk Control*, p. 12.

37 Roadhouse and Henderson, *Market Milk Industry*, p. 5.

38 B. L. Herrington, *Milk and Milk Processing* (New York: McGraw-Hill Book Co., 1948), pp. 167, 171.

39 *Ibid.*

40 P. Corash, Personal communication (Chief Milk Section, Dept. Health, New York).

41 *Report of the Milk Commission*, p. 1.

42 Bolduan, "Milk regulation."

43 *Ibid.*

44 Corash, Personal communication.

45 Herrington, *Milk and Milk Processing*, p. 218.

46 W. Longgood, "Cows milk shows DDT after spraying," *New York World-Telegram and the Sun*, June 3, 1957, p. 17.

21

Raising and Watering a City: Ellis Sylvester Chesbrough and Chicago's First Sanitation System

LOUIS P. CAIN

The engineers responsible for invention and mechanization in agriculture, manufacturing, and transportation are prominent historical figures, but few people are aware of the men who pioneered the sanitation systems so crucial to urbanization. As cities grew, their initial approaches to waste disposal and water supply proved unacceptable. As early as 1798 Benjamin Latrobe noted in his journal that the fresh groundwater which located the site of Philadelphia was befouled by the city's increasing population concentration. In Latrobe's opinion, Philadelphia's existing water-supply strategy was a major source of disease. Even before he assumed the responsibility for the city's new waterworks, Latrobe was convinced of the project's utility: "The great scheme of bringing the water of the Schuylkill to Philadelphia to supply the city is now become an object of immense importance, . . . though it is at present neglected from a failure of funds. The evil, however, which it is intended collaterally to correct is so serious and of such magnitude as to call loudly upon all who are inhabitants of Philadelphia for their utmost exertions to complete it."[1]

The emerging concentrations of population and manufacturing in the 19th century necessitated a reexamination of sanitation strategies. With urbanization, the haphazard approaches of the past could not guarantee pure water supplies and adequate waste disposal. Urban growth inevitably required the implementation of sanitation systems, and these systems, in turn, permitted further growth.

Students of Chicago's formative decades inevitably encounter the name of Ellis Sylvester Chesbrough; by studying Chesbrough, a student can focus on the truly unique character and contribution of Chicago's sanitation system. Chesbrough's works were the innovations most responsible for Chicago's unrestricted urban growth; they freed the city from the limitations imposed by an unfavorable natural topography. A flat, nonporous terrain, slightly elevated from Lake Michigan and the Chicago River, made drainage and absorption nearly impossible. In rainy weather, the topsoil became swamplike. Urban growth required a drainage system which could remove both surface water and household wastes. The natural depository for such a drainage system was Lake Michigan; however, the lake was simultaneously the city's natural water-supply source. Lake water had to be conserved if it was to be potable, and this meant it had to be protected from urban wastes. Fortunately, beginning in the 1850s, Chicago's city fathers recognized pollution as a serious threat to the city's health and took immediate action. This paper investigates how Chesbrough responded to Chicago's anomalous water-supply and waste-disposal needs in the 1850s and 1860s, and inquires into his engineering education to discover the antecedents of his innovative ideas.

I

Ellis Sylvester Chesbrough was born of Puritan ancestry in Baltimore County, Maryland, in July 1813. An unsuccessful business venture exhausted the family's means and suspended young Sylves-

LOUIS P. CAIN is Associate Professor of Economics, Loyola University, Chicago, Illinois.

Reprinted with permission from *Technology and Culture*, 1972, *13*: 353–372.

ter's education, and so, at nine years of age, he went to work. Between his ninth and fifteenth birthdays Chesbrough spent only a year in a classroom, but he did find time outside his counting-house duties to pursue his studies. Chesbrough acquired most of his basic education without the benefit of formal training or a regular teacher, and the same was true of his engineering education.

In 1828 Chesbrough's father took a job with a railroad engineering company employed by the Baltimore and Ohio Railroad Company. Through the father's influence, the son gained employment as a chainman with a similar company engaged in preliminary surveying work in and about Baltimore.[2] Chesbrough's company was under Lieutenant Joshua Barney, U.S. Army, and most of the engineers were army officers, many of them graduates of the U.S. Military Academy's practical, as opposed to theoretical, engineering course.[3] Chesbrough was fortunate in being affiliated with several of the army's most prominent engineers. In 1830–31 he worked as an assistant engineer to Colonel Stephen H. Long.[4] Near the end of 1831, Chesbrough joined the engineering corps of Captain William Gibbs McNeill, where he served immediately under Lieutenant George W. Whistler.[5]

The Panic of 1837 and the resulting depression dealt a hard blow to the country's internal improvement's bubble, and Chesbrough, like many other engineers, found himself out of work as the flow of funds dried up in the early 1840s. He went to his father's residence in Providence, Rhode Island, where, during the winter of 1842, he spent his leisure time in the workshop of a nearby railroad learning the practical use of tools. The following year he purchased a farm adjacent to one owned by his father in Niagara County, New York. His venture into farming was mercifully brief; after an unsuccessful year, Chesbrough gladly returned to engineering.

In 1846 Chesbrough was offered the position of chief engineer on the Boston Water Works' West Division. This position completed his engineering education. Up to this time, all his experience was related to railroad engineering, and he had mastered many civil engineering essentials, such as grading, tunneling, and surveying. Chesbrough was reluctant to accept the Boston position because he considered himself unacquainted with hydraulic engineering. His friends and Boston's water commissioners implored him to accept the position, and, after being assured John Jervis's counsel, Chesbrough assented.

There was good reason for Chesbrough to consider an association with Jervis valuable. Jervis had been active in every phase of engineering, particularly those dealing with hydraulics. Jervis was a product of the New York canal system and had learned hydraulic engineering on the job by working on the Erie Canal. In 1846 Jervis was appointed consulting engineer on the Boston Water Works, with Chesbrough the chief engineer. Jervis had the responsibility for designing both the Cochituate Aqueduct and the Brookline Reservoir; Chesbrough, the responsibility for supervising the execution of Jervis's plans.[6] In 1850 Chesbrough became sole commissioner of Boston's water works, and a year later, he became Boston's first city engineer.

The United States' early experience with internal improvements and the education of engineers coalesced in Chesbrough's career. He learned civil enginering from some of the army's most competent engineers. He learned hydraulic engineering from Jervis, perhaps the most competent engineer trained by the New York canal system. The education and experience which Chesbrough utilized in freeing Chicago from its topographical liabilities and in implementing an effective sanitation system grew out of his first-hand experience with many of the country's internal improvements.

II

In the early 1850s Chicago's random waste disposal methods led to a succession of cholera and dysentery epidemics. The Illinois legislature created the Chicago Board of Sewerage Commissioners on February 14, 1855, to combat what was generally conceded to be an intolerable situation.[7] The commissioners sought "the most competent engineer of the time who was available for the position of chief engineer."[8] Their selection, E. Sylvester Chesbrough, resigned his position as Boston's city engineer and came to Chicago.[9] Immediately after accepting the position, Chesbrough submitted a report in which he outlined his plan for a sewerage system designed to solve Chicago's drainage and waste-disposal problem.

His plan represents the first comprehensive sewerage system undertaken by any major city in the United States. He had learned about sewer construction, grading, and "building-raising" from different sources. Now he merged them and "pulled Chicago out of the mud."

Prior to Chesbrough's arrival, Chicago's sewerage commissioners solicited the public for plans and suggestions. Thirty-nine proposals were received, and, although the board claimed Chesbrough utilized many of these suggestions, he did not use any of the proposals in its entirety.[10] Chesbrough's task was to construct a sewerage system whose main objective was to "improve and preserve" the city's health. In his opinion, the existing privy vaults and drainage sluices were "abominations that should be swept away as speedily as possible," and that "to construct the vaults as they should be, and maintain them even in a comparatively inoffensive condition, would be more expensive than to construct an entire system of sewerage for no other purpose, if the past experience of London and other large cities was any guide for the future of Chicago."[11]

Chesbrough's 1855 report to the Board of Sewerage Commissioners made several references to the sewers of New York, Boston, and Philadelphia. Additionally, the report showed that Chesbrough was familiar, through his reading, with the sewers of London, Paris, and other European cities. It is important to remember, however, that not one U.S. city at that time had a comprehensive sewerage system, even though most had sewers. Consequently, Chesbrough had to rely on his training and intuition in assessing sewerage system alternatives.

Chesbrough's 1855 report considered four possibilities: (1) drainage directly into the Chicago River and then into Lake Michigan; (2) drainage directly into Lake Michigan; (3) drainage into artifical reservoirs to be pumped and used as fertilizer (sewage farming); and (4) drainage directly into the Chicago River, and then by a proposed steamboat canal into the Des Plaines River. Although this fourth possibility was the method which Chicago eventually adopted (the Chicago Sanitary District's Sanitary and Ship Canal), the city's 80,000 inhabitants in 1855 did not warrant the expense which this alternative involved.

Chesbrough recommended the first plan.[12] This is not to say he failed to realize that his preferred method was a potential health hazard, particularly during the warmer months, and might obstruct river navigation by making the waterways shallower.[13] Chesbrough discussed the objections to his recommended alternative:

> It is proposed to remove the first [health hazard] by pouring into the river from the lake a sufficient body of pure water into the North and South Branches to prevent offensive or injurious exhalations . . . The latter objection [obstruct navigation] is believed to be groundless, because the substances to be conveyed through the sewers to the river could in no case be heavier than the soil of this vicintiy, but would generally be much lighter. While these substances might, to some extent, be deposited there when there is little or no current, they would, during the seasons of rain and flood, be swept on by the same force that has hitherto preserved the depth of the river.[14]

Apparently, Chesbrough did not realize that spring freshets and floods might force the sewers' accumulations into the lake in such a way as to pollute the city's water supply. This is somewhat surprising, as the basic sanitation principle of the day was to locate the eventual sewage outlet as far from the water-supply source as possible.

Chesbrough had three objections to the second possibility, drainage directly into Lake Michigan. First, it would require a greater sewer length and, consequently, would incur greater cost. Second, he supposed that this plan would seriously affect the water supply, if any sewer outlets were located near the pumping station. At this time, Chicago's water-supply intake was located a short distance offshore at the Chicago Avenue lakefront, approximately one-half mile north of the Chicago River's mouth. Chesbrough did not elaborate on this objection. Third, he felt drainage into the lake would create difficulties in preventing sewer outlet injury during stormy weather, or snow and ice obstruction during winter.[15]

Sewer farming was rejected in part because of the uncertainty whether future fertilizer demand would be sufficient to cover distribution costs. Further, Chesbrough was uncertain as to both the needed reservoir capacity and the expense of building the necessary reservoirs. Finally, Chesbrough thought there would be a great health hazard created by foul odors emanating from sewage spread over a wide surface.

Chesbrough termed the use of a steamboat canal, not yet constructed to flush the sewage into the Des Plaines River, the fourth possibility, "too remote." Although he was aware of the "evils" which would result when raw sewage passed into Lake Michigan, Chesbrough felt it impossible to create an outlet to the southwest. Brown claims, however, that "he appears to have believed that this would be the ultimate solution of the sewerage problem," as, in fact, it was.[16]

> With regard to the fourth plan . . . which would divert a large and constantly flowing stream from Lake Michigan into the Illinois River, it is too remote a contingency to be relied upon for present purposes; besides the cost of it, or any other similar channel in that direction, sufficient to drain off the sewage of the city, would be not only far more than the present sewerage law provides for, but more than would be necessary to construct the sewers for five times the present population. Should the proposed steam-boat canal ever be made for commercial purposes the plan now recommended would be about as well adapted to such a state of things, as it is to the present.[17]

Certainly his plan was readily adaptable to such a scheme. The Sanitary District of Chicago was created in 1889 for the express purpose of implementing this fourth possibility. The Sanitary District then constructed the "proposed steamboat canal," which unquestionably was beyond the means of Chicagoans in 1855.

In December 1855 Chesbrough submitted his plan for Chicago's sewage disposal and drainage. Under this plan, all of the sewage of Chicago's west division, all the sewage of the north division except for the lakefront area, and about one-half the sewage of the south division was deposited in the Chicago River. This sewage passed from the river into Lake Michigan. The dividing line in the south division was State Street; the area east of State Street drained directly into the lake. As the area east of State Street was primarily residential, Chicago's business district was sewered into the river. This district, west of State Street, included the majority of Chicago's packinghouses, distilleries, and hotels. Thus, the river received large quantities of pollutants daily.[18]

The sewers themselves were outstanding phenomena. Brick sewers, three to six feet in diameter, were laid above the ground down the center of the street. Chicago's topography, being unusually flat, was unfavorable to sewer construction. The Chicago River banks were only two feet above the water level. Near the river's north and south branches, the ground level reached a maximum of 10 to 12 feet above the lake. In reality, the task of constructing underground sewers required raising the city.[19] From the beginning, Chesbrough insisted that a high grade was necessary for proper drainage and dry streets. Chicago lacked this high grade, and, thus, the decision to raise the city's level, concomitant with sewer installation, was one which solved the waste disposal and drainage problem in the context of Chicago's existing topography and future necessities.[20]

The Chesbrough plan called for an intercepting sewer system which emptied into the Chicago River. The sewers were to be constructed on the combined system; that is, they would collect sewage from both buildings and streets. This was consistent with the best contemporary thinking and practice. As sewer construction progressed away from the river, the streets had to be raised beneath the sewers. After the sewers were laid, earth was filled in around them, entirely covering them. The packed-down fill provided roadbeds for new, higher streets. These streets were rounded in the center, with gutter apertures leading to the sewer. Such streets would stay dry and could be paved, as contrasted to the mud which had plagued the city previously.

A second facet of Chesbrough's sewerage plan involved dredging the Chicago River. The river had been dredged previously, but it was still too small to handle the anticipated sewage load. Chesbrough planned to widen and deepen the river, as well as to straighten its meandering course. Contracts for this work had been let to the partnership of John P. Chapin and Harry Fox. It was Fox who suggested using the dredgings from the river as fill around the sewers.[21]

It is interesting to digress on the consequences of Chesbrough's plan to raise the city. Where vacant lots existed, they were filled to the new level. A few old frame buildings were torn down, and the lots filled. It proved relatively easy to raise frame buildings to the new level, if the owners could afford it. The city's newer buildings were brick and stone, however, and they were constructed on the old level. These newer buildings would not be torn down, and many of Chicago's homes and offices were to be left "in the hole." When new buildings and sidewalks were constructed on the higher level, Chicago increasingly became a city built on two levels.[22] Legal attempts to maintain the lower level were uniformly settled in favor of the city and its new level.[23]

The raising of brick buildings proved to be a difficult proposition. George Pullman, who later became famous for his "Palace cars," devised and instituted a method to raise brick buildings.[24] Pullman first used his method in connection with the Erie Canal enlargement of the 1850s, so Chesbrough would have known that the problems concomitant with raising the city's grade were surmountable. One of Pullman's biographers described his activities during those years:

> He made contracts with the State of New York for raising buildings on the line of the enlargement of the Erie Canal, which occupied about four years in their completion. At the end of that time, in 1859, he removed to Chicago, and almost immediately entered upon the work, then just begun, of bringing our city up to grade by the raising of many of our most prominent brick and marble structures, including the Matteson and Tremont Houses, together with many of our heaviest South Water street blocks. He was one of the contractors for raising by one operation, the massive buildings of the entire Lake street front of the block between Clark and LaSalle streets, including the Marine Bank and several of our largest stores, the business of all these continuing almost unimpeded during the process — a feat, in its class, probably without a parallel in the world.[25]

The Tremont Hotel was the first brick building which Pullman raised in Chicago. Soon his method was utilized to raise all Chicago's brick buildings from their former muddy level. The work required years. No one knows the cost, but it has been estimated at $10,000,000.[26]

In December 1856 the sewerage commissioners sent Chesbrough to visit several European cities in order to discover if their sewage disposal techniques were relevant to Chicago's needs.[27] Chicago was taking an open-minded approach to this question, and, evidently, the city was prepared to adopt an unconventional approach if it proved to be the best solution. The report of this trip, which Chesbrough submitted in 1858, represents one of the first sanitary engineering treatises.[28] Chesbrough visited and reported on the sewerage of Liverpool, Manchester, Rugby, London, Amsterdam, Hamburg, Paris, Worthing, Croydon, Leicester, Edinburgh, Glasgow, and Carlisle. He concluded that none of these cities furnished an exact criterion to judge the effects of disposing sewage directly into the Chicago River, but he felt their collective experience suggested that it probably would be necessary to keep the river free of sewage accumulations.

Chesbrough ended his report by relating the European experience to Chicago's sewerage needs. Two points which Chesbrough made in this concluding section are worthy of special mention.[29] The first is the experience of Worthing, "a small watering town on the southern coast of England." At one time this town of 5,000 had drained directly into the sea, "but owing to offensive smells caused by this practice, and the consequent injury to the reputation of town as a watering place, upon which its prosperity very much depends," Worthing decided to find an alternative sewerage scheme.[30] Chesbrough concluded that Worthing's experience "shows that the mere discharge of filth into the sea gives no security against its being cast back in a more offensive state than ever, especially when the prevailing winds are toward shore," and that this suggests "the possibility of creating on the lake shore as great a nuisance as would be taken from the river."[31]

Second, Chesbrough included a prophetic paragraph which could serve as a summary to Chicago's sanitary history for a half-century thereafter:

> Under these circumstances it seems advis-

> able to do nothing with regard to relieving the river at present, nor towards carrying out that portion of the plan which provides for forcing water from the lake into it, during the summer months. Should the Canal Company [the Illinois and Michigan Canal] not be obliged to pump enough during warm weather to keep the river from being offensive, it is understood that they would pump as much as they could for a reasonable compensation. This would furnish some criterion by which to judge of the probable effect of a still greater quantity driven in from the lake, according to the plan. The thorough [*sic*] cut for a steamboat canal, to the Illinois River, which the demands of commerce are calling more and more loudly for, if ever constructed, would give as perfect relief to Chicago as is proposed for London by the latest intercepting scheme.[32]

The Chicago River's south branch became quite polluted shortly after sewage was admitted into it. The Illinois and Michigan Canal's pumps, however, utilized south branch water to provide the canal's summit level, and, consequently, the pumps relieved a portion of the river's pollution load. The real significance of Chesbrough's statement lies in the fact that, as early as 1858, Chicagoans recognized the Illinois and Michigan Canal's sewage disposal potential.[33] In following years, the canal's pumps were used regularly to relieve the pollution load. Further, the canal itself was deepened and additional pumps were installed to increase the canal's capacity for handling sewage. Finally, the Chicago Sanitary District was formed in order to construct a new and enlarged canal to service Chicago's waste disposal needs, as Chesbrough had prophesied.

In 1861 the Board of Public Works was formed by incorporating the duties of the Board of Sewerage Commissioners, the Board of Water Commissioners, and other miscellaneous departments. Chesbrough was named chief engineer of this new board and, consequently, inherited the water-supply problem in addition to the waste-disposal problem. His inheritance was the "vicious circle" created by Lake Michigan's dual role as water supplier and eventual waste disposer.

III

Chicago's continued population growth through the decade of the 1850s, the new sewerage works, and the expansion of packinghouses and distilleries had increased the number of pollutants drained into the Chicago River. Lake Michigan soon became fouled by the river's influx, and Chicagoans began to complain of the public water supply's offensiveness and pollution. The existing water intake was a wooden pipe which extended a few hundred feet out into Lake Michigan, one-half mile north of the Chicago River's mouth. In 1859, one of Chicago's water commissioners "proposed to sink a wrought iron pipe . . . one mile out into the lake, to obtain the supply from a point which could not be affected by the river."[34] Chesbrough was asked to study and report on the commissioner's plan, and to do the same on "erecting additional pumping works, in such locality as shall secure a supply of pure water."

Chesbrough's report discussed several methods without making a specific recommendation. Even at this early date, however, he considered a tunnel under the lake to be the most desirable alternative. Chesbrough was not afraid to combine grading, tunneling, and hydraulic principles to create a new water-supply system. When he later offered plans for a lake tunnel, his innovative proposal drew considerable opposition at the start and unmitigated acclaim when it proved successful.

Shortly after its formation in 1861, the Board of Public Works adopted as its goal the acquisition of an unpolluted water supply. Consequently, the board requested Chesbrough to make a canvass of the various water-supply possibilities and to investigate several filtration methods. Chesbrough dismissed the existing filtration methods as inadequate; his studied opinion was that the tunnel method was the most desirable:

> The engineer of the Board [E. S. Chesbrough], after much doubt and careful examination of the whole subject, became more inclined to the tunnel plan than any other, as combining great directness to the nearest inexhaustible supply of pure water, with permanency of structure and ease of maintenance. The possibility, and, in the estimation of many, the probability of meeting

> insuperable difficulties in the nature of soil, or storms, or ice on the lake, were fully considered. One by one the objections appeared to be overcome, either by providing against them, or discovering that they had no real foundation.[35]

Chesbrough continued to explore the tunnel plan's potential. When he had worked out the details, a proposal was submitted to several engineers, all of whom considered the tunnel plan to be feasible. Nevertheless, the 1861 board was against adopting the project. After a new board was elected and additional soil examinations had been made, Chesbrough's water-supply tunnel plan was adopted. The new board reported:

> What is most to be desired by the city is, that the supply should be drawn from the deep water of the lake, two miles out from the present Water Works. . . . The careful investigation of the subject has satisfied us sufficiently to say, that with our present knowledge, we consider it practicable to extend a tunnel of five feet diameter the required distance under the bed of the lake, the mouth or inlet to such a conduit being the outmost shaft, protected by a pier [crib], which will be used in the construction of the tunnel.[36]

In their 1863 report, the Board of Public Works noted that three projects had been considered, any one of which would have afforded Chicago a healthier and better protected water supply. These were (1) a two-mile lake tunnel, (2) a filtering or settling basin, and (3) a one-mile lake tunnel located five miles to the north.[37] The board had two principal objections to the second plan. First, they commented:

> For settling and filtering the water from sediment, we are of the opinion that the basin would be found effective, and would continue to be so, but that for filtration it is not safe to rely upon it. There have been filtering basins of the character in other places. Some of them appear to have continued to work well during long use, and others have failed and become useless.[38]

Second, the board objected to the basin scheme because the water supply intakes would still be in the shallow water close to shore, and would not be located in a deeper point where the water was considered to be better.

Chesbrough's 1863 report acknowledged that the board had considered the three most promising possibilities and had rejected one; he was to assess the remaining two. Almost immediately he dismissed, on the grounds of greater cost, any project which required moving the existing water works, such as the board's third proposal:

> Other projects, such as erecting a new pumping works at Winnetka, or going to Crystal Lake and bringing a supply thence by simple gravitation, as is done for cities of New York, Boston, Baltimore, and Albany, have been considered, but their great cost, as compared with that of obtaining an abundant supply of good and wholesome water at points much nearer the city, is deemed a sufficient apology for not discussing their details here.[39]

Chesbrough concerned himself only with those plans which would bring water from a point two miles east of the existing Chicago Avenue Water Works, and there were two of these:

> Of the plans proposed for obtaining water from the lake, where it will be free from not only the wash of the shore, but from the effects of the river, two classes only have been considered; one, an *iron pipe with flexible joints*; and the other, *a tunnel under the bottom of the lake.*[40]

Although the cost of the iron pipe project was slightly less than the tunnel project, Chesbrough chose between them on other than an initial cost basis:[41]

> In consequence of the possibility of such a pipe being injured by anchors, by the sinking of a heavily loaded vessel over it, or by the effect of an unusual current in the lake moving it from its place, it has been thought preferable to attempt the construction of a tunnel under the bottom of the lake.[42]

His research had convinced him that the tunnel's construction would be less difficult than was generally supposed. Lill and Diversey's brewery, adjacent to the water works, was the site of artesian borings which showed that, between 25 and 100 feet deep, the ground at the lake shore was a clay which was also found on the lake bottom where the water was 25 feet deep. A tunnel could easily be constructed in this type of clay, if it were continuous. Chesbrough was confident that the clay was continuous, but he admitted he was uncertain whether beds of sand might not be interspersed with the clay.[43]

The lake shaft was to be formed by sinking iron cylinders to the desired depth. Chesbrough noted that this was not a difficult problem in that the pneumatic process had been successfully employed on "the Theiss bridge in Hungary, and the railroad bridge across the Savannah River. . . . and recently the Harlem bridge in New York."[44]

In giving cost estimates for the tunnel project's component parts, Chesbrough clearly showed the sources of his research. The principal source was the Thames tunnel, and Chesbrough noted that the first thoughts of most people were the great construction difficulties and "enormous" costs which had been encountered on the Thames project. He was quick to refute these thoughts and countered that "as we have every reason to believe, the clay formation here would shield us from such inroads of water as were met within the Thames tunnel operation."[45] In estimating excavation costs, Chesbrough made the same point: "There is good reason to believe that nothing in the soil here would be more difficult than that through which the sewers of London are sometimes tunneled."[46]

Chesbrough also used the Thames experience, plus that of the Boston Water Works tunnel, to estimate masonry costs. Cribs had been used principally in pier and breakwater construction, and Chesbrough based his crib cost estimates on figures which had been made for a proposed breakwater in Michigan City, Indiana, at the bottom of Lake Michigan.

After reaching his cost estimate for masonry and excavation, Chesbrough compared it with figures which had been reached for other major tunnel projects.[47] In particular, Chesbrough referred to reports from (1) the commissioner of the Troy and Greenfield Railroad, and (2) the Hoosac Tunnel. Included in the commissioner's report was the report of Charles Storrow, who had been sent to investigate European tunnels. Because the tunnels which Storrow had studied were for railroads, they were all much larger than the one which Chesbrough was planning. Therefore, Chesbrough estimated the cost of each tunnel had it been constructed with a five-foot width. From these estimates, he concluded that his cost estimate for the proposed water tunnel was reasonable.

The engineering achievement involved in constructing the water-supply system was no less significant than that represented by Chesbrough's sewer system. As conceived, the task was to dig a shaft near the lake shore to a depth significantly below the lake bottom and then burrow two miles beneath the lake. A similar shaft was to be dug at the lake end and was to be protected by a crib. The engineering problem was to connect the shore and lake points by a straight line 69 feet below the surface of Lake Michigan. Contemporary compasses could not be used since, below ground level, local attraction rendered them inaccurate. To a worker in the tunnel, the only place where the direction of the line drawn between the two shafts could be observed was at the top of either shaft. Consequently, when the engineers attempted to run the tunnel's axis parallel to this imaginary line on the lake's surface, they ran into difficulties affecting the turn from shaft to tunnel.[48]

When the lake shaft was completed, workers were lowered to begin burrowing westward to meet with the other workers burrowing eastward. The tunnel was sloped two feet per mile from the lake end to the shore so that it could be emptied should repairs prove necessary; the water would be shut off at the lake end. Although the methods were primitive — the tunnel was dug entirely by manual labor — it was claimed that the workers caused the two tunnel sections to meet within one inch of achieving a perfectly smooth wall.[49]

Chesbrough's engineering competence was coupled with a sense of economic reality, and these traits combined to insure the reputation he earned in Chicago. His 1863 report contained a section on "plans for improving the Chicago river." Chesbrough knew that moving the water-supply intake farther into the lake would not improve the river's offensive condition. In the 1855 sewerage report, he had argued that flushing canals would be necessary in both the north and south branches to purify the river, and he restated this position in several reports thereafter. By raising the issue once again, Chesbrough not only demonstrated the completeness of his approach, but also what one memorialist called "the characteristic firmness of conviction and modest persistence of Mr. Chesbrough."[50]

As before, Chesbrough's methodology was to enumerate and evaluate the possibilities for improving the river: (1) north and south branch flushing canals, (2) Des Plaines River diversion into the south branch, and (3) drainage southwest into the Illinois River Valley. The first was preferred because Chesbrough felt it was "undoubtedly feasible, would be completely under the control of the city, and there is every reason to believe [it] would be effectual."[51] He considered the second plan "defective" in that the Des Plaines River's flow was least when the Chicago River's pollution was greatest. Although Chesbrough correctly assumed that the third project would be the ultimate solution, he rejected it as "requiring much larger means than the Board can at present control."[52] Chesbrough's attention to Chicagoans' ability to pay established him as a practical man and lent credence to his innovative ideas. His consideration of a sanitary canal connecting the Chicago and Illinois Rivers indicates Chesbrough had learned that water-supply and waste-disposal problems are interdependent and must be solved simultaneously.

IV

Chicago is an urban center which had, and still has, serious water pollution problems. Lake Michigan's present pollution problem is primarily the result of industrial discharge in the Calumet and Indiana Harbor areas and the discharge of inadequately treated sewage by the North Shore Sanitary District (Lake County, Illinois) and several Wisconsin cities. Under normal circumstances, the Metropolitan Sanitary District of Chicago diverts the sewage and the treated effluent from Lake Michigan. Presently, Chicago is meeting its responsibility with respect to Lake Michigan pollution. On the other hand, both the Chicago River and the Illinois River valley are polluted because some industries in the Chicago area still discharge their wastes into the water and the Sanitary District falls short of 100 percent treatment. Approximately 10 percent of the sewage goes untreated at this time, but it is the district's stated objective to achieve 100 percent treatment in the 1970s. While these few sentences oversimplify a very complex situation, the outline is apparent. Chicago must seek outside help to reduce Lake Michigan pollution and the consequent threat to the city's water supply. Chicago and its Cook County suburbs, by themselves, could significantly reduce pollution in the Chicago, Des Plaines, and Illinois rivers.

When faced with Lake Michigan and Chicago River pollution in the 1850s and 1860s, Chicagoans had sought the best solutions available. Cost considerations had entered the argument only in deciding among equally effective methods; Chicagoans were not reluctant to pay the price necessary to secure sanitary conditions. They indebted the city through bond issues and themselves through tax assessments in order to finance these public works. Muddy streets and impure water were manifest physical representations of the city's problems, and solutions to these benefitted the city's residents, individually and collectively. The public's acceptance of an increased tax burden to finance these works must be viewed as public recognition of the problems' dimensions. If the city's water supply had not been conserved, and if the city's natural topography had not been improved, Chicago's urban growth would have been severely limited.

When the pollution problem is explored in a historical context, students will find that the objectives which Chesbrough sought — minimize pollution and obtain a pure water supply — are the same as today's objectives. Nineteenth-century engineers, however, were not faced with the imminent "death" of large bodies of water; they were faced only with protecting urban populations from polluted water supplies.

In studying Chesbrough's works in Chicago, one gets the impression that today's pollution problem is not the result of ignorance as to pollution's effects, but ignorance as to how deadly the pollution load has become. In many cases, techniques first utilized in the 1850s and 1860s are still used today. Although these techniques no longer solve the problems for which they were intended, their inadequacies did not become apparent until recently. Perhaps this is because the demands on these techniques were much less heavy during the earlier period than they now are. Perhaps it is because the engineers of Chesbrough's generation made such dramatic innovations that the declining effectiveness of these techniques and improvements just recently became evident to sanitary engineers and laymen. Or perhaps it is because the 20th-century sanitary engineers who recognize the problem are unable to communicate the necessity for action. While the technology and technicians have been available, an uninformed and apathetic public has not invested sufficient capital in pollution control. Whatever the case, through inaction, the cost of proper treatment has reached a price which may be greater than the public is willing to pay. Unfortunately, the 20th century has been unable to find a sanitary engineer with the same farsightedness in his method, and resoluteness in seeing his proposals adopted, as that characteristic of Ellis Sylvester Chesbrough.

NOTES

1 Benjamin Henry Latrobe, *The Journal of Latrobe* (New York, 1905), p. 98.

2 The engineering education of E. S. Chesbrough began in this company, and he quickly proved an apt student. See *Biographical Sketches of the Leading Men of Chicago*, written by the Best Talent of the Northwest (Chicago, 1868), p. 192; see also *Proc. Am. Soc. Civil Engrs.*, November 1889, *15*: 161.

3 See Daniel H. Calhoun, *American Civil Engineer: Origins and Conflict* (Cambridge, Mass., 1960), p. 38; and Forest Hill, *Roads, Rails and Waterways* (Norman, Okla., 1957), pp. 12 ff.

4 Of particular interest to Chesbrough's later career is the fact that Long had carried out extensive exploratory surveys in the West. In 1816 Long was asked to report to the federal government on the physiographic features in the region of a proposed canal between Lake Michigan and the Illinois River. Although it is only speculation, one wonders how much knowledge of Chicago's topographical peculiarities Long passed on to Chesbrough. It is known that Long prepared detailed reports of his visit to Chicago. See Richard George Wood, *Stephen Harriman Long* (Glendale, Calif., 1966).

5 The major supply of engineers developed from what Calhoun called "the persisting pattern of on-the-job training." The supply provided by the leading scholastic source, the U.S. Military Academy, and the leading civilian source, the New York State canal system, was insufficient. The engineers of that day were active builders; thus, some form of on-the-job training had to be inaugurated to increase the supply and meet the demand. What developed was a hierarchical engineering corps. Lacking any formal education, Chesbrough learned every phase of his job by working his way up the civil engineering hierarchy.

In addition to the books by Hill and Calhoun (see n. 3 above), other recent books which discuss the oral transmission of engineering knowledge are Stephen Salsbury, *The State, the Investor, and the Railroad: The Boston and Albany, 1825–1867* (Cambridge, Mass., 1967); Harry N. Scheiber, *Ohio Canal Era* (Athens, Ohio, 1969); and Ronald E. Shaw, *Erie Water West* (Lexington, Ky., 1966).

6 Chesbrough's role in the Cochituate works is mentioned in a study of the waterworks of Boston, New York, Philadelphia, and Baltimore by Nelson M. Blake (*Water for the Cities* [Syracuse, 1956]).

7 The board was empowered to (1) supervise the drainage and sewage disposal of Chicago's three natural divisions; (2) plan a coordinated system for the future; and (3) issue bonds, purchase lots, and erect buildings implementing their plan. The board's actions were made subject to the Chicago City Council's approval. The act is summarized in several works including G. P. Brown, *Drainage Channel and Waterway* (Chicago, 1894), p. 50.

8 A. T. Andreas, *History of Chicago from the Earliest Period to the Present Time* (Chicago, 1884), I, 191; Bessie Louise Pierce, *A History of Chicago* (New York, 1940), II, 330; Soper, Watson, and Martin, *A Report to the Chicago Real Estate Board on the Disposal of the Sewage and Protection of the Water Supply of Chicago, Illinois* (Chicago, 1915), p. 69, hereafter referred to as the *C.R.E.B. Report.*

9 It is quite possible that Jervis played a significant role in Chicago's choice, for during the early 1850s Jervis was professionally engaged in the Chicago area. Chicago's city fathers would have been aware of Jervis's engineering reputation, and it is probable that he was consulted regarding chief engineer candidates. Because he had worked with Chesbrough just prior to this, it is likely that Jervis gave Chesbrough an excellent recommendation.

In 1881 Chesbrough, serving as consulting engineer of the New Croton Aqueduct, employed Jervis, who discussed the work with Chesbrough daily. This indicates the esteem in which Chesbrough held Jervis, for Jervis was then 86 years old. Chesbrough, at 68 years of age, belonged to another generation.

10 Although the commissioners' report mentions the

public's proposals, it does not indicate what they were, or even which parts of Chesbrough's plan were adapted from these suggestions.

11 Brown, *Drainage Channel*, p. 53.

12 *Report and Plan of Sewerage for the City of Chicago, Illinois*, adopted by the Board of Sewerage Commissioners, Dec. 31, 1855, hereafter referred to as the *1855 Report.* Also quoted in *C.R.E.B. Report*, p. 71. Chesbrough had a systematic approach to costs, but a very general approach to benefits. This evidently was consistent with the approach adopted on other U.S. internal improvement projects. See Lawrence G. Hines, "The early nineteenth century internal improvement reports and the philosophy of public investment," *J. Econ. Issues*, December 1968, *2*: 384–392.

13 Chesbrough planned to pump sufficient lake water into the north and south branches of the Chicago River to flush offensive solid pollutants. He also proposed flushing the sewers as well. See reprinted article, Langdon Pearse, "Chicago's quest for potable water," *Water and Sewage Works*, May 1955, *3*.

14 *1855 Report.* Also quoted in Andreas, *History of Chicago*, I, 191.

15 *C.R.E.B. Report*, p. 72; Pearse, "Chicago's quest," p. 3.

16 Brown, *Drainage Channel*, p. 53. To be precise, the Sanitary District's Sanitary and Ship Canal was the last step in Chicago's adoption of the dilution method. Ultimately, Chicago's growth was sufficient to require sewage treatment in addition to dilution.

17 *1855 Report.* Also quoted in Brown, *Drainage Channel*, p. 55.

18 R. Isham Randolph, "A history of sanitation in Chicago," *J. Western Soc. Engrs.*, October 1939, *44*: 229; Richard S. Kirby and Philip G. Laurson, *The Early Years of Modern Civil Engineering* (New Haven, 1932), p. 234; George W. Rafter and M. N. Baker, *Sewage Disposal in the United States* (New York, 1894), pp. 169–170.

19 *C.R.E.B. Report*, p. 69.

20 The grade which the city council adopted was lower than Chesbrough advocated, but it was sufficiently high to permit the construction of 7–8-foot cellars. The council's decision was to raise the grade to 10 feet on streets adjacent to the river; Chesbrough's higher grade was rejected because the city fathers felt there would be difficulties in locating sufficient fill. See *C.R.E.B. Report*, p. 70.

21 *Biographical Sketches*, p. 482. Fox's company was responsible for almost every topographical improvement in the Chicago area. The company deepened the Chicago River, developed the Chicago Harbor, installed road and railroad bridges, dredged the Illinois and Michigan Canal, and then performed similar services throughout the Midwest.

22 Randolph, "Sanitation in Chicago," p. 229. For many years, some sewers lay wholly above the ground, at the same level or higher than adjoining buildings.

23 "Up from the mud: an account of how Chicago's streets and buildings were raised," compiled by Workers of the Writer's Program, W.P.A. in Illinois for Board of Education, 1941. The raising of cities was relatively common. It was pointed out to me that all of downtown Atlanta was "raised" by the construction of roadways.

24 *Ibid.*

25 *Biographical Sketches*, p. 472. See also Seymour Currey, *Chicago: Its History and Its Builders* (Chicago, 1962), Vol. III; and Stanley Buder, *Pullman: An Experiment in Industrial Order and Community Planning, 1880–1930* (New York, 1967).

26 Lloyd Wendt and Herman Kogan, *Give the Lady What She Wants* (Chicago, 1952), p. 57. Wendt and Kogan do not say how they arrived at this number, and give no reference. Pullman reportedly received $45,000 for raising the Tremont Hotel. At $45,000 per brick building, $10,000,000 will raise over 200 buildings. This is probably an overestimate of the number of buildings raised, but the large number of other expenditures, including Chicago River dredging and legal expenditures, suggest that the $10,000,000 figure is an underestimate.

27 *Report of the Results of Examinations Made in Relation to Sewerage in Several European Cities, in the Winter of 1856–57*, published in Chicago by the Board of Sewerage Commissioners (1858), p. 3, hereafter referred to as the *1858 Report.* See also Randolph, "Sanitation in Chicago," p. 229; Brown, *Drainage Channel*, p. 57.

28 *1858 Report*, p. 92. Chesbrough's memorialist in the *Proc. Am. Soc. Civil Engrs.* (November 1889, *15*: 162), unhesitatingly assessed the significance of Chesbrough's European trip report: "The importance of this report and the influence it exerted . . . can hardly be estimated. At the time the report was written, there was not a town or city in the United States that had been sewered in any manner worthy of being called a system. This being, perhaps, the first really exhaustive study which the subject had received on this side of the water, and Chicago being the first city to adopt a systematic sewerage system, the Chicago system soon became famous and Mr. Chesbrough, for twenty-five years, was the recognized head of sanitary engineering in this country." Modern usage would limit the term "sanitary engineer" to those men involved with water and

sewage treatment. Apparently, the American Society of Civil Engineers at that time considered a sanitary engineer to be a man involved with sanitation works. Thus, while Chesbrough was not concerned with sanitary engineering as that discipline is currently defined, he must be considered a precursor of the modern sanitary engineer and, in fact, was called one by his peers and contemporaries.

29 On this trip Chesbrough visited Zaardam, near Amsterdam, to investigate the possibility of using windmills to pump flushing water for Chicago's sewers; he decided in favor of steam pumps (*1858 Report*, p. 29).

30 *1858 Report*, p. 39.

31 *Ibid.*, p. 93.

32 *Ibid.*, p. 94.

33 Nevertheless, in 1863, the Board of Public Works issued a report on purifying the Chicago River. This is discussed in Brown, *Drainage Channel*, ch. 6. The report recommended the construction of flushing canals along the lines of Fullerton Avenue and Sixteenth Street. Therefore, although the Illinois and Michigan Canal's potential was realized, city officials evidently were not ready to pursue it.

34 Brown, *Drainage Channel*, p. 32.

35 Reported in Brown, *Drainage Channel*, p. 33.

36 *Second Annual Report of the Board of Public Works to the Common Council of the City of Chicago* (April 1, 1863), p. 5, hereafter referred to as *1863 Report*.

37 Cost estimates for each of the projects were as follows: 2-mile lake tunnel exclusive of light house, $307,552; a filtering or settling basin, $300,575; a 1-mile lake tunnel 5 miles to the north, $380,000 (*ibid.*, p. 9).

38 *Ibid.*, p. 8.

39 *Ibid.*, p. 39.

40 *Ibid.*

41 Chesbrough roughly estimated the iron pipe scheme to cost $250,000. The choice seems to have been made on the basis of expected cost. *Ibid.*, pp. 40–41.

42 *Ibid.*, p. 41.

43 *Ibid.*

44 *Ibid.* Originally, Chesbrough planned on four shafts.

45 *Ibid.*, p. 43.

46 *Ibid.*, p. 45.

47 Chesbrough estimated the cost to be $13.54 per linear foot. *Ibid.*, p. 48.

48 J. M. Wing, *The Tunnels and Water System of Chicago* (Chicago, 1874), p. 33.

49 *Ibid.*, p. 76.

50 *Proc. Am. Soc. Civil Engrs.*, November 1889, *15*: 162.

51 *1863 Report*, p. 57. Chesbrough was concerned with a definite planning period which seems to reflect a longer time than the Marshallian short run, and a shorter time than the Marshallian long run.

52 *Ibid.*

22

The Flamboyant Colonel Waring: An Anticontagionist Holds the American Stage in the Age of Pasteur and Koch

JAMES H. CASSEDY

Despite the dramatic European discoveries of the 1870s and 1880s in the medical sciences, the contagionist findings of the dawning age of bacteriology had little substantial impact upon the American medical profession or upon American sanitary practices until the 1890s and afterward. To be sure, occasional pioneer laboratory investigators like George Sternberg, Daniel Salmon, and Theobald Smith were active and were making significant contributions before 1890. Likewise, professors like William H. Welch and T. Mitchell Prudden were slowly spreading the news from Europe through academic circles. Also, a handful of far-seeing health officers like Charles V. Chapin of Providence and Hermann M. Biggs of New York were already looking into the potent implications of the newly proved germ theory for their day-to-day sanitary work. Yet, these pioneers did not find quick success or ready acceptance in the United States for their contagionist conclusions. On the contrary, for most of the last quarter of the 19th century it was the concept of anticontagionism which continued to hold the dominant position in the thinking of American doctors and sanitarians. In the period just preceding its complete eclipse, anticontagionism was enjoying its greatest vogue.[1]

The most conspicuous leader of American anticontagionism during this time was the colorful Colonel George E. Waring, Jr. (1833–1898). A persuasive publicist, Waring became the leading propagandist for the country-wide adoption of every kind of basic sanitary facility, private and public. An energetic and inventive engineer, he became one of the key individuals in the raising of sanitary engineering in the United States to the dignity of a profession. Not a physician, he nevertheless shaped American medical thinking of the period more than almost any doctor did.

Like Edwin Chadwick, Lemuel Shattuck, and certain other 19th-century sanitarians, Waring came into the public health movement by the side door, from an occupation in which he was not originally very much concerned with sanitation. Chadwick had first been a Poor Law bureaucrat, Shattuck a teacher and amateur genealogist. Waring started out as a farmer. After getting what training in agricultural chemistry and engineering was available in ante-bellum Poughkeepsie, New York, he toured Vermont and Maine lecturing upon scientific agriculture. Then, for a few years he was manager of Horace Greeley's farm at Chappaqua, New York. In 1857, when Frederick Law Olmsted and Calvert Vaux planned and started the construction of New York City's great Central Park, Waring joined their staff as an agricultural and drainage engineer. He stayed with this pioneer project through its virtual completion in 1861, at which time he was swept up in the Civil War. He spent four years as a cavalry officer in the Union army.

After the war Waring returned to his career as a scientific farmer, chiefly near Newport, Rhode Island. Elaborating upon his experience in this field, in a series of widely circulated technical books, he developed a reputation as an expert on scientific agriculture.[2] Waring also wrote popular horse stories.[3] As he began to enjoy a substantial income, he started going off on the European tours which were so fashionable. Then, in vivid travel accounts, which were published in *Scribners* and the *Atlantic Monthly*, he told stay-at-home Americans about the

James H. Cassedy is Historian, History of Medicine Division, National Library of Medicine, Bethesda, Maryland.

Reprinted with permission from *Bulletin of the History of Medicine*, 1962, *36*: 163–176.

things he had seen in Europe.[4] By the mid-1870s Waring was well-known to the American general reading public as well as to people in agricultural and engineering circles.

Waring's connection with the public health movement dates from the same immediate post-war period. Stimulated by his reading about the important achievements of English engineers and sanitarians since the 1840s, Waring gradually, as an adjunct to his work in agricultural drainage, became occupied with the whole broad range of problems associated with sanitary engineering. As his activities in this area multiplied, he found the most fertile sort of field for the exercise of both his engineering and his writing talents.

In 1867 Waring published the first of what would become a long list of popular and amazingly influential books, pamphlets, and articles upon various aspects of sanitation. This earliest sanitary publication from his pen, *Draining for Profit and Draining for Health*, was as strongly tinged with the materialism of the Gilded Age as it was with the idealism of the sanitary movement. With the work, however, Waring became established as a successful practical sanitarian.

To retain this reputation and to extend it still further, Waring had to be and was a persuasive sanitary salesman. One of his few failures in this capacity, however, came during this early period. In 1868 he acquired a financial interest in a British-designed earth closet. After getting his old friend Frederick Law Olmsted to help him make some modifications, Waring set about to sell it in the United States. Promotion of the earth closet involved making the most vigorous denunciation of the competing water closet. This Waring did by vividly painting the dangers to health from "sewer gas," the odor which often rose from defective water closets.[5] Despite his extensive propaganda, however, the earth closet did not have a large American sale. Rural people were satisfied with their privy vaults. On the other hand, those city Americans who were beginning to get away from the ancient privies were increasingly insisting upon water closets. This was particularly so as more water closets came on the market and as cities began to get adequate public water supplies. Waring, quickly sensing this trend, bowed to the inevitable and soon gave up his interest in earth closets.

With no apparent serious pangs of principle, Waring now shifted his sales argument so that, from being one of its most outspoken critics, he became the most fervent advocate in America for the universal adoption of the water closet. The important point for him now was not only that the privy vault had to go, but that the water closet had to be properly built and correctly installed. Broadening out quickly, Waring became an ardent crusader against all of the perils to health which were then thought to exist with the presence in the home of faulty bathroom plumbing and in the community of inadequate sewerage systems.

By the mid-1870s this crusade was having considerable influence. In 1875 and 1876 he published, in the *Atlantic Monthly* and *Scribners*, several series of popular articles on the sanitation and sewerage of houses and towns.[6] Henry I. Bowditch of Boston, himself among the most eminent of American sanitarians, was somewhat taken back by the "infinite gusto" with which Waring discussed such subjects on those traditionally polite pages.[7] But the readers of these magazines were convinced and shaken by this strenuous advocacy of sanitary works and better plumbing. In fact, as one highly qualified observer reported, Waring, in these articles, made New Englanders so vividly aware of the dangers to their health of sewer gas that they "feared it perhaps more than they did the Evil One."[8]

Sewer gas thus became to many Americans, as well as to many Europeans and Englishmen of the late 19th century, what miasmata had been to the people of many previous centuries. It came to be regarded as the source of virtually every communicable disease with the notable exception of smallpox. This was essentially the same traditional anticontagionist faith in the filth theory of disease and in environmental sanitation as that upon which Americans had relied since Noah Webster and Benjamin Rush had enunciated the principles before 1800. This was part and parcel of the same "sanitary idea" which Edwin Chadwick and Southwood Smith had devised in England in the 1840s. With cities becoming rapidly larger and progressively dirtier after the Civil War, and with the water closets of the day giving off as much odor as the privies, the anticontagionist sewer gas theory was highly plausible. In fact, as presented by the engineer-publicist Waring, it became as much a part of the armament of the late 19th century American anticontagionist as the "sanitary idea" itself or as the famous "groundwater theory" of disease of the great German scientist Max von Pettenkofer.

Waring's confident rationale of the causation of disease long carried more conviction for Americans than any of the arguments which the squabbling medical profession presented. In fact, during much of this period, a large part of that profession enthusiastically endorsed his views and accepted his leadership. This is not to say that Waring was an original thinker. Rather, he was the synthesizer and popularizer of the views of others. For example, from British medical literature and public health reports of the 1860s, he drew out material for a discussion of the so-called "filth diseases" which was widely circulated five years before John Simon elaborated his famous report on the same subject.[9] For this and other works, in order to bolster his attack on sewer gas (and, of course, to promote the sale of plumbing fixtures), Waring found some of his best arguments in the anticontagionist "pythogenic theory" of the prominent English clinician Dr. Charles Murchison.[10] In 1878, in order specifically to prove that typhoid fever was of spontaneous origin rather than contagious, Waring drew heavily not only upon the writings of Murchison but also on those of Chadwick and Pettenkofer. The resulting essay won for him the annual Fiske Fund Prize of the Rhode Island Medical Society.[11] Such an award, of course, reveals a great deal about the state of empirical medicine at that period. It also points up strongly the extent to which medical theory was then intertwined with the energetic but often dogmatic and a priori propagandizing of the engineer.[12]

In this 1878 essay, Waring argued persuasively, William Budd, Lister, and Koch notwithstanding, that there was "strong presumptive evidence of the correctness of Dr. Murchison's theory of a possible *de novo* origin," not only for typhoid fever but for almost all communicable diseases. He went on to trace disease outbreaks to such causes as a foul-smelling house drain or the proximity of a stagnant ditch. The poison itself, he said, might be due to "the exhalations of decomposing matters in dung-heaps, pig-sties, privy vaults, cellars, cesspools, drains, and sewers; or it may be due (according to Pettenkofer) to the development of the poison deep in the ground, and its escape in an active condition in ground exhalations." The remedy, of course, as he saw it, was obvious, particularly after the successes of the British sanitary revolution. This meant the removal of all of the sources of bad air, particularly through the installation of proper sanitary fixtures — drains, water closets, sinks, cesspools, sewers — all efficiently designed and provided with the elaborate valves necessary to keep sewer gas from coming up into houses. "Those more serious defects which come of ignorantly arranged plumbing work," Waring concluded, "are responsible not only for most of the zymotic diseases appearing in the better class of houses, but in like degree for the generally ailing condition of so many of those who pass most of their days and nights in these houses."[13]

The sanitation of the individual house which Waring advocated was, however, only part of the story. In order fully to prevent disease, according to the sanitary idea (which was also the ancient Hippocratean ideal of pure air, pure water, and pure soil), the entire community had to be cleansed. In the late 19th century several Americans were working on the problems this involved. Pioneers in the water purification experiments of these years included men like James B. Kirkwood of St. Louis, William R. Nichols of the Massachusetts Institute of Technology, the Lawrence investigators of slow sand filtration, and the Providence and Louisville investigators of mechanical filtration. In the evolution of modern sewage and refuse removal techniques, on the other hand, there were such important pioneers as Rudolph Hering of New York, Hiram Mills and his Lawrence associates, Samuel Gray and other Providence sanitarians — and Waring.

The sewerage systems of American cities before the Civil War almost without exception were haphazard and primitive affairs, little more than elongated open drains. This situation continued up to 1880 in most places, despite the development of scientific principles of sewer design and construction in England by Robert Rawlinson around 1850 and the beginning soon afterwards of modern systems in several large European cities. Engineers in Brooklyn, Chicago, Providence, and Boston had, by the 70s, drawn up good plans for sewers in those cities, but the construction of even these was hardly under way.[14] It took a yellow fever epidemic and the salesmanship of George E.

Waring to get American sewer construction really under way.

In 1878 the city of Memphis, Tennessee, was decimated by the worst of a series of devastating yellow fever epidemics. Out of a population of some 40,000 to 50,000, over half, who had heard the chilling news that the disease was coming up the Mississippi River, fled the city. Among those who stayed on, nearly all developed yellow fever, and around 5,000 died from it. Some sanitarians pointed to the catastrophe as an argument for stricter quarantine measures. Waring, however, was one of a number who saw the epidemic as proof that quarantine, which had been tried for years, was not the answer to yellow fever. Beyond any doubt, he pointed out, the reason for the epidemic lay in the incredibly filthy condition of the city, and the only way to prevent future devastation was to institute thorough measures of internal sanitation immediately.

During the wave of public horror which followed the epidemic, President Hayes appointed Waring as one of three special commissioners who were to cooperate with the newly established National Board of Health in devising a plan for the sanitary improvement of Memphis. Never at a loss, Waring was ready with a plan, and he lost no time persuading the rest of the commission and the board to accept it. He then hired himself out to the city of Memphis to carry out a large part of the plan, the building of a complete sewerage system. Waring's energetic carrying out of this project during 1880 was a dramatic demonstration of modern sanitary engineering in the service of the sanitary idea. It provided a powerful impetus to the launching of sewer construction projects in all sizes of communities across the United States.

The Memphis episode was a fortuitous element in Waring's sanitary crusade. Apart from this, however, the episode led to something of a controversy among American engineers as to the respective merits of the two principal kinds of sewerage systems. Waring was the champion of the "separate" system, such as he had installed in Memphis. Not original with Waring, the separate system had been advocated in England by Edwin Chadwick as early as 1842 as a sanitary necessity. During the 1870s, however, Waring had obtained the American rights to the system and had made certain modifications which he had patented. He thus had a substantial personal financial stake in this system, just as earlier he had had a stake in earth closets.[15]

The separate sewerage system, as opposed to the combined system, kept rain water apart from sewage and waste matter. Waring argued for the system such advantages as ease of ventilation, an absence of manholes, the use of smaller pipes, cheapness, and healthfulness.[16] Some other engineers argued equally forcefully the advantages of the combined system. When the argument came to a head in 1880, the American Public Health Association sent the respected engineer Rudolph Hering to Europe to investigate accepted European designs and principles of sewer construction. Hering's thorough report largely settled the controversy. It showed that combined systems were cheaper in densely populated areas such as large cities, while separate systems were cheaper in less settled areas. Technically and from the point of view of health, both were essentially sound.

Hering's report was an important factor in placing American sewer design from this time forward upon an increasingly rational basis. This did not mean, however, that Waring's interests suffered from the report. On the contrary, Waring had received much publicity for his separate or "Memphis" system, and he capitalized upon it to the full. He flooded the market with reports, brochures, and learned papers about the Memphis system and went as far afield as England to talk to sanitarians about his successes.[17] Presumably yellow fever, as a result of this work, had been banished from Memphis.

From this time on, Waring had more professional work than he could handle. He was in great demand as consulting engineer to sewerage projects, not only all over the United States but in Paris, The Hague, and other European cities. He was called in to advise on the sanitary condition of the White House. He was designated a special agent in charge of municipal social statistics for the Tenth Census.

Waring also played a prominent, if unenviable, part in the ill-fated National Board of Health. Elected secretary of that body, he had early recognized the danger to the board from the bitter opposition of Dr. John Hamilton of the Marine Hospital Service. When Congress met in 1884 to decide whether or not to continue the board, Waring testified vigorously in its behalf and against Hamilton's opposition to federal sanitary activity. But Hamilton had played his hand well in getting congressional support, and in this fight he turned out to be the stronger of the two. Never adequately supported, never fully understood by the democracy, and too far ahead of its times, the board was now allowed by Congress to pass out of existence.[18]

In and out of Newport, Rhode Island, during these years, Waring occasionally found time in which to experiment. In one of his experiments which had some significance, he pointed out the role which aeration could play in the processing of sewage.[19] But Waring did not fit well into the part of the patient, careful researcher. More than experimentation, he liked direct action of the sort that he had known ever since his cavalry service in the Civil War. He also liked to associate with the great and near great.

In Newport, therefore, he reveled in his role as sanitary shepherd for the vacation villas of the wealthy tycoons of American business and finance. His exact position was that of Consulting Engineer of the Sanitary Protection Association of Newport. This was a private group, founded in 1878, whose members subscribed for regular expert sanitary inspection and maintenance for their estates. It was an unusual private sanitary initiative, one which was taken in the absence of adequate public sanitary facilities. Waring did much, through his prestige as well as his actual participation, to make the organization a success. Although it had a European model, it was the first of its kind in the United States. During the 1880s and '90s, private groups in a number of other American cities — Brooklyn, Lynn, Trenton, Montreal, and Savannah, among others — followed this Newport initiative and founded similar cooperative sanitary organizations.[20]

Whatever sort of project Waring turned his hand to, he got things done, because he was a forceful and energetic person. He was a man of ingenuity and daring who was completely at home among the strongwilled individualists of these late 19th-century decades. He was also a man who had much of the showmanship and not a little of the sense of civic responsibility which Theodore Roosevelt was already beginning to display. All of these traits were displayed in abundance from 1895 to 1898, when Waring was Commissioner of Street Cleaning for New York City under the anti-Tammany administration of Mayor Strong. As commissioner, Waring aggressively and quickly changed New York streets from among the dirtiest in the world to among the cleanest. To do this, he first formed an advisory committee of civic-minded citizens to help him survey the conditions and to advise him as to remedies. Then he set out to reorganize his department in order to raise its morale and efficiency. He took the personnel out of politics, put them all into white duck uniforms, and then put them on a career basis, with a for then novel Board of Arbitration to settle routine employee problems. He renovated the department's street-cleaning and garbage-collecting equipment. To obtain efficiency in his operation, he insisted that New Yorkers separate their refuse into three categories: garbage, ashes, and rubbish. Finally, in the East Side slum areas, he organized dozens of boys' and girls' clubs, whose members were to promote the city's cleanliness by reporting rubbish thrown into the streets and by themselves conducting cleanups of school yards and tenements. The children met in weekly meetings, wore special badges, and marched proudly with the regular street-cleaning battalions in the annual parade of New York's "white wings" or "white angels," an event which Waring had begun.

Some of these innovations did not last beyond Waring's term as Street Commissioner. The basic changes, however, constituted a permanent improvement of New York's street cleaning and garbage collection services. This provided a notable example for other cities and towns across the United States.[21]

Waring cleaned up the streets of New York in the name of health, just as his previous work had been in the name of health. To the anticontagionists of the day, he had long since become the highest type of hero of his age, the "apostle of cleanliness, the scourge of dirt."[22] For them, what he had done in New York was an essential step in applying the sanitary idea to the city. They followed him all the way in his Chadwickian belief that any kind of filth, anything that was dirty, was a dangerous source of possible disease and must be removed.

There were also others in New York during the 90s who were concerned with the prevention of disease. But these persons did not approach the problem through street cleaning. These others were contagionists who were caught up in the early enthusiasm of the age of bacteriology. T. Mitchell Prudden was one of the teachers who was showing the new generation of medical students the dangers of germs. Hermann M. Biggs was fighting tuberculosis through anti-spitting ordinances, careful medical inspection, and adequate hospitalization. William H. Park had been devising laboratory tests to determine the presence in individuals of the germs of diphtheria. In 1893 the New York City Department of Health built a diagnostic laboratory so it could make these tests on a routine basis. It also began to manufacture the new antitoxin to try to prevent and cure diphtheria.

All of these activities were beginning to undermine the position of New York anticontagionists. But New York was a large place. There was still plenty of room, during the 1890s, for both camps, for both beliefs. In fact, this was true not just in New York but everywhere, at least as long as yellow fever remained a mysterious disease apparently caused, so far as anyone could tell, by spontaneous generation in filth. The resolution of this mystery soon after 1900 constitutes an ironic final commentary upon Waring's career.

In 1898, with the return of Tammany Hall to power in New York City, Waring was out of a job. This was the year of the Spanish-American War. After the cessation of hostilities in Cuba, the United States army commanders were gravely concerned with dangers from yellow fever to the troops who would for several years have to occupy Havana and other cities of the island. To meet this serious threat from disease, the army enlisted an outside commission of experts to select camp sites and make suggestions for their proper sanitation. The commission was also charged with making a thorough investigation of the sanitary condition of Havana and other Cuban cities and recommending the measures necessary to stamp out yellow fever and other communicable diseases.

Waring was chosen chairman of the commission and went to Cuba early in October of 1898. In his short stay of just under three weeks he learned everything that he wanted to know. It was, of course, no news to anyone that Havana was one of the filthiest cities in the western hemisphere. Waring merely confirmed that there were virtually no sewers; that garbage, rubbish, and feces were thrown freely into the streets; that public markets were nauseatingly foul; that house privies were so neglected that their contents frequently flowed over into yards and wells; that the street cleaning department had virtually no money; and that there was no systematic plan for garbage collection or disposal. He noted that there was a good water supply to the city but that there were extensive marshes which promoted bad malarial conditions.

To Waring, the answer to these conditions was an obvious one. For the sum of ten million dollars, he said, he could eliminate yellow fever from Havana. He would construct a complete sewerage system, pave all of the streets, drain all of the marshes. He would build a municipal garbage incinerator, establish sanitary markets and abattoirs, eliminate all privy vaults, and introduce water closets universally. He would reorganize the department of public cleansing and put it upon an efficient basis.[23]

His survey completed, Waring left Cuba before the end of October. On the way back to the United States he wrote up the first draft of his report and recommendations. The day after his arrival in New York he fell ill. Four days later, he died of yellow fever.

Many people mourned Waring's untimely end. One observer argued that he had been a victim of American expansionism. Another wrote, still more aptly, that "his death at the hands of the king of dirt diseases gives a mournful but most impressive emphasis to the lesson which he taught so earnestly of the kinship of dirt and disease."[24] Feeling much the same way as this second commentator, the army commanders in Cuba acted quickly upon Waring's recommendations. Everything that he had considered necessary for the health of the troops was done. In the process Havana was changed in a few months from one of the dirtiest into one of the cleanest cities in the Americas. It was a transformation which excited the admiration of the world. It was widely hailed, moreover, as a great triumph for the anticontagionist viewpoint, for the sanitary idea. The success of Memphis was clearly being repeated in Havana.

Unfortunately for the partisans of anticontagionism, despite all that had been done, yellow fever remained rampant in Havana. As never before, people began to realize that, despite its many salutary effects, cleanliness by itself was not the answer. The army now had to start all over again. This time, however, it chose a totally different kind of approach. Now it was the Yellow Fever Commission, under the laboratory-oriented Major Walter Reed, which moved in. Quickly, the commission sifted the available facts and theories, and ultimately it took up the little-regarded mosquito hypothesis of Carlos Finlay. Inevitably, new heroes, who exposed themselves alternately to filth and to mosquito bites, were made in the control wards of the commission. And, inexorably, the participants moved forward to a conclusion. Filth as such was shown to play no causative role in the disease. Instead, the mosquito known as the stegomyia was correctly singled out and proven to be the carrier of the yellow fever poison. Finally, then, it was up to William Crawford Gorgas and his engineers to search out and destroy every breeding place of the stegomyia. This done, yellow fever was eradicated and the American forces were safe in Havana.[25]

Even before the Reed Commission's findings were published, alert and scientifically trained health officers of the new era (Charles V. Chapin of Providence stood out among them) were already proclaiming "the end of the filth theory of disease."[26] But the commission's work drove the "coffin nail" into the remnants of the anticontagionists' belief. After 1900, no great new champion of the filth theory emerged in the United States to take Waring's place. The laboratory researchers and scientific public health men of the age of bacteriology in a few years enjoyed an almost complete dominance in national public health circles. The filth theorists who remained, a dogmatic and narrowly unprogressive minority for the most part, could only mutter ineffectually and fade into the backwash of the public health movement. There, at local levels, as Martin Arrowsmith would find out, they delayed the spread of the new scientific doctrines and techniques for some years. But they would never emerge from the backwash. Waring had died just in time, while he still had valid reason to think that he was right. His followers found themselves in the untenable position of holding inflexibly to an idea which had been shown to be only half right. Filth in the form of human excrement certainly caused disease, but the laboratory men pointed out that there was no direct connection between infectious disease and such general dirty things as decaying potatoes, bad smells, untidy streets, or trash in vacant lots.

With his view discredited, Waring quickly came to be remembered by the laboratory men chiefly as one of those who, despite the more accurate knowledge about the infectious diseases which flowered after 1875, had still clung to the crude ideas of an earlier age.[27] In the far-sweeping age of bacteriology, the engineer could no longer influence medical theory as Waring had done unless he were also a precise laboratory scientist.

Most of the laboratory men of the early 20th century could not see that Waring, like his master Edwin Chadwick and the other filth theorists, had in fact made a great contribution to mankind in carrying through with the sanitary idea. They could not see that the insistence upon sewers, pure water, water closets, and clean streets for our cities was a major civilizing influence. During the early reign of the laboratory men, the vague general approach to disease through the eradication of dirt on the basis of a priori reasoning was considered to be imcompatible with the precise a posteriori approach of specific measures for particular diseases.[28] It would be 20 or 30 years or more before health officials could begin again to see value to the public health in both approaches. With such a revised perspective, there would be a better chance, perhaps, for an effective social medicine to take hold.

NOTES

1 This is by no means an original finding. The student of this subject will already be familiar with articles by such authors as Erwin Ackerknecht and Phyllis A. Richmond.

2 *Elements of Agriculture*, originally published in 1854 as a "book for young farmers," was reissued in 1868. In 1869 Waring published a revision of W. S. Courtney's, *The Farmers' and Mechanics' Manual. Waring's Book of the Farm*, which first appeared in 1877, went through several editions. In 1881, he published *The Saddle Horse*, a training and riding guide.

3 *See*, for instance, *Whip and Spur* (1875), *Ruby* (1883), and *Vix* (1883).

4 As subsequently published in book form, these included *A Farmer's Vacation* (1876), *The Bride of the Rhine* (1878), and *Tyrol and the Skirt of the Alps* (1880).

5 G. E. Waring, Jr., *Earth Closets: How to Make Them and How to Use Them* (New York: Tribune Association, 1868); and *Earth Closets and Earth Sewage* (New York: Tribune Association, 1870).

6 These articles were quickly collected and published in book form: *The Sanitary Drainage of Houses and Towns* (New York: Hurd and Houghton; Cambridge, Mass.: Riverside Press, 1876), was the most influential and went through several editions. Others included *The Sanitary Condition of City and Country Dwelling Houses* (New York: D. Van Nostrand Co., 1877) and *Village Improvements and Farm Villages* (Boston: J. R. Osgood & Co., 1877).

7 Henry I. Bowditch, *Public Hygiene in America* (Boston: Little, Brown, 1877), *passim*.

8 Charles V. Chapin, "Science and public health," in *Papers of Charles V. Chapin, M.D.*, (New York: Commonwealth Fund; London: Oxford Univ. Press, 1934), p. 50.

9 Waring, *Earth Closets and Earth Sewage, passim*; John Simon, *Filth Diseases and Their Prevention* (Boston: J. Campbell, 1876).

10 Murchison's most famous work was *A Treatise on the Continued Fevers of Great Britain* (London: Parker, Son, and Bourn, 1862).

11 Waring, "The causation of typhoid fever," in *First Annual Report of the State Board of Health of the State of Rhode Island* (Providence, 1879), pp. 159–173.

12 Almost 20 years later Waring was still accorded an honored place in American medical circles. In 1896, for instance, he delivered the "annual address in medicine" at Yale University, a talk on the subject of "The proper disposal of sewage."

13 Waring, "Causation of typhoid fever," pp. 159, 161, 163, 172.

14 For further historical details on these developments, see Rudolph Hering, "Sewage and solid refuse removal," in *A Half Century of Public Health*, ed. M. P. Ravenel (New York: American Public Health Association, 1921), pp. 181–196; G. W. Fuller et al., "Historic review of the development of sanitary engineering in the United States during the past one hundred and fifty years: a symposium," *Tr. Am. Soc. Civil Engrs.*, 1928, *92*: 1207–1324; and W. P. Gerhard, "A half century of sanitation," *Am. Architect & Bldg. News*, 1899, *63* (Nos. 1209, Feb. 25; 1210, March 4; 1211, March 11): 61–63, 67–69, 75–76.

15 Gerhard, "A half century of sanitation," p. 67.

16 Waring, "The sewering and draining of cities," *Public Health: Papers and Reports*, 1880, *5*: 35–40.

17 Gerhard, "A half century of sanitation," *passim*.

18 For a further account of this controversy, see Wilson G. Smillie, *Public Health: Its Promise for the Future* (New York: Macmillan, 1955), pp. 337–338.

19 Kenneth Allen, "Remarks," in Fuller et al., "Historic review," p. 1294; also Waring, *The Purification of Sewage by Forced Aeration* (Newport, R.I.: F. W. Marshall, 1895).

20 See Horatio R. Storer, "Sanitary protection in Newport," *Public Health: Papers and Reports*, 1881, *6*: 209–216.

21 For details of Waring's work in New York, the reader may consult the various meagre biographical sources, most important of which are the following three articles: "George E. Waring, Jr.," *D.A.B.*, XIX, 456–457; William Potts, "George Edwin Waring, Jr.," obit. in *The Charities Review* (N.Y.), 1898, *8*: 461–468; and Albert Shaw, *Life of Col. George E. Waring, Jr.* (New York: Patriotic League, 1899). Despite its title, the Shaw pamphlet is far from a thorough biography. Rather, it consists of a short (10 page) tribute, together with excerpts from several newspaper obituaries. More valuably, however, it includes a résumé of Waring's uncompleted report on Havana, together with a short paper written by Waring in 1897, "New York, AD 1997 — a prophecy." This last is a short but interesting projection into the future, somewhat in the tradition of *Utopia, New Atlantis*, or more particularly, Benjamin Richardson's *Hygeia: A City of Health*, which had been having a considerable vogue for two decades among both contagionists and anticontagionists.

22 Quoted in Shaw, *Life of Col. Waring, Jr.*, p. 31. Also see Potts, "George Edwin Waring, Jr.," p. 462.

23 For details of Waring's report on Havana, see résumé in Shaw, *Life of Col. Waring, Jr., passim*.

24 Quoted, *ibid.*, pp. 30, 31.

25 For the full dramatic story of the Reed Commission and its work, there is still no better source than Howard Kelly, *Walter Reed and Yellow Fever* (New York: McClure, Phillips & Co, 1906).

26 Charles V. Chapin, "The end of the filth theory of disease," *Popular Science Monthly*, 1902, *60*: 234–239.

27 *Ibid.*, p. 239.

28 See James H. Cassedy, "Dr. Charles V. Chapin and the modern public health movement" (Ph.D. dissertation, Brown Univ., 1959), ch. 17.

Hygiene

The importance of personal hygiene in maintaining good health is beyond dispute today. The great majority of early Americans, however, rarely bathed and showed little appreciation for fresh air, sunlight, or exercise. Their eating habits, including the consumption of gargantuan amounts of meat, kept many stomachs continually upset. Fruits and most vegetables seldom appeared on the table, and butter or lard often saturated the food that did appear. It is no wonder that one writer called dyspepsia "the great endemic of the northern states."

In the 1830s Sylvester Graham launched his popular health crusade. To preserve health, Graham advocated subsisting "entirely on the products of the vegetable kingdom and pure water," while abstaining from all harmful activities like drinking, smoking, and masturbating. Since stimulating substances were thought to arouse the sexual passions, the adoption of a bland, meatless diet seemed the best way to control these unwholesome urges. Graham lectured throughout the country, winning a large following among those Americans who had lost faith in the more traditional methods of preserving health. Above all he sought to establish hygiene on scientific principles, as James C. Whorton points out in his essay on vegetarianism, the central plank in Graham's platform.

For health reformers, cleanliness ranked next to meatlessness. Graham himself recommended a sponge bath every morning upon rising or, better still, the "exceedingly great luxury" of standing in a tub and pouring a tumbler of water over the whole body. At the time, according to Harold Donaldson Eberlein, even the most fastidious Americans saw little reason for a healthy person to bathe all over. But despite Graham's efforts, and the availability of bathtubs with attached plumbing after the 1820s, the notion of regular bathing caught on slowly. A survey conducted in 1877 for the Michigan state board of health revealed that, although the "better" classes customarily took a weekly bath, among mechanics and farming families "the regular and systematic use of the bath has not come into general appreciation."

A third concern of health reformers was women's fashionable clothing, which was often both morally and physiologically objectionable. Fashionable layers of long skirts and petticoats, sometimes weighing as much as fifteen pounds, swept floors and streets, while vise-like corsets tortured midriffs into exaggerated hourglass shapes, resulting in frequent fainting and internal damage. About 1850 a New York woman, Elizabeth Smith Miller, broke with fashion and donned a short skirt over pantaloons. Her unusual attire attracted little attention until she met Amelia Bloomer, who began advocating the costume in her temperance magazine. For a short time a number of prominent feminists wore the so-called "Bloomer," but its greatest popularity came in the Midwest, where reformers continued to promote it into the 1870s.

Whatever the merits of these specific 19th-century reforms, Graham's movement did focus considerable attention on the intimate relationship between health and life-style, a relationship for which 20th-century science has accumulated a large body of evidence. Although concern for health sometimes relates more to fad than science, people who do not abuse their bodies live demonstrably longer and healthier lives than those who do.

23

"Tempest in a Flesh-Pot": The Formulation of a Physiological Rationale for Vegetarianism

JAMES C. WHORTON

As if the presidential campaign of 1860 were not momentous enough, the eminent hydropath Russell Trall complained to a Philadelphia audience that neither Lincoln, nor Douglas, nor the other contenders had yet "broached any subject so vitally important to the voters, as that of beef *versus* bread, hog *v.* hominy, mutton *v.* squash, . . . [or] chicken *v.* whortleberries."[1] From any other assembly, the charge would have drawn only hoots and laughter, but Trall was speaking before the American Vegetarian Society, many of whose members had been engaged for up to a quarter of a century in the struggle against a form of slavery which they thought was the most degrading and ruinous of all — that imposed by the appetite for flesh food. This conflict, to be sure, was ancient, but during the 1830s through the 1850s a new strategy had been imposed, a new emphasis which was reflected in the title of Trall's address, *The Scientific Basis of Vegetarianism.* Historically Pythagoreans, the 19th century's preferred synonym for vegetarians, had relied on religious and philosophical principles to carry the battle against beef and mutton, with the evidence of science being given a place only in the rear guard, if at all. But when the American Vegetarian Society was founded in 1850, the list of resolutions adopted, while including religious and humanitarian statements, began with the declaration that "comparative anatomy, human physiology, and . . . chemical analysis . . . unitedly proclaim . . . that not only the human race may, but *should,* subsist upon the productions of the vegetable kingdom."[2]

This reordering of priorities was the consequence of the evaluation of diet made by the health reform or Grahamite movement of America's Jacksonian era.[3] Sylvester Graham (1794–1851), Presbyterian minister turned lecturer turned hygiene crusader, stumped throughout the northeastern and New England states during the 1830s and 1840s, urging a regimen of unrefined flour, daily exercise, cold baths, hard mattresses, loose clothing, and tight morals. Those who rallied about Graham were mostly laymen, but a number of physicians also joined the cause. Most prominent among the physicians were William Alcott (1798–1859), who was also an educator of note and the most active publicist among health reformers, and Reuben Mussey (1780–1866), a well-known surgeon and professor first at Dartmouth College at Hanover, New Hampshire, and then at Miami Medical College in Cincinnati, Ohio. Alcott, Mussey, and others in the crusade differed with Graham and with one another on occasional points of hygiene, but overall their ideas were sufficiently close to justify the period's use of "Grahamism" to denote health reform.

By whichever name, the movement was to be largely absorbed by the 1850s into the irregular medical system of hydropathy. In this way the health reform program came to be espoused by hydropathic practitioners such as Russell Trall (1812–1877), a New Yorker who had earned the M.D. degree, but had then become disenchanted with heroic drug therapy and turned to water treatment and hygiene.[4] There was thus variety in this band of lay and medical students of physiology, but the group as a whole, with the possible exception of Mussey, could only appear to professional physiologists and the majority of regular physicians as a bunch of meddling amateurs.

JAMES C. WHORTON is Associate Professor, Department of Biomedical History, School of Medicine, University of Washington, Seattle, Washington.

Reprinted with permission from the *Journal of the History of Medicine and Allied Sciences*, 1977, *32*: 115–39.

These were the men, however, who advanced vegetarianism in the United States to the point where it emerged from general health reform as a distinct hygienic movement in its own right in the 1850s. But even then, and to a degree ever after, vegetarianism was dominated by the philosophy of Grahamism. It was a philosophy with the surface appearance of a hodgepodge of enthusiasms — for scientific progress, Christian perfectionism, romantic primitivism, and educational innovation especially — and which seemingly contradicted the reformers' insistence that living should be kept simple. Nevertheless, in practice it operated quite smoothly. The determinants of hygienic good or evil were simply two: the conviction, drawn from the writings of the renowned French physician François Broussais, that overstimulation, producing a local irritation which can spread through the nervous system to affect any area of the body, is the seat of all disease; and the reformers' understanding of Christian morality. Grahamites shared the contemporary confidence of the agreement between science and religion, and went beyond even temperance advocates and sanitary reformers in their assertion that health and morality must be related. Health reformers perceived such deep mutual reinforcement between physiology and Christianity that they fully expected scientific issues to be susceptible to moral analysis. Their "Christian physiology" was an interpretation of the latest physiological data in such a way as to demonstrate that good hygiene always conforms with Christian behavior.[5]

For no aspect of hygiene was this demonstration more important than for diet. Grahamites recognized food as the most frequent stimulant of the body, and regarded meat as especially stimulating. At the same time they believed certain Old Testament passages denied flesh as food for man, and that the New Testament's spirit was irreconcilable with the brutality of the slaughterhouse. Vegetable diet was thus identified as the fundamental reform, the one which must precede all others, and which would ultimately lead to not just physical renewal but to social and religious elevation as well. In the end, health reformers carried the contemporary optimism about human perfectibility to the extreme by proclaiming hygiene to be the key to the Kingdom of Heaven. Since vegetarianism was the key to hygiene, the demonstration that the most humane of diets was also the most healthful was imperative. The whole gospel of hygienic regeneration rested upon this point.

Scientific objectivity in this demonstration was impossible. Grahamites saw themselves not as active scientists but as educators, as interpreters of science to the public. Their investigations were not conducted in the laboratory but in the library where they combed the literature of physiology for information relevant to practical hygiene. Directed by the faith that hygiene harmonizes with morality, they selected two types of experiments and ideas as worth publicizing. First, those which clearly indicated the superiority of vegetable diet could be advertised at face value. Second, those which seemingly denied this superiority had to be reassessed and shown invalid. This use of science as grist for an ideological mill by people generally lacking in advanced physiological study stirred the wrath of physiologists and physicians. The result was a series of exchanges aptly characterized by one participant (of nom de plume Emancipated) as "a tempest in a flesh-pot!"[6] As was unintentionally implied, the tempest did not constitute a major chapter in the history of physiology, but its examination may serve to define further the character of the health reform movement. Nowhere is the determination to have the new science ratify the New Testament clearer than in the early formulation of a physiological rationale for vegetarianism.

As the name "Pythagoreans" suggests, vegetarianism has an ancient history, but its assumption of the status of a movement which aroused much public interest and made some conversions predates health reform by only a few decades."[7] After having languished for centuries, vegetarianism was reinvigorated in the late 1700s by the stimulus of humanitarianism. Especially in England was the concern for fellow man extended to fellow creature, and blended with a romantic sentimentality which at times made vegetarian appeals embarrassingly maudlin. The title of the first of these appeals effectively described the orientation of virtually all pre-Grahamite vegetarian literature: *The Cry of Nature: or, an Appeal to Mercy and to Justice, on Behalf of the Persecuted Animals*.[8]

The argument for the humaneness of vegetable diet was often buttressed in such works with references to scripture, particularly to Genesis 1:29, which seemed to state clearly that the original diet appointed for humankind by God did not include flesh.[9] Such passages could, in fact, promote a primarily religious vegetarianism, and it was in this form that the Pythagorean diet was introduced to America. The Bible Christian Church, a fundamentalist sect originating in England at Manchester in the early 1800s, held to vegetable diet as the only one sanctioned by scripture. In 1817, a minister in the church, William Metcalfe, led a band of Bible Christians to Philadelphia and began preaching vegetarianism to the American public. Metcalfe is supposed to have influenced Graham to give up flesh food, though greater significance might be attached to the influence Graham and Alcott exerted on Metcalfe. Under their tutelage he came to place nearly as much weight on the physical as on the spiritual wickedness of flesh food. In advanced years he even completed a homeopathic medical education to gain expertise in the physiology of diet.[10]

Metcalfe's progress symbolized the transformation of vegetarianism from a moral to a physical preoccupation, but the process began much earlier. There was a great outpouring of popular literature on hygiene in the 18th and early 19th centuries, and while it is true that the bulk of the advice on diet was quantitative, urging control of the amount of food, there were occasional attempts to draw qualitative distinctions favorable to a vegetable diet. Two figures did particular service in this line: the Falstaffian London physician George Cheyne, whose publications in the 1830s and 1840s revealed how the more digestible and less inflammatory vegetable diet had salvaged the "crazy Carcase" he had abused in youth;[11] and William Lambe, a London practitioner of the early 1800s, who regarded animal food as a "habitual irritation." Lambe also insisted on the argument which became the cornerstone of vegetarianism's physiological edifice, that the human body lacks the carnivore's claws, teeth, and short intestinal tract and therefore must have been designed for a herbivorous diet.[12]

The reception given these ideas by his medical colleagues, Lambe admitted, was a contempt that was "immeasurable," yet there were some laymen who reacted favorably. No doubt some converts overreacted, presaging the readiness of Grahamites to blame all the evils of the world on flesh food. England's irrepressible poet Percy Shelley excelled here, including in his indictment of meat the charge that it was responsible for the bloody excesses of the French Revolution. Shelley nevertheless had also devoted considerable time to the study of natural science, including chemistry, anatomy, and medicine, and acknowledged the usefulness of these for his case. Some of his most romantic praise of vegetable diet was in tribute to its physical benefits: "Above all, he [the vegetarian] will acquire an easiness of breathing . . . with a remarkable exemption from that powerful and difficult panting now felt by almost everyone after hastily climbing an ordinary mountain."[13]

Realistically, the uphill battle had to be fought by vegetarians, for Cheyne and Lambe, even Shelley, notwithstanding, the overwhelming force of medical belief was on the side of a flesh diet. It was general opinion among hygienists that the stimulus of meat was essential for strength and endurance, that animal food was more easily digested than vegetable, and that food already "animalized," hence closer in nature to human flesh, could be more easily assimilated.[14] In the minds of nearly all writers on health, the danger of meat seemed only to be excess quantity. The ancient watchword of hygiene — temperance — still so dominated thought that quantitative considerations strongly subordinated qualitative ones. Gluttony, no matter what the food, seemed the great abuse, and though too much meat was believed injurious because of its tendency to produce plethora and internal putrefaction, the total elimination of meat seemed unphilosophical extremism. Dietitians, quite simply, were inclined to agree with the wit who jeered,

> "Abstain from flesh!" . . . Pythagorean,
> Feed *thou* on *pulse* — *roast beef* feed we on.[15]

Clearly, however strong a case one might build against flesh-eating on philosophical, religious, or humanitarian grounds, so long as physiology indicated that meat was required for health, vegetarianism could not be conscientiously supported or even seriously considered. And while this burden of proof had been recognized before the 1830s, no vegetarians had shouldered it so eagerly or made it so central an element of strategy as the health reformers were to do. The new thrust of vegetarianism was identified by Alcott in response to a confession sometimes made by the more liberal physiologists, that it was *possible* for adequate vitality to be achieved on a vegetable diet. "We do not ask him to grant more," Alcott gloated. "If man is as well off on vegetable food as without it, we have moral reasons of so much weight to place against animal food . . . sufficient to lead to its rejection."[16] This announcement of the moral superiority of vegetarianism contained an implication which veiled the animating bias of health reform reasoning. It suggested that the morality of diet must wait upon the determination of its healthfulness, and that the slaughter of animals must be accepted if flesh is found physically essential. But the deck was already stacked against flesh-eating. Alcott's confidence flowed from his awareness that a meat diet was immoral and that the laws of physiology could not conflict with those of morality since they had the same author. To defend an immoral diet as physically superior would be to brand God a bungler. This preconception of nature impelled the health reformers to demonstrate more than the physiological equality of a vegetable with a mixed diet. God would not compromise in His creation, and if a fleshless regimen were morally best, it must be physically best. Could humankind be healthfully omnivorous? "Indeed, strange that the Creator . . . should have so signally failed to adapt the organization of his creatures to the purposes of his *wisdom* as displayed in his word."[17] Could a meat eater be Christian? "How," came the reply, "can a man serve God with a stomach full of grease?"[18] The religious need to establish vegetarianism as physiologically *better* than a meat diet is what spurred health reformers to their dietetic exaggerations and peculiar readings of physiology, and what made their disagreements with physiologists a tempest instead of a more reasoned scientific debate.

The agitation of vegetarians was further insured by the refusal of most physiologists to take them seriously. It seemed the dietetic system was being judged by the eccentricities of its proponents, rather than by its scientific merits, and a spirit of stubborn defiance was kindled by the personal affronts delivered by physiologists. In truth, raillery was more common than reason in criticisms of the vegetable regimen, and lay and medical journals alike had much merriment at vegetarians' expense. "Emasculation is the first fruit of Grahamism," charged one; among the "lean-visaged cadaverous disciples" of Graham, revealed another, "the gentlemen resemble busts cut in chalk," the ladies "mummies preserved in saffron"; a Grahamite was described by a third observer using frontier dialect.

> [He] looked like a full-blown bladder arter some of the air had leaked out, kinder wrinkled and rumpled like, and his eyes as dim as a lamp that's living on a small allowance of ile. He puts me in mind of a pair of kitchen tongs, all legs, shaft and head, and no belly; a real gander gutted looking creature, as hollow as a bamboo walking cane, and twice as yaller.[19]

Such insults were doubly painful for being partly true, as most health reform devotees had adopted the system to treat their invalidism, and not all had recovered very quickly. Nevertheless, some fine examples of strength and endurance had been produced by the vegetable diet, and to deny these was to display ignorance of the true characteristics of a healthy body. Vegetarians appeared emaciated only because flesh eaters were plethoric, "portly gentlemen, with forms that might have shamed Jack Falstaff, and visages which would provoke the envy of a turkey-cock."[20] In one of the impracticable thought experiments of which he was so fond, Graham submitted that "if a very fat man, in the enjoyment of what is ordinarily considered good health, and a lean man in good health," be confined and left to starve, "the lean man will lose in weight much more slowly, and live several days longer than the fat man."[21] The hope of vengeance behind this experiment was but scantily disguised; elsewhere the need to retaliate for meat eaters' calumnies found unrestrained expression. A list of the kinds of people who ought to use animal food included not just "those who wish to become corpulent," and "those who wish to have their fluids continually in a half-putrid state," but also "idiots," and "those who wish to become stupid, like idiots."[22] If dietary dogmatism was likely in view of the rigidity of the health reformers' guidelines for theorizing, it was made inevitable by their desire for personal vindication.

The combination of physiology and pique was evident from the opening of hostilities between the two groups of dietitians. In 1835 the Boylston Medical Committee's prize was awarded to a New

Hampshire physician, Luther Bell, for his essay discussing "What diet can be selected which will ensure the greatest probable health and strength to the laborer in the climate of New England?" At the outset, Bell admitted he was writing to counter the "schemes of Pythagorean or Utopian dreamers," and at the conclusion proposed that the mixed diet of most New England laborers was quite healthful, containing "no grand errors" and requiring "no radical change."[23] In reaching these standard judgments, however, Bell had deviated from the usual justification for a diet including meat. The traditional argument was that while human teeth and alimentary organs were closer in structure to those of vegetable eaters than to those of flesh eaters, they were nevertheless identical to neither; man "preserves a medium between the complicated apparatus of herbivorous, and the simple apparatus of carnivorous animals, and is, therefore, *omnivorous*."[24] Bell regarded this as quibbling on one point and missing a more significant one. Human anatomy was too close to that of frugivorous animals to allow classification as intermediate. "But the only conclusion which ought to be drawn from this similarity is, that he is designed to have his food in about the same state of mechanical cohesion, requiring about the same energy of masticatory organs as if it consisted of fruits, etc. alone."[25] In other words, anatomy indicated what it was possible to eat, not what was necessary, and for humankind the possibilities were almost limitless. The distinction overlooked by vegetarians comparing human anatomy to animals' was that man was more than an animal. He possessed the faculty of reason which would not have been bestowed by God except to be used. Through the application of reason to the art of cookery, many kinds of foods, animal as well as vegetable, could be rendered masticable by frugivorous teeth. Thus the natural diet of man consisted of any food which his reason could adapt to his body, and he must indeed be considered omnivorous.[26]

As high as was their regard for human reason, vegetarian casuists could not accept such a conclusion. Reason was the gift of God, but so was free will, so reason could be abused. Underlying reason was a basic set of laws and instincts of self-preservation which defined humankind's fundamental nature; and reason, to be *natural*, must be used in accord with these laws and instincts. The romantic vegetarians from the beginning of the 19th century had argued from a similar feeling when maintaining that since the sight and smell of raw flesh were repulsive to man, they were not natural for him. The health reformers would only have added that to make the flesh more appealing through cookery was to set reason against instinct, to use it unnaturally. A general statement of the health reform understanding of the relation of reason to human nature was offered by Graham in a quick reply to Bell's essay:

> We possess, to some extent, the physiological *capability* of adapting ourselves to conditions and things to which we are not *naturally* adapted; and we possess the rational and voluntary powers of adapting many things to our *use*, which are not *naturally* fitted for us; nevertheless all departure from the constitutional laws of our nature, in the exercise of these *capabilities*, is always, and necessarily, attended with commensurate injury to our physiological interests.

And there was much evidence in addition to anatomy to demonstrate that man was "*naturally* a fruit- and vegetable-eating animal."[27]

The anatomy lesson alone sufficed for proof, and at the risk of belaboring the point it must be urged that anatomical and other evidence was never separated from a scriptural context. "What was an orang, a chimpanzee, or a gorilla made for?", Mussey pondered.

> In reply it may be asked; for what more probably than to present to man a standing attestation to the truth and the value of the dietetic lesson given him in Paradise; to demonstrate to him that an animal with an organization like his own in relation to food may subsist exclusively on the eatables granted to himself in Eden, and yet enjoy enduring health and an adequate amount of activity and strength.[28]

Imitation of the orang was thus a *natural* use of reason, one in accord with God-given instinct. An example of an unnatural use would be the phenomenon so frequently pointed to by physiologists as proof of human omnivorousness. Bell cited with approval the common observation that since humanity covered the globe and thrived on a nearly infinite variety of animal and vegetable products, it must have been "designed by infinite wisdom" to subsist on a mixed diet.[29] On the contrary, vegetarians responded, since flesh food was never intended by infinite wisdom, inhabitants of the Arctic and other barren regions where flesh was the only available food must be there by choice and not by divine design, and must have used their reason wrongly. As Alcott moralized, "Man has no right to reside in northern regions till he can carry the climate . . . along with him [i.e., carry along the agriculture of temperate climes]."[30] Ultimately such arguments were but insoluble wranglings over nature versus nurture, though Bell's essay is important for drawing out the contrasting attitudes toward the nature of man which lay behind the dietetic dispute. Bell also served to intensify the more strictly physiological debate over vegetarianism.[31] From this time forth the conflict which was mostly generated by vegetarians was steady, and health reformers kept constant watch for signs of unnatural reasoning by physiologists.

Vegetarians' reasoning was done within an up-to-date scheme of atomistic biology that was nevertheless pliable enough to meet moral demands. They were in complete agreement with the orthodox view that nutrition was the result of "all parts of the human body undergo[ing] an internal motion, which has the double effect of expelling the molecules which are no longer needed as components of the organs, and of replacing them by new molecules."[32] Two aspects of this perennial renovation of the body were seen by vegetarians as having fundamental importance for health: the quality of the particles supplied by the food, and the rate of molecular turnover. Since meat products decomposed more rapidly than vegetables, and meat chyle was quicker than vegetable chyle to putrefy, it was clear which foods supplied the best particles — vegetables must have "greater purity and a more perfect vitality."[33] Further, as animal systems carried waste molecules from their own tissue renovations — molecules which had "become worn out, effete, dead and putrid" — flesh foods actually contained particles of poison.[34]

The resistance of particles to decay also suggested a second virtue of vegetable food, the slowness of replacement of its atoms. In health reform thought, strict obedience to all the laws of hygiene would be manifested not just by perfect health at all ages, but by a greatly protracted life span. Antediluvian longevity was assumed as the norm from which humankind had degenerated, and if longevity was to be regained, each stage of development of the body from infancy through childhood, etc., would have to be retarded. Only when the child took a hundred years to become a man could ideal health be claimed, and since maturing was but a process of molecular exchange, the slower this exchange, the healthier and longer lived the individual. The mechanics of life were simple: "a man may not inaptly be compared with a watch — the *faster it goes the sooner it will run down*."[35]

This fear of fast living directed the response to one of the longest standing nutritional assumptions of conventional physiology, and the misconception which most exasperated vegetarians. The opinion that meat was required for strength and stamina was a standard item in texts on diet.[36] Grahamites countered this belief with innumerable examples of vigorous vegetable eaters, and even an argument to support the claim of the herbivorous rhinoceros to the title of "king of the jungle"![37] But a more telling strategy was their effort to show that flesh, as unnatural food, actually brought on debility instead of imparting strength. Declarations to this effect were rarely substantiated,[38] but the reasoning was more significant than the statement. Again one sees the influence on physiology of Christian morality, with flesh eating being condemned in the process. Meat had long been appreciated as more "stimulating" than vegetables, the high specific dynamic action of animal foods being crudely recognized as a "digestive fever." This stimulating power of flesh was generally regarded by physicians as both its contribution and its danger to health: a certain degree of stimulation was required, but, as the orthodox physiologist John Ayrton Paris warned, "a diet of animal food cannot . . . be exclusively employed. It is too highly stimulant; the springs of life are urged on too fast; and disease necessarily follows."[39] For health reformers, such an admission seemed to damn flesh food altogether. Their reading of Broussais, as suggested previously, had established a fear of stimulation which made them regard any feeling of physical excitement as a sign of disease. By their definition, "stimulation" was a pathological process.

> Those effects which are called *stimulant*, *tonic*, etc., are in reality the evidence of the *resistance* which the vital powers make to the injurious or impure substance, and not, as is commonly supposed, the action of the article on the system. The *feeling of strength* is increased, for the reason that the energies of the system are roused into unnatural intensity of action to defend the vital machinery; and the reason that a depression of power is always experienced afterwards, is because the vital energy had been expended, uselessly wasted, in the struggle.[40]

Furthermore, the excessive stimulation of meat accelerated the body's molecular transformations and thereby shortened life, or, as Alcott phrased it, "the system . . . is inevitably worn into a premature dissolution, by the violent and unnatural heat of an over-stimulated and precipitate circulation."[41]

Alcott immediately added that the cool vegetable diet "has a tendency to temper the passions," thus revealing again the unity of morality and physiology. Broussais's pathology was undoubtedly adopted in part because it catered to the health reformers' moral dread of stimulation. If immoral, unchristian behavior were the product of depraved, uncontrollable appetites, then any stimulus to these appetites should be removed. Mussey was being somewhat restrained when he advised that "every degree of unnecessary excitation of the organic actions must be regarded as a departure from the highest health, and the increased irritability of the nerves dependent on disease will give rise to peevishness, despondency, and selfishness."[42] The same consideration of "excitation" drove Trall to a more typical charge, that:

> There is no delusion on earth so widespread as this, which confuses stimulation with nutrition. It is the very parent source of that awful . . . multitude of errors which are leading the nations of the earth into all manner of riotous living, and urging them on in the road to swift destruction. This terrible mistake is the primal cause of all the gluttony, all the drunkenness, all the dissipation, all the debauchery in the world — I had almost said, of all the vice and crime also.[43]

The need to suppress stimulation made the condemnation of flesh food on physiological grounds essential — hence, the twofold significance of references to meat as "the brandy of diet."[44]

Unnatural stimulation was also at the basis of the attack on what vegetarians regarded as a second misconception about their diet, the belief that it was less digestible than animal food. The traditional assumption that similarity of composition made the transformation of meat into human flesh relatively easy still held sway.[45] This commonsense argument had been recently reinforced by the numerous experiments performed by the U.S. army surgeon William Beaumont on the stomach of Alexis St. Martin, a French-Canadian trapper afflicted with a gastric fistula. Beaumont's experiments seemed to demonstrate that "generally speaking, vegetable aliment requires more time, and probably greater powers of the gastric organs, than animal."[46] Bell had cited Beaumont's conclusion in his Boylston essay defending a mixed diet, so the question of digestibility was not one which the Grahamites could ignore. The experiments might be simply dismissed out of hand as inapplicable, since they had been performed on a diseased instead of a normal stomach.[47] But to do that would be to pass up a golden occasion to demonstrate the conflict between flesh and physiology. Thus the very first issue of the *Graham Journal of Health and Longevity* carried the opening installment of a long series of extracts from Beaumont's book, extracts designed to "prepare the reader's mind for the reviewer's notes."[48] In the meantime the American Physiological Society, a health reform organization, was corresponding with Beaumont "to see on what terms St. Martin would come to Boston and submit to further and perhaps more perfect investigations."[49] The effort to obtain St. Martin came to naught, but the language of the request betrayed the vegetarian attitude toward the work already done by Beaumont. It was by implication imperfect, and when the long-promised review by Graham appeared, it explained why Beaumont was not a "truly scientific physiologist."[50] By Graham's analysis, Beaumont's great failing was to think that physiology could be reduced to chemistry, and to treat chymification as a chemical, rather than a vital, process. Graham was a vitalist in the mold of Bichat; he admitted that the body was composed of the same atoms as inorganic matter, but he asserted that unique laws existed for the arrangement of the atoms. He regarded life as a "forced state" of constant conflict between the vital power and the more primitive affinities of unorganized matter. And he despised the presumption of modern chemists who tried to quantify the variable phenomena of life. If physiology were subject to chemistry then the tables of chymification times of various foods which Beaumont had compiled could serve as an accurate guide, and the foods "which passed through the stomach in the shortest time, . . . whether it be soused tripe, pig's feet, or whatever else,"[51] could be regarded as the most easily digested. But in fact, digestion was accomplished by vital force, which acted against, not through, chemical force. Therefore, the digestibility of an item was to be measured not by the time but by the energy expended in dissolving it. If experience showed the body to be weakened more by flesh food than by vegetables, then flesh could hardly be considered more digestible, no matter how quickly it passed through the stomach. And what was the digestive fever, if not a sign of the abnormal exertion of vital force in the digestion of meat? For that very reason "they who subsist principally on animal food . . . always feel more stupid and dull during gastric digestion, and feel a much greater degree of exhaustion."[52] Again stimulation was identified as pathological, and in such a way as to turn Beaumont's data against him; "it may [therefore] be regarded as a general law, that those kinds of food, appropriate for man, which *naturally* pass slowly through the stomach, are digested with the least vital expense and . . . are most conducive to the general welfare of the system."[53] Digestibility, Graham thus suggested, with a curious quantification of vitality, is directly and not inversely proportional to the time of digestion. Other health reformers followed Graham's lead, and the principle of "slow digestion is good digestion" became an axiom of vegetarianism.[54]

Digestibility dovetailed with nutrition in the vegetarian construct, for if vegetables took longer to pass through the digestive tract, it must be because they contained a greater quantity of nutritive matter to be absorbed.[55] This was a congenial conclusion apparently validated by analytical chemistry. Virtually every presentation of vegetarianism during the health reform period included a table derived "from the works of Percy, Vaquelin [*sic*] and other distinguished analystical [*sic*] chimests [*sic*]"[56] which demonstrated many vegetables to be much more concentrated nourishment than meat. Accepting the ancient belief in a single nutritive substance, "aliment," and using analyses of the water content of various uncooked foods, vegetarians were able to suppose that wheat, 15 percent by weight of water, contained 85 "nutritive parts" per 100. Rice was thus 90 percent aliment, lentils 94 percent, sugar 95 percent, and tapioca 98 percent. Butcher's meat held an enfeebling 35 nutritive parts per 100, and milk only 20 parts. The prevalent idea that meat was highly nutritious was shown to be fallacious, an error caused by mistaking stimulation for nutrition.[57] Furthermore, the higher nutritive value of vegetables reinforced the demand for moderation at the table; in this sense, vegetable gluttony could be even more injurious than flesh gluttony, and the quantity eaten had to be carefully restricted.[58]

Insistence on the nutritional superiority of vegetables to meat, at first glance an effective tactic, nevertheless led vegetarians into a clumsy situation. It seemed to conflict directly with another cherished belief, that of the *innutritiousness* of vegetable diet. Vegetables had long been recognized as bulkier items than meat, as promoters of free bowel movement. Presumably this was because vegetables contained much matter which was not absorbed and therefore was not nutritious. From the beginning vegetarians defended their diet as a mixture of nourishing with much non-nourishing matter. This was the advantage of unbolted Graham flour over white flour, for instance. The necessity of such a mixture was argued on the basis of the experimental work of the great French physiologist François Magendie. One of the first questions to activate the animal chemistry of the early 19th century was that of the origin of the large quantities of nitrogen in animal tissue. Particularly with regard to herbivores whose diet contained relatively small proportions of nitrogen, there was much speculation as to whether the diet could supply all the nitrogen needed and what internal processes of "animalization" might transform non-nitrogenous food into flesh, or whether some amount might be absorbed from the atmosphere.[59] The 1816 experiments of Magendie were intended to settle the dispute. Feeding dogs on diets of sugar and water, olive oil and water, and butter and water — all nitrogen-free rations — he found that the animals invariably sickened and died. Magendie's conclusion that "the nitrogen which is found in the animal economy is in great part extracted from the food"[60] was correct, but was not fully demonstrable at the time. Pure fibrine, albumen, or gelatin, all high in nitrogen, also failed to maintain life, so that Magendie's work might be subject to at least a second interpretation.[61] A number of reputable physiologists argued that Magendie's experiments "merely prove that an animal cannot be supported by highly concentrated aliment."[62] Vegetarians embraced this interpretation eagerly,[63] as it made the bulkiness of vegetable diet more healthful than concentrated animal food. For the most part they ignored the question raised by their concurrent use of analytical tables showing vegetable foods to be more than twice as nourishing as meat. When they did turn to it, the contradiction was easily resolved by maintaining that highly nutritious foods like bread must be tempered by low nutrition foods such as potatoes, beets, and turnips.[64] The claims, usually presented separately, that the virtue of vegetables lay, on the one hand, in their concentrated nutrition and, on the other, in their dilute nutrition suggest an attempt to get the most out of diverse chemical and physiological data with the hope that neophytes would not detect the contradiction.

The deceit soon became unnecessary, for the remarkable sophistication which animal chemistry acquired in the 1840s made the tables of "nutritive parts per hundred" obsolete, and also presented new challenges to vegetarians. Associated with the opinion that Magendie had shown nothing more than that concentrated food is inadequate was the belief that at least some of the nitrogen of the body was derived from the atmosphere. The careful experiments performed by Jean-Baptiste Boussingault in the late 1830s and early 1840s refuted this theory and demonstrated that all tissue nitrogen, even in herbivorous animals, is obtained from food.[65] The subsequent demand by physiologists that a nourishing diet must contain considerable amounts of nitrogenized foods was intensified by the pronouncement of Justus von Liebig, the most respected authority on animal chemistry, that muscular motion can be produced only by protein oxidation.[66] Health reformers thus felt constrained to prove that their relatively low protein diet did in fact supply sufficient nitrogen. Actually there remains good reason to question whether Grahamites did consume adequate protein. Ignorant of essential amino acids and the mixed vegetable diet necessary to obtain these, and intent on eating sparingly of only one or two dishes per meal, the conscientious health-reform vegetarian (if he eschewed milk, as many did) might have easily inflicted protein deficiency upon himself.[67] At the time the objection evoked only amused disbelief. "The purely herbivorous animals derive their growth and strength from vegetable food . . . *their* systems are supplied with azote [nitrogen] without eating animal food; why may not man's system be supplied in the same way?"[68] But if the fact of healthy animal life on a vegetable diet was obvious, the explanation was less than certain. Several approaches to explaining it were tried, the most direct being to deny the pertinence of the chemical data. Alcott toyed with this idea, submitting that the argument that since body tissues contain nitrogen they must be supplied with food containing much nitrogen was akin to the syllogism "Lime enters into the composition of the bones; mortar contains lime, therefore we must eat mortar."[69] The mystery of how low nitrogen foods could form high nitrogen tissues, however, invited a more frank vitalism, and Graham disputed most loudly the legitimacy of animal chemistry. In response to Magendie's demand for azote in the diet, Graham said simply, "It is not in the power of chemistry in the least possible degree, to ascertain what substances the alimentary organs of the living animal body require for the nourishment of the body, nor from what chemical elements the organic elements are formed."[70]

As had occurred among orthodox physiologists, the majority of health reformers were turning away from such attempts to shield the science of life entirely from chemistry. If nitrogen were present in the body, it must have been ingested. Those who doubted the ability of vegetables to supply all the required nitrogen continued to argue for absorption of the element from the atmosphere,[71] but from the early 1840s forward, vegetarians preferred to support the position that all body nitrogen was extracted from the food, and extracted most efficiently and safely from vegetable food. Their inspiration for this point might seem an unlikely one, for Justus von Liebig eventually marketed an extract of beef as a health food. In his epoch-making *Animal Chemistry* of 1842, Liebig presented information which struck vegetarians as precisely the chemical evidence they needed. The nitrogenized constituents of the food of herbivorous animals — vegetable fibrine, albumen, and caseine — were, he pointed out, "identical in composition with the chief constituents of blood, animal fibrine, and albumen."[72] The proteins required by the animal body existed ready-made in plants and needed only to be absorbed. Even carnivores obtained their protein ultimately from vegetable sources, and thus one might say "the animal organism is a higher kind of vegetable."[73] Vegetarians fastened onto these paragraphs as proof that not only did vegetables contain sufficient utilizable protein for health, but that the vegetable protein, even if identical in composition to animal protein, was better. It was more natural, reasonable, and healthful, being eaten directly after its production rather than after an unnecessary, expensive, and contaminating passage through an animal body.

> Do we not take materials fresh from nature when we wish to build a substantial, beautiful and durable mansion, instead of taking down some other edifice to build from its rubbish? So also in vital architecture, let us build up our earthly tabernacles by materials taken freshly from nature, and then we shall find ourselves possessed of sound and durable bodies.[74]

The new form of nutrition table that developed in the wake of Liebig's classification of foods as "plastic" and "respiratory," or "blood forming" and "heat forming," indicated in a less moralistic way that vegetable diet was both adequate and preferable for meeting the nitrogen needs of the body. Meat contained more protein than most foods, but according to the statistics of the time, less than peas, beans, and lentils. Nor did low protein content mean that a food was not nourishing, for what some vegetables lacked in the blood-forming principle, they made up in the heat-forming one. A mixed vegetable diet might thus be regarded as much better balanced than flesh food, and even "flesh-eating physiologists" might recognize that wheat flour had the best combination of plastic and respiratory compounds for human nutrition.[75] This recognition, important in itself, launched the vegetarian assault on still another popular myth about the need for meat.

The warm fullness that follows a heavy flesh meal had long suggested the use of animal food to resist cold weather. Northern voyagers in particular insisted that fat meat was required for their survival.[76] Health reformers viewed this in the same light as the belief that alcohol was needed to withstand cold: in both cases, they argued, the warmth was a temporary effect of an enervating stimulus, and not a lasting, protective heat. The error persisted, however, and according to vegetarians was encouraged by Liebig. Thousands, Alcott claimed, had heard of the German chemist's emphasis on the consumption of respiratory foods to maintain body heat and of his analyses showing animal fat to be rich in carbon and hydrogen, and "hastily concluded that animal food was indispensable to the highest health." They were strengthened in this notion by popular medical lecturers who attacked vegetarianism with the charge "that vegetable food will not sustain man in cold climates."[77] Liebig did observe that inhabitants of frigid zones ate enormous quantities of flesh, and sometimes tallow candles, and might even guzzle train oil safely, as such amounts of carbon and hydrogen were necessary to generate their body heat.[78] But he also showed that 4 pounds of starch contained as much potential body heat as 13 pounds of meat, and at least implied that arctic peoples could live more efficiently on vegetable products, if they could get them.[79] Vegetarians caught the implication, and found in Liebig's statistics proof that vegetables were superior as respiratory food, in addition to being better plastic food. When measured in uncooked foods, the heat-producing matter of fat meat was found to be considerably less than that of the grains, and nearly identical to that of peas and beans. "Is it necessary to eat beef, for the sake of its 51 or 52 percent of the heat-forming principle — when the vegetable kingdom affords it in ample quantity and proportion?"[80] And "proportion" was the key word. Vegetables were *balanced* foods, containing large separate reservoirs of flesh-forming and heat-forming principles. But flesh eaters, according to Liebig, had to produce much of their body heat by the oxidation of plastic foods, or rather, of their own tissues, thus accelerating the rate of metamorphosis of their body parts.[81] By health-reform logic, flesh was not just an inefficient foodstuff, but by hastening the molecular processes of life, it hastened the approach of death. In a much larger sense than Liebig intended, vegetarians agreed that restriction to a flesh diet, or even a mixed one, "is characteristic of the savage state."[82]

That vegetables were the only satisfactory foods for the civilized Christian state was the ultimate point intended by vegetarians' formulation of a physiological rationale. In succinct form, the rationale maintained that human anatomy as designed by God was herbivorous; vegetable atoms were more stable and more slowly cycled through the body than those of meat; vegetables were sufficient for strength without being pathologically "stimulating"; vegetables were more digestible and contained more nutritious matter for both tissue maintenance and heat production. Vegetarians congratulated themselves for the service of enlightenment they had performed.

> Nature's Dietetic laws lay hid in Night,
> Let Vegetarians be to give us light.
> Or in other words,
> Mankind in the dark ages were mostly
>   Carnivorous,
> But now the light shines, let us all be
>   Frugivorous.[83]

Throughout the period of revelation of Nature's Dietetic Laws, Grahamites had also been working to lay a solid empirical foundation for their rationale. Collecting histories of individuals from the antediluvians to their contemporary Amos Townsend, a graminivorous bank cashier who could "dictate a letter, count money, and hold conversation with an individual, all at the same time, with no embarrassment,"[84] and histories of cultural groups from the ancient Roman legions to the contemporary southern slaves, whose "bodily powers are well known,"[85] vegetarians compiled a great corpus of testimonials exemplifying the extraordinary health and longevity attainable on a vegetable diet. These cases were considered by Grahamites to be their experimental evidence,[86] and it must be observed that they were as subjectively interpreted as was physiological theory. The vegetarians' eagerness for living proof of the advantages of their system could move them to accept testimonials which flew in the face of physiology. Even the editors of the *American Vegetarian* considered remarkable the 1850 case history of a man who starved away his dyspepsia on a diet of three Graham crackers and a gill of water a day. After steadily losing weight for two months, he claimed to have begun to gain weight, adding as much as half a pound a day, "or nearly three times as much as the whole weight of my food; . . . though I never in my life, came to the table with a better appetite, I was never better satisfied with my meals, when they were finished."[87]

Even dismissing this hoax, it is valid to say that testimonial evaluation was so uncritical as to make anecdotes admissible as proof. But when their opponents showed the same laxity, vegetarians pounced on the blunder. Did consumptives sent to the Rocky Mountains recover on an all-flesh diet? If so, it was because the patients "were also compelled to be almost continually in the open air, enduring healthful and invigorating exercise . . . had they added to these a pure and well-regulated vegetable diet their recovery would have been rendered more certain and complete."[88] The first point, at least, was fairly taken, but what of the many cases of flesh eaters who also indulged in spirits, or tobacco, or opium, or all of these, and still lived to advanced years? "If here and there one of them lasts till old age, it is by virtue of an iron constitution."[89] The prejudice of health reformers was perhaps never clearer than in such statements, unless it were in the apologies for vegetarians who died young. To note the most prominent example, the announcement of the death of Graham at the less-than-advanced age of 56 was prefaced with the assurance that "there is nothing, when we take into view his whole history, *his peculiar constitution* and habits which militates against . . . the superior healthfulness of a well-selected vegetable diet."[90] Graham had inherited a weak frame and had occasionally strayed from his own teachings; at least the former explanation might be given for any vegetarian who expired too soon. The health reformers could thus have their cake and eat it too, and did so with intemperate zeal. There was no limit to the number of times vegetables were absolved of blame by a frail constitution, and flesh forbidden credit by an iron one.

It might appear that the violence done to logic and to science by vegetarians was too clumsily masked not to be recognized, and that the physiological plea to reject flesh would have been inconsequential. Yet the testimony of conversion that fills the pages of vegetarian literature rings with sincerity. "Light — the light of physiology — has flashed in upon my mind, sufficient to emancipate me from the dreadful thralldom I so long endured."[91]

Most of such testimony also resounds with the mid-19th century's pietistic confidence in the unity of the moral and natural worlds, and it might be anticipated that, as this confidence waned through the later 1800s, the physiological argument would lose much of its force. But while the public grew somewhat less receptive to the equation of hygiene with humaneness, and vegetarians themselves less set on identifying true physiology with Christianity, the insistence on the superior healthfulness of a vegetable diet has never been relinquished.[92] There would thus appear to be a predisposition to believe that simple, bloodless food must be best for the body, springing from some deeper soil than the Evangelicalism which provided immediate inspiration and guidance for health reform physiology. Vegetarianism in Graham's day and since has been profoundly affected by the tension between primitive longing for the natural and modern enthusiasm for science, by what Lovejoy has called the "crisis" of primitivism.[93]

Historians of the idea of primitivism have directed attention to the persistence in European culture of the belief that the human race has degenerated from an original state of perfect happiness and accord with nature. Vegetable diet and physical vigor have commonly been cited as virtues of that "golden age."[94] But during the course of the 18th century the primitivist determination to abandon the artificial luxuries of civilization and return to an untainted state of nature came to be challenged by the Enlightenment's faith in human progress and its zeal for exploiting science to this end. An unprecedented volume of appeals to imitate the simpler past was met by dreams of creating a complex future, and the pull of each was so strong as to impose a Janus-like distortion in many minds. Primitivism and progressivism came to be frequently combined, the same author now pleading for the rejection of modernity, then arguing that the restitution of past glory must be guided by an understanding of modern science.

Health reformers and later vegetarians were deeply disturbed by the artificiality of life encouraged by industrial science, and looked backward to Eden as the natural environment, one in which undefiled instincts directed people's living habits. Yet in considering how to return appetites to their natural purity, they were unable to ignore the recent revelations of science, and the promise these held for the education of man in the laws of his natural condition. Science as revealed nature could make future humankind as natural as original man; but it would not make him as simple. With knowledge of science, humanity would possess a sophistication and power which would place man well above the original state. In this confused situation, the primitive condition came to appear both ideal and outmoded, one which had to be restored but also improved. Alcott had to instruct readers that vegetable diet and other proper hygiene would bring about not a mere return to nature, but rather "a gradual ascent to nature. Man's nature is intended . . . to include art, and to be affected and modified by science . . . in making our ascent up the mount whence we have fallen, it is by no means necessary that we should return to barbarism."[95]

Such misgivings about the joys of Eden without science point to the difficulty of that passage from traditional modes of thought to new ones which marked the early 19th century. It reveals the struggle many waged with Rousseau's paradox, that of man being the only creature possessing powers beyond those needed for self-preservation, yet being made miserable by the superfluity.[96] Health reform in general, and its vegetarianism in particular, were nothing less than an attempt to remove this misery by the creation of a science which was not just Christian, but *natural*, a blending of reason with instinct. However much one deplores health-reform vegetarians' self-serving interpretations of physiology, they must be commended for their efforts to resolve a great modern dilemma, the question of how to use science to improve the human condition without alienating man from nature in the process.

NOTES

1 Russell Trall, *The Scientific Basis of Vegetarianism* (Philadelphia, 1860), p. 2.

2 "Proceedings from the convention," *Am. Veg.*, 1851, *1*: 1–10, p. 6.

3 The best treatments of the health reform movement are: R. Shryock, "Sylvester Graham and the popular health movement, 1830–1870," in *Medicine in America: Historical Essays* (Baltimore, 1966), pp. 111–125; H. E. Hoff and J. F. Fulton, "The centenary of the first American Physiological Society founded at Boston by William A. Alcott and Sylvester Graham," *Bull. Hist. Med.*, 1937, *5*: 687–734; W. B. Walker, "The health reform movement in the United States, 1830–1870" (Ph.D. dissertation, Johns Hopkins, 1955); S. W. Nissenbaum, "Careful love: Sylvester Graham and the emergence of Victorian sexual theory in America, 1830–1840" (Ph.D. dissertation, Univ. of Wisconsin, 1968); J. Blake, "Health reform," in *The Rise of Adventism*, ed. E. Gaustad (New York, 1974); Ronald Numbers, *Prophetess of Health: A Study of Ellen G. White* (New York, 1976), pp. 48–76.

4 For biographical information on Trall and hydropathy, see H. Weiss and H. Kemble, *The Great American Water-Cure Craze* (Trenton, N.J., 1967), pp. 80–88.

5 J. Whorton, "'Christian physiology': William Alcott's prescription for the millennium," *Bull. Hist. Med.*, 1975, *49*: 466–481.

6 "Emancipated," "Dietetic charlatanry, again," *Graham J. Hlth. & Long.*, 1837, *1*: 274.

7 Nissenbaum, "Careful love," pp. 35–58, offers a survey of the history of vegetarianism to 1830. A general history of vegetarianism which focuses on England, but gives some attention to the United States, is Charles Forward, *Fifty Years of Food Reform* (London, 1898).

8 J. Oswald, *The Cry of Nature* (London, 1791). Other prominent works of the kind included George Nicholson, *On the Primeval Diet of Man . . . On Man's Conduct to Animals* (Poughnill, England, 1801); Joseph Ritson, *An Essay on Abstinence from Animal Food, as a Moral Duty* (London, 1802); and J. F. Newton, *The Return to Nature, or, A Defence of the Vegetable Regimen* (London, 1811).

9 The meaning of this, and other biblical passages, had already been exhaustively debated in the 18th century. See James MacKenzie, *The History of Health and the Art of Preserving It*, 2nd ed. (Edinburgh, 1759), pp. 44–50.

10 J. Metcalfe, *Memoir of the Rev. William Metcalfe, M.D.* (Philadelphia, 1866); W. Metcalfe, "Rev. William Cowherd," *Am. Veg.*, 1854, *4*: 69–72; William Alcott, "Bible Christians," *Lib. Hlth.*, 1840, *4*: 69.

11 G. Cheyne, *An Essay on Health and Long Life*, 8th ed. (London, 1734), p. xvi. For biographical information on Cheyne, see R. Siddal, "George Cheyne, M.D.," *Ann. Med. Hist.*, 1942, 3rd series, *4*: 95–109; H. Viets, "George Cheyne, 1673–1743," *Bull. Hist. Med.*, 1949, *23*: 435–452; K. Kelleher, "The gout doctor. George Cheyne, M.D. (1671–1743)," *Practitioner*, 1971, *206*: 416–421.

12 William Lambe, *Additional Reports on the Effects of a Peculiar Regimen in Cases of Cancer, Scrofula, Consumption, Asthma, and Other Chronic Diseases* (London, 1815), pp. 90, 127, 131, 147, 172. Also see B. Hill, "Vegetables and distilled water. William Lambe, M.D. (1765–1847)," *Practitioner*, 1965, *194*: 285.

13 Percy Shelley, *A Vindication of Natural Diet* (London, 1884), pp. 16–17, 27.

14 B. Lynch, *A Guide to Health through the Various Stages of Life* (London, 1744), p. 178; B. Faust, *The Catechism of Health* (London, 1832), p. 40; Anthony Willich, *Lectures on Diet and Regimen*, 3rd ed. (New York, 1801), pp. 209–222; William Kitchiner, *The Art of Invigorating or Prolonging Life*, 5th ed. (London, 1824), p. 10; William Lawrence, *Lectures on Physiology, Zoology, and the Natural History of Man* (Salem, Mass., 1828), p. 187; MacKenzie, *History of Health*, p. 18; Thomas Graham, *Sure Methods of Improving Health and Prolonging Life*, 3rd ed. (London, 1833), pp. 4–6.

15 Quoted in William Wadd, *Comments on Corpulency* (London, 1829), p. 142.

16 William Alcott, *Vegetable Diet: As Sanctioned by Medical Men and by Experience in All Ages* (Boston, 1838), p. 165.

17 W. Metcalfe, "Bible doctrine," *Lib. Hlth.*, 1840, *4*: 159. For similar sentiments, see L. Coles, *Philosophy of Health* (Boston, 1857), p. 64.

18 Letter to editor, *Graham J. Hlth. & Long.*, 1838, *2*: 317. Another correspondent recognized that Grahamism "is in fact Bibleism." Simeon Collins, letter to editor, *Graham J. Hlth. & Long.*, 1837, *1*: 5. Also see J. C. Jackson, "Christianity and the health reformation," *Water-Cure J.*, 1858, *26*: 82–84.

19 W. W., "Some facts and logic respecting dietetics," *Boston Med. & Surg. J.*, 1836, *14*: 169; editor, "Dietetic charlatanry; or the new ethics of eating," *N.Y. Rev.*, 1837, *1*: 336–351, pp. 339, 341; editor, "Vegetable diet," *Water-Cure J.*, 1849, *8*: 93. Also see C. Ticknor, *The Philosophy of Living* (New York, 1836), pp. 46, 53; "Dr. Alcott's work on diet," *Boston Med. & Surg. J.*, 1839, *19*: 220–222, 282; editor, "A desultory dissertation on dietetics," *U.S. Mag. & Democ. Rev.*, 1849, *24*: 343. Normally rather relaxed in their observation of the rules of logic, vegetarians seized on the irrelevancy of *ad hominem* criticisms: e.g., editor, "Vegetarian convention," *Water-Cure J.*, 1856, *22*: 86.

20 "Emancipated," "Dietetic charlatanry," *Graham J. Hlth. & Long.*, 1837, *1*: 257–259, p. 258.

21 S. Graham, *Lectures on the Science of Human Life*, 2 vols. (Boston, 1839), I, 340.

22 William Alcott, "Eating animal food," *Lib. Hlth.*, 1841, *5*: 120.

23 Luther Bell, "Dr. Bell's prize dissertation on diet," *Boston Med. & Surg. J.*, 1836, *13*: 303. Bell did suggest that the proportion of animal food in the New England diet was often too large and should be reduced, but he was strongly opposed to elimination of meat.

24 F. Magendie, *A Summary of Physiology*, 2nd ed. (Baltimore, 1824), p. 178. Also see Lawrence, *Lectures on Physiology*, a work which clearly influenced Bell's analysis.

25 Bell, "Dr. Bell's prize dissertation," p. 248.

26 *Ibid.*, pp. 248–249. J. A. Paris, *A Treatise on Diet*, 5th ed. (London, 1837), pp. 8–11, offers a similar argument.

27 S. Graham, "Remarks on Dr. Bell's prize essay," *Boston Med. & Surg. J.*, 1835–36, *13*: 332. Graham, *Human Life*, I, 418–439; II, 16–18 and 80–86, gives further detailed attention to the interactions between human reason, appetite, and moral power. Also see William Alcott, "Man omnivorous," *Lib. Hlth.*, 1837, *1*: 20–27; and H. Clubb, "Vegetarianism," *Water-Cure J.*, 1854, *18*: 105.

28 Reuben Mussey, *Health: Its Friends and Foes* (Boston, 1862), p. 175.

29 Bell, "Dr. Bell's prize dissertation," pp. 251–252; Jonathan Pereira, *A Treatise on Food and Diet*, 2nd ed. (New York, 1847), p. 286. General acceptance of this opinion is evident from its occurrence in Paris, *Diet*, p. 128; William Carpenter, *Principles of Human Physiology*, 4th ed. (Philadelphia, 1852), p. 380; Ticknor, *Philosophy of Living*, pp. 34–36; Robley Dunglison, *On the Influence of Atmosphere and Locality . . . Constituting Elements of Hygiene* (Philadelphia, 1835), p. 213; Edward Hitchcock, *Dyspepsy Forestalled and Resisted* (Amherst, Mass., 1830), p. 99.

30 William Alcott, "Vegetarianism in Ohio," *Am. Veg.*, 1852, *2*: 35. Also see Alcott, "The Arctic regions," *Lib. Hlth.*, 1838, *2*: 260.

31 The *Boston Medical and Surgical Journal* was kept busy for months printing the angry exchanges between Bell and Graham and their supporters. Even the question of the relation of Grahamism to insanity was thoroughly aired. *Boston Med. & Surg. J.*, 1835–36, *13*: 379–382, 396–398, 408–409; *ibid.*, 1836, *14*: 22–28, 29–31, 38–46, 87–96, 103–108, 139–141, 166–172, 199–201, 266–271, 319–322, 338.

32 F. Magendie quoted by J. Fruton, *Molecules and Life: Historical Essays on the Interplay of Chemistry and Biology* (New York, 1972), p. 401.

33 Alcott, *Vegetable Diet*, p. 230, is but one of many places where this argument is presented.

34 O. May, "Is meat poisonous?", *Water-Cure J.*, 1856, *22*: 102; also Trall, *Vegetarianism*, p. 10.

35 D. Cambell, "Stimulation," *Graham J. Hlth. & Long.*, 1837, *1*: 291. Also S. Graham, *Human Life*, I, 480–481, II, 148; William Alcott, *The Laws of Health*, 2nd ed. (Boston, 1859), pp. 2, 17; Alcott, "Renovation of the body," *Teacher of Health*, 1843, *1*: 243–247.

36 For examples, see Paris, *Diet*, p. 134; Andrew Combe, *The Physiology of Digestion*, 4th ed. (Edinburgh, 1842), p. 139; Calvin Cutter, *A Treatise on Anatomy, Physiology and Hygiene*, 2nd ed. (Boston, 1852), p. 139.

37 Graham, *Human Life*, II, 186.

38 Vegetarians were correct in pointing out that many animals were already diseased at the time of slaughter; they were especially fond of Graham's analogy of the stomach of a flesh eater being like a "potter's field" where the dead of all diseases were buried. *Ibid.*, p. 375.

39 Paris, *Diet*, p. 133.

40 R. Trall, footnote in J. Smith, *Fruits and Farinacea: The Proper Food of Man*, 2nd ed. (New York, 1854), p. 171. Also Graham, *Human Life*, II, 148; and William Alcott, "What shall we eat?," *Moral Reformer*, 1836, *2*: 245–248.

41 William Alcott, "Animal and vegetable food," *Lib. Hlth.*, 1840, *4*: 221.

42 Mussey, *Health*, p. 232.

43 Trall, *Vegetarianism*, p. 10. Also see letter to editor, "Is cleanliness a virtue?," *Graham J. Hlth. & Long.*, 1839, *3*: 92; Graham, *Human Life*, II, 18, 338–354; Coles, *Philosophy of Health*, p. 65; William Alcott, "Eating flesh and licentiousness," *Am. Veg.*, 1853, *3*: 141–142; C. de Wolfe, "The anticipated results of vegetarianism," *Am. Veg.*, 1852, *2*: 10. One may even find quasi-atomic interpretations of the effects of meat upon character. T. Nichols, letter to editor, *Am. Veg.*, 1851, *1*: 55; and G. Taylor, "The

philosophy of diet," *Water-Cure J.*, 1855, *19*: 128.

44 W. Metcalfe, "Reasons for being a vegetarian," *Am. Veg.*, 1851, *1*: 74.

45 Paris, *Diet*, p. 131. Also Combe, *Physiology of Digestion*, pp. 143–144.

46 W. Beaumont, *Experiments and Observations on the Gastric Juice, and the Physiology of Digestion* (Plattsburgh, N.Y., 1833), p. 36. This opinion was repeated on pp. 46–47, 144, and 275, and was adopted by other physiologists, e.g., Combe, *Physiology of Digestion*, pp. 138, 143–144; and Ticknor, *Philosophy of Living*, p. 59.

47 William Alcott, "Notices of publications," *Moral Reformer*, 1836, *2*: 260.

48 D. Cambell, "Gastric experiments — fourth series," *Graham J. Hlth. & Long.*, 1837, *1*: 187.

49 *Ibid.*, p. 225. For the history of the American Physiological Society, see Hoff and Fulton, "The centenary."

50 Graham, "Review of Beaumont's experiments," *Graham J. Hlth. & Long.*, 1837, *1*: 262–264, p. 264.

51 *Ibid.*, p. 270. The best presentation of his vitalism is in Graham, *Human Life*, I, 62–83; I, 291–294, and II, 110–112, offer his vitalistic theory of digestion, which has been used to supplement the Beaumont review in the discussion above. Nissenbaum, "Careful love," pp. 75–81, discusses the influence of Bichat on Graham.

52 Graham, *Human Life*, II, 112.

53 Graham, "Review of Beaumont's experiments," *Graham J. Hlth. & Long.*, 1837, *1*: 269–270, p. 270.

54 D. Cambell, "Quantity of food — regulation of appetite," *Graham J. Hlth. & Long.*, 1839, *3*: 77; William Alcott, "Experiments on digestion," *Lib. Hlth.*, 1840, *4*: 124.

55 J. Wright, "Meat," *Am. Veg.*, 1851, *1*: 43.

56 D. Cambell, "What is nourishing?" *Graham J. Hlth. & Long.*, 1838, *2*: 159. In spite of their vitalism, Grahamites used chemical data when it agreed with their position.

57 One attempt to clarify this point was made by S. Graham, "Answer to five important questions," *Graham J. Hlth. & Long.*, 1837, *1*: 233–237, p. 236.

58 Cambell, "Quantity of food," p. 77.

59 F. Holmes, "Elementary analysis and the origins of physiological chemistry," *Isis*, 1963, *54*: 50–81, pp. 61–63, 71–72, places this problem within the context of the growth of analytical organic chemistry. Also see Fruton, *Molecules and Life*, pp. 398–399.

60 F. Magendie, "Mémoire sur les propriétés nutritives des substances qui ne contiennent pas d'azote," *Ann. Chim. Phys.*, 1816, *3*: 75.

61 Pereira, *Food and Diet*, p. 19; J. J. Muller, *Elements of Physiology*, 2nd ed. (Philadelphia, 1843), pp. 331–333; Smith, *Fruits and Farinacea*, p. 149.

62 Paris, *Diet*, p. 180; also Beaumont, *Experiments*, p. 39; and Dunglison, *Influence of Atmosphere*, p. 284.

63 William Alcott, "Objections to animal food," *Moral Reformer*, 1835, *1*: 278.

64 William Alcott, "Bread too nutritious," *Moral Reformer*, 1836, *2*: 219.

65 R. Aulie, "Boussingault and the nitrogen cycle," *Proc. Am. Phil. Soc.*, 1970, *114*: 435–479, esp. pp. 449–451.

66 J. von Liebig, *Animal Chemistry* (Cambridge, Mass., 1842), p. 233.

67 Some indication of ideal vegetarian meals may be obtained from William Alcott, "Variety in our meals," *Moral Reformer*, 1836, *2*: 316–317; Alcott, "Advantages of simplicity in diet," *Lib. Hlth.*, 1841, *5*: 297–312; Alcott, "Is there carbon in flesh-meat?", *Am. Veg.*, 1851, *1*: 214–215, p. 215.

68 William Alcott, "Is animal food necessary because of the azote it contains?," *Lib. Hlth.*, 1838, *2*: 175–176.

69 *Ibid.*, p. 175.

70 Graham, *Human Life*, I, 542–543: also Graham, "Answer to five important questions," p. 233.

71 Smith, *Fruits and Farinacea*, pp. 136–137.

72 Liebig, *Animal Chemistry*, p. 47.

73 *Ibid.*, p. 48.

74 L. Hough, "Address," *Am. Veg.*, 1851, *1*: 22–24, p. 23. Also see R. Mussey, "Letter," *Am. Veg.*, 1851, *1*: 194–195; William Alcott, "Flesh meat in vegetables," *Teacher of Health*, 1843, *1*: 291; and W. Metcalfe, "Why do you not eat flesh meat?", *Am. Veg.*, 1852, *2*: 30, for a few examples of the enthusiasm of vegetarians for this feature of Liebig's work.

75 Carpenter, *Human Physiology*, p. 379. William Alcott, "Vegetable food to give heat," *Am. Veg.*, 1892, *2*: 163, refers to Carpenter as a "flesh-eating physiologist" in taking note of his praise for bread.

76 W. Sweetser, *A Treatise on Digestion* (Boston, 1837), pp. 133–134.

77 William Alcott, "Vegetarianism in Ohio," *Am. Veg.*, 1852, *2*: 34. L. Hough, "Dr. Wieting vs. vegetarianism," *Am. Veg.*, 1851, *1*: 49. Also see Trall, *Vegetarianism*, p. 9.

78 Liebig, *Animal Chemistry*, p. 21. Hough, "Address," p. 48, shows that this observation of Liebig's was used in antivegetarian arguments.

79 Liebig, *Animal Chemistry*, pp. 74, 288.

80 William Alcott, "Is there carbon in flesh-meat?", *Am. Veg.*, 1851, *1*: 214. Also see Alcott, "Does animal food give more heat than vegetable food?" *Am. Veg.*, 1851, *1*: 69–71. The old and new forms of nutrition tables could even be combined to make a doubly impressive case for vegetarianism. T. Nichols, "Dietetics," *Water-Cure J.*, 1850, *10*: 89.

81 Liebig, *Animal Chemistry*, pp. 73–75.

82 *Ibid.*, p. 75.

83 E. Thomas, "For the *American Vegetarian*," *Am. Veg.*, 1854, *4*: 131.
84 Alcott, *Vegetable Diet*, pp. 75–76.
85 *Ibid.*, p. 265.
86 *Ibid.*, p. 166.
87 J. Robinson, "Starving the dyspepsia," *Am. Veg.*, 1850, *1*: 154.
88 D. Cambell, "Opinion of Professor Alban G. Smith," *Graham J. Hlth. & Long.*, 1838, *2*: 54–56, p. 56.
89 Such "refutations" of the safety of meat are frequent in health reform literature; this example is from one of the most comprehensive discussions of the question by William Alcott, "Living at the expense of life," *Lib. Hlth.*, 1837, *1*: 342.
90 S. Hunt, "Death of Sylvester Graham," *Am. Veg.*, 1851, *1*: 187 (italics mine). Also see R. Trall, "Biographical sketch of Sylvester Graham," *Water-Cure J.*, 1851, *12*: 110.
91 William Alcott, "Causes of human suffering," *Lib. Hlth.*, 1838, *2*: 240–243, p. 241.
92 For a concise presentation of the modern physiological rationale of vegetarianism, see J. de Langre, "The physical cost of fleshfoods," *Veg. World*, 1975, issue 4, p. 8.
93 A. Lovejoy, "Foreword" to L. Whitney, *Primitivism and the Idea of Progress in English Popular Literature of the 18th Century* (Baltimore, 1934), p. xv.
94 *Ibid.*; G. Boas and A. Lovejoy, *Primitivism and Related Ideas in Antiquity* (Baltimore, 1935); G. Boas, *Essays on Primitivism and Related Ideas in the Middle Ages* (New York, 1966); R. Walker, *The Golden Feast: A Perennial Theme in Poetry* (London, 1952).
95 W. Alcott, *Lectures on Life and Health; or, the Laws and Means of Physical Culture* (Boston, 1853), p. 226.
96 J. J. Rousseau, *Émile* (London, 1780), p. 45.

24

When Society First Took a Bath

HAROLD DONALDSON EBERLEIN

Think of an America without bathtubs! And you would not have to think very far back. Indispensable as we now regard it, the bathtub in which one could get "wett all over at once" has been in fairly common use scarcely a full century; in some parts of the country, indeed, the bathtub era falls well short of the century mark. The supremacy of washbowl and pitcher yielded but slowly to the vogue for new-fangled "contraptions"; there was much obstructive prejudice to overcome. Even after popular opinion in Philadelphia, Boston, and New York grudgingly accepted the bathtub as an accessory of respectability, the "Saturday night" inhibition often restricted its use to weekly ablutions. Not 40 years ago, one good woman in Philadelphia, whose family had just met with "unexpected financial prosperity" and moved into a fashionable city neighborhood to a house with *two* bathrooms, told an admiring visitor she was so excited about the unwonted bathing splendor and convenience she could hardly wait for Saturday nights to come round! Later still, a Philadelphia family of high social standing and two bathrooms decided they needed only one of them; the daughters kept their ballgowns, laid out full length, in the upstairs bathtub!

All this may be humiliating to cleanliness-boosters who like to proclaim the U.S.A. the bathtubbiest country in the world, and would fain boast a long, honorable past for that present distinction. But it will temper pride and beget livelier thankfulness for bath and shower blessings if we recall the trials and tribulations through which we have reached our current state of grace as the best-washed nation on earth. This compliment the London *Times* paid several years ago, when it published a discursive analysis of cleanliness statistics, giving America first place, Japan second, and England third.

England fell to third rank — notwithstanding proverbial British solicitude for bathing — largely on the basis of bathtub and shower distribution. Anyone who has had to face the ordeal of a clammy hat-bath (filled over night) on a chill November morning, or go unbathed, will give a sympathetic chuckle at England's award to *third* place. Recollections of old English country houses with one or, perhaps, two baths at most; the matutinal wait for a shy little housemaid's or a valet's knock and summons, "Bath's ready, sir"; and then the hasty scramble in dressing gown and slippers to reach the distant bathroom before somebody else popped into it, make one endorse the slogan "a bath for every bedroom."

But England is heaven in the matter of baths compared to rural France or sundry other parts of the Continent, where getting a bath at any time, but especially in winter, is a real achievement, even now. *Par exemple*, a right reverend Monsignor, a chaplain in World War I and billeted one winter in a French village, relates a ludicrous experience. He wanted a bath and addressed himself to the local *curé*. M. *le Curé* threw up his hands with a shocked "*Mon Dieu, en hiver!*" Then, remembering that all Britons were half-mad, he called his housekeeper to gratify this strange whim. A wine barrel sawed in half she placed near the kitchen fire. Into it, a dipperful at a time, she ladled water from a large cauldron. Taking the Scriptural injunction "watch and pray" quite literally, M. *le Curé* sat by with his breviary to superintend the performance. When the Monsignor stepped into the barrel and began to trickle the tepid water over himself with a sponge, the *curé* was convulsed. The Monsignor felt more respectable afterwards, anyhow. It was a

---

HAROLD DONALDSON EBERLEIN (1875–1964) was an authority on the history of Philadelphia.

Reprinted with permission from the *Pennsylvania Magazine of History*, 1943, *67*: 30–48.

bit more comfortable than some of the early morning baths of his Yorkshire boyhood days; he and his brother sat in tin hat-baths while a groom sprinkled them with cold water out of a big garden watering pot. The Monsignor's French bath recalls an anecdote recently recounted by a medical friend. During World War I, the doughboys in his company had to bring him their letters to censor. In one of them he was amazed to read "the French had chain-stores, just the same as in America, only they all seemed to belong to a Mr. Bain who specialized in baths. Whenever you went into a village and found Mr. Bain's name over a door, you could always get a bath"!

In the face of inertia and prejudice, the initiative and perseverance it took to form our present bathing habits and build our national reputation for cleanliness, entitle the first promoters of bathtubs and showers to everlasting gratitude and respect. At the risk of being thought cranks, they did a patriotic service and eventually made society bath-minded. Incidentally, when American society first really took a bath is not merely a matter of academic interest; the whole situation is full of intimate humor.

As early as the 17th century folk of the "better sort" went to "take the waters" at "baths." New England had its springs and wells that attracted favorable attention; so had Maryland and Virginia, before the last of the Stuarts ascended the throne. In Pennsylvania, the springs in Chester County and Bucks drew their clientele of fashionable Philadelphia visitors as early as the second decade of the 18th century. A little later, certain seaside places on the Jersey coast became the objectives of brief holiday visits for those Philadelphians who fancied salt air and sea bathing, for there were, to be sure, a few hardy souls who liked to swim in rivers or bathe in the surf, if the water was right, and the air was right, and the sun shone brightly. If we judge by the bulk of written or printed evidence of the period, the main object in swimming was *exercise* (highly approved by B. Franklin); resulting cleanness, a secondary consideration (when considered at all), was incidental. Perhaps we ought rather to say it was often *accidental*, if we assume the element of "intention."

All this while, visitors to the inland spas almost invariably confined their "taking the waters" to drinking copiously (with Spartan resolution if the "waters" were nasty); bathing externally was "a horse of another color" and needed some exceptional urge. To the average person in good health an all-over bath was not at all a necessity, not even a desideratum. He considered a visit to one of the advertised springs or bathing places an occasional lark, to be attended by sundry diversions and amusements and, of course, enticing food and drink; he was quite ready to accept the old Roman idea of concomitant entertainment, take in the side shows, consume the food and drinkables, and then generally omitted the bath! It makes one think of the old couplet,

"Mother, may I go in to swim?"
"Yes, my darling daughter.
Hang your clothes on a hickory limb,
But don't go near the water!"

A few sybaritic voluptuaries might, at sufficient intervals, indulge in the extreme luxury of an all-over bath, but it was not a thing to be mentioned any more than it would be nowadays for a person to boast of bathing in a tubful of milk or champagne. A bath might, indeed, be a real punishment — like the wetting administered scolds in the ducking-stool, or "keel-hauling" refractory sailors; again, it might be an inconvenient penance prescribed by the family doctor. Although, perhaps, Benjamin Franklin's famous copper slipper-bath that he imported from France was not exactly a penitential device, the philosopher frequented it to allay a disorder of his increasing age. Being eminently practical-minded, he rigged up a bookrack on the instep of the slipper and assuaged the tedium of bathing by reading as he soaked. The receipted bills for his bath thermometers are still preserved in Philadelphia in the library of the American Philosophical Society. While he was sitting in a similar slipper-bath, Charlotte Corday killed Marat, and Napoleon is pictured in a tub of the same kind.

Common indifference to complete synchronous ablution provokes sharp comment from Charles Brockden Brown, in the early 19th century (*vox clamantis in eremo*), in one of his notes to his translation of Volney's book on American soil and climate, published in Philadelphia in 1804. Alluding to our hot summers, he speaks of the vast numbers who pass through a long life

> amidst all these heats, clothed in cloth, flannel and black fur hats and lying on a feather bed at night, drinking nothing but wine and porter and eating strong meats three times a day, and never allowing water to touch any part of them but their extremities for a year together.

It makes one itch and swelter to think of it! Some of the more austere religionists viewed the bath as a frivolous amusement, a sinful luxury; as such, it was a diversion for sober godly folk to eschew. Such a thing as our notion of a daily bath for the sake of comfort as well as cleanliness entered the heads of few. When Mary Baker Eddy, in *Science and Health*, wrote: "Washing should be only to keep the body clean, and this can be done with less than daily scrubbing the whole surface," she was voicing only a slightly belated antipathy to the bathtub.

Personal cleanliness in polite society, after all, has been a matter of varying standards through the ages. The Romans loved to bathe and were clean throughout nearly the whole social scale; only the lowest city rabble and the *pagani* were unwashed. In the Middle Ages, on the other hand, there was an accepted connection between dirt and holiness; vermin and sanctity were by no means strangers, witness the hegira of "inhabitants" that crawled out of St. Thomas à Becket's clothing after his murder. According to the chronicler:

> The vermin boiled over like water in a simmering cauldron, and the onlookers burst into alternate weeping and laughter.

The "odor of sanctity" must have been a sickening stench.[1] Louis XIV, although he hated it, had to use strong scent on his handkerchiefs because the great ladies and gentlemen of his Court were definitely malodorous, thanks to their dislike of soap and water; they considered Madame eccentric because she liked to bathe. Madame de Sevigné, writing to her daughter, notes the "curious fact" that "we wash our hands, but never wash our feet"! In the reign of Louis XV, we know that the courtiers had an ill-developed ablutionary sense, to say the least.

In 17th-century France, England, and America, the louse, who flourishes only where there is personal uncleanliness, though not exactly a cherished pet, was a recognized member of the social system. Shakespeare probably voices the limit of easy-going tolerance when he makes Sir Hugh Evans say,

> It is a familiar beast of man and signifies love.

Ordinarily M. *le Pou* incurred active disapprobation. Samuel Pepys complains that he had to go to his Westminster barber's "to have my Periwigg he lately made me cleansed of its nits, which vexed me cruelly that he should have put such a thing into my hands." When George Washington copied his "Rules of civility" in his fourteenth year (that was in 1746), he wrote, "Kill no vermin, as Fleas, lice, tics, etc. in the sight of others."

Later in the 18th century, when ladies of quality wore their hair dressed over towering "drums," and often kept their coiffures in place for four or five days on end, and even longer — both because of the scarcity of hairdressers, and also the time, labor, and expense involved — they now and again complained in hot weather of "rancid heads," and small wonder, smeared with pomatum and grease as their pates were. Small wonder, either, that their scalps beneath these lofty confections of greased hair and ribbons often itched agonizingly so that they sought relief by inserting silver louse-scratchers — very like short meat-skewers; they occasionally turn up in antique shops, one of the "elegancies of uncleanliness" — and pursuing the unwelcome guests. In France, there was a precise etiquette of scratching. Reboux, describing the education of a princess of France in the middle of the 17th century, writes,

> One had carefully taught the young princess that it was bad manners to scratch when one did it by habit and not by necessity, and that it was improper to take lice or fleas or other vermin by the neck to kill them in company, except in the most intimate circles.

If French princesses of the blood royal were thus minutely instructed before whom it was or was not permissible to hunt and kill lice, we may be sure of two things — elsewhere in exalted society there were codes of louse-etiquette also, and there were lice to hunt and kill. The closed season was presumably short and intermittent.

By the end of the 18th century, the louse was

taboo in the "highest circles" and had been relegated to the polls of the "lower orders." Whenever redemptioners or other bound servants, white or black, entered the family's service, Elizabeth Drinker, of Philadelphia, notes in her *Diary* the pains she was at to have them scrubbed and disinfected, and their clothing burned if necessary. Here is a sample entry, in October 1794:

> We discover'd a day or two ago, that black Scipio had contracted acquaintance while in Jail, that was realy too disgusting to be easy under . . . Sall, after a strict scruting found three, which was three too many to be born with, the difficulty was, he had no change of raiment, linnen excepted, I had him strip'd, and wash'd from stem to stem, in a tub warm Soap suds, his head well lathered and when rinc'd clean, pour'd a quantity spirits over it, then dress'd him in Girl's cloaths, 'till his own could be scalded &c, he appear'd rather diverted, than displeas'd.

Rum infused with larkspur was a valued exterminant, and larkspur used to be in demand on southern plantations to rout "boogers" from the heads of the blacks.

M. *le Pou* doesn't like soap and water. Had there been sufficient bathing, he wouldn't have been as much in evidence at the end of the 18th century as he was, even among humbler folk. Unpleasant as it may be to admit it, it is undeniably true that in the 17th and 18th centuries many highly-respected persons were definitely untidy, or worse, and had at least casual acquaintance with objectionable parasites. This would not have been so had society in general taken bathing more seriously.

The impetus towards better standards of cleanliness had mixed origins. There were the owners of springs or wells, to which, rightly or wrongly, valuable medicinal properties were attributed; they tried to exploit the waters for profit and offered various attractions to draw the public thither. There were progressive individuals, or sometimes communities, who took advantage of natural local conditions favorable for swimming to establish baths and showers, more or less as a seasonal amusement but with quasi-cleanliness intent. And there were fastidious persons who always looked with favor on bathing and, being blessed with inventive ingenuity and initiative, from the mid-18th century onward they made independent efforts to contrive for themselves and their families suitable bathing facilities in advance of the customary "inadequacies" of their day. Their stimulating example was not wholly lost on the communities in which they lived, although it seems to have taken an unduly long time for their support of the "gospel of soap and water" to make a measurable public impression.

One of the earliest instances of stressing the desirability of really bathing at medicinal springs occurred in 1765, when Bathtown or Bath, in the Northern Liberties of Philadelphia, attracted some attention. As already pointed out, people were ready enough to *drink* the waters; to *bathe* in them, the public had to be enticed by the bait of food and entertainment, and there was always the likelihood of their taking the bait and not the bath. John White, "living near the new Bath," advertised that he humbly proposed, with his wife's assistance, "to accommodate the ladies and gentlemen with breakfasting on the best tea, coffee, cream, etc., which articles may also be had in the afternoon." After mentioning some kind of Turkish bath and noting other attractions, mostly of nonaquatic nature, however, he hopes the "salutary purposes which the founder intended" (which meant actually *bathing*) would now be "effected." The founder was that enlightened and public-spirited physician, Dr. John Kearsley. One should add that tradition says William Penn knew of the spring and had some notion of establishing a bath there. One more point, that, to the score of Penn's wise vision.

Despite the well-meant efforts to make Philadelphians bathe, Bathtown seems to have enjoyed only a passing vogue. For that degree of cleanliness indispensable to ordinary decency, society obstinately clung to washbowl and pitcher. People of means and a taste for elegancy often had Nanking china bathtubs — large round affairs, about 21 inches in diameter, with straight or slightly inward-sloping sides, and about 6 or 7 inches deep — like that of Dr. William Smith, the first provost of the University of Pennsylvania. These handsome blue-and-white porcelain bathtubs, raised on low wooden stands, about 18 or 19 inches high, permitted considerably more splashing than an ordinary washbowl on a much higher washstand. Modern antique hunters sometimes imagine they were intended for exceptionally capacious punch receptacles, for goldfish, or else for jardinières — the writer has seen them used for the latter purpose — but they were really the most luxurious of the bedroom appointments for bathing in that day. People still living remember them as bedroom accessories in their Philadelphia childhood homes. Really cleanly, fastidious persons mastered an adroit washcloth and bowl technique. There were adepts in this technique surviving well into the present century. To one such old lady — she was very clean but abhorred bathtubs and never got into one — an irreverent member of the younger generation suggested giving an ink eraser for a Christmas present as a possibly useful toilet adjunct.

Trenton had a public bath as early as 1771 for, when the Drinkers were there on a visit from Philadelphia, Elizabeth writes in her *Diary*:

> June 30, 1771: First day; . . . H. D. went into the Bath this mor^g . . . S. Merriott Sen. Molly Hall, Anna Humber; and Self, went this Afternoon into ye Bath, I found the shock much greater than I expected; . . .
>
> July 1: . . . took a ride this Morn^g. to ye Bath, had not courage to go in.

By July 4, however, she had screwed up her courage to the sticking point for "at 11 °Clock I went into ye Bath; with Fear and trembling, but felt cleaver[2] after it." Public baths at this time, whether swimming, plunge, or shower, apparently were open only during warm or mild weather, as we see by an announcement in the New York *Royal Gazette*, April 18, 1778:

> Bathing Machine, Upon the plan of those used at Margate, and other Wateringplaces in England, is to be established on the North River near Vauxhall by June 1. The subscription price is a guinea a season, or five shillings a bath. . . . It is to be open from June 1 to the end of September from 6 A.M. until 12 noon.

The "Bathing Machine, Upon the plan of those used at Margate," finally got started two months late. It is not recorded how New Yorkers took to it. We may be thankful the fashion didn't continue indefinitely and become national.

By 1794, the vogue for summer "bathing" as a frolic had grown apace amongst New Yorkers. In his *Travels*, Henry Wansey records what was evidently the forerunner of Coney Island:

> June 29. I made another excursion into Long Island, with a gentleman of New York; we crossed at nine in the morning, at Brooklyn Ferry, with our horses, and rode through Flat Bush to Gravesend, near the Narrows, where there is a beautiful view of the sea and all the shipping entering the harbour. A Mr. Bailey, of New York, has just built a very handsome tea-drinking pleasure house, to accommodate parties who come hither from all the neighbouring ports; . . . it seems parties are made here from thirty or forty miles distance, in the Summer time. . . . So much company resort to this pleasant island on each fine Sunday, from New York and other places, as to keep four large ferry boats, holding twenty persons each, in constant employ.

The expressed intention of Mr. Bailey "also to have bathing-machines, and several other species of entertainment," as well as the "handsome tea-drinking pleasure house," however, would seem to indicate that the holiday-makers still felt distinct hesitancy about really going into the water and getting wet without the inducement of a contraption (the "other species of entertainment" thrown in for good measure) to make the unwonted occasion a more thrilling adventure. Bathing, for the sake of the bath, still lacked the element of spontaneous enthusiasm.

Equally considerate of the prevalent "hydrophobia," and equally diplomatic in promising additional enticements to lure the public so that the obligation to bathe should not be too pressing, was the advertisement of the Harrogate waters and baths in the Philadelphia papers of 1784. The obliging Boniface who kept the inn at Harrogate (then about four miles outside the city) praised the properties of the waters, duly attested by the most eminent physicians; mentioned the "houses erected over the Harrogate waters" with "two showers baths and two dressing rooms" and also, at "the Chalybeate spring," the "convenient bath for plunging or swimming"; but he laid especial emphasis of both space and verbiage on the garden, which "is in excellent order, and additional improvements made to render it agreeable and pleasant," and the fact that he "is determined to keep the best of liquors of all kinds." Likewise, the type didn't let the reader forget that "breakfasts, dinners, tea, coffee and fruits of all kinds may be had at the shortest notice, and also excellent accommodations for boarding and lodging." Harrogate eventually became popular as a public garden, numbering frequent concerts and exhibitions among its attractions.

That people were gradually becoming bath-minded, or at least bath-conscious, appears from a letter John Jones wrote Franklin in April 1785, seeking the illustrious Doctor's advice about what was evidently a contemplated business venture. Jones had "long entertained a high opinion of the utility of bathing" and was "desirous of seeing the practice of it brought into general use in this country." He intended to have "a building erected where the different kinds of baths," including Russian vapor baths, might be "commodiously united"; he hoped to have Franklin's suggestions about plan and other practical details before proceeding. Another evidence of dawning bath-consciousness crops up in such cooperative community efforts as that mentioned by Elizabeth Drinker, on a visit to Downingtown, in Pennsylvania, in September 1798. A bathhouse had been built "by a subscription in this neighbourhood." The bathhouse was locked, but Mrs. Drinker "could discern through the keyhold, the Bath, the Pump &c."

During the last two decades of the 18th century, enough public baths came into being to show that at least the idea of bathing, *versus* total dependence on washbowl and pitcher, had taken root, however infrequently the more progressive members of the community might practise it. Besides the various baths and gardens established in Philadelphia — then the wealthiest and most luxurious as well as the most conservative city in the country — there were noteworthy bathing opportunities in New York, then, as always, forward-looking. In 1782, Henry Ludlam advertised a "bathing house for the use of ladies which he has erected in his yard on the North River, adjoining Powles Hook Ferry." In 1792, Nicholas Denise announces that he

> has just established, though at great expence and under M. Boucher's directions, a very convenient Bathing House, having eight rooms, in every one of which Baths may be had with either fresh, salt, or warm Water . . . .

This seems to be the first instance of warm water at a public bath. In 1797, Abel F. Fisher opened a "Tea Garden and Bathing House," where also there were warm and cold, salt and fresh, baths. Bathing, however, still had to be assiduously advertised.

The pioneers of bathing *at home* contrived divers ingenious expedients to secure the occasional luxury of a real bath. However clumsy, inadequate, and inconvenient we should now consider their devices, we owe them gratitude for their initiative and the example they set. So far as we know, they were all persons of acknowledged position and anything they might do was bound ultimately to have weight with public opinion. In striving to gratify their own personal desires for cleanliness, they set a soap-and-water fashion that eventually benefitted all ranks of society. The earliest of these domestic equipments date from the latter part of the 18th century.

At Rose Hill Manor, near Frederick, in Maryland, the home of Governor Thomas Johnson from 1794 to 1819, is what is said to be the first bathtub in the state. A great stone basin, about eight by five feet, and four feet deep, stands in a little stone house at one side of the main dwelling. This room — for it is really nothing more — was heated by charcoal stoves. Tradition says that on Monday mornings the slaves filled the tub with water and then let it temper in the heat of the stoves till Saturday night, when the governor took his bath.

Another early garden bathhouse the Honorable St. George Tucker devised at his home in Williamsburg about 1796.

> Like Thomas Jefferson, with whom he corresponded frequently, he was always inventing mechanical contrivances of every sort. He turned the little dairy house by the well in the Tucker House yard into a bathroom far surpassing in luxury anything of which Williamsburg could boast for the next hundred years.

Beside the well house, close to the converted dairy, a channelled stone was raised on two posts. Water from the well buckets was poured into the hollowed stone and ran thence by a lead pipe, which divided in two and poured into each of the two copper bathtubs in the old dairy. These coffin-shaped copper tubs were raised from the floor and there was room enough under each to insert two or three braziers to warm the water. A great-grandson of St. George Tucker, now living in the house, distinctly remembers at least one of the braziers, and also the lead pipe, bits of which he abstracted as a lad to make shot for his "slappy." We constantly encounter reticence and timidity amongst the first feminine bathtub bathers. Mrs. St. George Tucker was no exception. Henry Tucker, writing to his father (then away from home) in June 1796, says: "Mama has taken a bath and enjoyed it very much though at first she was quite frightened."

It was evidently deemed the proper thing to have the bath in a small separate building outside the house. Taking a tub bath was a nasty, splashy business and would only mess up the tidy rooms of the house. Besides, when there was no room in the house provided for them, the bathtub contrivances would have been unsightly. And then there was the lack of piping or drainage to get rid of the water afterwards. In 1796, at The Highlands, in the Whitemarsh Valley, Anthony Morris built a beautiful octagonal spring and bathhouse. The "bathing room" is on the upper floor and has a handsomely executed fireplace and other woodwork. The early tradition of detached bathhouses in the garden, and the inconvenience and unsightliness likely to be occasioned in the house by a tub, probably had something to do with the feeling that seems unquestionably to have existed later, when there was no real reason for it — namely, that it was *infra dig.* to have a bathtub in the house, not quite nice, and that really respectable people did not do it. At any rate, at or about the time that Nicholas Biddle was making his 1830 addition to Andalusia, he built a separate bathhouse about 60 feet away from the kitchen wing. He then procured from Italy a deep white marble bathtub, about the size of a generous horse trough, and much like an old Roman sarcophagus in appearance. When he wished a bath, the servants carried out pails of hot water and filled the sarcophagus. It is now in the garden and makes an ideal abode for goldfish.

Old Philadelphia diaries, account books, and letters afford many enlightening details about 18th-century bathing habits and, as Philadelphia was the wealthiest and most luxurious colonial metropolis, it had the best of whatever there was. To Joseph Carson, merchant and shipowner, belongs the credit for having the first shower bath on record in Philadelphia. On December 23, 1790, he paid 4 pounds, 15 shillings for it. Whether he had it put up outside his house or installed within is not chronicled. We have more light on the shower-bath experiences of the Drinker family. They were progressive folk as well as bath-minded and, in 1798, they had a shower bath set up in the back-yard of their town house. On July 31, 1798, Elizabeth Drinker writes in her *Diary*:

> Nancy pulled the string of ye Shower bath again this even^g^. she seems better reconciled to it. — ye water has stood some hours in the Yard, which alters the property much, she goes under ye bath in a single gown and an Oyl cloath cap, — her maid Patience and our Sally went into the bath box together, used ye same water with a little added to it — it was a fine frolick for them. . . .

Although the shower was installed in 1798, it was not until July 1, 1799, that Mrs. Drinker herself became "reconciled" to it and conquered her timidity. On that date she inscribes in her *Diary*:

> Nancy came here this even^g^. she and self went into the Shower bath. I bore it better than I expected, not having been wett all over at once, for 28 years past.

A shower bath installed in the Pennsylvania Hospital about the same time was supposed to have an especially beneficial effect upon insane patients. In structure, the shower bath of the late 18th century apparently resembled a modern telephone booth. Some seem to have been placed in old Boston houses about this period. (The Bostonians evidently did not put them in the backyard as the Drinkers did.) The bather entered and closed the door, while an assistant outside mounted a stepladder and poured water into a sieve-like receptacle on top. (The Drinker shower had a chain to pull that released the water from the overhead cullender.) The water ran out through a hole in the bottom of the shower box and into another receptacle put there to catch it. The idea of water dribbling from an overhead channel or box on the bather was not new — old illustrations show that the Swiss had such contrivances in the 16th century — but the enclosing box was a modern improvement that ensured privacy to the bather and kept the sloppiness of the operation within bounds.

What really gave a marked impulse to the spread of bathing habits among the more modern-minded element of the community was the appearance, about the turn of the century, of "bathing tubs" and, soon afterwards, the establishment of fairly adequate municipal water systems in the different cities of the eastern seaboard. The "bathing tubs" were elongated ovals in shape, about seven feet long by two-and-a-half feet wide, made of wooden staves like the oldfashioned round washtubs, and had one end brought up in a high arch — the whole effect rather suggestive of a mummy case. The Drinkers bought one of these in 1803 and often lent it to "neighbours who had illness in their homes." For this wooden creation, "lined with tin and painted . . . with Castors under y^e^ bottom and a brass lock to let out the water," they paid $17.

On January 27, 1801, Philadelphia's municipal water supply was turned on — other cities got piped water at subsequent intervals — and one of the French émigrés, Joseph Simon by name, opened a public bathhouse, near Third and Arch streets, where his patrons could bathe in permanently fixed bathtubs equipped with running water and drains. It is encouraging to know that he had sufficient custom to continue his enterprise for more than 20 years, when he retired with a competency and sold out his baths to a successor. His customers, however, were not always frequent in their attendance. Mrs. Drinker says, in July 1806:

> My husband has been twice in the french man's bath and William once this Summer — It is a little more expensive but much less trouble for the men, than getting it [the "bathing tub"] ready at home. . . .

For economy of time and labor, the "bathing tubs" at home sometimes got used at one filling by a succession of bathers. To quote Elizabeth Drinker once more, on August 6, 1806, she chronicles:

> I went into a warm bath this afternoon, H. D. [Mr. Drinker] after me, because he was going out, Lydia and Patience [the maids] went into ye same bath after him, and John [manservant] after them — If so many bodies were clensed, I think the water must have been foul enough . . . . [Bacterial apprehension still nonexistent!]

When Robert Sutcliff, an English Friend, landed in New York at the end of July 1804, the very next day his friends took him to see a recently established public bathhouse as one of the notable "sights" of the town. In his journal, under date of "7th Month 31st, 1804," he writes:

> This morning I was conducted by my companions to one of the Public Baths kept in the city of New York. These Baths are upon a plan I had not seen before. On each side of a long and spacious passage, is a range of small rooms, in each of which is a Bath sufficient to accommodate one person; with suitable Conveniences for dressing and undressing. On the side of each Bath are two brass cocks, the one furnishing warm and the other cold water; so that the bather may have the water at what temperature he pleases. There is also a valve, by means of which, if there is more than is pleasant, he may let part of it out. Some of these Baths are made of white marble; and are so constructed that a person may lie down or sit in them. So grateful it is to remain a considerable time in them, in the warm season of the year, that it is a common practice for bathers to take books [detestable habit] with them to read while they thus indulge themselves in the Bath. There are also Baths in a different part of the house set apart for females.

Note that Sutcliff — probably taking his cue from his American friends — speaks of bathtub bathing as a luxury, an "indulgence," an agreeable warm weather diversion, not a daily necessity, the year round.

Even with well-appointed public bathhouses and running city water readily available, the idea of frequently getting "wett all over at once" for the sake of cleanliness, and the satisfaction of feeling well-groomed, seems to have taken hold of only a small minority of the public. The "man in the street," and also plenty who would resent that classification, had to be urged and coaxed to bathe. Taking a bath ought to have a pretext or an excuse. On June 1, 1824, in a newspaper advertisement trumpeting the innovation as the last word in modern luxury and elegance (but stressing luxury), the proprietor of the Worcester [Massachusetts] Coffee House plainly implies this reluctant attitude when he

> INFORMS his Friends and the Public generally, that he has recently added to the former *Convenience* of his Establishment, a commodious BATHING HOUSE, in separate apartments for Ladies and Gentlemen, where Visitors may be at any time accommodated with WARM AND COLD BATHS, in a perfectly retired and convenient situation. Pure Spring Water is now brought through Pipes, for the use of his House and to supply his Baths; this Luxury, in a hot and dusty season, together with an ever-flowing SODA FOUNTAIN, the choicest of Liquors, a well filled Larder, and indefatigable endeavors to render his House pleasant and agreeable to his Customers, he flatters himself will insure a continuance of Public Patronage.

The "ever-flowing SODA FOUNTAIN" is a blandishment to cajole visitors into trying the novelty; the "perfectly retired and convenient situation" (probably in the basement, where the earliest hotel bathing arrangements were usually placed) suggests the furtiveness of a speakeasy, where the surreptitious bather will not be found out and exposed to ridicule as an extravagant sybarite and a sissy, or one of the "gentler sex" accused of "indelicacy" in letting it be discovered that she was taking a bath.

About five years later, when the epoch-making Tremont House in Boston opened its doors to the public, October 16, 1829, there was no deprecatory tone in the announcement that among its "numerous superiorities" there were eight "bathing rooms" in the basement "adjoining the housekeeper's apartments, the laundry and the larder." The Tremont was the pioneer "luxury hotel" of America, in fact, the first in the world. Educational intent as well as business instinct actuated its promoters, and they saw no occasion to adopt an apologetic attitude about their basement bathing establishment. It was as good as any the most up-to-date plumbing skill could then compass; it was an important feature in the hitherto unknown policy of "luxury and maximum service to patrons" they were just inaugurating. Another of the Tremont's "superiorities" was that every bedroom had a washbowl and pitcher, and free soap! This, while one could still say of the country in general that

> a few innkeepers . . . had a supply of bowls and pitchers and would send one up to a guest's room, with a supply of water, on request, but it seems to have been a service grudgingly granted. In most of the inns of that period the guest could wash himself before breakfast and at other times in the barroom, or, if at a country inn, he could wash in the kitchen or at the backyard pump.[3]

In May 1836, when the Astor House in New York opened as the *dernier cri* in hotel luxury and splendor, it proclaimed with almost brazen effrontery its 17 basement "bathing rooms" and two showers. The public was getting used to bathing announcements, even getting used to the occasional sight of bathtubs.

Little by little, forward-looking persons were overcoming the inertia about bathing and were installing bathtubs in their houses, in spite of the conventional semi-disapprobation of such gadgets. It is encouraging to know of the 401 baths in Philadelphia reported by the Watering Committee in 1823, but the names of the enlightened and courageous owners have not so far been discovered. The first private Philadelphia bathtub with attached plumbing of which we have definite record, Henry Carey, the publisher, installed in his town house in 1826. From about 1829 onwards, plumbers advertised bathtubs and shower baths, and presumably their advertisements met with some response, however limited. Many of these illustrated advertisements appear in the Philadelphia directories of the period.

If a tub bath was no longer to be reckoned in one of the four categories previously noted, nevertheless with most persons it was still infrequent enough to be counted something of an event. The comparatively few bathtubs so far installed in private dwellings and the convenience of public bathing establishments favored such enterprises as the Philadelphia Baths that William Swaim, of "Panacea" repute, opened in 1828. The advertisement quotes Count Rumford's observations on the beneficial effects of bathing and cleanliness, and assures prospective patrons that there are

> apartments for each of the sexes, having several and separate entrances; the best female attendance being provided for the service of the ladies . . . every provision has been made for shower bathing, so that the latter salutary application may be enjoyed at pleasure, by means of appropriate contrivances under the complete control of the individual who employs it.

A contemporary description, in equally highfalutin language, characteristic of the time, tells us that

> the northern section, which comprises a double range of bathing rooms, an ample shower bath, and a suite of parlours, all well furnished, is appropriated exclusively to ladies; the southern section is for the accommodation of gentlemen. Here also are two ranges of bathing rooms, a bar room, and a reservoir, twenty-six feet by ten, in which the water is tempered by steam, and may be raised to the height of six feet. . . . The bathing vessels [the writer means bathtubs], fifty in number, are composed either of Italian marble finely wrought, or copper ingeniously plated with Banca tin.

There was a swimming teacher in the "swimming room" to teach the "natatory art" in perfect security and "without hazard." With such "elegant" surroundings, it was becoming a fashionable fad to bathe. Swaim's baths prospered.

For his aid in bringing about the gradual change in public sentiment towards bathing, instead of dependence on washbowl and pitcher, Sylvester Graham — the Graham for whom bread and crackers are named — deserves grateful recognition. As early as 1830 he started his crusade for health reform, and insistence on frequent bathing — "in very warm water at least three times a week" — was one of the cardinal points of his program to achieve his "*mens sana in corpore sano*" ideal for the American public. His efforts produced widespread effects; Graham organizations of one sort or another and Graham publications started up all over the country, and Graham principles and practices were thoroughly discussed. How timely was his advocacy of frequent bathing appears when the Boston *Moral Reformer*, in 1835, quotes a "young man of great promise" who inquires of the editor: "I have been in the habit during the past winter of taking a warm bath every three weeks. Is this too often to follow the year round?"[4]

About 1844 — only two years after the appearance of the mythical "first American bathtub" in Cincinnati, according to the hoax perpetrated by Mr. Mencken — came the first private baths in hotels, destined to play an increasingly potent role in the program of "luxury and maximum service" now being adopted by hotelkeepers throughout the country. About 1835 the Philadelphia Common Councils had tried to pass an ordinance prohibiting tub bathing between November 1 and March 15. In 1845, Boston had actually proscribed bathing in winter except upon medical advice, while Virginia, some time before, had imposed a tax of $30 a year on every bathtub brought into the state, and up to almost the middle of the century popular opinion held it actually dangerous to bathe in a tub during the winter months. But by 1850, between the large city hotels and multiplying bathing establishments, aided all along by a rapidly developing system of the best plumbing in the world, for both public and domestic equipment, bathing came to be almost a craze.

To bathe was the smart thing to do. Those who didn't take a bath, at reasonable intervals at least, just weren't "in it." Baths of all kinds — Turkish, mud, galvanic, Russian, Swedish, and what not — sprang into existence and were well patronized at all hours of the day and night. At many of the public baths, the old diverting etceteras were not forgotten — "one could get mint juleps to drink while sitting in a bathtub" — but they were now definitely minor considerations; the bath was the thing.

Thus, by the mid-19th century — the discouraging ordeals and laborious mechanical inconveniences of bathing now things of the past — bathing had come into its own as a recognized social institution. Thanks to hotelkeepers, bathing-house proprietors, and skillful plumbers, a fashion had been set. Society in general had at last taken a bath and daily bathing had become a cardinal virtue.

NOTES

The author desires to acknowledge his obligations to Jefferson Williamson, *The American Hotel* (Knopf, 1930): Cecil Drinker, M.D., *Not So Long Ago* (Oxford Univ. Press, 1937); Hans Zinsser, *Rats, Lice and History* (Little, Brown & Co., 1935); Howard W. Haggard, M.D., *Devils, Drugs and Doctors* (Harper's, 1929); Mary Haldane Coleman, *St. George Tucker; Citizen of No Mean City* (Dietz Press, 1938); Helen Urner Price in *National Historical Magazine*, June 1940, and sundry diaries and early books of travel: also to Joseph Carson, Edward Carey Gardiner, Dr. Francis R. Packard, Edward Robins, Lawrence J. Morris, Richard H. Shryock, Dayton Voorhees, E. Milby Burton, of the Charleston Museum, William Sumner Appleton, of the Society for the Preservation of New England Antiquities, Clarence S. Brigham, of the American Antiquarian Society, Miss Elizabeth C. Litsinger, of the Enoch Pratt Free Library, all of whom furnished valuable data, and to Berthold A. Sorby, of the New York Public Library, who called attention to many useful references.

1 During the Middle Ages and Renaissance there were bathing and swimming opportunities aplenty, public or otherwise accessible; opposition from the Church arose, not from any ecclesiastical approbation of uncleanliness *per se*, but from the opinion (not altogether unjustified) that the usual bathing facilities and practices were accessory to immorality. The annals of ceremonial ablutions disclose appalling indifference and ignorance with respect to sanatory considerations.

2 This "v" is correct, not a misprint for "n." Cleaver" was her way of spelling "clever." She would not have admitted feeling "cleaner." "Clever" was a rather favorite Quaker word, and when Mrs. Drinker said she felt "clever," she meant "bucked up."

3 Williamson, *The American Hotel.*

4 Richard H. Shryock in *Miss. Valley Hist. Rev.*, 1931, *28*: 172.

Reform

America's urban health problems reached frightening proportions during the middle years of the 19th century. Mortality rates in cities like New York, Boston, and Philadelphia rose alarmingly, as infectious diseases raged out of control. Hoards of immigrants crowded into ill-ventilated tenements and basement hovels, while workers of all ages toiled long hours in stifling sweatshops. Although Americans living below the subsistence level were the most vulnerable, the public health movement arose primarily from concerns of the middle and upper classes.

Among the many factors motivating public health reformers in the 1840s was pietism, described by Charles E. Rosenberg and Carroll Smith-Rosenberg. This evangelical dedication to helping others, also evident in contemporary temperance and abolitionist crusades, often gave public health reform a religious flavor.

The American movement also benefitted from the English experience with sanitary reform, although our country's political institutions created unique problems. Gert H. Brieger describes the political struggle in New York to establish a permanent, effective board of health, which culminated in 1866 with the creation of the Metropolitan Board of Health, the first of its kind in America. Within a year of its birth this organization successfully met its first challenge in reducing the death rate during a cholera epidemic.

Following New York's lead, other cities and states established their own boards, and for a brief period, from 1879 to 1883, there was even a National Board of Health. But the public health movement generally remained a municipal or state affair, led by public-spirited physicians, sanitarians, engineers, nurses, and various philanthropic groups. By the 1870s their efforts seemed to be paying off, as urban death rates declined and allocations for public health stabilized.

The movement generally failed to reduce infant mortality until the early 20th century. Maternal mortality stayed high for even longer. As Joyce Antler and Daniel M. Fox point out, childbirth remained dangerous for mothers until the 1940s. The successful movement to make maternity safe illustrates how 20th-century reformers dealt with a major health problem.

25

Pietism and the Origins of the American Public Health Movement: A Note on John H. Griscom and Robert M. Hartley

CHARLES E. ROSENBERG AND CARROLL SMITH-ROSENBERG

In 1842 Robert M. Hartley, a pious and charitable New Yorker, helped found the New York Association for Improving the Condition of the Poor. That same year John H. Griscom, M.D., City Inspector, submitted to New York's Common Council an elaborately critical report on the city's sanitary condition. These two events initiated the first more-than-episodic public health movement in any American city; there is a distinct continuity in men and ideas between these events in 1842 and the better-known public health agitation of the 60s.

During the decades before the Civil War, New York seemed the filthiest and least healthy of American cities. In the 1840s and early 1850s the two New Yorkers most concerned with the need for reforming such baleful conditions were the abovementioned John H. Griscom and Robert Hartley — the first a name familiar to students of the history of public health, the second very likely unknown. These men were in some ways dissimilar: one was a physician, the other a businessman turned innovator in social welfare; one a Quaker, the other an orthodox Presbyterian. In other ways they had much in common. For the medical historian, their most pertinent similarity lies in both having become involved in public health reform as a result, essentially, of their response to an intense pietism widespread in their generation.

That evangelical religion had a broad impact in ante-bellum America has become a historical commonplace.[1] It is the intention of this paper to suggest that such spiritual dedication played an important role in helping to create a concern for health conditions in the nation's cities. The vast majority of respectable urban Americans — including physicians — found no great difficulty in ignoring the medieval filth and misery which surrounded them. English and French crusaders for public health reform found only a handful of North American advocates before the late 1850s. The motivations which inspired America's pioneer sanitarians cannot therefore be explained alone in terms of European influences or as an inevitable, almost instinctive, rejection of intolerable conditions. The following pages attempt no comprehensive study of either Hartley or Griscom, but hope only to suggest the place of religious motives in shaping their dedication to social reform — as such pietistic convictions did in inspiring the work of virtually every urban philanthropist in this period.

I

To historians of American public health and American urban history, John H. Griscom is known primarily as the author of an eloquent pamphlet describing the *Sanitary Condition of the Laboring Population of New York* (1845).[2] Yet this is only a small part of his efforts in the cause of public health. Beginning with his tenure as New York's City Inspector — the community's principal health officer — in 1842 and culminating with his presidency of the Third National Quarantine and Sanitary Convention in 1859, Griscom labored constantly to alert his fellow New Yorkers to the need for sanitary reform. Griscom was for a number of years almost alone among New York physicians in his crusade.[3] This reformist impulse was indeed so atypical in the medical world of the

---

CHARLES E. ROSENBERG is Professor of History at the University of Pennsylvania, Philadelphia, Pennsylvania. CARROLL SMITH-ROSENBERG is Associate Professor of History, University of Pennsylvania, Philadelphia, Pennsylvania.

Reprinted with permission from the *Journal of the History of Medicine and Allied Sciences*, 1968, *23*: 16–35.

1840s that it seems logical to explain Griscom's involvement in public health matters not in terms of his role as a physician, but in terms of his being his father's son.

The senior John Griscom was a Quaker educator and philanthropist who exemplified in his long career of benevolence a characteristically American respect for science and learning coupled with an intense pietism. Griscom was born in 1774 into an established Quaker family in New Jersey. He studied briefly in Philadelphia, then turned to secondary school teaching in Burlington, New Jersey. Griscom was remarkably successful, and at the invitation of a number of wealthy New Yorkers he moved in 1807 to the emerging metropolis and began to conduct a private school. This was the beginning of more than a half-century of ceaseless benevolence.[4] In addition to his teaching, Griscom was, for example, instrumental in founding the House of Refuge for destitute and vagrant children and a Society for the Prevention of Pauperism — as well as a half-dozen similar philanthropies. He was very much a part of New York's interdenominational evangelical establishment; though a Quaker, he worked closely with Methodists, with Episcopalians, with Presbyterians, to found and manage some of the city's most ambitious charities.[5]

In one area, however, Griscom's activities were quite individualistic. He was fascinated by science generally and chemistry specifically. The Quaker schoolmaster was one of the first Americans successfully to attempt the popularization of chemistry; he spoke at schools and lyceums, to mechanics groups, and gave public lectures.[6] Such scientific proselytizing implied no concession to materialism. Quite the contrary: Griscom's world was of a piece and the study of nature could, he assumed, only illuminate God's greatness. Griscom assumed indeed that any and all learning must inevitably have a spiritual effect. "It seems to me almost an axiomatic truth," he explained, "that sound learning and science do, by a natural law, gravitate towards virtue."[7] And as a man of piety he never shirked his duty of serving as an evangel of science, helping to make his fellow Americans at once more learned and moral.

Griscom soon became one of the handful of respectable New Yorkers alarmed by the misery of so many among the city's poor. In his work with school-age children and especially as a result of his years with the House of Refuge and the Society for the Prevention of Pauperism, Griscom accumulated detailed knowledge of the conditions in which his less fortunate fellow New Yorkers lived. With such broadly social concerns, and in a society in which scientific knowledge was uncommon, Griscom was gradually drawn into areas which seem to the 20th-century reader specifically medical. In 1822, for example, he became embroiled — as a reigning expert on chemistry and thus on disinfection — in debate over the best means of preventing the spread of yellow fever. In similar fashion, Griscom was called upon to act as an adviser on ventilation.[8] Yellow fever, ventilation, science education, and, most important, the condition of the poor — these were to be the central concerns in the life of his physician son.[9]

John H. Griscom was born in 1809 and attended his father's New York school. Not surprisingly, with the elder Griscom so well connected in New York's scientific and philanthropic circles, the younger traveled the path of accepted success in New York medicine. He attended several full sessions of the Rutgers Medical College, where his father served as Professor of Chemistry and Natural Philosophy, and studied successively under two eminent preceptors, John D. Godman and Valentine Mott. After the final collapse of the Rutgers School in 1830, Griscom attended the University of Pennsylvania School of Medicine, graduating in 1832. While he was still a medical student, he had been a walker in the New York Hospital. Returning to New York from Philadelphia, he was awarded an appointment at the New York Dispensary. In 1842 Griscom was also made attending physician at the Eastern Dispensary and a year later received a coveted appointment as attending physician at New York Hospital. Griscom was a founding member of both the New York Medical and Surgical Society and the New York Academy of Medicine. When the academy was organized in 1847, Griscom served on five of its committees the first year, an unmistakable indication — as both common sense and political scientists tell us — of establishment membership.[10]

In addition to his responsibilities as a practitioner, Griscom found time to express a passion for intellectual improvement similar to that which had marked his father's career. The younger Griscom began in the late 1830s to devote a good deal of time to popular education in physiology and hygiene. He wrote several school texts, and soon began to offer public lectures. Fundamental improvement in the health of Americans would depend ultimately, he always held, upon disseminating the truths of hygiene at all levels throughout the community; there was no subject so important and so unfortunately neglected in the curriculum. "The general introduction of this subject," he wrote in 1844, "as a branch of school learning, would, I hesitate not to say, have a greater meliorating influence upon the human condition, than any other." Griscom also believed that hygiene and physiology had a spiritual as well as material content. What subject, for example, could more effectively demonstrate to children their total dependence upon the Lord and the need for obeying His admirably contrived laws? "Indulgence in a vicious or immoral course of life," Griscom assured his young readers, "is sure to prove destructive to health."[11] An understanding of anatomy and physiology would, moreover, in addition to preserving health and morality, draw the mind upwards towards the Contriver of this marvelous "animal mechanism."

Griscom drew habitually upon arguments from design. New York's mortality rates, for example, could not be a normal part of God's world; could He have planned so inefficient a system? A goodly portion of the sickness which afflicted men, Griscom argued, resulted not from some mysterious and ineluctable dispensation of Providence, but from man's own ignorance. (And in the moral calculus of the Griscoms, sin and ignorance unimproved were hardly distinguishable.) Were men only to utilize properly the fresh air, the pure water, the intelligence granted them by the Lord, they would escape unnecessary sickness and premature death. Yet air, water, food — the necessities of life — became all too often the channels through which disease attacked. "Left to the care of nature herself," Griscom lectured, "these would be far less frequently, to man, the sources of disease; but by his own wilfullness and intermeddling, and sad to say, by his own ignorance, he creates the poison which he presents to his own lips."[12] Like many of his contemporaries, Griscom emphasized the unnatural quality of city life, the essentially more healthful — because more natural — life of the savage. One need only compare the rude health of the American Indian with Griscom's wan and narrow-chested fellow New Yorkers.[13] The contrast was easily explained: the savage lived a simple life, in unthinking harmony with the bounties supplied abundantly by the Lord. The ignorance and cupidity of civilized man, on the other hand, everywhere polluted the sources for a healthful life.

This emphasis was consistent with Griscom's essentially optimistic and melioristic tone; civilized life was not inevitably or necessarily unhealthy. To remedy its evils, one need only apply knowledge already available; ventilation was a case in point. The true fault lay not in the existence of cities as such, but in man's obstinate failure to use his intelligence in making city life as healthy as it might be. In this sense, Griscom was certain, such neglects were culpable, an affront to God. "Cleanliness," he noted in 1850, "is said to be 'next to godliness,' and if, after admitting this, we reflect that cleanliness can not exist without ventilation, we must then look upon the latter as not only a *moral* but *religious* duty." What was needed, Griscom urged, was a "*sanatory* regeneration of society."[14]

But, it may be objected, all these arguments were quite commonplace, formulae so traditionalistic that it would be unsafe to assume from them any overwhelming degree of pietism in their user. This may, to some extent, be conceded; but Griscom's lasting significance does not rest upon the formal content of his writings. His historical reputation is based on the Quaker physician's tenacious commitment to bettering the living conditions of deprived New Yorkers. For this was a period when such concerns were atypical in the medical profession, when the filling of public health posts was often a badge of professional inadequacy or second-rate careerism. It does not seem likely that the well-connected Griscom was simply an opportunist seeking notoriety and the sinecure of a political appointment.[15] And if this is not the case, the only apparent motivation for his untiring concern was religious — for a truly secular humanitarianism was still essentially alien to Griscom's time and social class. Even in his explicitly detailed appeals for public health reorganization, Griscom displayed a persistent tone of moral concern, a guiding dependence upon moral imperatives in shaping his understanding of individual behavior and the place which such reform might play in the upgrading of civic virtue.

Most famous of these appeals is his *Sanitary Condition of the Laboring Population of New York*, delivered in December of 1844 as a public lecture and published soon after. (This pamphlet was in its turn an expansion and elaboration of remarks Griscom had appended to his 1842 report as City Inspector).[16] The Quaker physician emphasized the contrast between the city's essentially healthful physicial setting and its disgracefully high mortality rate. There was an ummistakable connection between New York's excessive premature deaths and the miserable condition of the city's tenements. Most deplorable was the plight of thousands who inhabited underground apartments, prey to cellar dampness — even flooding — and poor ventilation. As he describes such conditions, Griscom's decorous prose suggests the emotional impact of the squalor he has seen. "It is almost impossible," he explained, "when contemplating the circumstances and conditions of the poor beings who inhabit these holes, to maintain the proper degree of calmness requisite for thorough inspection, and the exercise of a sound judgment, respecting them."[17] The only solution lay in the use of the state's regulatory powers; New York City needed a board of health endowed with broad powers and staffed by properly trained medical men.[18] Griscom reiterated such arguments for two decades — at legislative hearings, in journal articles, at meetings of the New York Academy of Medicine and the American Medical Association.

Public health reform would result not only in healthier New Yorkers, but in more moral and law-abiding ones. John H. Griscom's world, like his father's, was an organic one. Physical health and living conditions, morality and religion were a tightly knit series of causes and effects. The cellar resident, no matter how pious or industrious at first, could not long remain a productive, church-going member of society. Damp, ill-ventilated apartments soon brought disease, depressed vital energies, and, inevitably, the "moral tone" as well. Unemployment, neglect of person and God soon followed. Such debilitated slum-dwellers turned then to alcohol for the physiological stimulation lacking in their unhospitable environment; the picture of the filthy, drunken, immoral pauper was complete. "From a low state of general health," Griscom explained,

> whether in an individual or in numbers, proceed diminished energy of body and of mind, and a vitiated moral perception, the frequent precursor of habits and deeds, which give employment to the officers of police, and the ministers of justice. . . . The coincidence, or parallelism, of moral degradation and physical disease, is plainly apparent to an experienced observer.[19]

How, for example, could man's innate love of modesty and decorum manifest itself in New York's reeking tenements? Was it surprising that incest, prostitution, and venereal disease should thrive in districts where families had to perform all their biological functions in one small and crowded room? Just as man has an innate feeling for morality, he had an instinctive feeling for order and cleanliness; but, Griscom asked, how could these homely virtues be encouraged in such circumstances? Rents were so high and accommodations so shoddy that even with a steady job and the best of will, working men found it almost impossible to find decent quarters for their families.[20] Man's natural capacity for virtue, like his natural state of health, was every day corrupted — by individual sin and ignorance and by the inequities of social organization.

And the atmosphere, the most universal of God's blessings, was, lamentably, in cities everywhere polluted. Not only did a vitiated atmosphere deplete the slum-dweller's vital powers, it served as a medium for the spread of disease. Epidemic and "miasmatic" diseases — cholera, yellow fever, malaria — were, of course, presumed to be spread through the atmosphere. Griscom believed, however, that even those diseases normally assumed to be contagious might in confined circumstances also be air-borne. "The contagious viri of small-pox, measles, scarlet fever, and all others of that class," Griscom explained, "are also admitted to be communicated through the intermedium of the atmosphere. . . ."[21] The more contaminated the atmosphere, the more concentrated the infectious principle — and the more likely one was to contract it. In crowded tenements all these circumstances coincided; diseases normally noncontagious might often become so, while the slum-dwellers, with vital energies chronically reduced by breathing such vitiated air, succumbed readily whenever they were unfortunate enough to come in contact with "contagious viri." It was only to be expected that Griscom should have emphasized the evils of a vitiated atmosphere and the need for improved systems of ventilation in his calls for reform.[22] Not only was ventilation a fashionable cause, it provided a scientifically reassuring vehicle for Griscom's need to instruct and improve.

Griscom could at first muster scant support in his attempts to gather data on slum conditions and in demanding their reform. Both in his 1842 report as City Inspector and in his *Sanitary Condition of the Laboring Population* Griscom relied heavily upon the testimony of missionaries of the New York City Tract Society. For they, with the city's dispensary physicians, were the only emissaries of respectable society to the tenement districts in which the poor lived and died.[23] Griscom's dependence upon the help of city missionaries indicates not only something of his personal ties, but something of the origins of a growing awareness of slum conditions among proper and articulate New Yorkers. It is no accident that public health reformers in this generation spoke so often and so casually of the need for health missionaries and the distribution of health tracts. The reviewer of Griscom's *Sanitary Condition* in the *New York Journal of Medicine* actually suggested, by way of conclusion, that it be reprinted and distributed by the City Tract Society.[24] In ideas, in actions, in associations, Griscom consistently displayed the pietistic origin of his concern for public health.

In subsequent years, as increasing numbers of physicians became interested in public health problems, this motivating pattern of religiously oriented humanitarianism persisted. Stephen Smith and his wife, for example, were both active in the affairs of the American Female Guardian Society, an organization occupying a "left-wing" position in the evangelical united front. John Ordronaux, another prominent writer on public health matters, urged in his 1866 anniversary discourse to the New York Academy of Medicine that the American Tract Society print and distribute health tracts among the poor:

> Let the poor be taught that there is religion in cleanliness, in ventilation, and in good food; let them but once be induced to put these lessons into practice, and we may rest assured their spiritual culture and moral elevation will be rendered all the more easy and certain.

"Disease, like sin," he explained, "is permitted to exist; but conscience and revelation on the one hand, and reason and science on the other, are the kindred means with which God has armed us against them."[25]

II

More influential than Griscom in illuminating the misery and sickness which existed in New York of the 1840s was his contemporary, Robert M. Hartley. Hartley was a man of great vigor and tenacity — and, as a principal organizer and longtime director of the New York Association for Improving the Condition of the Poor, is ordinarily considered the shaper of America's first protosocial welfare agency. One of the most significant of Hartley's accomplishments was his leadership of the association's pioneer involvement in tenement and public health reform, an involvement which in point of time exactly paralleled Griscom's.

Despite Hartley's self-consciously pragmatic attempts to professionalize charity, the history of the A.I.C.P. and Hartley's own life illustrate how directly the origins of his social activism were rooted in the evangelical enthusiasm of his youth. Robert Milham Hartley was born in England in 1796 and came to the United States as a three-year-old with his merchant father. The family settled in western New York state, in an area known to historians and contemporaries as the Burned-Over district, for the intensity of the religious revivals which swept through it. Like his father, young Hartley went into business, making a mercantile career in New York City. But as in the case of many of his contemporaries, the competitive urgings of commerce did not fill his life. As a boy, Hartley experienced a conversion to evangelical Protestantism and even before arriving in New York City, while still a clerk in upstate New York, he organized prayer meetings and crusaded for proper Sabbath observance. Soon after moving to New York City, Hartley became active in the affairs of his Presbyterian church, serving as an elder and assuming leadership in the church's program of house-to-house missionary visiting. Hartley also began to play an active role in the work of the New York City Tract Society. In 1829 he helped organize the New York City Temperance Society and in 1833 became its corresponding secretary and agent. Hartley was instrumental in formulating the latter society's policy of total abstinence — a novelty at a time when temperance still meant only temperance.[26]

The perfectionism implied in Hartley's advocacy of total abstinence was a characteristic of the late 1820s and early 1830s, a period of increasingly millennial enthusiasm. Hartley's spiritual life was informed by this intense pietism throughout his career, even when dedicated as an older man to ostensibly secular goals (as the rational distribution of charity and the construction of model tenements). Fortunately for the historian, Hartley kept a diary which demonstrates clearly the continuity of his spiritual commitment. The entry for October 15, 1845, for example, reads:

> Revised a plan for the press, long under consideration, to remodel all the city dispensaries so as to distribute the physicians and the medical depots generally over the city. And now, O my soul, how hast thou this day withstood the assaults of an evil world? Answer ere thou sinkest to the insensibility of sleep, as under the searching eye of him with whom thou has to do.

And that for March 19, 1856:

> I am, on a review, much dissatisfied with my labors to-day. I have done but little of that I designed to do. Truly I am an unprofitable servant; yet God mercifully forbears to punish. O for a higher wisdom than my own to direct the labors of my calling! At evening attended a sanitary lecture at the Cooper Institute. To-day my mind has been pervaded with a deep seriousness, and a desire to dwell on spiritual things.

Such sentiments were habitual with the one-time merchant who could, by 1856, nevertheless write that sanitary reform was "the basis of most other reform in this city." There was not, nor could there be, any conflict between Hartley's vigorous pragmatism and intense pietism; the spiritual energies of his youth had been gradually rechanneled so as to shape and motivate his career of overtly secular benevolence. His pious activism had always to be maximized; it could alone placate his consciousness of sin and spiritual imperfection. "My failures," Hartley wrote when past 70, "I believe were less owing to insuperable difficulties, than to my lack of earnestness and energy."[27] The contemplative life had few appeals for the pious in Jacksonian America.

These spiritual compulsions and the slum contacts they engendered had made Hartley and a number of like-minded evangelicals aware of their city's unsavory health conditions well before the formation of the A.I.C.P. in 1842. By the mid-1830s, for example, the New York City Tract Society, of which Hartley had been a member since 1827, began with New York's other city missions to take notice of the sickness and poverty encountered by their missionaries and volunteer tract distributors. Conditions already bad were harshly exacerbated by the panic of 1837 and the lengthy depression which followed; with growing frequency, the annual reports of these evangelical societies lamented in detail the misery of the city's slums. It had begun to seem increasingly unlikely that the souls of the poor could be saved while their bodies remained in such wretchedness.[28] Hartley's temperance work too, though it may seem today a moral, if not moralistic, concern, drew him increasingly into an understanding of the brutal facts of slum life.

It was, indeed, through temperance that Hartley first became involved with a specific public health problem. New York's infant mortality rate was remarkably high — and by the mid-1830s, Hartley had become aware of what he considered a central role played by contaminated milk in swelling these dismaying statistics. He was particularly indignant when investigations showed that a good portion of the city's milk supply came from animals closely confined in filthy and unventilated stalls, and — worst of all — fed exclusively on distillery swill. In the winter of 1836–37, Hartley wrote a series of articles exposing these evils, and in 1842 a full-length treatise on the subject.[29]

Hartley's discussion of the milk problem displays a characteristic 19th-century mixture of pragmatic scientism, religious metaphor doing duty as medical logic, and unmistakable piety. Arguments from Liebig nestle comfortably against those drawn from moral imperative and providential design.

Hartley appealed, as did Griscom, to the ultimate value of the natural — read godly — in condemning the unhealthfulness of the milk produced in such grossly unnatural conditions. Cows kept without exercise, in filthy and unventilated stables, without room even to turn about, fed on hot and reeking swill — such animals could be expected to live but a short time and to produce milk as foul as their own conditions and diet. Could men of good will fold their arms and blame the death of so many innocents upon some inscrutable and unavoidable dispensation? "Can such be the purpose of the benevolent Creator?" Hartley, like Griscom, asked fellow New Yorkers.

> Is so large a number of His rational offspring born with such feeble powers of vitality that life necessarily becomes extinct on the threshold of existence? Such conclusions, being inconsistent with the teachings of his Word and Providence, must be rejected as impious and absurd.

And to an activist like Hartley, the conclusion was unmistakable: no truly pious New Yorker should purchase milk from this tainted source. "Can you continue so, and feel that you have discharged your duty to God, to your families and to the community? Are you not bound by the most powerful obligations to wash your hands from all participation in so great an evil?"[30]

It takes no great sophistication to discern the moralism, the temperance zeal in Hartley's overtly pragmatic concern for pure milk. And one could, indeed, make a great deal of the function played by images of pollution, of unnatural alcohol defiling that most natural of foods, God's pure milk (as one could with Griscom's discussion of the manner in which men violated the air they breathed).[31] Their habitual dependence upon such emotion-laden metaphors does not prove Hartley or Griscom to have been pious obscurantists; they were simply utilizing a traditional idiom in rationalizing and dramatizing a deeply held philanthropic commitment. (This was in a period, it must be recalled, when existing etiological knowledge seemed only to underscore the unity between moral and medical truths expressed by such time-honored images and admonitions.) The distinction between that which we regard as pragmatic environmentalism and that which we dismiss as mere moralism is, in regard to the public health movement of the 1840s and 50s, far more confusing than enlightening. Both styles of thought supplemented each other, interacting with the energies of pietism to motivate and broaden the concern of a man like Hartley with the human problems of his city.

Hartley's interest in public health only began with his crusade for pure milk. As corresponding secretary and agent of the A.I.C.P., Hartley soon involved himself and the association he guided in a varied group of measures aimed at improving the health of New Yorkers. For Hartley, like Griscom, assumed that man could be neither provident nor moral without health. As one surveys American cities in the 1840s and early 1850s, it soon becomes apparent that the A.I.C.P. had indeed the most coherent and far-seeing public health program of any benevolent group — while medical societies still concerned themselves only marginally with such matters.

The association's managers were certain of the means by which the city's health conditions could be improved; the provision of decent housing was an indispensable first step. As early as 1846, only two years after the organization had begun independent life, its directors voted to form a committee to investigate New York's slums. The committee issued its report the following year; the city's tenements, they concluded, were utterly inadequate to the preservation of either human health or Christian morality. Echoing Griscom's arguments of 1842, the association's committee contended that New York's crowded, filthy, and ill-ventilated tenements eroded not only good health and moral standards, but also self-respect and religious sentiment. Man, a weakened creature at best, needed a decent environment in order to preserve his industriousness, cleanliness, and morality. This environment, the committee reported to their fellow New Yorkers, could not be found in the city's ever-widening slums. The committee concluded by warning the association firmly: if they hoped to reduce the amount of poverty in New York and improve the morale of the poor, they must first reform tenement conditions.[32]

> Great value should be attached to this much-desired reform, seeing it lies at the basis of other reforms; and as the health and

> morals of thousands are injured or destroyed by the influence of circumstances around them, an improvement of the circumstances in connection with other appropriate means, afford the only rational hope of effectively elevating their character and condition, and of relieving the city from numerous evils which now exist.

Following European precedents, Hartley and the association turned first to private investment. Model tenements could be constructed, buildings which would provide light and air and still bring a 6 percent return to the Christian capitalists who, it was hoped, would finance their construction. Despite years of effort, however, and the launching of one substantial experiment, these plans never came to fruition.[33] By the mid-1850s, the association, still dedicated to the amelioration of tenement housing, had turned largely to legislative solutions; only the power of the state could end the worst of such abuses — and thus allow the possibility of physical and moral regeneration.[34]

Most notably, the A.I.C.P. sponsored an ambitious study of New York's housing conditions, a study far more detailed than Griscom's earlier report. The committee presented a detailed, ward-by-ward description of New York's slums. A model of lucidity for its time, this document remained until the mid-60s a source of data for American housing reformers and public health workers.[35] Throughout the 1850s, in legislative investigations, in medical articles and reports, in the activities of the New York Sanitary Association and the National Quarantine and Sanitary Conventions, the findings of the A.I.C.P. played a significant role in demonstrating the need for improved housing in safeguarding the health of the city's working population.[36]

In their broad concern for New York's "dependent classes," the A.I.C.P. did not limit its health program to demands for housing reform. It endorsed an eclectic range of public health measures, including the provision of medical care for the indigent. No sooner, indeed, had the A.I.C.P. been founded than it began to investigate the health of the poor and the adequacy of medical care available. In 1845, even before the appearance of its first annual report, the Association published Hartley's *A Plan for the Better Distribution of Medical Attendance*, a proposal for the increased provision of out-patient care. Within six years, the A.I.C.P. established two new medical dispensaries. Association visitors worked closely with dispensary physicians, bringing them to the sick poor, even distributing medicines from central depositories. Throughout the 1850s and 60s, the A.I.C.P continued to concern itself with such practical health needs. In 1852 it opened a Bath and Wash House, where for a minimal charge (imposed to prevent pauperization of the users) the poor could bathe and wash their clothing. This was New York's first public bath. In 1862, as well, the association's legislative efforts at last won a state law regulating the production and sale of milk. During these same years the A.I.C.P. also supported such general public health measures as the improvement of the city's sewers, the regulation of slaughter houses and bone-boiling establishments, and the prevention of tenement dwellers from keeping pigs, goats, and cows in their apartments. It fought among a growing number of allies and with final success — in 1866 — to secure an effective, professionally staffed metropolitan Board of Health.[37]

III

The preceding pages have not sought to contend that all Americans who called in the 1840s and 50s for public health reform were "secularized" evangelists, but rather to argue that a certain number, especially among this pioneer generation, found a central motivation for their driving activism in a pervading spirit of millennial piety. English example and influence were certainly influential, indeed crucial; the writings of Hartley and Griscom reflected again and again their familiarity with contemporary English public health appeals. Yet the question remains: why were these men — unlike the great majority of their medical contemporaries — so receptive to the ideas of the pioneer English sanitarians? The only plausible explanation lies, we have suggested, in their religiously based commitment to saving and helping the unfortunate, in their assumption that an intimate relationship existed between environment, health, and morals.

Perhaps, finally, it might be argued that "pietistic" or "evangelical" is not quite the right word to describe the motivations of men so different as the orthodox Hartley and the Quaker Griscom. And it must be confessed that they differed markedly in their attitude toward the poor and the poverty both sought to alleviate. (Griscom, for example, was at heart an environmental determinist, concerned far more with the implacably forbidding conditions of the slum than with the sins of those who inhabited them. Hartley, on the other hand, never escaped the conviction that original sin was the ultimate cause of all human misery, despite his understanding of the environmental factors which seemed often to cause and always to exacerbate the demoralization of poverty).[38] Yet these individual differences suggest all the more unmistakably the overarching commonality of feeling which bound Griscom and Hartley together, an urgent need to help and in helping to convert — whether one understands the term conversion in the narrowly orthodox sense of predestined salvation, or in the humanistic sense which characterized the Griscom family's millennial faith in education, in science, and in moral improvement. It meant, in operational terms, a need to reach out to the disadvantaged, an inability to tolerate wrongs which might through one's efforts be ameliorated.

NOTES

1 The now-classic discussion of the influence of pietism in American history is that by H. Richard Niebuhr, *The Kingdom of God in America* (New York: Harper & Bros., 1937). W. G. McLoughlin has provided a more recent synthetic discussion of "Pietism and the American character," *Am. Quart.*, 1965, *17*: 163–186. The present study uses the term "pietism" within a specifically Christian context; McLoughlin employs the term in a much broader sense, to describe almost all behavior dictated in any way by moral imperatives. Among the most influential of recent monographic discussions of the social effects of pietism in ante-bellum America are Whitney Cross, *The Burned-Over District. The Social and Intellectual History of Enthusiastic Religion in Western New York, 1800–1850* (Ithaca: Cornell Univ. Press, 1950); T. L. Smith, *Revivalism and Social Reform in Mid-Nineteenth-Century America* (New York and Nashville: Abingdon, 1957).

2 *The Sanitary Condition of the Laboring Population of New York. With Suggestions for Its Improvement. A Discourse (with Additions) Delivered on the 30th December, 1844, at the Repository of the American Institute* (New York: Harper & Bros., 1845). Compare the discussion of this pamphlet by George Rosen, *A History of Public Health* (New York: MD Publications, c. 1958), pp. 237–239. Rosen contends (p. 238) that "this study already contains in essence the principles and objectives that were to characterize the American sanitary reform movement for the next 30 years."

3 This generalization is based partially on a search for items of public health concern in half a dozen American medical journals between 1843 and 1847. The comparative lack of concern is unmistakable and emphasized by the English origin of many of those items found directly relating to public health. We should like to thank Steven J. Peitzman, a student at the University of Pennsylvania, for his help in this search. With the 1850s, the interest of American physicians began to increase.

4 The most important source of information for Griscom's life is the memoir by his son: J. H. Griscom, *Memoir of John Griscom, LL.D., Late Professor of Chemistry and Natural Philosophy; with an Account of the New York High School; Society for the Prevention of Pauperism; the House of Refuge; and Other Institutions. Compiled from an autobiography, and other sources* (New York: Robert Carter and Brothers, 1859). Cf. E. F. Smith, "John Griscom," *D.A.B.*, VIII, 7. The manuscript division of the New York Public Library contains an important collection of Griscom's incoming correspondence. For the background of Quaker pietism and benevolence, see S. V. James, *A People among Peoples: Quaker Benevolence in Eighteenth-Century America* (Cambridge, Mass.: Harvard Univ. Press, 1963).

5 Formal theological positions were remarkably unimportant in comparison with the common dedication of such men to spiritual activism and social improvement. Griscom, a Quaker, could write of Thomas Chalmers, a Scotch Presbyterian: "It would be difficult to name any writer of the past or present century, entitled to a higher rank . . . as a defender and expounder of theological truth." *Memoir*, p. 379. Chalmers was, significantly, a pioneer in social welfare as well as a prominent theologian and popularizer of natural theology.

6 A recent student of science in Jeffersonian America has described Griscom's chemical lectures as atypically successful and long-lived. J. C. Greene, "Science and the public in the age of Jefferson," *Isis*, 1958, *49*: 20.

7 From a letter of Griscom's, Aug. 27, 1847. *Memoir*, p. 365. Cf. Jos. Murray, Jr., to Griscom, Feb. 13, 1817, Griscom Correspondence, NYPL.

8 On ventilation, see Henry Vethake to Griscom, Nov. 27, 1819; Jacob Bigelow to Griscom, Oct. 29, 1822, Griscom Correspondence. On Griscom's yellow fever interests, see James Hardie, *An Account of the Yellow Fever Which Occurred in the City of New York, in the Year 1822 . . .* (New York: Samuel Marks, 1822), pp. 51, 71; New York City, Board of Health, *A History of the Proceedings of the Board of Health, of the City of New York, in the Summer and Fall of 1822 . . .* (New York: P. & H. Van Pelt, 1823), pp. 230–242. As early as 1807, David Hosack had written to Griscom, asking for an explanation of factors effecting putrefaction and their possible relationship to disease etiology. Hosack to Griscom, Oct. 23, 1809, Hosack Letter-Book, Rare Book Room, New York Academy of Medicine.

9 Unfortunately, there seem to have survived almost no documents illustrating the younger Griscom's personal life. Perhaps most significant in illuminating Griscom's spiritual life is his careful memoir of his father; its tone leaves little doubt of the son's pietistic orientation. There are a half-dozen Griscom letters in the Gulian Verplanck Papers at the New-York Historical Society. The Municipal Archives and Records Center, 38 William Street, contains many documents signed by Griscom in the papers of the Commissioners of Emigration; these are, however, routine notations relating to the bonding of handicapped immigrants. (Griscom was "secular agent" of the Commissioner from 1848 to 1851.) A search of the rough minutes and Filed and Approved Papers of the Common Council at the archives disclosed no materials relating directly to Griscom's tenure as City Inspector.

10 Philip Van Ingen, *The New York Academy of Medicine. Its First Hundred Years* (New York: Columbia Univ. Press, 1949), p. 20. Van Ingen also notes that Griscom was among the first group of trustees elected when the Academy was chartered (p. 43). For other biographical material, see S. W. Francis, *Biographical Sketches of Distinguished Living New York Physicians* (New York: George P. Putnam, 1867), pp. 45–59; [Philip Van Ingen], *A Brief Account of the First One Hundred Years of the New York Medical and Surgical Society* ([New York]: Privately printed, 1946), p. 43, which notes that Griscom resigned from the society as a protest against the expulsion of Horace Green; "John H. Griscom (1809–1874)," *Dictionary of American Medical Biography*, ed. Howard A. Kelly and Walter Burrage (New York and London: D. Appleton Co., 1928), pp. 501–502; "New York Medical and Surgical Society. First 100 years. Biographies. Vol. II.," Rare Book Room, New York Academy of Medicine, pp. 475–484. This typed sketch is the most detailed account available of Griscom's life.

11 "Our Creator afflicts us with diseases," Griscom elaborated, "that we may know how frail and dependent we are. But he has also given us a knowledge of the laws which regulate our growth, and our lives, so that by attending to them, and living purely and uprightly, we may avoid those diseases, in a great degree." Griscom, *First Lessons in Human Physiology; To Which Are Added Brief Rules of Health. For the Use of Schools*, 6th ed. (New York: Roe Lockwood & Son, 1847), pp. 132–133. A principal motive in his writing of texts for the study of such comparatively novel subjects, Griscom explained to parents, "has been the desire to render the study of our frames subservient to moral improvement, by furnishing the young reader with incontestible evidence of a Great First Cause." *Animal Mechanism and Physiology; Being a Plain and Familiar Exposition of the Structure and Functions of the Human System . . .* (New York: Harper & Bros., 1839), p. vii. All of Griscom's specific appeals for public health reform called at least in passing for efforts to raise the level of public knowledge; he urged, for example, at one point the establishment of a "Hygiological Society" to be composed of physicians and laymen and dedicated to the spread of hygienic truths. *Anniversary Discourse. Before the New York Academy of Medicine. Delivered in Clinton Hall, November 22d, 1854* (New York: R. Craighead, 1855), p. 52.

12 Griscom, *Improvements of the Public Health, and the Establishment of a Sanitary Police in the City of New York* (Albany: C. Van Benthuysen, 1857), p. 3. Such seemingly primitivistic appeals to the contrast between the health of the rural, even savage, life and urban conditions are to be found in virtually all of Griscom's writings. Like natural theology itself, such ideas were almost universal at this time. For a discussion of the emotional resonance in this period between the idea of sin and the unnatural, virtue and the natural, see C. E. Rosenberg, *The Cholera Years: The United States, 1832, 1849, and 1866* (Chicago: Univ. of Chicago Press, 1962), p. 132 and *passim.*

13 In addition to his frequent reiteration of the standard warnings of his generation against tightly-laced corsets and alcohol, Griscom wrote books on the problems of ventilation and — in amusingly apocalyptic tones — the evils of tobacco. *The Use of Tobacco, and the Evils, Physical, Moral, and Social, Resulting Therefrom* (New York: G. P. Putnam & Son, 1868); *The Uses and Abuses of Air: Showing Its Influence in Sustaining Life, and Producing Disease . . .* (New York: Redfield, 1850).

14 Griscom, *Uses and Abuses of Air*, pp. 137 n, 143.

15 Such allegations were made in editorials in D. M. Reese's *American Medical Gazette*, accusing Griscom of a 20-year dedication to the hope of feeding from the "public crib." "That consumption hospital," *ibid.*, 1857, *8*: 112–113; "Medical politics," *ibid.*, 113. Van Ingen's history of the New York Academy of Medicine notes Griscom had been involved in reprimanding Reese for allegedly unethical conduct. Van Ingen, *New York Academy of Medicine*, pp. 90–91, 115–116. An anonymous reviewer was also harshly critical of an 1842 pamphlet by Griscom on spinal deformity, implying that it was the work of a quack and written to attract "business." *N.Y. Med. Gaz.*, 1842, *2*: 179–182. This is the only evidence we have found indicating that Griscom may have been inspired by sordid motives.

16 New York City, *Annual Report of the Interments in the City and County of New-York, for the Year 1842, with Remarks Thereon, And a Brief View of the Sanitary Condition of the City* (New York: James Van Norden, 1843). This report had been ordered printed in "four times the usual number." The source of Griscom's political influence in 1842 and thus the explanation of his appointment as City Inspector is, in the absence of manuscript evidence, obscure.

17 Griscom, *Sanitary Condition*, p. 8. Like many of his contemporaries, Griscom habitually emphasized the economic gains to be realized through public health reform; one feels, however, that such hard-headed appeals were simply arguments and rationalizations for a more basic humanitarian commitment.

18 There was no American equivalent of the Chadwickian hostility to physicians among lay advocates of public health. Griscom based all of his proposals upon the impossibility of any but physicians properly fulfilling the duties of a health officer; in keeping with his emphasis was Griscom's assumption that existing medical knowledge was adequate to the explanation and thus prevention of a good portion of the sickness which burdened the city. In 1842, Griscom outlined his essential organizational point of view in regard to New York's Board of Health. New York City, Board of Aldermen, *Communication from the City Inspector, Recommending a Reorganization of the Health Police*, April 24, 1843. Doc. No. 111, pp. 1314–1320.

19 The first portion of this quotation is from Griscom, *Sanitary Condition*, p. 1, the second from Griscom's *Annual Report for 1842*, p. 173.

20 Griscom was also consistently critical of both the exploitive behavior of many of the city's property-holders and the culpable failure of many among the wealthy to ventilate their mansions and observe moderation in eating and drinking — all sins more deserving of condemnation than the almost involuntary misdeeds of the poor. Cf. *Sanitary Condition*, p. 20.

21 Griscom, *Uses and Abuses of Air*, p. 92. The etiological position assumed by Griscom — quite common in the 1840s — was termed by contemporaries "contingent-contagionism," the conviction, that is, that many infectious diseases were contagious only in such confined quarters as hospital wards and slum apartments. This belief provided an excellent vehicle for the expression of social criticism as well as explaining some of the logical dilemmas implicit in either contagionism or noncontagionism.

22 It is tempting, moreover, to interpret Griscom's rejection of early ideas of the specific and particularate etiology of epidemic disease within the same humanitarian framework. Like many other public health leaders of his first generation — Edwin Snow of Providence and H. G. Clark of Boston, for example — Griscom found it difficult to modify his earlier emphasis upon the importance of local conditions in creating the necessary environment for epidemic disease. For an emphasis upon local causes implied a system in which man's own actions and volitions were the ultimate and most meaningful cause of the pestilence which afflicted him; to place the blame for an epidemic upon some impersonal and specific contagion — as John Snow seemed to do in the case of cholera — was to create an etiological scheme in which Griscom's habitual demands for environmental reform would be deprived of their immediacy. In 1866, for example, Griscom argued that the presence of cholera on a ship in quarantine was due not to some specific and unavoidable contagion, but to the ship's filthy condition. If the ship had been equally filthy and there had been no cholera influence present, ship fever would have resulted; if the ship had been clean there would have been neither cholera nor typhus. Griscom, "The where, the when, the why, and the how, of the first appearance and greatest prevalence of cholera in cities," *Bull. N.Y. Acad. Med.*, 1866, *3*: 6–26, and his comments at page 49–50. His bias in favor of an etiology which justified sanitary reform is equally apparent in his discussion of yellow fever; he argued, for example, that it was of little practical significance whether the city's filthy docks and slips had given rise to yellow fever or simply provided "a richly manured soil in which the germs of that disease, introduced from abroad, would grow with redoubled vigor, . . . It is enough to know that such conditions are inimical to human life, and should never be permitted." *A History, Chronological and Circumstantial, of the Visitations of Yellow Fever in New York City . . .*

(New York: Hall, Clayton & Co., 1858), p. 21. Cf. Rosenberg, *The Cholera Years*, p. 196.

23 For the testimony of these city missionaries, see *Sanitary Condition*, pp. 24–38; New York, *Annual Report of Interments, 1842*, pp. 167–171. More than a few prominent New York clergymen became active in medical and public health affairs — Henry Bellows, for example, and William Muhlenberg (Bellows, of course, directed the Sanitary Commission during the Civil War, while Muhlenberg founded St. Luke's Hospital.) Cf. Ann Ayres, *The Life and Work of William Augustus Muhlenberg* (New York: Harper & Bros., 1880); W. Q. Maxwell, *Lincoln's Fifth Wheel: The Political History of the United States Sanitary Commission* (New York: Longmans, Green & Co., 1956). Perhaps most professional in his career as city missionary-*cum*-public health expert was S. B. Halliday, active for a half-century in the saving of souls and the improvement of health conditions. It is quite clear that the original motivations for Halliday's concern with environmental reform — nurtured during decades of work for a succession of New York religious charities — lay in his conversion during the revivalistic enthusiasm of the early 1830s. Cf. S. B. Halliday, *Lost and Found; or Life Among the Poor* (New York: Blakeman & Mason, 1859); Carroll S. Rosenberg, "Protestants and Five Pointers: The Five Points House of Industry, 1850–1870. *N.-Y. Hist. Soc. Quart.*, 1964, *48*: 347 and *passim*. The relationship between the city mission movement and the growing demand for environmental reform is a complex one. For a more detailed account, see: Carroll S. Rosenberg, "Evangelicalism and the New City. The city mission movement in New York, 1812–1870" (Ph.D. dissertation, Columbia Univ., 1968).

24 *N.Y. J. Med.*, 1845, *4*: 30. In a city with a paucity of institutional structure and organizational models, it was natural that Griscom should have drawn upon the personnel and pattern of activities of the city missions — just as he depended upon the city's dispensaries. In almost all his proposals for board of health reorganization, Griscom suggested that the dispensary physicians, the only medical men who understood tenement conditions, be made district health officers.

25 John Ordronaux, *Prophylaxis, an Anniversary Oration Delivered before the New York Academy of Medicine, Wednesday, Dec. 19th, 1866* (New York: Bailliere Brothers, 1867), pp. 16, 68.

26 Both in his purely evangelical work and in his temperance agitation, Hartley was a consistent advocate of the need for methodical house-to-house visitation; it was such visiting which, for the first time, brought numbers of middle-class New Yorkers into contact with slum conditions. The basic source for Hartley's life is a *Memorial of Robert Milham Hartley. Edited by his son, Isaac Smithson Hartley, D.D.* (Utica, N.Y.: Printed, not published, 1882). The preceding paragraph is synthesized from his detailed biography. For evaluations of Hartley's place in the development of American social welfare, see R. H. Bremner, *From the Depths. The Discovery of Poverty in the United States* (New York: New York Univ Press, c. 1956), pp. 35–38; Roy Lubove, "The New York Association for Improving the Condition of the Poor: the formative years," *N.-Y. Hist. Soc. Quart.*, 1959, *43*: 307–27. The most important source for Hartley's ideas and activities are the annual reports of the A.I.C.P. for its first three decades; there are also some valuable surviving manuscript sources — including the minutes of the association's Board of Managers — at the Community Service Society, 105 E. 22nd Street, New York. For the city mission background of Hartley's early work and the significance both practical and theological of house-to-house visiting, see Carroll S. Rosenberg, "Evangelicalism and the New City."

27 Hartley, *Memorial*, pp. 229, 288, 297, respectively for the quoted passages. These are typical of many similar entries.

28 The institutional history of the A.I.C.P., like Hartley's personal biography, demonstrates an evolution from pietistic beginnings to a more secular benevolence. Though ordinarily considered a pragmatic — if in some ways moralistic and status-oriented — response to urban conditions, the association actually began as an outgrowth of the New York City Tract Society. This organization had, by the early 1840s, found itself so preoccupied with the economic needs of the poor that its managers feared their primary objective of converting all New Yorkers to evangelical Protestantism might be lost in the demands of day-to-day meliorism. Hence their establishment of a separate organization, the A.I.C.P., to deal with the material ills of the poor. (John H. Griscom was a member of the association's first executive committee, as well as serving as a volunteer visitor and committee member for his district.) Though the A.I.C.P's object was not formally the salvation of souls, the moral and psychological views of poverty entertained by the spokesmen of this new organization were identical with those expressed for many years by New York's evangelical leaders. For a detailed treatment of these developments, see Carroll S. Rosenberg, "Evangelicalism and the New City," chs. 6, 10. The founding of the A.I.C.P. by the Tract Society can be traced in the archives of the latter group, now the New York City Mission Society, 105 E. 22d Street.

29 R. M. Hartley, *An Historical, Scientific and Practical Essay on Milk as an Article of Human Sustenance; with a Consideration of the Effects Consequent upon the Unnatural Methods of Producing It for the Supply of Large Cities* (New York: Jonathan Leavitt, 1842).

30 *Ibid.*, pp. 235, 331. Cf. pp. 29–30, 128, 144–145, 208, 212, 232. Hartley's argument from design was, of course, a commonplace in this generation, among physicians as well as laymen and the clergy. This was vigorously illustrated by Dr. A. K. Gardner, a prominent specialist in diseases of women and children, when testifying at a hearing in 1858 and recalling the condition of swill-fed cows he had seen: "And I drew the conclusion that they were not in a state of nature; and the next conclusion that I drew was, that cows not in a natural condition, could not give milk of a natural character. . . . I then considered that if God made the milk in a certain way, that it could not be improved upon; and if any milk was totally opposite from the natural milk, God's milk, that it must be totally wrong." New York City Board of Health, *Majority and Minority Reports of the Select Committee of the Board of Health, Appointed to Investigate the Character and Condition of the Sources from Which Cow's Milk Is Derived, for Sale in the City of New York* (New York: Charles W. Baker, 1858), pp. 169–170.

31 For an important discussion of the background of such images of "infection" and the gradual and complex secularization of this concept, see Owsei Temkin, "An historical analysis of the concept of infection," in *Studies in Intellectual History* (Baltimore: Johns Hopkins Press, 1953), pp. 123–147, esp. pp. 139–144. See also the discussion of the interaction between scientific thought and religious values provided by L. G. Stevenson in two significant articles: "Science down the drain. On the hostility of certain sanitarians to animal experimentation, bacteriology and immunology," *Bull. Hist. Med.*, 1955, *29*: 1–26, esp. pp. 3–4n.; and "Religious elements in the background of the British anti-vivisection movement," *Yale J. Biol. & Med.*, 1956, *29*: 125–127.

32 New York Association for Improving the Condition of the Poor, *4th Annual Report*, 1847, p. 23; *3rd Annual Report*, 1846, p. 22.

33 R. H. Bremner has written an account of the A.I.C.P.'s one substantial experiment in this area: "The big flat: history of a New York tenement house," *Am. Hist. Rev.*, 1958, *64*: 54–62. Cf. A.I.C.P., *5th Annual Report*, 1848, pp. 18–19; *10th Annual Report, 1853*, pp. 26–27; Board of Managers, Minutes, April 10, 1854, Community Service Society.

34 It was always assumed, of course, that such reforms would have an inevitable spiritual effect. At the eleventh annual meeting of the A.I.C.P., for example, the influential clergyman T. L. Cuyler, made this point of view explicit in praising the association's just-completed housing report. "The sanitary statements of the Report," he proposed, "show that where cleanliness and ventilation are neglected, disease and mortality are proportionately increased. And where the body is unclean, and the dwelling wretched, there is commonly a correspondingly moral degradation. . . . Sanitary reform," Cuyler urged, "is intimately connected with the spread of true religion. The dwellings of the poor are to be looked after as well as their souls," N.Y.A.I.C.P., *11th Annual Report, 1854*, p. 6. The other principal speaker at this meeting was the Reverend Henry Bellows, later — as we have noted — prominent for his work with the Sanitary Commission during the Civil War. Both Cuyler and Bellows were also active in the New York Sanitary Association.

35 N.Y.A.I.C.P., *First Report of a Committee on the Sanitary Condition of the Poor in the City of New York* (New York: John F. Trow, 1853). Though less famous than the Shattuck Report of 1850, this document seems to have been quoted with equal frequency in the dozen years after its publication. Also revealing is the detailed discussion of this report the succeeding year in the association's *11th Annual Report, 1854*, pp. 19–29. Hartley, who wrote all the association's annual reports, significantly began his discussion with a quotation from Thomas Chalmers: "That all our sufferings and evils (so far as they exceed those inseparable from a finite and imperfect nature) may be traced to ignorance or neglect of those laws of nature which God has established for our good, and displayed for our instruction." *Ibid.*, p. 19. Beginning with the mid-1850s and through the establishment of the Metropolitan Board of Health in 1866, the A.I.C.P. reports regularly called for state intervention in New York's housing and sanitary affairs.

36 Long-time A.I.C.P. supporters were, for example, influential in the New York Sanitary Association (founded 1859), though the association itself was modeled after the British Health of Towns Associations, while similar ties existed between the A.I.C.P. and the Citizens' Association. For a discussion of the events leading to the passage of the Metropolitan Board of Health Bill and the place of these organizations, see G. H. Brieger, "Sanitary reform in New York City: Stephen Smith and the passage of the Metropolitan Health Bill," *Bull. Hist. Med.*, 1966, *40*: 407–429. [See pp. 359–373 in this book.] For an example of the prominence of A.I.C.P. findings in contemporary public health debate, see New York State, Senate, *Report of the Select Committee Appointed to Investigate the Health Department of the City of*

New York. In Senate, Feb. 3, 1859. Document No. 49 [Albany, 1859]. The committee's conclusions simply echo the Hartley-Griscom position in calling for state action and in blaming much of the city's pauperism and ill-health on poor housing, pp. 13–16.

37 N.Y.A.I.C.P., *A Plan for Better Distribution of Medical Attendance and Medicines for the Indigent Sick, by the Public Dispensaries in the City of New York* (New York, 1845). On dispensaries see A.I.C.P., *8th Annual Report, 1851*, pp. 20–22; *9th Annual Report, 1852*, pp. 38–39. The two dispensaries were the DeMilt and the Northeastern. There was some controversy as to how much the A.I.C.P. actually had to do with the DeMilt Dispensary after Hartley arranged the meetings which led to its establishment. DeMilt Dispensary in the City of New York, *25th Annual Report, 1875*, pp. 25–28. More relevant, however, is the philanthropic career of F. E.Mather, a prominent New Yorker and president of the DeMilt Dispensary for its first quarter-century. He became involved in such public health matters through the A.I.C.P. and later served as president of the New York Sanitary Association and attended the National Sanitary and Quarantine Conventions. On public baths, see N.Y.A.I.C.P., *9th Annual Report, 1852*, pp. 39–40. N.Y.A.I.C.P., *19th Annual Report, 1862*, pp. 54–58, reprints the text of the act against adulteration of milk. For the history of the Society for the Ruptured and Crippled, see *ibid.*, 38–43; Fenwick Beekman, *The Hospital for the Ruptured and Crippled. A Historical Sketch . . .* (New York: Printed, not published, 1939). Hartley took a personal interest in the establishment of the Presbyterian Hospital and served for eight years as its secretary. *Memorial*, p. 484.

38 Griscom retained his formal adherence to the Society of Friends, "whose tenets," he explained late in life, "are regarded by me as most in accordance with Scripture teachings, as the most liberal in sentiment, and most truly democratic in practice of all sects." Francis, *Biographical Sketches*, p. 54. We have been unable to determine whether Griscom was an orthodox or Hicksite Quaker. His humanitarian environmentalism is, indeed, Griscom's most significant — and endearing — characteristic. He even blamed poor ventilation for the sluggish behavior of school children who normally received the rod instead of the fresh air they actually needed. *Uses and Abuses of Air*, p. 51. Hartley is consistently harsher than Griscom in his social and individual judgments — a harshness intensified by his rigid Manchestrian views.

26

Sanitary Reform in New York City: Stephen Smith and the Passage of the Metropolitan Health Bill

GERT H. BRIEGER

I

"Frenzy in the South," proclaimed the bold headline of the *New York Times* on March 10, 1865. These were the last days of the long and bitter struggle, and New Yorkers welcomed the news. Each day they read about Grant and Sheridan in Virginia and of Sherman's impressive march up through the Carolinas. On March 16, however, a different subject dominated the first two pages of the paper. Instead of the usual fare of war news, the *Times* provided its readers with the testimony of Dr. Stephen Smith presented before a joint committee of the New York State Legislature. He had given evidence about the sanitary conditions of New York City and on the urgent need for new health laws. Smith gave a stinging indictment of the municipal authorities responsible for the public health and described the miserable conditions of the city's streets and tenements. This testimony, based on a massive effort by a large group of reform-dedicated physicians, was the culmination of years of effort by numerous citizens of America's major metropolis.[1]

The horrible conditions which existed at the close of the Civil War were not peculiar to New York or to that period. As Ford has pointed out, the relationship between cellar-dwellings and disease production in New York had been discussed as early as the 1790s.[2] In 1820 David Hosack told the medical students of the College of Physicians and Surgeons that the filth in various parts of the city was marked and that amelioration could probably not be achieved without the aid of the state legislature.[3] Benjamin W. McCready, in 1837, pointed to poor housing and insufficient space as a major source of ill-health among the workers.[4] In 1842, John H. Griscom, one of the truly important figures in the story of sanitary reform, appended to his annual report of the City Inspector's office a pamphlet entitled "A Brief View of the Sanitary Condition of the City," in which he described living conditions and the destitution and misery of cellar-dwellers. He urged upon the Common Council the necessity of better housing laws.[5]

In December 1844, Griscom delivered a discourse at the American Institute which he published during the next year as *The Sanitary Condition of the Laboring Population of New York*. He reported the health problems which faced many tenement-dwelling New Yorkers, and he urged "SANITARY REFORM." He was anxious to profit from the experience of English and French sanitarians, and their influence is evident in the text as well as the title.[6]

Griscom was one of the first to show that the system of subtenancy and the rental extortions of the sublandlord were among the principle causes of misery of so many of the city's poor. This system enabled the owner of one or several houses to rent them to a sublandlord, who in turn divided them into as many apartments as possible. He then extracted as much rent as he could, often from helpless immigrants. By making few repairs and providing little maintenance he realized a great profit. Often he owned the local store as well and fixed prices at relatively high levels. The working classes were virtually restricted to lower Manhattan because there was no means of inexpensive, rapid transportation which would have freed them from the packed tenement conditions.[7]

GERT H. BRIEGER is Professor and Chairman, Department of the History of Health Sciences, University of California, San Francisco, California.

Reprinted with permission from the *Bulletin of the History of Medicine*, 1966, *40*: 407–429.

Griscom also clearly described the evils of cellar-dwellings, often soggy and lacking ventilation. Many of the cellar-apartments were below sea level. When high tides came, the rooms were submerged! During heavy rains, the streets drained into the cellars. The cellar-dwellers, or Troglodytes as they were often called, lived and slept on planks suspended well above the floors.

In contrast to McCready, who seems to have practiced and taught medicine in comparative quiet, Griscom continued active agitation for improved public health laws. He was one of the first to stress that the physicians in the public dispensaries of the city would be ideally suited for the jobs of health wardens or sanitary inspectors.[8] He was the first witness before the Select Committee of the New York Senate appointed in 1858 to investigate the health department of New York City. He then sat with the committee during its interrogation of over 20 witnesses, often interjecting lively questions and barbed remarks.[9]

This committee was appointed to investigate the "assertion that great defects exist, and great improvements are practicable in the health department and sanitary laws of the city of New York."[10] Three major questions were asked: (1) Whether the allegations were true that New York had a higher ratio of mortality than other large cities. (2) If true, what were the causes of this excess mortality. (3) What were the possible remedies.[11]

Almost unanimously the witnesses gave an affirmative answer to the first question. As to the causes, this report established what was to become a constantly recurring refrain. Almost all the witnesses ascribed the excessive mortality to overcrowded tenement houses, improper light, ventilation, and food, filthy streets, insufficient sewerage, and an almost total lack of a regularly constituted and effective department of health.

Contrary to the arguments put forward by the City Inspector, Mr. Morton, the committee stated that a properly constituted health department would require the talents of the best educated men, well versed in the recent advances of medical science. Not since 1844 had a physician been City Inspector. "A man when he wants his watch repaired," argued Dr. John McNulty, "does not take it to a shoemaker. . . ."[12]

The City Inspector and his men disagreed. Mr. Richard Downing, Superintendent of Sanitary Inspection, claimed that knowledge of the law, not medicine, was necessary. It did not require medical knowledge, he said, to smell an odor or to recognize a filthy street.[13] Mr. Morton added his feeling that physicians would not do the job; they would think it undignified to "go running through tenement houses and sticking their noses down privies, to see if they were healthy or not. . . ."[14]

For two years prior to the Senate committee's investigation, the leading medical society, the New York Academy of Medicine, petitioned the legislature for modifications of the health laws. In 1856 the academy sent a memorial to Albany which stated that "a large portion of the annual mortality of this city results from diseases, whose causes are more or less within our control, but which are totally unchecked by any public administration of proper sanitary precautions, and that from this neglect, in addition to a very great and unnecessary loss of life, the city and State endure an incalculable detriment to their commercial and moral interests."[15] No bill was passed at the 1857 session.[16] Nor was a renewal of the petition successful the following year.

In the meantime, however, the legislature did pass the Metropolitan Police Bill, in 1857, an important model and precedent for future health legislation. By transferring to state control the city's police force, the Republican state legislature created a new police district comprising the counties of New York, Kings, Richmond, and Westchester. The Board of Police was to consist of five commissioners, plus the mayors of New York and Brooklyn. New York's Mayor Fernando Wood resisted the new law and kept control of his original municipal force — most of whom had voted for him on the Democratic ticket. Only after rioting in the streets with the municipal faction, the arrest of Mayor Wood, and the use of the state militia, did the Metropolitan Police finally win their right to act as the city's legally constituted guardians of the peace.[17]

A recent historian of this episode pointed out how the situation was complicated by a growing political and social cleavage between New York City and the rest of the state.[18] Each mayor, in his annual messages of the succeeding years, used the argument that local problems, such as sanitation, should be kept under local control. Thus the sanitary reform measures, suggested repeatedly between 1856 and 1866 by the leading physicians of New York, took on increasingly complex political overtones. Health bill advocates found themselves fighting, not only for good health and efficient sanitary administration, but against political corruption and the control of Tammany Hall over the city.[19]

In the meantime, the New York Sanitary Association had been founded in January 1859. The members immediately took up the fight for the health bill before the legislature, then in session. John Griscom and Elisha Harris were officers of the group, and Stephen Smith, Joseph M. Smith, and Peter Cooper were among the members of the council.[20]

That winter the association impressed upon the legislators the urgent need for a health bill. They used established arguments: New York's ratio of mortality was greater than that of most cities in the United States and western Europe; those diseases which most contributed to this mortality were due to the absence of proper sanitary administrations and were just those diseases thought to be preventable; New York had three separate health authorities, none of which functioned properly. These were the Board of Health, composed of the Mayor, Aldermen, and Councilmen and rarely in session; the Commissioners of Health, including the Mayor, the Presidents of the Boards of Aldermen and Councilmen, the Resident Physician, and Health Officer of the Port; and the City Inspector's Department.[21] The Sanitary Association pointed out that there were about 112 individuals directly and indirectly supposedly concerned for the health of the people, but "that there is not one who feels it to be required of him to take note of, or to use any effort whatever to check the immense amount of disease. . . ."[22]

Once again the story was the same. Their bill failed to pass.

By the end of 1860, the Sanitary Association could say that its meetings had been well attended and that it considered itself a permanent organization. It continued to act as a lobby group in Albany. The membership increased to over 250, representing the professions of law, medicine, education, and divinity.[23]

As late as 1862 the group continued to hear interesting papers, but the pressures of the war seem to have caused a cessation of its activities sometime in that year.[24]

While I have concerned myself primarily with matters of the public health, problems of personal health were not ignored. The sanitarians had the twin aims of improving the health laws and of educating the people, especially the poor, in the ways of proper hygiene. This, indeed, was also the aim of the numerous philanthropic organizations that flourished in New York at mid-century. The popular magazines and the newspapers often contained articles on health or advice on matters pertaining to diet or epidemics. One author, in 1856, thought that Americans should be the healthiest people in the world. If they were not, it was due to the hectic pace of life, with too much work and too little play.[25]

Medical teachers did not neglect the subject of hygiene, although often admitting that, in this area, ". . . the profession of medicine has hitherto grievously failed"[26] — this, even though the medical profession had expended an incredible amount of time and talent upon the subject of public and private hygiene in the quarter century before the Civil War.[27] And so, too, many doctors believed that hygiene and not quarantine was the true law of health.[28]

II

When the *New York Journal of Medicine* ceased publication in 1860, Stephen Smith shifted his editorial chair to the newly established *American Medical Times*, and he began four years of vigorous crusading in a large variety of areas. The older journal had contained few editorial comments in its bimonthly numbers, while its successor, a weekly, published lengthy editorials in every issue. In his writings he concerned himself with the role of medicine and the medical profession in society, including frequent expositions on wartime problems.[29]

Since Smith was a New Yorker, and because his journal was published in that city and presumably found most of its readers there, he usually devoted himself to local sanitary problems — primarily the need for legislative reform and the necessity for vigorous action on the part of the medical profession. In his first editorial in the new journal he set forth many of the precepts he planned to follow. He singled out the subject of hygiene to receive vigilant and faithful attention.[30] In the third number he elaborated on these ideas and stated his intention periodically to examine the more important questions relating to sanitary and quarantine systems of American cities and particularly the role and duty of the medical profession.[31] Despite the potential usefulness of his public health editorials nationally, he consistently focused on New York City.

During the summer of 1860 things looked bleak indeed. The country was threatened by division, political feelings ran high, and local sanitary problems continued to increase. More and more immigrants had to be fed and housed as each month passed. Smith shared the pessimistic mood of late summer when he noted that amidst legislative corruption it was not at all certain that improved health laws could be obtained: "And such are the necessities of the people, such the jeopardy of life and health as well as commercial interests, that our population cannot safely await the good time coming, when good laws and municipal reform shall effect the sanitary improvements now demanded. From various quarters the question comes up — What shall be done?"[32]

His answer was clear: he believed that more pressing than questions of quarantine were those relating to civic hygiene. More attention had to be devoted to municipal sanitary arrangements, especially to those of New York.[33]

The cause of sanitary reform moved forward slowly during the Civil War. Although official population figures showed a slight decrease in the 1865 census as compared with 1860, the city's municipal problems became worse.[34] Stokes noted that the city's growth during the war had been checked, but not stopped entirely. Fewer buildings were erected and the misery of crowded tenements grew. The increase in production and the resultant higher wages probably did elevate the general standard of living, but often prices increased too so the poorest classes were left with a net loss.[35] The poor did not share in the profits of rising real estate values and the general business expansion — in fact these things operated to their disadvantage. The increase in luxury which "struck every observer" falls short of describing the condition of more than half of the population — the tenement dwellers.[36]

Although wages rose, prices rose faster. Eggs, 15 cents in 1861, rose to 25 cents by the end of 1863; potatoes went from $1.50 to $2.25 per bushel during the same period. The increase in wages was generally about 25 percent, or less than half the increase of prices.[37]

Citizens interested in sanitary reform worked on through the war years. They helped introduce a bill into the state legislature each winter, but it failed to pass with each succeeding session. The daily papers and popular journals continued to clamor for both municipal and sanitary reform, building up to quite a pitch in the year prior to the success of 1866 — the Metropolitan Health Bill.

The medical press was also active, especially the influential *American Medical Times*. Others, besides Stephen Smith, participated in the effort; but it is on Smith's role I wish to focus. I should note that his work in the early 1860s was of much broader scope than my emphasis on sanitation would indicate.

Prior to 1864, Smith's efforts in behalf of a Metropolitan Health Bill were confined chiefly to the numerous editorials praising each bill, exhorting his fellow physicians to exert influence upon the legislature, and bemoaning the lack of a properly constituted health department in the city.

In December 1860, he asked: Will the next legislature provide a sanitary code for the city?[38] He pointed out that more than a fourth of the state's population resided in New York and Brooklyn. He noted that it was widely acknowledged that these million and a quarter people were "living under one of the most corrupt and corrupting municipal governments in the civilized world, and that reform without the interposition of State legislation is impractical." To call the existing Health Department by that name was a misnomer. "It does little for health, but much for disease and death."[39]

Early in 1861, Smith aimed his editorial guns in a violent attack on the City Inspector, who was to become a favorite target for the next five years.[40]

The City Inspector was really the only active health official in New York. It is true that there was a Physician of the Port and a Resident Physician, who, with the Mayor and Presidents of the Boards of Councilmen and Aldermen, constituted a

Commission of Health. In fact, however, in matters other than quarantine, it was mainly the City Inspector and his 44 health wardens who looked after the sanitation of the city.[41]

In his report for 1860, the inspector, Mr. Daniel E. Delavan, a two-year incumbent in the post, claimed a healthy condition for New York when compared to European cities.[42] What problems there were he attributed mainly to immigrants. His report admitted many of the sanitary problems of New York and he gave some reasons for them. In the first place, he was very critical of the medical profession for their failure to cooperate in the proper registration of vital statistics. Thus he noted the paradox of "opposition among the very class whose leading spirits have been most active for some years past in this city in urging the cause of sanitary reform."[43] He admitted to the filthy condition of the streets, stating that the Common Council had removed $50,000 from his budget and that in November 1860 money for street cleaning ran out; 300 miles of paved streets was a lot to sweep.[44] Mr. Delavan also was opposed to having the state legislature do for the citizens what they could best do for themselves. With a final thrust aimed at those working for reform, he said, "Nor is it necessary for the further efficiency of this department that it should become the nursery of students of medicine. . . ."[45]

Smith dealt harshly with this report. He noted that it contained ". . . its usual variety of loose and often absurd statements in regard to the public health, and deductions, the result of the most profound ignorance of sanitary science."[46] He objected mostly to the assertion that New York was a healthy city. The ratio of 1 death in 36 of its population made the mortality rate the highest of civilized cities.

Early in 1862, Smith bemoaned the singular indifference, which he felt was evident in the city, toward the fearful living conditions of most of its people.[47] The *Medical and Surgical Reporter* of Philadelphia agreed and said that the Augean stable had to be cleansed and a Hercules of sanitary science was needed to do the job.[48]

In February 1862 Smith became more optimistic about the possibility of a health bill. There was good evidence at last that a reorganization of the health department was to take place. Perhaps he saw a turning point in the road to victory when he noted that, "the question which is presented this winter is not, Shall there be a reform, but, What shall be its character?"[49]

Optimism was short-lived. In early May he began an editorial plaintively announcing the adjournment of the legislature without the enactment of a health bill. The metropolitan concept introduced into the proposed bill was distasteful to the mayor. Smith decided that Mayor Opdyke had really joined the "Ring" and thereby had aided the defeat of "this most righteous measure."[50]

Others, too, "confessed to a very great disappointment" at the failure of the bill. The *Medical and Surgical Reporter* entitled its editorial, "Health Bills and a Diseased Body Politic." "Politicians, those curses of our country . . ." doubtless were to blame, said the *Reporter*.[51] And so again New York was left to its own sanitary devices, devices that were due to receive shocking public description and denunciation in the succeeding few years.

In what had become a cycle of editorial moods, Smith seemed most discouraged toward the end of 1862. It was an extremely busy year for him, personally. Besides the weekly editorial writing and editing of the *Medical Times*, he wrote a manual for military surgeons, used in the Civil War; he continued active teaching and practice at the Bellevue Hospital and its new Medical College, where he was the first Professor of the Principles of Surgery; and he served a stint in the military hospitals of Virginia as an acting assistant surgeon. But the sanitary reform of New York was still a pressing concern for him.

In November he wrote that prospects for a bill seemed discouraging, that many had been led to believe that subsequent efforts would lead nowhere and hence should be abandoned indefinitely. Smith disagreed. While thousands of New Yorkers were dying annually of what he firmly believed were preventable diseases, and while half the city's population lived in the cheerless, sunless, and airless tenements, it was unthinkable to yield in the struggle. Ceaseless agitation would be required. His feelings were perhaps neatly summed up when he noted in November of 1862, "we should not, however, lose sight of the fact that we are striving to accomplish a reform which in importance and in magnitude rises superior to all civil, social, religious, or political questions of the time."[52] Allowing for the exaggeration and zeal of the reformer, this statement still, I believe, illustrates the extent of his commitment to sanitary reform, especially in view of the state of the nation's political and economic health.

He described the efforts he envisioned from legislative enactments: First, they should protect the citizen, especially the impoverished one, from disease and thereby lengthen life; second, they would develop a strong and healthy generation of citizens; and third, all health reforms would add greatly to the sum of human happiness. So fully impressed was he with the importance of sanitary reform that he felt, even though the prospect of success was not as great as it had been the year before, "we ought to put forth increased energy instead of relaxing our efforts."[53]

Public apathy was a major obstacle in the path of sanitary reform. This unconcern was as prevalent in much of the medical profession as it seems to have been in the general public. Numerous writers appealed to the educated, the rich, the influential, to raise their voices in protest. *Harper's Weekly* noted, for instance, "There is certainly no city in the world where intelligent and decent people surrender themselves to a band of knaves with such good humor as in New York."[54] The *Medical Times* noted that: "The country is horrified when a thousand fall victims in an ill-fought battle, but in this city 10,000 die annually of diseases which the city authorities have the power to remove, and no one is shocked."[55]

December 12, 1863, marked a turning point. On that day a group of the leading lawyers and merchants of the city, including Peter Cooper, John Jacob Astor, Jr., August Belmont, and Hamilton Fish, formed the Citizens' Association. They were organized "for purposes of public usefulness."[56]

At an association meeting two months later, a committee was formed to solicit from the medical profession the "fullest and most reliable information relative to the public health." Shortly, 24 of the city's leading medical men received a letter from the association — among them: Valentine Mott, Willard Parker, Stephen Smith, John H. Griscom, Elisha Harris, Austin Flint, Frank H. Hamilton, and Gurdon Buck.

Only a week later, on March 9, the physicians answered the committee's request for information. The doctors pointed out that although New York with its many natural advantages ought to be one of the healthiest cities, the exact reverse was the case. They believed the high mortality rate was a reliable index of the city's miserable health conditions. They provided comparative statistics: mortality in New York was 1 in every 35.7 of the population, while in Philadelphia it was 1 in 43.6, in Boston 1 in 41.2, and in Hartford as low as 1 in 54.8. The city fared poorly in comparison to London and Liverpool as well. They pointed to Lyon Playfair's figures in Great Britain, which showed that for every death there were at least 28 cases of illness.[57]

In the meantime, the Citizens' Association busied itself with the task of lobbying for the health bill then being considered in Albany. Representatives appeared before the legislature on March 15 and 16, only to meet resistance from both Democratic and Republican members. The former regarded the sweeping measures proposed under a metropolitan, nonpolitical health department as being aimed at their friends, which indeed it was. The Republicans were reluctant to interfere in city affairs, thereby hurting their chances in the upcoming presidential election that fall. The members of the Citizens' Association found, according to Stephen Smith, that to many members of the legislature, "the death of five thousand citizens was not so serious as the possibility of a presidential defeat."[58]

It must have been clear, at this point, to the Citizens' Association and the friends of sanitary reform, that what they really needed was a set of clear and extensive facts about the health conditions of the city — facts that would overcome the inertia of some legislators and facts which would once and for all clearly disprove the data which the City Inspector's Office had for so long been bringing to Albany to controvert any proposal for better laws.

A Council of Hygiene and Public Health was formed in April within the Citizens' Association. Its president was Joseph M. Smith, a prominent physician and writer who had made a monumental study of the epidemics of New York State.[59] Elisha Harris, a close friend and neighbor of Stephen Smith, was made secretary. The council consisted of 16 physicians, many of whom had been recipients and signers of the letters noted above.[60]

To gather the necessary facts about the true

health and sanitary conditions of New York and its three-quarters of a million residents, an extensive survey was planned. This survey was organized and directed primarily by Stephen Smith.[61] It was to become, according to numerous commenters, the most complete sanitary survey ever made, and certainly an important landmark in the history of public health in America.

The survey began early in May, got under full swing by July, and was completed by mid-November.[62] The city was divided into 31 districts, each inspected thoroughly by a physician. It was intended, by means of the survey, to arrive at "positive knowledge of the amount of preventible disease existing in New York, the location of insalubrious quarters, the peculiar habitats of typhus, smallpox, . . . and the conditions on which the alarming prevalence of these diseases depend."[63] A month later, in late July, Smith noted, "It is nothing less than a full and accurate inquiry into the causes of disease in this city by competent medical men."[64] And thus it should also be credited as a landmark in the history of epidemiology.

Although there were numerous etiological theories current in 1864, in the sanitarians' view the environment played the most important part, especially the so-called localizing causes, or those which promoted the prevalence of disease in particular localities. Each of the 31 inspectors reported on his district and described his findings mainly in terms of cleanliness and filth.[65]

The inspectors were, for the most part, young physicians who were employed by one of the public (charity supported) dispensaries of the city. They were ideally qualified, for their patients mostly came from the poorer districts; moreover, they had had experience in visiting the tenements. They were given only token compensation ($40 per month) for their labor. Their reports, charts, maps, and diagrams filled 17 folio volumes. On his return from his work on behalf of the U.S. Sanitary Commission, Dr. Harris edited the 360-page report and added a 143-page introduction. The report was published in April 1865. The reviews of the book were uniformly laudatory, and many pointed out the great importance of the survey and the *Report* for the future of sanitary government in New York.[66]

The *Report* has been frequently cited in discussions of American public health and of housing problems. Indeed, it deserves to be ranked very high among primary documents, not only in the history of public health reform but in epidemiology as well. Furthermore, it affords an extremely detailed look at some aspects of the way of life in each of the wards of New York in 1864, and it should be of great interest in the study of urban history.

Epidemiology has been defined as "the study of the distribution and determinants of disease prevalence in man."[67] According to this concept, then, the *Report* belongs among the most important of 19th century epidemiological studies. It contains graphic, statistical, and descriptive information on population, number and size of tenement houses, prevailing diseases, schools, churches, stores, slaughter-houses, factories, brothels, drinking establishments, sewerage, streets, and topography.

Its impact was manifold. Certainly it did not "drop stillborn from the printer's hand," as had been the case with the Shattuck *Report* 15 years earlier. Instead, as Kramer has pointed out for the Chadwick *Report*, it was a document that was alive; it aroused indignation and wonderment; it had emotional appeal beyond its intellectual content. And it led to effective legislation.[68]

Besides the descriptions of overflowing privies with their nauseous odors, garbage, offal, ashes, and generally dirty streets, the inspectors also wrote about slaughterhouses, fat- and bone-boiling establishments, and stables, all dispersed among the tenements. The streets were the main focus of complaint from the magazines and newspapers of the day as well. Youngsters, it is said, could easily earn nickels by standing along Broadway and sweeping a path through the muck for those who wanted to cross.[69] On Thirty-ninth Street, the inspector reported that blood and liquid animal remains flowed for two blocks from a slaughterhouse to the river.[70] Another great source of nuisance was the wooden garbage box. These usually rotted, allowing liquid contents to flow out. It seems they also provided a ready source of wood for political bonfires.[71]

Occasionally the survey itself was responsible for immediate improvements. In parts of the third district the inspector noted progress with each succeeding visit he made.[72]

It was armed with the data from this comprehensive epidemiological study of New York City that Stephen Smith appeared before the legislature in Albany on February 13, 1865. The report had not yet been published, but Smith in his testimony, to which I alluded at the opening of this paper, quoted widely from it. He spoke before the joint committee of the Senate and Assembly, presided over by Andrew D. White. The committee had already heard testimony from Mr. Dorman B. Eaton on the legal aspects of the proposed bill.[73] Smith told them that he and the Citizens' Association had been inspired and aided by the work of similar organizations in Great Britain, notably the Health of Towns Association.

He further told the legislators that the best method of arriving at a complete understanding of the existing causes of disease was by a house-to-house inspection. Since it was disease that was the object of study, it could only have been carried out properly by sufficiently trained men, viz., physicians.

He described conditions in general terms of cleanliness, stating that the degree of public health of a town was to be measured by its cleanliness and that in no way was the sanitary government of New York to be commended. He called the City Inspector's department a "gigantic imposture." The 22 health wardens and an equal number of assistants were grossly ignorant of sanitary matters, but that was to be expected in view of their backgrounds, since they were liquor store owners, local politicians, stonemasons, and carpenters. Not only were they ignorant of medical matters, but Smith also accused them of unwillingness to visit houses where known cases of disease existed. He told of one health warden who sent for an attendant of a smallpox patient in an upper room. Ordering the attendant not to approach too closely, he then advised: "Burn camphor on the stove, and hang bags of camphor about the necks of the children." Smith then asked the members of the Senate and Assembly:

> To what depth of humiliation must that community have descended, which tolerates as its sanitary officers men who are not only utterly disqualified by education, business, and moral character, but who have not even the poor qualification of courage to perform their duties?

He ended his long testimony with the recommendation that New York heed the experience of other large cities in establishing a well-organized health board. That board, he opined, should be independent of politics and above partisan control. Furthermore the board must combine administrative ability with a knowledge of disease and its prevention. For this reason he felt that the composition of the board should include medical and nonmedical members. His testimony, although well organized and at times forceful as well as eloquent, was not original. It represented the consensus of most of his coworkers. It is to his credit, however, that the problems of sanitary reform were continually held up before the medical profession through his editorials in the *American Medical Times* and now were brought before the general public, with the aid of the *New York Times*. Equally to his credit was it that he had helped to write the medical portion of the proposed bill and, together with Dorman B. Eaton, a lawyer and a keen student of sanitary laws, had drafted the final version.

Why the *Times* hesitated for over a month before publishing his speech I cannot explain with certainty. It is entirely possible that when the testimony was given on February 13, the prospect of legislation was bright; but that by March 16, when the *Times* printed the speech, the bill was already in dire straits.[74] Henry Raymond and the *Times* were deeply committed to a health reform measure, as is attested by frequent editorials during the winter of 1865 and again during the next session in 1866. It may well be that the *Times* felt that publication of the facts would serve to bring pressure to bear upon the reluctant legislators.[75] That it did not achieve this result is a matter of record. But now the issues and the facts were clearly before the public. Because part of the Citizens' Association survey was published in the *Times* it achieved a wider public circulation for writing on the subject of sanitation than had ever been the case before. This was a milestone in New York history.

Unfortunately, Smith's testimony in February, its publication in March, and the subsequent appearance of the printed *Report* were not enough to sway the lawmakers in Albany. Frequent editorials in the *Times*, the *Tribune*, and the *Citizen*, a weekly paper founded by the Citizens' Association in 1864, did not seem to help either.

On January 16, 1865, the *Times* noted that

typhus and smallpox were running rife. The "ignorant men called 'Health Wardens'" were receiving annually an aggregate of nearly $50,000, but in the opinion of the newspaper, "The only persons who are doing anything for the public health are the agents of the Citizens' Association."

On March 3, the *Tribune* reported the continuing discussion in Albany and the testimony that had been given for the bill by the members of the Citizens' Association and against it by Francis I. A. Boole, the City Inspector; Lewis A. Sayre, the resident physician; and Cyrus Ramsey, the Registrar in the City Inspector's department. According to the *Tribune*, Ramsey attempted ineffectually to controvert the statements made by Smith, Eaton, and the friends of reform. The *Tribune*, somewhat incredulously, noted that Ramsey was driven to extremes in support of the existing corrupt system when he even went so far as to ridicule the idea that cleanliness was an important source of health.[76]

As March progressed, the *Times* pointed out that the Democratic members in the legislature hung together on every question, but not the Republicans. The health bill had, despite pleas from many sides, once again become a political and partisan issue.[77] The *Tribune* said, "To lose the rich *placer* of the City Inspector's department is to cut the winds of scores of active workers, whose only duty is to sign the payrolls and work for the party that gives them fat sinecures."[78]

On April 12, three days after Appomattox, the bill finally came out of committee into the House. Two days later, amid "perfect bedlam," it was defeated. Most New Yorkers, however, were probably much too dazed and saddened to read the account from Albany on the morning of April 15. The headline that day proclaimed "Awful Event."[79] It is not likely that in the days following the tragic and shocking death of Lincoln, those who had labored so hard that year for a health bill had any time for grief on its account.

In 1865 cholera threatened New York again, and the press of the city became increasingly alarmed over the prospects of another epidemic. The summer passed, however, and with a sigh of relief those concerned felt that with the approaching cold season the city would be safe, at least temporarily. But the need for legislative action became more acute.[80]

On November 9, the *Nation* claimed that New York was nearly as filthy as the Asiatic towns from which the cholera came.

> It is awful yet comical to learn that the Board of Health, which at such a crisis ought to reign supreme, is such a disreputable body that, nobody having the power to adjourn it if once organized, the Mayor is afraid to call it together.[81]

The *Times*, a day later, noted that the Mayor considered the cholera the lesser of the two evils, and so left the Board alone.[82]

As 1866 opened, Mayor John T. Hoffman, a Tammany leader, stated in his first message to the Common Council that the Board of Commissioners of Health, would be "able to accomplish all that may be required of it." He was against a metropolitan bill, and he used the old argument that such a bill would be an interference with the municipal rights of New York.[83] The *Times* retorted that the only branches of the city government managed with honesty were Central Park, the Police Department, and the charities on Blackwell's Island — all created by the state legislature. As for the *Times*, it felt that, "We would prefer to live under a 'Legislative Commission' to dying prematurely and painfully under the pure Democratic rule of a city constituency."[84]

All through January and February the *Times*, and occasionally the *Tribune*, continued to press for a bill. After a complicated fight between the Senate, which passed a bill including the names of four physicians who were to be commissioners, and the Assembly, which wanted to allow the governor to name the members of the board, the whole thing was nearly scuttled once again.[85] Success was finally achieved on February 15. The Assembly passed an amended bill allowing the governor to name the commissioners. With the aid of an impassioned speech by Senator Andrew D. White, using some of the testimony Stephen Smith had presented the previous year, the Conference Committee of the two houses settled their differences and received assurances from Governor Fenton that none of his appointments would be on a political basis.[86] On February 21, 1866, the *Times* felt that the final victory for a health bill was not to be passed over without public notice. The dedicated physicians and philanthropists who, for ten years, had come each winter to Albany received due praise.

The official date of passage was February 26, and the title of the law was "An Act to Create A Metropolitan Sanitary District and Board of Health therein for the Preservation of Life and Health and to Prevent the Spread of Disease."[87]

The law, which in essence had been drafted by Stephen Smith and Dorman B. Eaton the year before, created a health department for the metropolitan area of New York. The new Metropolitan Board of Health, as it was called, was given extremely broad powers to make laws, to carry them out, and to sit in judgment of them, all at the same time. Questions of constitutionality would soon arise.[88]

The general implications of this bill of 1866 are several. It was undoubtedly a major triumph in the history of public health, as noted by Rosen.[89] Locally it served to give a great city the beginning of really effective sanitary government, carried out by professionals. Furthermore, as a major piece of reform legislation it may have been one of the beginning moves against a thread of corruption so strong that it was not broken until the Tweed "Ring" was finally deposed in the early 1870s. The Reverend Samuel Osgood may have had the health bill in mind when he said:

> Careful legislation, with intelligent suffrage and a city government more on the plan of the national, and taking from the Common Council its temptations to base jobs, will set us right, and free us from being subject to the dynasty of dirt and sovereignty of sots.[90]

On a broader scale, the sanitary reform of New York City had several more specific results. In the first place it was the first comprehensive health legislation of its kind in the United States, and later it was to serve as a model for numerous local and state bills. In this respect too the reform movement seems to have united the sanitary interests of numerous physicians and laymen alike. Sanitary science was becoming a specialty in this country, as in Europe. The work in New York also led to the formation of the most important national health group, the American Public Health Association. Stephen Smith, who was one of the prime movers in its founding and its first president, gave credit to his work for the Metropolitan Health Bill and later as a commissioner on the board for providing the inception of the A.P.H.A. in 1872.[91]

Finally, the sanitary reform work in New York also played a role in the changing status or image of the physician and of medicine as a whole. Kramer has noted that before public health could be undertaken, medicine had to put its house in order.[92] But the reverse may have been even more the case: Effective sanitary legislation and the organization of competent health departments played a great part in helping medicine to reestablish the much needed order in the house.

NOTES

A portion of this paper was presented to The Johns Hopkins Medical History Club, March 14, 1966, and at the Hixon Hour, University of Kansas Medical Center, April 18, 1966. It is part of a larger project, a biographical study of Stephen Smith, in which I am presently engaged. See *Bull. Hist. Med.*, 1965, *39*: 85.

This investigation was supported by U.S. Public Health Service Training Grant number 9T1-LM-105-06.

1 Smith had presented the evidence to the legislative committee on Feb. 13, 1865. It was published in the *New York Times* a month later and was reprinted in Stephen Smith, *The City That Was* (New York: Allaben, 1911), ch. 4. The latter version contained only very minor changes.

2 James Ford, *Slums and Housing, with Special Reference to New York City, History, Conditions, Policy*, 2 vols. (Cambridge, Mass.: Harvard Univ. Press, 1936), I, 17–204. Ford describes many of the early health ordinances. The amount of space he has devoted to sanitary matters is an indication of the close relationship of health and housing. There are a number of other works that deal with health conditions and sanitary laws prior to 1866. A few examples are Susan Wade Peabody, "Historical study of legislation regarding public health in the states of New York and Massachusetts," *J. Infect. Dis.*, 1909, Suppl. No. 4, 156 pp.; Charles F. Bolduan, "Over a century of health administration in New York City," *Department of Health Monograph Series*, No. 13, 1916; John Blake, "Historical study of the development of the New York City Department of Health," typescript, *c.* 1952, 128 pp.; Charles E. Rosenberg, *The Cholera*

Years, The United States in 1832, 1849, and 1866 (Chicago: Univ. of Chicago Press, 1962); George Rosen, "Public health problems in New York City during the nineteenth century," *N.Y. St. J. Med.*, 1950, *50*: 73–78; and Howard D. Kramer, "Early municipal and state boards of health," *Bull. Hist. Med.*, 1950, *24*: 503–509.

I should also say at the outset that the city did have a health organization during the years prior to the Metropolitan Health Bill of 1866. A history of the department is in the process of being compiled by Professor John Duffy, who will give in great detail what I have perhaps too much simplified in this paper. [Editors' note: Since the original publication of this article, Duffy's book has been published: John Duffy, *A History of Public Health in New York City*, 2 vols. (New York: Russell Sage Foundation, 1968–1974).] It was the "felt reality" of the time, however, according to many physicians, that New York did not indeed have a health department worthy of that name. *Reports, Resolutions, and Proceedings of the Commissioners of Health of the City of New York For the Years 1856–1859* (New York: Clark, 1860), reveals that meetings were frequent, sometimes even daily, but that mostly they dealt with quarantine matters and occasionally with removal of nuisances.

3 David Hosack, "Observations on the means of improving the medical police of the city of New York," in *Essays on Various Subjects of Medical Science*, 2 vols. (New York: Seymour, 1824), II, 9–86.

4 Benjamin W. McCready, *On the Influence of Trades, Professions, and Occupations in the United States, in the Production of Disease*, ed. Genevieve Miller (Baltimore: Johns Hopkins Press, 1943), pp. 41–45.

5 John H. Griscom, *Annual Report of the Interments in the City and County of New York for the Year 1842, with Remarks Therein, And a Brief View of the Sanitary Condition of the City* (New York, 1843). See also Lawrence Veiller, "Tenement house reform in New York City, 1834–1900," in *The Tenement House Problem*, ed. Robert W. DeForest and Lawrence Veiller, 2 vols. (New York: Macmillan, 1903), I, 71–75, in which Veiller has included long quotes from Griscom.

6 Not only were New Yorkers influenced and inspired by the work of the Parisian and London sanitarians, but there were frequent allusions to the mortality rates in these cities, as compared to New York. New York usually fared second best. See also "Health. New York versus London," *Hunt's Merchant's Magazine*, 1863, *48*: 120–124; and "Health of New York, Philadelphia, and Baltimore, for 1860," *Am. Med. Monthly*, 1861, *15*: 312–316. It was especially galling to New Yorkers that the over-all mortality rate of the United States was far lower than that of England (15 per 1000 *v.* 23 per 1000) yet in New York City it was much higher (36 per 1000). See *Report of the Committee on the Incorporation of Cities and Villages, on the bill entitled "An Act concerning the Public Health of the counties of New York, Kings, and Richmond,"* New York State Legislature, Assembly Doc. No. 129, 1860.

7 The problem of tenements and housing reform has been fully dealt with by others. The role of housing in sanitary reform was a central one. See for instance, Ford, *Slums and Housing*; DeForest and Veiller, *The Tenement House Problem*; Gordon Atkins, *Health, Housing, and Poverty in New York City 1865–1898* (Ann Arbor: Edwards, 1947), which includes a good discussion of the sanitary reform of 1866. Roy Lubove, *The Progressives and the Slums* (Pittsburgh: Univ. of Pittsburgh Press, 1962), also deals with the formation of the Metropolitan Board of Health.

8 John H. Griscom, "Improvements of the public health, and the establishment of a sanitary police in the city of New York," *Tr. Med. Soc. St. N.Y.*, 1857, pp. 107–123.

9 *Report of the Select Committee Appointed to Investigate the Health Department of the City of New York*, New York State Legislature, Senate Doc. No. 49, 1859.

10 *Ibid.*, p. 1.

11 *Ibid.*, p. 3.

12 *Ibid.*, p. 52.

13 *Ibid.*, pp. 156–157.

14 *Ibid.*, p. 174.

15 New York State Legislature, Assembly Doc. No. 129, p. 1.

16 Not only was the bill refused, but, to add to the problems of sanitation, the City Inspector was at that time given supervision of street cleaning. As the New York Sanitary Association pointed out later, this was added to his already grossly neglected sanitary duties. *Reports of the Sanitary Association of the City of New York* (New York, 1859), p. 7.

17 See Denis T. Lynch, *"Boss" Tweed, the Story of a Grim Generation* (New York: Boni and Liverwright, 1927), pp. 187–199; Samuel A. Pleasants, *Fernando Wood of New York* (New York: Columbia Univ. Studies in History, Economics and Public Law, No. 536, 1948), ch. 5; James F. Richardson, "Mayor Fernando Wood and the New York Police force, 1855–1857," *N.-Y. Hist. Soc. Quart.*, 1966, *50*: 5–40.

18 Richardson, "Mayor Fernando Wood," p. 6.

19 Those interested in sanitary reform seem to have been well aware of their enemies. Stephen Smith frequently described corrupt practices such as the bribery to which the Tammany-controlled City Inspector's Office allegedly resorted. The 1857 bill had been "effectually defeated by the paid agents of corrupt officials who succeeded, at a late period of the session, in sequestering or destroying all traces

of the bill, both manuscript and printed." *Am. Med. Times*, 1860, *1*: 423. It must also be noted that the friends of sanitary reform early realized that a health department with jurisdiction merely over New York, and not including Brooklyn or the other surrounding communities, would have been of little avail. The large interchange of people each day made the metropolitan concept a necessity. See "New York Health Bills," *Am. Med. Times*, 1862, *4*: 70–71. For a brief, general description of New York City government see Seth Low, *New York in 1850 and in 1890* (New York: New-York Historical Society, 1892).

20 N.Y. Sanitary Association, *Report*. Elisha Harris must have been everybody's favorite secretary. He held that job in the Sanitary Association, and later in the Council of Hygiene, the U.S. Sanitary Commission, and the American Public Health Association. See also, Wilson G. Smillie, *Public Health, Its Promise for the Future* (New York: Macmillan, 1955), pp. 289–290.

21 N.Y. Sanitary Association, *Report*, pp. 11–13.

22 *Ibid.*, p. 13.

23 *Second Annual Report of the N.Y. Sanitary Association* for the year ending December 1860 (New York, 1860), pp. 1–23.

24 Louis Elsberg's "The domain of medical police," *Am. Med. Monthly*, 1862, *17*: 321–337, was delivered before the Association. This concept of medical police was a prominent idea in the writings of John Griscom too. See George Rosen, "The fate of the concept of medical police 1780–1890," *Centaurus*, 1957, *5*: 97–113. Actually the term "sanitary police" might be more applicable to the goals of the New York sanitarians. According to Shattuck, in the term "medical police," cure of disease is implied; while in the idea of "sanitary police" prevention is stressed. Lemuel Shattuck, *Report of the Sanitary Commission of Massachusetts 1850* (repr.; Cambridge, Mass.: Harvard Univ. Press, 1948).

25 [Robert Tomes], "Why we get sick," *Harper's Monthly*, 1856, *13*: 642–647. The author noted that, "A host of diseases of the heart, the brain, nerves, and stomach, which exhaust the doctor's skill and fill his pockets, came in with modern civilization. To these diseases the Americans are far more subject than any other people . . . ," p. 642.

26 Frank H. Hamilton, "Hygiene," *N.Y. J. Med.*, 1859, 7: 60–74, p. 60. Hamilton, a renowned surgeon, had been Stephen Smith's teacher and preceptor and remained a close friend in later years.

27 *Ibid.*, p. 63.

28 "Quarantine and Hygiene," *North Am. Rev.*, 1860, *91*: 438–491, p. 491.

29 Although Elisha Harris and George Shrady were assistant editors, I have ascribed the editorials to Smith, throughout. Harris actually resigned in 1861 because of increasing work with the U.S. Sanitary Commission. Shrady apparently did most of the reports of medical society meetings. Furthermore, Smith published many of the editorials in his book *Doctor in Medicine and Other Papers on Professional Subjects* (New York: Wood, 1872), thereby claiming authorship for those included. In various letters to his wife, to be dealt with in a future study, Smith complained of the wearying task of his weekly editorials. In this paper I am concerned only with those editorials that dealt with sanitary reform.

30 *Am. Med. Times*, 1860, *1*: 15. Howard D. Kramer, "The beginnings of the public health movement in the United States," *Bull. Hist. Med.*, 1947, *21*: 352–376, gives Smith and the *American Medical Times* a great deal of credit for bringing about reform, p. 375. Also Kramer, "Early municipal and state boards."

31 "Our sanitary defences," *Am. Med. Times*, 1860, *1*: 46–47.

32 *Ibid.*, p. 100.

33 *Ibid.*, 1861, *2*: 47–48.

34 For a general discussion see Emerson D. Fite, *Social and Industrial Conditions in the North During the Civil War* (New York: Macmillan, 1910), p. 229.

35 I. N. Phelps Stokes, *The Iconography of Manhattan Island*, 6 vols. (New York, 1895–1928), III, 736–756; Milledge L. Bonham, Jr., "New York and the Civil War," in *History of the State of New York*, 10 vols., ed. Alexander C. Flick (New York: Columbia Univ. Press, 1933–1937), VII, 99–135.

36 Allan Nevins, *The Evening Post, A Century of Journalism* (New York: Boni and Liverwright, 1922), p. 364.

37 Fite, *Social and Industrial Conditions*, p. 184. Also Edgar W. Martin, *The Standard of Living in 1860* (Chicago: Univ. of Chicago Press, 1942), contains many useful data.

38 "Health laws," *Am. Med. Times*, 1860, *1*: 423–424.

39 *Ibid.*

40 "Health of New York in 1860," *Am. Med. Times*, 1861, *2*: 63–64.

41 See *Proceedings of a Select Committee of The Senate . . . Appointed to Investigate Various Departments of the City of New York*, New York State Legislature, Senate Doc. No. 38, Feb. 9, 1865. In this 612-page report, which dealt only with the City Inspector's department, there is a wealth of information. Testimony revealed the buying and selling of jobs and the incompetence of the health wardens. The duties of the 22 wardens and an equal number of assistants were to report nuisances, inspect buildings, privies, and cesspools, report all diseases, and to prevent

accumulation of garbage and offal on the streets and sidewalks (p. 345). Several health wardens admitted they did not go personally to see cases of disease. They generally admitted that some smallpox existed and "a few fevers," when in fact smallpox, typhus, typhoid, cholera infantum, and scarlatina were widespread (pp. 455–456). Several of the wardens also admitted that they "devoted" a month's pay — but usually claimed ignorance of the fact it was used to aid defeat of health bills in Albany (pp. 462, 467).

42 *Annual Report of the City Inspector . . . for the Year Ending December 31, 1860* (New York: Board of Aldermen, Doc. No. 5, 1861), p. 10.

43 *Ibid.*, pp. 16–17.

44 *Ibid.*, pp. 19–22.

45 *Ibid.*, p. 60.

46 *Am. Med. Times*, 1861, *2*: 63.

47 "Sanitary legislation," *Am. Med. Times*, 1862, *4*: 28–29.

48 *Med. & Surg. Reptr.*, 1862, *7*: 349–351.

49 "New York health bills," *Am. Med. Times*, 1862, *4*: 70.

50 "Failure of the health bill," *ibid.*, pp. 250–251.

51 *Med. & Surg. Reptr.*, 1862, *8*: 124–125.

52 "The prospect of health-reform in New York," *Am. Med. Times*, 1862, *5*: 276.

53 *Ibid.*, p. 277.

54 *Harper's Weekly*, 1863, *7*: 786.

55 "Sanitary interests in New York," *Am. Med. Times*, 1863, *6*: 21–22.

56 For a description of the founding of the Citizens' Association see Edward C. Mack, *Peter Cooper, Citizen of New York* (New York: Duell, Sloan, Pearce, 1949), ch. 19. See also the *New York Citizen*, Aug. 13, 1864.

57 These two letters may be found in *Report of the Council of Hygiene and Public Health of the Citizens' Association of New York, Upon the Sanitary Condition of the City* (New York: Appleton, 1865), pp. ix–xiii.

58 "Citizens' Association and health reform," *Am. Med. Times*, 1864, *8*: 200. Also at the beginning of 1864 there was an investigation into the affairs of the City Inspector's department. Smith published excerpts from a letter written by Thomas N. Carr, who had been superintendent of street cleaning. Carr said that New York simply had no sanitary department worthy of the name. He felt that the only concern the City Inspector had was for the streets. Carr continued: "On an examination of the annual sanitary reports of England or France, the mind is astonished by the vastness of research, investigation, and scientific elaboration which these reports contain, and yet, strange to say, street cleaning, instead of being the all absorbing feature of these documents, is not even mentioned." *Am. Med. Times*, 1864, *8*: 57.

59 Joseph M. Smith, "Report on the medical topography and epidemics of New York," *Tr. A.M.A.*, 1860, *13*: 81–269.

60 In 1865 Smith became the secretary. For the names of the members of the council, see the first part of the introduction to the *Report*.

61 The evidence concerning Smith's role lies mostly within his own writings, especially *The City That Was*. Charles F. Chandler, however, also gave Smith credit for organizing the survey. See *Stephen Smith, Addresses in Recognition of His Public Services on the Occasion of His Eighty Eighth Birthday* (New York: New York Academy of Medicine, 1911), p. 19, in which Chandler, then an old man himself, noted, "This work was organized and supervised to its completion by Dr. Stephen Smith." In 1864 Joseph M. Smith, the president of the council, was 75 years old. Elisha Harris, the secretary, was mainly occupied by the U.S. Sanitary Commission.

62 *New York Times*, March 16, 1865, or *The City That Was*, p. 57.

63 *Am. Med. Times*, 1864, *8*: 307. The *New York Tribune*, June 3, 1864, had great praise for the efforts of the Citizens' Association.

64 *Am. Med. Times*, 1866, *9*: 47.

65 There is a long discussion of etiological factors in disease in the introductory portion of the *Report*, pp. xlvii–lxviii. See also Richard H. Shryock, "The origins and significance of the public health movement in the United States," *Ann. Med. Hist.*, 1929, *1*: 645–665, especially pp. 650–652; Charles E. Rosenberg, "The cause of cholera: aspects of etiological thought in nineteenth century America," *Bull. Hist. Med.*, 1960, *34*: 331–354 [see pp. 257–271 in this book], and his *The Cholera Years*; and John Simon, *Filth Diseases and Their Prevention*, 1st Am. ed. (Boston: Campbell, 1876).

66 The *New York Times* on July 7, 1865, said: "No volume of intenser interest has ever seen the light in this city. . . ." See also *Nation*, 1865, *1*: 250; *Am. J. Med. Sci.*, 1865, *100*: 419–428.

67 Brian MacMahon, Thomas F. Pugh, and Johannes Ipsen, *Epidemiologic Methods* (Boston: Little, Brown, 1960), p. 3.

68 Kramer, "Beginnings," pp. 361–362. There were occasional descriptions of living conditions among the poor in the general press. See, for instance, Samuel B. Halliday, *The Lost and Found; or Life Among the Poor* (New York: Blakeman & Mason, 1859). Halliday was a member of the N.Y. Sanitary Association. Soon after the survey of the Citizens' Association was published there was a vivid article in the *Nation* by Bayard Taylor, entitled "A descent into the depths," 1866, *2*: 302–304. Although I have focused attention on the two societies in which

Smith played a role, this is not to say that they were the only ones active in sanitary reform at this time. The A.I.C.P. and the various missions and tract societies were also active. The A.I.C.P. *Report* for 1853 contains a long discussion of sanitary needs. Its founder and leading spirit, Robert M. Hartley, was well known for his crusade against swill milk. See Roy Lubove, "The New York Association for Improving the Condition of the Poor: the formative years," *N.-Y. Hist. Soc. Quart.*, 1959, *43*: 307–327; and Atkins, *Health, Housing, and Poverty*. Carroll S. Rosenberg's "Protestants and Five Pointers: The Five Points House of Industry, 1850–1870," *N.-Y. Hist. Soc. Quart.*, 1964, *48*: 327–347, describes New York's most notorious slum and efforts toward amelioration. Also Allan Nevins has drawn attention to the reformers in his "The golden thread in the history of New York," *N.-Y. Hist. Soc. Quart.*, 1955, *39*: 5–22.

69 Israel Weinstein, "Eighty years of public health in New York City," *Bull. N.Y. Acad. Med.*, 1947, *23*: 221–237.

70 *Citizens' Association Report*, pp. 261–262.

71 *Ibid.*, p. 285; and *Annual Report of the City Inspector . . . for the Year Ending December 31, 1861* (New York: Board of Alderman, Doc. no. 4, 1862), pp. 21–23.

72 *Citizens' Association Report*, p. 42.

73 Smith, *City That Was*, p. 46; Andrew Dickson White, *Autobiography*, 2 vols. (New York: Century, 1905), I, 107–110. White reported the oft-quoted testimony of one of the city's health wardens, who, when asked the meaning of the word "hygiene," answered that it referred to bad smells arising from standing water. White also sat on a Senate committee during the investigation of the City Inspector's department early in 1865. Despite the pleas of the Citizens' Association, City Inspector Boole was not dismissed. See Stokes, *Iconography*, V, 1912; and Senate Doc. No. 38, 1865, p. 467. Eaton's testimony was given Feb. 2, 1865, and was published by "Friends of the Bill" later that year. Together with an appendix, his remarks take up 56 printed pages. *Remarks of D. B. Eaton, Esq., at a Joint Meeting of the Committees of the Senate and Assembly* (New York: Nesbitt, 1865).

74 On March 10 and 11, 1865, the *Times* noted that opposition was brewing from quarters formerly friendly to the bill. The paper warned that delay in passage of the bill was dangerous, so late in the session. Smith gave a great deal of credit to Henry J. Raymond, editor of the *Times*, calling him an ardent reformer. *City That Was*, p. 173.

75 That some of the legislators were impressed by the testimony was attested to by at least one member of Smith's audience. After hearing the description of sweatshop conditions in the tenements and of clothing, in the process of manufacture, draped over cribs of children with active smallpox, one of the committee supposedly said to Smith: "Why I bought underwear at one of those stores a few days ago, and I believe I have got smallpox, for I begin to itch all over." *City That Was*, p. 156. It should be stressed that this episode was 46 years in the past when the book was published.

76 Ramsey was a physician but seems to have been completely under Tammany sway. Lewis A. Sayre was the Resident Physician of New York, as well as a leading teacher of orthopedic surgery. His difference of opinion with the members of the Citizens' Association seems, on the surface, to have been on intellectual grounds. Smith, who was a fellow faculty member of Sayre's at Bellevue, had once called the latter's job (as Resident Physician) a sinecure. *Am. Med. Times*, 1862, *4*: 252. It is, of course, quite possible that Sayre's own vested interests prompted his belief in the status quo. His salary was about $5,000 per year.

77 *New York Times*, March 20, 1865.

78 *New York Tribune*, March 20, 1865.

79 *New York Times*, April 13, 15, 17; *New York Tribune*, April 15. The *Times* on April 17 noted three reasons for the defeat of the bill: Several Union (Republican) members were absent owing to illness; several others were unwilling to create another commission for the Governor; and, City Inspector F. I. A. Boole had spent nearly the whole winter in Albany, armed with sufficient funds to kill the bill. This occurred in an Assembly in which the Republicans had a majority of 24. For a discussion of Boole, see Gustavus Myers, *The History of Tammany Hall* (New York: Boni and Liverwright, 1917), pp. 205–208. An informative discussion of the state political situation at this time may be found in Homer A. Stebbins, *A Political History of the State of New York 1865–1869* (New York: Columbia Univ. Studies in History, Economics and Public Law, No. 55, 1913).

80 *New York Times*, Oct. 31, Nov. 9, 1865; *Nation*, 1865, *1*: 609.

81 *Nation*, 1865, *1*: 577.

82 Quoted by Rosenberg, *Cholera Years*, p. 186. See also Smith, *City That Was*, p. 166.

83 The speech is printed in the *New York Times*, Jan. 3, 1866.

84 *Ibid.*, Jan. 7, 1866.

85 *Ibid.*, Feb. 7, 1866.

86 *Ibid.*, Feb. 16, 20, 1866.

87 *Laws of New York, 1866*, Ch. 74 (reprinted by Bergen & Tripp, Printers, 1866).

88 Smith described Eaton's role and his activities in other spheres in chapter 6 of *The City That Was*. This

book, incidentally, was dedicated to the memory of Dorman B. Eaton. Eaton was perhaps best known for his work in civil service reform. See Ari Hoogenboom, *Outlawing The Spoils: A history of the Civil Service Reform movement, 1865–1883* (Urbana: Univ. of Illinois Press, 1961). Eaton was credited by Smith with having written the legal aspects of that bill. Eaton's views can be seen in his "The essential conditions of good sanitary administration," *Reports and Papers, American Public Health Association*, 1874–1875, *2*: 498–514. He was a student of English sanitary law and patterned the New York bill on what he had learned in England. See Dorman B. Eaton, *Sanitary Regulations in England and New York* (New York: Amerman, 1872). See also Stephen Smith, "Development of American public health endeavor," *Am. J. Public Hlth.*, 1915, *5*: 1115–1119; Stephen Smith, "The origin and organization of the Department of Health of the City of New York," *Med. Rec.*, 1918, *93*: 1115–1117; and his "The history of public health, 1871–1921," in *A Half Century of Public Health*, ed. M. P. Ravenel (New York: A.P.H.A., 1921), pp. 1–12; especially pp. 4–10 deal with the Metropolitan Health Bill.

89 George Rosen, *A History of Public Health* (New York: MD, 1958), p. 247.

90 Samuel Osgood, *New York in the Nineteenth Century* (New York: New-York Historical Society, 1866), pp. 40–41. See also a review of numerous documents of the Citizens' Association, including the *Report of the Council of Hygiene*, by James Parton, "The government of the City of New York," *North Am. Rev.*, 1866, *103*: 413–465. Deserving more work is an analysis of those who were involved in the health reform movement. What were their backgrounds, their motives, and how large a part did they actually play? Also, how was the health reform movement, if indeed one can call it a movement at all, related to other reforms and reformers of the time? Health legislation played an important role in the general amelioration of the urban environment and in the development of cities. This too is an aspect of 19th-century public health that deserves much more study. See particularly Charles N. Glaab, *The American City, A Documentary Study* (Homewood: Dorsey, 1963). Also Arthur M. Schlesinger, "The city in American history," *Miss. Valley Hist. Rev.*, 1940, *27*: 43–66, and Blake McKelvey, *The Urbanization of America 1860–1915* (New Brunswick: Rutgers Univ. Press, 1963).

91 Stephen Smith, "American public health endeavor," p. 1117. Eaton and Elisha Harris were also active in the early work of the A.P.H.A.

92 Kramer, "Beginnings," p. 370.

27

The Movement toward a Safe Maternity: Physician Accountability in New York City, 1915–1940

JOYCE ANTLER AND DANIEL M. FOX

Until the 1940s, childbirth was, for most American women, a time of great danger and apprehension. Each year during the two decades after 1915, approximately 15,000 women perished from causes related to childbirth. Only tuberculosis accounted for more deaths among women in the child-bearing years. The number of puerperal deaths, moreover, merely suggested the total loss of life in childbirth, for the deaths of many women with preexisting chronic conditions were frequently assigned not to puerperal causes but to the diseases that preceded their pregnancies. "As far as her chance of living through childbirth is concerned," wrote Dr. Josephine Baker, an authority in maternal and child health, the United States was near being "the most unsafe country in the world for the pregnant woman."[1] Many thousands of other women survived pregnancy with severe disability and lowered health status.

Although the issue of maternal mortality was the subject of many studies, conferences, and papers after 1915, it was not until the middle 30s, with the publication of a report on maternal mortality by the New York Academy of Medicine, that an effective strategy for its reduction came to be widely adopted. As we shall see, the startling facts produced by that report, together with the academy's unusual tactic of seeking maximum publicity in the lay press for its findings, galvanized the medical profession into action, and led to widespread reform of obstetric practice in New York and other cities. The report has consequently been regarded as an important contributory factor in the marked decline of maternal mortality rates that occurred throughout the nation after 1935.

By the 1920s, the high rates of puerperal mortality in the United States attracted urgent attention. Because maternal death threatened family stability, it was seen as an even greater social loss than infant mortality, a problem to which health professionals had much earlier directed their attention. Saving mothers' lives, furthermore, was an issue which cut across the birth control controversy of the time, uniting conservative and liberal physicians and lay reformers. Safeguarding pregnancy rather than avoiding it became a central motive in the campaign to reduce the risk of childbirth.

While puerperal mortality rates in the United States remained stationary over a long period of time, mortality from most other diseases had shown marked decline. Spectacular improvements in medical science and technology, particularly in the field of prevention, occurred in the last decade of the 19th century and the first decades of the 20th. From 1890 to 1915, deaths per 100,000 in the U.S. Death Registration Area were reduced from 252 to 148.8 in tuberculosis, from 186.9 to 82.9 in pneumonia, from 97.8 to 15.7 in diphtheria and croup, and from 46.3 to 12.4 in typhoid fever.[2] The death rate from causes incidental to bearing children, however, showed no improvement. In 1890, the maternal death rate per 100,000 population was 15.3; in 1915, it was 15.2, while a year later it had risen to 16.3.[3] In spite of the introduction of prenatal supervision, wider dissemination of aseptic technique, and the increasing incidence of hospitalization for delivery, little progress was made in reducing the maternal death rate after 1915. Maternal mortality in the U.S.

Joyce Antler is with the Department of History, State University of New York at Stony Brook.

Daniel M. Fox is Professor of Humanities in Medicine and Assistant Vice President for Academic Affairs, Health Sciences Center, State University of New York at Stony Brook.

Reprinted with permission from the *Bulletin of the History of Medicine*, 1976, *50*: 569–595.

Registration Area never went below 61 per 10,000 births, the 1915 figure, prior to 1936.[4] In contrast, after 1915 infant mortality from practically every cause was reduced by 40 percent, from 99.9 per 10,000 live births in 1915 to 60.1 in 1934.[5]

No matter what statistical procedure was used, the United States maintained a high rate in comparison with other nations. In 1930, it ranked last out of 25 nations, its rate more than double that of Sweden, Denmark, Finland, Holland, Italy, Japan, and Uruguay.[6] Though mortality rates were not absolutely comparable among the various nations, studies showed that differences in statistical procedures or in methods of assigning causes to deaths did not explain the United States' exceedingly high rate.[7]

The stable rates of puerperal mortality threatened medical self-esteem. Physicians acknowledged that approximately one-half to three-quarters of puerperal deaths were caused by infection, toxemia, and hemorrhage, diseases considered controllable through adequate supervision during pregnancy and appropriate technique in labor and delivery.[8]

The failure to reduce maternal mortality rates produced lively debates within the medical community. Indeed, the problem of maternal mortality was amongst the most controversial public health problems of the day, generating heated arguments concerning the nature and conduct of obstetrics. Yet, in spite of the recognition of the problem, no clear consensus on the reasons for the high death rates emerged. Speculations involved a wide range of causes, including the lack of adequate prenatal care, pernicious midwifery, incompetence of general practitioners, poor obstetrical training of medical students and nurses, the low status and fee scale of obstetrics in contrast to general medicine and surgery, the expansion of indications for operative interference together with the more regular use of anesthesia, the absence of clinical material for training and lack of scientific interest in obstetrics, as well as its separation from gynecology, abortion and illegitimacy, falling birth rates, and finally, modern feminism, with its demand for technical-medical aids to achieve quick and painless labor.[9] Running through the debate was a fundamental question whose resolution would be decisive in shaping the future pattern of obstetric practice: Should childbirth be viewed mainly as a natural, physiological process, usually resulting in spontaneous delivery and which, under appropriate supervision, could be managed by nonphysician attendants? Or was the more useful perception that it was a dangerous, and sometimes pathological, condition, frequently necessitating radical operative intervention, which required the attendance of skilled physician practitioners throughout?

I

Medical interest in maternal health had been relatively slow to develop.[10] The prevention and control of illness and death of mothers and children was the most neglected of all public health services, Grace Abbott, director of the U.S. Children's Bureau, once commented.[11] Public responsibility for the securing of maternal and child health services in the U.S. lagged behind European initiatives. New York City in 1908 became the first governmental unit at any level to establish a division of child hygiene concerned solely with maternal and child health; ten years later, similar bureaus existed in only a handful of states.

The publication of mortality statistics by the U.S. Census Bureau in 1906 had first called attention to the prevailing high infant and maternal mortality. Over the next decade, health reformers interested in maternal and child welfare centered their efforts on the eradication of infant mortality. Services to childbearing mothers consisted primarily of limited, sporadic antepartum care for pregnant women, provided in an attempt to reduce the high infant death rate.

A 1917 report by Dr. Grace Meigs of the Children's Bureau, the first of its several studies of maternal mortality, was credited by several physicians with awakening the medical profession to an awareness of the severity of the problem of puerperal death.[12] The Meigs report characterized childbirth in the United States as suffering from an "unconscious neglect due to age-long ignorance and fatalism," and emphasized, assembling relevant statistics, that thousands of women died in childbirth from preventable causes.[13] The road to improvement, the report declared, was for women themselves to demand better care.

The passage of the Maternity and Infancy Act of 1921 (Sheppard-Towner Act), which marked the definite recognition of maternal mortality as a public health problem, was largely the work of a national woman's lobby. The legislation, drawn up by the Children's Bureau as a direct response to conditions revealed in its study of infant and maternal deaths, provided federal grants to states for fostering health services to mothers and children. The organization of state maternal and child health units followed. Thousands of prenatal and infant care programs initiated under these state divisions were developed.[14] While the Sheppard-Towner Act had little effect on maternal mortality rates before it lapsed in 1929, it aroused great public interest in maternity, enabling many women to learn what to ask and expect of their physicians, and alerting the medical profession to their demands.

By the 1920s, largely because of the impetus provided by the Sheppard-Towner program, prenatal care had become the favorite strategy of health reformers (though not of the medical profession generally) interested in maternal welfare.[15] But a minority of obstetricians, including the influential George Kosmak, editor of the *American Journal of Obstetrics and Gynecology*, began to question commonly held assumptions about the effectiveness of prenatal care in reducing maternal mortality.[16] They believed that while antepartum care helped diminish such accidents of pregnancy as toxemia, the leading cause of puerperal death — infection — occurred during and shortly after labor, and was more closely related to obstetric practice at these times than to the care of the expectant mother.

The definition of good obstetrics was, however, in contention. For many years, the untrained, poorly regulated midwife had borne the brunt of complaints about the low level of American obstetrics. Midwives delivered a significant proportion of American babies in 1915, approximately 40 percent nationwide (30 percent in New York City). In 1930, the nation's 47,000 midwives were responsible for 15 percent of births, though in some states, primarily in the South, they delivered 40–50 percent of babies.[17] Though they were required to register with local health departments in the majority of states, only a few states required licensing as a prerequisite for registration, and even these had minimum educational qualifications for licensure. Many unlicensed, unregistered midwives practiced without supervision of any kind. Educational opportunities for midwives were almost totally lacking: in the United States, there were only two schools, one in New York and one in Philadelphia, that trained midwives.[18]

According to widely held medical opinion, the use of incompetent midwives by low-income families was responsible for the high rates of maternal mortality. By the 1920s, however, the declining number of midwives in large cities threatened the easy correlation of puerperal mortality with their attendance. Moreover, the lowest mortality rates were frequently found in cities with the highest percentage of births attended by midwives.[19] In states where childbirth was completely in physician hands, like New Hampshire, Vermont, and Oregon, maternal death rates were as high as the national average.[20] Finally, maternal mortality was lower in all European countries (except Scotland) than in the United States, although at least one-half and usually more than 80 percent of births in these nations were attended by midwives, as compared to only 15 percent in the Unitded States (in 1930).[21]

Many medical observers considered the general practitioner the great danger in obstetrics.[22] According to this view, the G.P. took on obstetric work as a loss leader to acquire the medical practice of the patient's family, but gave it as little time and attention as possible because fees for obstetric cases were low. Hurried and under great pressure, the young practitioner would frequently resort to techniques he had little skill in performing in the interest of hastening labor. While it was usually agreed that general practitioners were suitable attendants for normal confinements, the absence of specified standards for obstetric specialization permitted them free access to more complicated cases of abnormal labor, despite their lack of training and experience. Furthermore, the G.P.'s constant contact with infectious diseases treated in his routine practice increased the chances of puerperal sepsis. "Obstetrics," it was said, "is the general practitioner's specialty."[23]

Part of the problem lay in the low status accorded to obstetrics among medical specialties. Obstetrics was considered the least appreciated branch — the "Cinderella" or "stepdaughter" — of medicine. Practitioners did not receive as complete a training in obstetrics as they did in medicine and surgery. Medical students were given at least twice and often five times as many hours in general surgery as in obstetrics, although most general practitioners spent twice as much time in obstetric care as surgery. Because childbirth had historically been seen as a natural function, the public at large thought the obstetrician's accomplishments less than those of his surgical colleagues in gynecology. Since females originally practiced it, obstetrics was conceived of as "hardly a man's job," which could apparently be mastered by inspiration after the observation of a small number of cases.[24] Even the leading figure in early 20th-century American obstetrics, J. Whitridge Williams of Johns Hopkins, annually apologized to medical students for the long association of his discipline with ignorant midwives.[25] That maternal mortality was lowest, however, in countries in which medical schools gave the longest and most complete undergraduate training in obstetrics did not fail to attract attention, and most reformers concluded that any improvement in obstetrics would have to follow curriculum revision directed toward securing more hours of obstetrical training.

The great increase in radical, or operative, obstetrics after 1915 appeared to be a primary cause of rising puerperal mortality, counterbalancing lives saved as the result of the introduction of asepsis and improved prenatal care. Forceps delivery, previously uncommon, was now practiced routinely for fetal as well as maternal indications. Caesarian sections, performed in the past only for definite indications like contracted pelvis and obstructed birth canal, had been extended to almost all complications of pregnancy and labor, including patient convenience. In many hospitals, one-quarter to one-half of all deliveries were performed by forceps, Caesarian sections, or version, a trend no doubt accelerated because surgical deliveries commanded fees twice those for spontaneous births. Economic factors also prevented the physician from spending time waiting for women to deliver spontaneously, another reason for the upsurge in surgical delivery. Experts believed, nevertheless, that 90–95 percent of all pregnancies were capable of being delivered by normal means. They pointed out that the lowest maternal death rates in the world were those of Holland, Sweden, and Denmark where at least 95 percent of births were spontaneous.[26]

The great increase in hospitalization of parturient women and the easy accessibility of anesthesia were cited as factors leading to increased, rather than decreased, maternal mortality, because they fostered surgical intervention. In the early 1930s, 56–85 percent of all live births in the ten largest U.S. cities took place in hospitals. Though hospitalization had advantages for the pregnant woman, it exposed her to infections and led, said some observers, to the "often false feeling of security of the operating room" and thus to unnecessary and dangerous operations.[27] The popularity of in-hospital surgical interventions, moreover, influenced the training of interns, so that while artificial deliveries were stressed, the importance of the physiology of labor and of conservative obstetrics was ignored.

The departure from the traditional "watchful expectancy" of obstetrics in favor of routine surgical delivery was based on a conception of labor as "decidedly pathologic" and the idea that the modern woman, a "neurasthenic product of civilization," stood suffering with less fortitude than her forebears, demanding anesthesia and even Caesarian section to escape its dangers and pains. The patient herself was regarded as a cause for the high puerperal death rates almost as frequently as were midwives and G.P.'s. Her self-indulgent demands for a quick and painless labor — a result, it was said, of modern life-styles, education, and magazine publicity — forced physicians against their will into a "reign of operative terror," where anesthesia inhibited the normal contractions of labor and made intervention imperative.[28] "American obstetrics," said one critic to a convention of the American Medical Association in 1936, "seems to be becoming a competitive practice to please American women in accordance with what they read in lay magazines."[29]

Although some women physicians supported the use of anesthesia to relieve childbirth suffering, they generally opposed routine surgical delivery. Many believed that the solution to the problem of maternal mortality lay in the assumption of obstetric practice by female doctors, who, they believed, were more sensitive to the needs of patients during childbirth, a position rigorously denied in the male-dominated discussion of maternal mortality. The superiority of female doctors in childbirth, they believed, was clearly indicated by the low maternal death rates of women's hospitals staffed by female physicians.[30]

Abortion and birth control, finally, were recognized as causes of increased maternal mortality. The desire to limit family size or to terminate growing numbers of unwanted out-of-wedlock pregnancies, some physicians claimed, resulted in large numbers of maternal deaths from intentional abortions, neutralizing gains made from improved obstetric practice.[31] Falling birth rates, furthermore, meant an increasing number of older primiparas who were less resistant to puerperal accidents, and hence, greater maternal mortality.[32] Birth control advocates, on the other hand, recognized that abortion deaths contributed to maternal mortality, but modified the argument. According to their view, the chief reason for the high death rates was the unwillingness of many women of impaired health or desperate economic circumstances to bear children, and their consequent resort to illegal abortion, frequently ending in death.[33]

II

New York City had long maintained a tradition of leadership in obstetrics and child welfare. The first effort to regulate midwife practice in the United States was undertaken in New York City in 1906; the following year, the first organized attempt to provide prenatal services to mothers began when the New York Association for Improving the Condition of the Poor engaged several nurses to visit mothers in tenement homes to instruct them in infant hygiene and "prevent infant deaths by caring for the mothers before the babies were born."[34] In 1908, the nation's first Bureau of Child Hygiene was established in the New York City Department of Health, and in 1911, the first school for midwives opened at Bellevue.

New York City had just begun to reorganize its system of maternal and obstetric care in 1915 following a study by a committee of New York physicians appointed by the then Health Commissioner, Dr. Haven Emerson, to analyze the conditions of childbirth in Manhattan, and their relation to the deaths of infants under one month of age. The committee, finding that many such deaths were caused by lack of prenatal care and poor care at the time of delivery, recommended that the city be divided into zones, in each of which would be established a maternity center where mothers could come for prenatal care. As a result of the study, the first maternity center in the United States was formed by the Women's City Club of New York in 1917, its work later taken over by the Maternity Center Association, founded the following year, which organized 30 prenatal clinics throughout the city. Later the association discontinued sponsorship of the prenatal clinics in favor of complete and intensive care for all phases of the maternity cycle at one model center. More than any other single agency, the Maternity Center Association developed and demonstrated a model for a community maternity service, and through its institutes for public health nurses and other educational work, stimulated other communities to establish similar services.[35]

Despite its superior health services and record of accomplishment in obstetrics and child health, New York City's puerperal death rate in 1930 was barely a percentage point lower than the national average. While the city's infant mortality rate had declined from 85.4 deaths per 1,000 live births in 1920 to 50.9 in 1933, its rate of maternal mortality had in fact increased from 5.33 per 1,000 live births in 1921 to 5.98 in 1932. The Public Health Relations Committee of the New York Academy of Medicine had been aware of the city's high puerperal death rate since 1917, when at the urging of Dr. George Kosmak, a subcommittee was appointed to gather data on maternal mortality in New York. When this study, based on hospital questionnaires, as well as a successive study which utilized Health Department statistics, failed to produce accurate results, a new plan to study the public health problems of obstetrics in New York was suggested by Drs. Kosmak and Ralph W. Lobenstine at the request of the Public Health Relations Committee. The committee then appointed a Subcommittee on Maternal Mortality, consisting of Dr. Frederic E. Sondern, chairman, and Drs. Philip Van Ingen, Benjamin P. Watson, and Ransom S. Hooker. The subcommittee decided to undertake a survey based on a direct, personal inquiry of puerperal deaths, to begin January 1, 1930, and continue for three years, running concurrently with the deaths. An Obstetrical Advisory Committee, chaired by Dr. Watson, and with Kosmak, John O. Polak, and Harry Aranow as members, was appointed. Ransom Hooker was chosen director of the study. The work of gathering and tabulating the material was performed by two women physicians, Dr. Marynia Farnham and Dr. Elizabeth Arnstein, and several registered nurses. Dr. Farnham, along with Kosmak, wrote much of the final report. The New York Obstetrical Society provided an initial loan, and the Commonwealth Fund provided funds for the completion of the study.[36]

Kosmak and Watson, both prominent New York obstetricians deeply concerned about the problem of maternal mortality, were active and influential members of the Obstetrical Advisory Committee. Kosmak was president, in 1930, of the New York Obstetrical Society, and in 1932, of the New York County Medical Society, and edited the *American Journal of Obstetrics and Gynecology*. His long-standing interest in the problem of maternal mortality was related to his vigorous, orthodox Catholic opposition to birth control and the belief that, to maintain the birth rate, pregnancy had to be made desirable through elimination of the fear of childbirth. A medical as well as social conservative, Kosmak questioned trends toward hospitalization of all confinements, routine surgical delivery and anesthesia, and the widespread promotion of prenatal care as the remedy for maternal mortality. After a 1927 trip to Scandinavia, which impressed him with the excellent results obtained from carefully supervised midwife practice, he retreated from his former antipathy to midwifery, and began to consider the trained midwife as a possible participant in a reformed system of obstetric care.[37]

Watson, Professor of Obstetrics and Gynecology at Columbia University, had trained in Scotland, taught and practised in Canada, and participated in a survey of maternal mortality in Scotland in 1925. His account of an outbreak of puerperal infection at Sloane Hospital in 1927 received national publicity, although it discomforted many in the profession. Like Kosmak, he espoused a conservative obstetrics, questioning the routine hospitalization of obstetric patients. However, he was more definitive in recommending a system of trained nurse-midwives as part of a professional hospital team to handle normal deliveries, a decidedly minority opinion in the medical profession.[38] A third member of the Advisory Committee, John O. Polak of the Long Island College Hospital, was an exponent of the value of home deliveries.

The methodology employed in the New York investigation was adopted from a Children's Bureau Study of maternal mortality in 15 states in 1927–1928 (published in 1933), the first thorough clinical study of large numbers of maternal deaths, and involved an analysis of individual case records supplemented by a personal interview with the attending physician. Each week during the period of the survey, the New York City Health Department forwarded to investigators copies of all death certificates which named a puerperal condition as primary or contributory, or which stated the existence of pregnancy. Within one month of each death, while circumstances were fresh in the minds of attendants, interviews were conducted with everyone who attended the patient at any time during pregnancy, delivery, or the puerperium. Investigators had access to all written hospital records.

The Obstetric Advisory Committee, in consultation with investigators, then examined each case to determine the true cause of death and whether the death was preventable, using as the criterion for an avoidable death whether the "best possible skill in diagnosis and treatment which the community could make available" had been applied. Responsibility for a preventable death was assigned either to the attendant — physician or midwife — or to the patient herself. If every possible precaution had been taken by the patient and attendant, and if the delivery had been properly carried out, the death was considered nonpreventable. Accounts of the quality of care were correlated to the patient's economic status, which was determined from housing data; and information on hospital procedures, standards and personnel was gathered by questionnaire.[39]

The benefit of clinical methodology was demonstrated by the finding that the usual reporting methods which relied on vital statistics routinely filed with departments of health resulted in a high margin of error, 17.8 percent. In the case of abortion, the disparity between the actual and reported cause of death was 34.7 percent, and for septicemia, 29.2 percent.[40]

The outstanding finding of the study was that in

the total series (2,041 deaths) nearly two-thirds (65.8 percent) of all deaths were judged to be preventable had the patient received proper care. By cause, 77.1 percent of deaths from induced abortions, 75.1 percent of deaths from septicemia, 76.1 percent of deaths from hemorrhage, and 87.1 percent of deaths following accidents of labor were considered avoidable. For all the preventable deaths, responsibility lay with the physician in 61.1 percent of cases, with the patient in 36.7 percent, and with midwives in only 2.2 percent. Following operative delivery, 76.8 percent of deaths were considered avoidable, a higher percentage than in the total series, with responsibility assigned to the physicians 86.8 percent of the time. Physician responsibility for preventable deaths was divided almost equally between faults of technique, 50.9 percent, and errors of judgment, 49.1 percent, suggesting a "surprisingly high degree of actual technical incompetence" and "a lack of respect for operative undertakings."[41]

By cause, the largest proportion of deaths (25.0 percent) was due to septicemia; next in importance were deaths from abortion (17.5 percent).[42] Almost half the deaths in the entire series (45 percent) had followed operative delivery. The mortality rate for operative delivery was found to be five times that for spontaneous delivery (10.5 to 2.0). Caesarian sections, although they represented only 2.2 percent of total deliveries in the series, constituted a remarkable 19.8 percent of total deaths (excluding deaths from abortions and extrauterine pregnancies).[43] Anesthesia was the direct cause of death in 20 cases, but was administered to 87.7 percent of patients whose death was attributed to operative shock. (Noting the close association between anesthesia and operative delivery, the report warned against the casual use of anesthesia for the "mere alleviation or the entire elimination of pain."[44])

For hospital deliveries, the death rate was more than two times that for deliveries in homes (4.5 to 1.9), where about 30 percent of all births took place, leading the committee to suggest a reexamination of attitudes toward home confinement.[45] There was no difference in the result of home deliveries by physicians or by midwives, even though only one-third of the midwives interviewed were found to be truly competent. The death rate for deliveries by midwives who had contact with 5.4 percent of patients in the series was, at 1.6 per 1,000 live births, 64 percent lower than the general series rate of 4.5 per 1,000 live births.[46]

Data on hospital practice throughout the city, collected by questionnaire, showed that the proportion of preventable deaths was significantly lower in municipal (34.2 percent) than in either voluntary (49.1 percent) or obstetric (51.4 percent) hospitals, a finding the committee attributed to the fact that the percentage of Caesarian sections performed in municipal hospitals was less than one-half that in obstetric hospitals and little more than one-half that for voluntary hospitals. The report concluded that no adequate control of voluntary or proprietary hospitals was maintained in the city.[47]

Finally, the risk of death in pregnancy was found to be highly correlated with economic status, race, and nativity. The highest puerperal death rate was found among the least-favored group, the lowest among the most privileged, although the white-collar class showed a higher rate than the less well-off artisan group, which relied on free care provided by municipal and voluntary hospitals.[48] For Negro women and foreign-born women, the data, however disturbing, followed customary curves: the death rate for black women was twice as great as for white women; the rate for foreign-born women from all puerperal causes greatly exceeded that for native-born women.[49]

From these statistical findings, the committee concluded that the death rate of women in childbirth in New York was unnecessarily high because of the following reasons: (1) *Inadequate and improper prenatal care.* In almost 60 percent of the cases examined, the patient failed to seek prenatal care, and where it was sought, the attendant frequently failed to provide it. (2) *High incidence of operative interference during labor.* Frequently operations were performed for the wrong indications, at improper times, and without an appropriately trained attendant. (3) *The attendants' incapacity in judgment or skill.* Here, errors included the failure to provide proper prenatal care, frequently incorrect prognosis and improper conduct of delivery, the lack of consultation, and the failure to maintain proper asepsis. (4) *Inadequate hospital standards.* These included improper physical equipment;

lack of appropriate labor and delivery facilities; failure to carry out isolation; use of operating rooms as delivery rooms; the performance of major operative procedures by unsupervised residents or junior members of attending staffs without consultation with chiefs; the failure of many proprietary hospitals to exercise staff supervision. (5) *Midwife incompetence.* The training of midwives, many of them elderly, illiterate, foreign-born women, was frequently insufficient, and there was no attempt to evaluate qualifications for licensure.[50]

The committee's recommendations for changes in methods of obstetric practice included: education for the public as to the necessity of prenatal care, the dangers of operative delivery, and the relative safety of home delivery, with the more active participation by physician organizations in lay education through press, radio, and publications; improved training of medical students, including prolonged graduate study for specialization, and of hospital internes; the confinement of nonspecialist practitioners to normal cases, requiring frequent and early consultations with highly trained specialists; improved hospital facilities and supervision of staff, including stricter control of proprietary hospitals, the appointment of qualified obstetricians as staff directors, the maintenance of separate obstetric delivery rooms, the observation of rules for asepsis, especially masking, and stringent isolation; and finally, improved training and supervision of better qualified midwives.[51]

While the committee had found many midwives poorly trained, it concluded that, since the results of their practice were as good as those obtained by physicians under comparable circumstances, the midwife was an "acceptable attendant for properly selected cases of labor and delivery" and should have a position in any scheme for providing for maternity care. "In face of the pressing problem of assuring proper care for all women at an outlay that is not prohibitive," it reported, "she has proven her value." The medical profession must accept the midwife as "one of its adjuncts," an "ally" in reducing childbirth morbidity and mortality. "There must be a readiness to cooperate with her."[52]

The report left no doubt as to the major source of the high puerperal death rate:

> Sixty percent of all deaths which could have been avoided have been brought about by some incapacity in the attendant. . . . Most are plainly the results of incompetence. Prevention in this field will mean increasing the respect of the physician for the gravity of obstetrical operations and educating him to a greater caution in attacking problems which are properly the field only of the highly trained obstetrician. . . . .
>
> The hazards of childbirth in New York City are greater than they need be. Responsibility for reducing them rests with the medical profession.[53]

Despite its greater detail and more elaborate methodology, the conclusions of the New York study were similar to those of recent surveys elsewhere in the United States and abroad. Studies of maternal deaths in Britain and Scotland, a study of puerperal mortality in Massachusetts and one in Cleveland, the 15-state Children's Bureau study and reports presented to the White House Conference on Child Health and Protection called by President Hoover pointed to the conclusion that maternal mortality was preventable, and was related to such factors as lack of prenatal care, operative interference by incompetent attendants, inadequate and improperly supervised institutional facilities, poorly trained, unregulated midwives, as well as contributing negligence of patients and their families.[54] The remedies, too, were similar: education, standards, and obstetrical restraint. What distinguished the academy report from other studies were: a precise and detailed clinical methodology which provided indisputable evidence about preventability; the undisguised attribution of blame for preventable deaths to the medical profession; and an acceptance of trained midwives and home delivery in normal obstetrical cases, contrary to general medical opinion. Most important, the academy deliberately and effectively publicized its findings through an unusual media release that was designed to attract attention and precipitate controversy within the medical profession.

The report received wide medical and lay attention. Before the report, published by the Commonwealth Fund in November 1933, was reviewed in any medical journal, the Medical Information

Bureau of the academy released to the lay press a carefully worded summary of it entitled, *Why Women Die in Childbirth.*[55] The findings, especially the responsibility assigned to physicians for many preventable deaths, were given prominent attention in more than 300 newspapers in 30 states. "When a doctor attacks another doctor," the *Nation* editorialized, "it is time for the general public to take notice."[56]

Despite the committee's matter-of-fact approach, the assignment of responsibility to the medical community was controversial. The New York Obstetrical Society, an original sponsor of the study, filed a formal complaint with the academy, whose council had approved the committee report by a unanimous vote, protesting this publicity.[57] The medical societies of Queens, Bronx, and Albany counties also protested the method of publicity.[58] Many physicians, as was customary when the profession was embarrassed, suggested sinister motives.

A subcommittee of the academy's Public Health Relations Committee, composed of two former academy presidents, Dr. S. W. Lambert and Dr. J. S. Hartwell, was appointed to report on the press release and the Obstetrical Society's protest against it. The committee concluded that the abstract had been released by the Medical Information Bureau in accordance with academy bylaws, and that much criticism of the method of publicity arose from the decision to postpone reviewing the report in the medical press until after publication of the book and lay articles about it. It found that the release did provide an accurate summary of the report's findings, and that its much-criticized caption, *Why Women Die in Childbirth*, described the study appropriately. The committee defended the deliberate publicity, concluding that the saving of even one mother's life was more important than medical prestige. Unfavorable criticism arose, the academy spokesmen declared, from the "startling nature of the facts" themselves, which provoked fear that the revelations would do harm to physicians. Minimizing the seriousness of the situation would, they countered, open the profession to the charge of shielding itself from attack.[59]

The Obstetrical Society counterattacked, appointing its own committee to report on the academy abstract. While the target ostensibly was the manner of publicity, in fact the society committee attacked the major interpretations of the report itself. It argued, first, that preventability was an imprecise concept (the obstetricians preferred the term "controllable"), which might result in unfair lawsuits for malpractice. Secondly, it argued that the report distorted the facts in assigning midwives only 2.2 percent of preventable deaths, since midwives attended a small proportion of deliveries out of the total series. (The true percentage of preventable mortality, it suggested, was 75 percent in midwife-attended cases compared to 68 percent for the physician group.) Licensing any additional midwives was opposed, for as long as the midwife was permitted to practice, "obstetrics will never be elevated to the position it rightly deserves." Home delivery, furthermore, was not safer than delivery in well-organized hospitals. Surgical interventions then performed under proper indications by skilled personnel were "merciful" and "life-saving." Caesarian section was one of the "greatest blessings" to modern women. Proper administration of anesthesia was "essential," "valuable," and "humane."[60]

At its April meeting, the Obstetrical Society endorsed the committee's report, and authorized its immediate release to the lay press in an abstract titled *How Childbirth May Be Made Safe.*[61] Dr. Benjamin Watson, chairman of the Obstetrical Advisory Committee to the academy study, promptly resigned his office as first vice-president of the Obstetrical Society in protest.[62] Kosmak also resigned from the society's council, and refused to publish either the society's transactions concerning the academy study, or its abstract, in the *American Journal of Obstetrics and Gynecology.* The issue was purely a local one, he wrote the society's secretary, for which there would be no national audience.[63]

The academy strategy of maximum publicity achieved the intended political effect. Medical associations in cooperation with the Health Department acted with unaccustomed speed to eliminate obstetric mismanagement and carry out the recommendations of the report. The New York Obstetrical Society offered the services of its newly formed Maternal Advisory Committee to the city Health Commissioner, and most of the county medical societies appointed their own subcommittees on maternal welfare.[64] An Advisory Obstetric Council to the Departments of Health and Hospitals, with Kosmak as general secretary, was appointed to make a citywide survey of obstetric facilities, methods and personnel, and submit recommendations. As a consultant to the Bureau of Child Hygiene, Kosmak also assisted in the development of a prenatal program for the city.[65] By 1938, Dr. Watson, who had resigned as vice-president of the Obstetrical Society during the controversy, became its president.

Several months after the report was published, Kosmak presented the political analysis which justified the deliberate publicity to a meeting of the Obstetrical Society itself.[66] The failures revealed by the study, "were the shortcomings of medical men" which could be corrected only by the profession. The report did not threaten the 70 obstetric specialists who were society members, but rather, the 4,000 practitioners of medicine in New York who necessarily performed the bulk of its obstetrics. The most important task in correcting the situation was to restrict the G.P. The society should therefore present a united front in support of the academy report, and not allow its criticisms of it to be used by G.P.'s against it. As for the midwife, "like it or not" she was "an institution and we simply must make the best of it and must provide for improvement" until a substitute could be found. Trained midwives, Kosmak asserted, were superior in skills and ability to the student nurses to whom hurried doctors regularly entrusted the care of their hospitalized maternity patients.

Some weeks later, Kosmak addressed a special meeting called by the New York Academy of Medicine to discuss "the constructive aspects" of its report.[67] He spoke of the problem of the general practitioner and of the poorly supervised interne and junior staff member, who, because of the absence of standards, "could do things in obstetrics which he would not be tempted to do in other fields of medicine." Kosmak admitted that the imposition of restraints through "self-imposed regulations" of medical agencies might be interpreted as "interference with the legal rights of a licensed physician" but he believed such action would do much to reestablish public confidence and "thus react favorably rather than otherwise" on medical practice.

Kosmak endeavored to enlist wide community and lay support of mortality review in the belief that the securing of a safe motherhood was a collective responsibility to be carried out at the local level. The strategy of maximum exposure undertaken by the academy to publicize its report reflected this view. Physicians were to provide leadership through the establishment of committees to survey and evaluate local data, Kosmak explained, but a wide segment of the community — nurses' groups, women's clubs, and allied professions and agencies — had to be actively engaged in order to act upon the data. Only through intense community involvement ("community control," as Kosmak phrased it) could the tide of maternal mortality be reversed and an "obstetric conscience" created. Self-regulation at the local level, furthermore, could prevent the introduction of some degree of federal control of medical practice, a possibility which Kosmak, a staunch opponent of state intervention in medicine, greatly feared.[68]

The methods expounded by Kosmak produced successful results in a short period of time. Maternal mortality in New York City declined by 45 percent in the five years following publication of the report.[69] While several factors may have contributed to the reduction, New York City's positive experience helped establish mortality review as an important preventive tool in curbing puerperal death.

III

The analysis of maternal deaths proceeded in several other cities, where, as in New York, initial studies led to the establishment of permanent committees mandated to conduct continuous reviews of obstetric practice. The results of the New York study were publicized extensively by agencies like the Maternity Center Association of New York. Many cities and counties began to study their maternal deaths and to formulate inclusive plans for the care of mothers and babies. Along with the New York model, Philadelphia's maternal mortality committee became a prototype for a mortality review mechanism widely adopted across the country. In 1930, the Philadelphia County Medical Society appointed a maternal welfare committee, under the chairmanship of Dr. Philip Williams, to investigate obstetric conditions in the city. Patterning its three-year survey directly after the New York Academy study in an attempt to determine causes of death, whether preventable, and where responsibility lay, its conclusion — that the major blame for the city's high death rate rested primarily with the medical profession, with midwives a negligible factor — repeated the New York findings.[70]

After the completion of the study, the Philadelphia committee decided to continue its analysis of maternal deaths through a cooperative program developed between hospital obstetric staffs and the County Medical Society. The committee expanded its membership to include representatives from maternity departments of all Philadelphia hospitals as well as interns, residents, social workers, and other interested parties. Under Dr. Williams' guidance, and without fear of malpractice suits, maternal deaths were carefully analyzed in an "open monthly forum" to assess responsibility for blame.

The monthly seminars revealed the practice of "much bad obstetrics," according to Dr. Williams, and corrective measures, particularly to prevent unnecessary obstetric surgery by unqualified staff, were taken. Hospitals accepted new rules specifying obligatory consultations before Caesarian section as well as techniques in labor, delivery room, and nursery, and redefined staff privileges.[71]

As a result of the monthly review meetings, an "obstetric conscience" was created in Philadelphia. An excellent description of how the committee achieved this result was provided by Dr. Thaddeus Montgomery, a participant in the Philadelphia committee. "At first," he wrote,

> no very noticeable effect upon maternal mortality was observed, but as the years passed and the activities of the Committee became more widely recognized, a subtle change of attitude took place. Hospital staffs became zealous in the analysis of their own obstetric fatalities. . . . The occurrence of a maternal death became a calamity to be carefully studied by the institution in which it occurred. . . . Gradually physicians began to feel that in the conduct of obstetric delivery they were not free agents to act as they would, but that the medical opinion of the city was looking over their shoulders to see that they gave to each patient the best that modern obstetric practice had to offer. Consultation in different situations was expected, and "acrobatic" obstetrics became taboo — no longer to be tolerated.[72]

The work of this committee resulted in a dramatic decline in maternal deaths, a result which Williams believed preceded improvement caused by the widespread use of antibiotics, sulfa drugs, and blood banks. From 1931 to 1940, the rate of maternal mortality in Philadelphia dropped by almost two-thirds (from 68 per 10,000 live births to 23).[73] So highly successful was its work, in fact, that the Obstetrical Society established similar mortality review committees to investigate problems of stillbirths, fetal deaths, and premature births, where further problems of obstetric mismanagement had been revealed. Similar gains took place in other large cities, and in fact, throughout the United States as a whole, although it seemed that the rate of maternal mortality decreased more quickly and substantially in states like New York, Pennsylvania, Connecticut, Rhode Island, and New Jersey, where cooperation and self-criticism reached its peak.

By the end of the 30s, many more maternal mortality review committees had been formed by state and county medical societies in cooperation with hospitals and health departments. Their establishment stimulated healthy rivalry among communities jealous of their progress in the field, each vying with the others to show lower mortality figures from year to year. Following the procedure developed in New York and Philadelphia, each maternal death was carefully studied and analyzed, in open meetings, to determine how the death might have been prevented and who was at fault. The process deterred unnecessary and dangerous procedures by unqualified attendants, and by case discussion reinforced the need for expert obstetric consultation when problems arose. Descendants of these committees, in most states and many local areas, are today major participants in peer review in cases of maternal mortality and morbidity.[74]

IV

The establishment of maternal mortality review committees was one aspect of a vast expansion in maternal welfare work that took place in the 1930s. By the end of the decade, many communities had active maternal welfare agencies engaged in a wide variety of educational, preventive, and regulatory work, including mortality review. Many experts correlated the rapid reduction of maternal mortality after 1935 with these activities.[75] Our data suggest, however, that cause and effect are more complicated.

After remaining stationary for so many decades, the puerperal death rate had begun to fall in the early 30s, though rather slowly. After 1936, the decline accelerated. From 1930 to 1936, the United States maternal mortality rate fell 15 percent (from 6.7 to 5.7 per 1,000 live births), or approximately 3 percent a year. In the years 1936–1938, the rates fell 12 percent annually (from 5.7 to 4.2). The comparative rate of decrease was 14 percent in the years 1930–1935, 35 percent in 1935–1940, and in the 1940s, 74 percent.[76]

During the decade after 1933, when the New York Academy's report was published, the maternal death rate in the United States declined by 60 percent, almost double the rate of reduction for infant mortality, which decreased 31 percent.[77] The decline in maternal mortality rates, moreover, was not paralleled by decreases in rates of other important causes of death. By 1949, the maternal mortality rate for the entire United States was less than one maternal death per 1,000 live births, comparing favorably with the lowest rates obtainable abroad. The change had occurred in every part of the country — in 1949, even the highest state rate (2.4) was about one-half the lowest rate in 1933 (4.3 per 1,000 live births) — and had affected rates from every cause of puerperal mortality.[78] Maternity mortality was no longer a serious nationwide problem, even if rates remained relatively high in particular areas.

Although the decline in maternal mortality rates in the 1930s appears to have been most dramatic in places like New York and Philadelphia where the greatest medical and civic activity to control obstetric practice occurred, the reduction in maternal mortality in the United States was so widespread that it cannot be comfortably accounted for by increased maternal welfare services and improved obstetric care alone. Moreover, maternal mortality rates fell sharply in the same period of time throughout the world. Beginning about 1936, maternal mortality dropped sharply in the United States, Switzerland, the Union of South Africa, Mexico, Scotland, New Zealand, the Irish Free State, Australia, Canada, England, and Wales. Within seven to eight years, the rate had been reduced by half in many of these nations.[79]

There is at present no satisfactory explanation for the change occurring with such apparent uniformity among countries so obviously disparate, and with such varying levels of medical care and services.[80] For the United States, several contributory causes can be suggested.

Advances in medical knowledge and techniques were of major importance, particularly the development and use, after 1933, of antibiotics, sulfonamides, and blood and blood substitutes. The beginning of the sharpest declines in maternal mortality rates coincided with the wider adoption of these measures, although rates had started to fall even earlier. Furthermore, the reduction in puerperal mortality was not limited to deaths due to infection and to hemorrhage, shock, and trauma, those causes most affected by use of the new drugs and blood substitutes.

Better training and the institutionalization of obstetrics as a specialty improved obstetric practice. Beginning in 1930, when the American Board of Obstetrics and Gynecology was established, there was a considerable expansion of educational and training programs in obstetrics for general practitioners and explicit standards for certification of specialists. Other notable educational efforts were those of the American Committee on Maternal Welfare, and in midwifery, the Maternity Center Association of New York, and the Frontier Nursing Service in Kentucky.

Improved hospital facilities for obstetric care governed by published and increasingly well-enforced standards and an expansion of prenatal services reduced the risks of puerperal death. Minimum standards established by the American College of Surgeons and by the American Hospital Association helped promote better hospital regulations for asepsis, stricter supervision of house staff, and the isolation of obstetric departments. Hospitalization for confinement increased more than 100 percent in the ten years after 1933 (from approximately 35 percent to 72 percent of all births), and for the first time was not associated with higher rates of puerperal death. Expansion of prenatal care facilities, aided by funds provided in the Social Security Act of 1935, helped create improved antepartum services throughout the country.

Increased public awareness of pregnancy and

childbirth also helped foster a safer maternity. During the 1930s, long-standing taboos against public discussion of pregnancy and childbirth were broken. The Maternity Center Association's national campaign of public information played a crucial role in this development: it conducted institutes for 15,000 public health nurses throughout the United States on pregnancy and childbirth, and sponsored exhibits at the Chicago and New York World Fairs which were seen by hundreds of thousands. The landmark film "Birth of a Baby," produced under the auspices of the American Committee on Maternal Health, was widely shown. The educational work of thousands of local health departments also helped foster a greater knowledge of the need for adequate prenatal, intranatal, and postnatal care for mothers.

Although it is impossible to measure their comparative contributions with any degree of precision, all of these factors played some role in reducing the high level of maternal deaths to a fraction of their previous toll. A major econometric study of maternal mortality conducted in 1950 concluded that for the first time in history a large nation like the United States had pushed its puerperal death rate slightly under the apparently irreducible minimum of one maternal death per 1,000 live births. Seeking an explanation for this finding, the authors compared maternal deaths by cause in 1933 and 1948, assigning three major reasons for the decline — better prenatal care, introduction of antibiotics and other drugs, and improved medical care of pregnant women (intra- and post-natal), involving more adequate physician training and skills. The reduction in mortality rates, they concluded, indicated that the "improved training and the increased skill of the physician are by far the most important factors."[81] Improved physician ability, which affected all classes of puerperal death, each of which had shown reduction, was thus the key variable in the decline of puerperal mortality.

Better training and physician skills were, to an extent which is unfortunately unmeasurable, effected by education and peer review. Many leading physicians were persuaded that maternal mortality review played a major role in improving physician skill and maintaining accountability during these years. One participant, in a comment typical of many others, observed that he "learned more obstetrics by sitting on the Maternal Welfare Committee in Chicago" than in all his other efforts in 40 years of medicine.[82] Dr. Philip Williams of Philadelphia also commented on the efficacy of continuing year-round obstetric mortality review, as opposed, for example, to institutes and seminars conducted by county medical societies, as a method of extramural graduate education for local physicians and general practitioners.[83]

V

Much of the credit for institutionalizing the review committee as a self-regulatory device goes to the landmark report of the New York Academy of Medicine, whose competent and thorough fact-finding served as an indictment and challenge to physicians, stimulated other investigations across the nation, and demonstrated a viable strategy for self-regulation within the profession.[84]

While the academy report succeeded in providing a mechanism for reform and regulation in obstetrics, its own prescriptions for the direction of change were largely avoided. Although conservatism in obstetrics was a by-product of the report and the many maternal mortality reviews it engendered, the Committee's cautious endorsement of a maternity scheme based on home confinements of normal pregnancies under the care of trained midwives as well as physicians became almost immediately irrelevant. In the five years after publication of the report, hospitalization of maternity patients in New York City increased by 30 percent to 91 percent of all births. Accompanying this change was a decline in the number of midwives in the city from 863 to 280, and a decrease in midwife-attended births from 10 percent in 1933 to 2 percent in 1938, a product of stricter regulation by the Department of Health and the closing of the Bellevue School of Midwifery.[85] Similar changes were taking place on the national level.[86]

The possibility of a basic shift towards a system based on the assumption that birth was not pathologic no longer existed. The 1930s represented a transition period in American obstetrics. By the end of the decade, childbirth had been made safer, but it had advanced irrevocably toward a technological focus. Potentially dangerous medical and surgical practices continued, today affecting infants more often than mothers, though under conditions of greater physician accountability. The New York Academy of Medicine's report on maternal mortality marked a point in time when another option seemed available. The immediate problem — the waste of women's lives in childbirth — was solved. The underlying issue remained.

NOTES

Presented to the 50th anniversary meeting of the American Association for the History of Medicine, Philadelphia, Pennsylvania, May 2, 1975.

1 Josephine Baker, "Maternal mortality in the United States," *J.A.M.A.*, 1927, *89*: 2016.

2 Society of the Lying-In Hospital of the City of New York, *Maternity: An Educational Survey of a National Problem* (New York, 1923), p. 6.

3 *Ibid.*

4 The urban rate, moreover, was consistently higher than the rural, not being less than 64 since 1915, or less than 70 since 1917, with a peak of 96 in 1918 and a rate of 74 in 1932. For nonwhite women, maternal mortality in 1915 was 106. In 1932 it was 98, the only year in which the 1915 rate improved. Fred L. Adair, "Maternal, fetal and neonatal morbidity and mortality," *Am. J. Obst. & Gynec.*, 1935, *29*: 389.

5 Robert M. Woodbury, "Infant mortality in the United States," *Ann. Am. Acad. Polit. & Soc. Sci.*, 1936, *188*: 96.

6 In infant mortality, however, the U.S. ranked seventh, both in 1919–1921, with a rate of 82.3, and in 1929–1931, with rate of 64.6. Jacob Yerushalmy, "Infant and maternal mortality in the modern world," *Ann. Am. Acad. Polit. & Soc. Sci.*, 1945, *237*: 134–141.

7 Elizabeth C. Tandy, *Comparability of Maternal Mortality Rates in the United States and Certain Foreign Countries*, U.S. Children's Bureau Pub. 229 (Washington, D.C.: Government Printing Office, 1935).

8 See, for example, White House Conference on Child Health and Protection, *Obstetric Education* (New York: The Century Co., 1932), p. 49.

9 Significant works on maternal mortality during this period include Grace L. Meigs, *Maternal Mortality — from All Conditions Connected with Childbirth in the United States and Certain Other Countries*, U.S. Children's Bureau Pub. 19 (Washington, D.C.: Government Printing Office, 1917); George Clark Mosher, "Maternity morbidity and mortality in the United States," *Am. J. Obst. & Gynec.*, 1924, 7: 294–298, discussion, 326–330; Austin Flint, "Responsibility of the medical profession in further reducing maternal mortality," *Am. J. Obst. & Gynec.*, 1925, *9*: 864–866; Susan Coffin et al., "Maternal mortality in Massachusetts," *J.A.M.A.*, 1926, *86*: 408–413; Robert Morse Woodbury, *Maternal Mortality: The Risk of Death in Childbirth and from All Diseases Caused by Pregnancy and Confinement*, U.S. Children's Bureau Pub. 158 (Washington, D.C.: Government Printing Office, 1926); Lee K. Frankel, "The present status of maternal and infant hygiene in the United States," *Am. J. Public Hlth.*, 1927, *12*: 1209–1217, discussion, pp. 1217–1220; Henry Jellett, *The Causes and Prevention of Maternal Mortality* (London: J. & A. Churchill, 1929); J. V. De Porte, *Maternal Mortality and Stillbirths in New York State, 1915–1925* (Albany: New York State Department of Health, 1928); Matthias Nicoll, Jr., "Maternity as a public health problem," *Am. J. Public Hlth.*, 1929, *19*: 961–968; Louis I. Dublin, "Mortality among women from causes incidental to childbearing," *Am. J. Obst. & Dis. Women & Children*, 1918, *78*: 20–37; "The risks of childbirth," *Forum*, 1932, *87*: 250–284; White House Conference on Child Health and Protection, *Fetal, Newborn and Maternal Morbidity and Mortality* (New York: D. Appleton-Century Co., 1933); Edward S. Brackett, "Observations on the problem of maternal mortality," *New Eng. J. Med.*, 1934, *210*: 845–51.

10 On the development of maternal and child health services in the United States, see John Blake, *Origins of Maternal and Child Health Programs* (New Haven: Department of Public Health, Yale Univ. School of Medicine, 1953); and William M. Schmidt, "The development of health services for mothers and children in the United States," *Am. J. Public Hlth.*, 1973, *63*: 419–427.

11 Cited in George Clark Mosher, "The problem of mother and child," *Med. Woman's J.*, 1927, *34*: 217.

12 See, for example, Robert de Normandie, "Medical men and maternal mortality," *Woman Citizen*, December 1926, pp. 20–22.

13 Meigs, *Maternal Mortality*, p. 5.

14 For a representative description of maternity education programs established during the Sheppard-Towner period, see Florence McKay, "What New York State is doing to reduce maternal mortality," *Am. J. Obst. & Gynec.*, 1925, *9*: 704–708. Also see J. Stanley Lemons, "The Sheppard-Towner Act: progressivism in the 1920s," *J. Am. Hist.*, 1969, *55*: 776–786.

15 The importance of prenatal care as a factor in maternal health was established in a landmark study by John Whitridge Williams of Johns Hopkins in 1915

(J. Whitridge Williams, "The limitations and possibilities of prenatal care," *J.A.M.A.*, 1915, *64*: 95–101). Williams understood, as many of his contemporaries did not, the close connection between prenatal care and good obstetric care in hospital settings.

16 Kosmak testified before the Committee on Interstate and Foreign Commerce of the 70th Congress that Sheppard-Towner activities concentrated unnecessarily on prenatal care. See Nicoll, "Maternity as a public health problem," p. 965. This view was confirmed some years later in a clinical study conducted at Yale University Medical School under the auspices of the American Public Health Association. The study concluded that "quality of delivery service is probably a greater factor than any other, including prenatal care, in the improvement of the outcome of maternity and the lessening of maternal mortality." See Margaret Tyler, J. H. Watkins, and H. H. Walker, *Report on the Evaluation of Prenatal Care* (New Haven: Institute of Human Relations, Yale Univ. School of Medicine, 1934).

17 Palmer Findley, *The Story of Childbirth* (Garden City, N.Y.: Doubleday Doran, 1933), p. 127, and *Obstetric Education*, p. 204.

18 Woodbury, *Maternal Mortality*, p. 78.

19 Dr. Julius Levy of New Jersey's Bureau of Child Hygiene showed for example that, in 1921, four of the largest cities, Newark, New York, Baltimore, and Cleveland, each with more than 25 percent of births attended by midwives, had lower rates of maternal mortality than Boston, with a highly organized medical system, a well-educated general public, and only 2.5 percent of births delivered by midwives. Julius Levy, "Maternal mortality and mortality in the first month of life in relation to attendant at birth," *Am. J. Public Hlth.*, 1923, *13*: 89.

20 Baker, "Maternal mortality in the U.S.," p. 2017.

21 *Obstetric Education*, p. 96. European midwives, however, particularly in the Scandinavian countries, received lengthy and intensive training in obstetrics.

22 See, for example, comments by Drs. Davis, Speidel, Polak, and Lanford, in Mosher, "Maternal morbidity and mortality," pp. 295, 326; Dublin, "The risks of childbirth," p. 281; and Findley, *The Story of Childbirth*, p. 325.

23 George Gray Ward, "Our obstetric and gynecologic responsibilities," *J.A.M.A.*, 1926, *87*: 1.

24 On the status of obstetrics, see B. P. Watson, "Can our methods of obstetric practice be improved?" *Bull. N.Y. Acad. Med.*, 1930, *6*: 647–663; Mosher, "Maternal morbidity and mortality," pp. 295–296; and Nicoll, "Maternity as a public health problem," p. 966.

25 *Dr. Williams' Obstetrics, 1897–1898*; Rufus I. Cole MSS (Health Sciences Library, State University of New York at Stony Brook).

26 See the report of E. D. Plass, "Forceps and Cesarean section," in *Fetal, Newborn, and Maternal Morbidity and Mortality*, pp. 215–247. Also see J. Whitridge Williams, "A criticism of certain tendencies in American obstetrics," *N.Y. St. J. Med.*, 1922, *22*: 493–499; Rudolf W. Holmes, "The fads and fancies of obstetrics: a comment on the pseudoscientific trend of modern obstetrics," *Am. J. Obst. & Gynec.*, 1921, *2*: 225–237, and discussion, pp. 297–397; Ward, "Our obstetric and gynecologic responsibilities," pp. 1–3; Watson, "Can our methods of obstetric practice be improved?" p. 655; and Flint, "Responsibility of the medical profession on further reducing maternal mortality," p. 866.

27 *Obstetric Education*, p. 18.

28 Examples of this attitude are found in Joseph de Lee, "Obstetrics vs. midwifery," *J.A.M.A.*, 1934, *103*: 308; Findley, *Story of Childbirth*, pp. 53–54, 196–197; George Clark Mosher, "Ten years of painless childbirth," *Am. J. Obst. & Gynec.*, 1932, *3*: 142–143. Also see the comments of Dr. Ray Lyman Wilbur, quoted in Helene Huntington Smith, "The case for anesthesia," *Delineator*, 1932, *125*: 50.

29 The critic was Dr. Buford Garvin, cited in "Pains of childbirth," *Time*, May 25, 1936, 36.

30 See, for example, the statement of Dr. Bertha Van Hoosen, head of the Department of Obstetrics at Loyola University, quoted in Rosine Wistein, "Maternal mortality: a comparative study," *Med. Woman's J.*, 1932, *39*: 29, and "Maternal mortality" (editorial), *ibid.*, p. 66. On the low puerperal death rates of women's hospitals, see Maude Glasgow, *The Subjection of Woman and the Traditions of Men* (New York: Maude Glasgow, 1940), 232–233.

31 Adair, "Maternal, fetal, and neonatal morbidity and mortality," p. 387.

32 "Maternal mortality," *Med. Times & Long Island Med. J.*, May 1934, 157.

33 Lydia Allen de Vilbiss, "A proposed method for reducing the maternal mortality rate," *Med. J. & Rec.*, 1930, *132*: 391–392; and Helen Miller, "Contraception as a means of conserving maternal health," *Birth Control Rev.*, 1929, *13*: 281–282.

34 Iago Galdston, *Maternal Deaths — the Ways to Prevention* (New York: The Commonwealth Fund, 1937), p. 7.

35 Maternity Center Association, *Annual Report, April 1918–Dec. 31, 1921* (New York, 1921), pp. 13, 20–21, 24; *45th Annual Report & Log 1915–1963 of the Maternity Center Association* (New York, 1964), *11*: 1–7.

36 New York Academy of Medicine, Committee on Public Health Relations, *Maternal Mortality in New*

York City: A Study of All Puerperal Deaths, 1930–1932 (New York: The Commonwealth Fund, 1933), pp. ix–xii. Dr. Polak died while the study was in progress, and was replaced by Dr. Charles A. Gordon.

37 George W. Kosmak, "Sensible standards for proper obstetric care," *J. Med. Soc. N.J.*, 1930, *27*: 331–335; "Results of supervised midwife practice in certain European countries," *J.A.M.A.*, 1927, *89*: 2009–2012; "Community responsibilities for safeguarding motherhood," *Public Health & Nursing*, 1932, *26*: 292–299; B. P. Watson, "In memoriam: George William Kosmak," *Tr. Am. Gynec. Soc.*, 1955, *78*: 233–234; and Howard C. Taylor, Jr., "Memorial for Dr. George W. Kosmak," New York Obstetrical Society MSS (New York Academy of Medicine). Collection hereafter referred to as N.Y.O.S. MSS.

38 Watson, "Can our method of obstetric practice be improved?" pp. 656–663.

39 On methodology, see N.Y.A.M., *Maternal Mortality in New York City*, pp. 11–13.

40 *Ibid.*, p. 17.

41 *Ibid.*, p. 32–38.

42 *Ibid.*, p. 54, and Ransom S. Hooker, "Maternal mortality in New York," *The Health Examiner*, 1933, *3*: 13.

43 N.Y.A.M., *Maternal Mortality in New York City*, pp. 126, 130, 137.

44 *Ibid.*, pp. 115–116.

45 *Ibid.*, pp. 139–140.

46 *Ibid.*, pp. 195–198.

47 *Ibid.*, pp. 181–182.

48 *Ibid.*, pp. 151–152.

49 *Ibid.*, pp. 163–167. Caesarian section as a cause of death, however, was more frequent among white women (20.5 percent), than Negro women (14.7 percent). *Ibid.*, p. 131.

50 *Ibid.*, pp. 213–216.

51 *Ibid.*, pp. 216–221.

52 *Ibid.*, pp. 209–212.

53 *Ibid.*, pp. 49, 222.

54 See U.S. Department of Labor, Children's Bureau Pub. 223, *Maternal Mortality in Fifteen States* (Washington, D.C.: Government Printing Office, 1934); Robert Bolt, "Maternal mortality study for Cleveland, Ohio," *Am. J. Obst. & Gynec.*, 1934, *27*: 309–313; J. Parlane Kinloch, *Maternal Mortality: Report on Maternal Mortality in Aberdeen, 1918–1927* (Edinburgh: Scottish Board of Health, 1928); as well as studies by Coffin et al. and the White House Conference on Child Health and Protection. Also see James Young, "Maternal mortality studies," *Am. J. Obst. & Gynec.*, 1936, *31*: 198–212.

55 N.Y.A.M., Medical Information Bureau, "Why women die in childbirth," Nov. 20, 1933.

56 "Hazards of childbirth," *Nation*, 1933, *137*: 612.

57 Draft of letter from New York Obstetrical Society to Dr. Bernard Sachs, president, N.Y.A.M., Dec. 4, 1933, N.Y.O.S. MSS.

58 Philip Van Ingen, *The New York Academy of Medicine* (New York: Columbia Univ. Press, 1949), p. 445.

59 *Report of Subcommittee on Publicity of Maternal Mortality Report* (New York: N.Y.A.M., Public Health Relations Committee, 1934).

60 *Report of the New York Obstetrical Society to Review the Maternal Mortality Report of the Public Health Relations Committee of the New York Academy of Medicine* (New York: N.Y.O.S., 1934).

61 *How Childbirth May Be Made Safe* (New York: N.Y.O.S., 1934).

62 Benjamin P. Watson, Sect. New York Obstetrical Society, to Hervey Williamson, April 11, 1934, N.Y.O.S. MSS.

63 George W. Kosmak to Hervey Williamson, April 12, 1934, and June 15, 1934, N.Y.O.S. MSS.

64 Hervey Williamson to John L. Rice, N.Y.C. Commissioner of Health, March 14, 1934, N.Y.O.S. MSS.

65 John L. Rice, *Guarding the Health of the People of New York City, Preliminary Reports for 1934–1936* (New York: N.Y.C. Department of Health, 1936), p. 36; *50 Years of Better Health for New York's Mothers and Babies, 1908–1958* (New York: N.Y.C. Department of Health, 1958), p. 16.

66 N.Y.O.S., *Transactions of Proceedings*, Feb. 13, 1934, pp. 41–45, N.Y.O.S. MSS.

67 *Constructive Aspects of the Maternal Mortality Report of the New York Academy of Medicine* (New York: N.Y.A.M., 1934), pp. 1–9.

68 Kosmak, "Community responsibilities for safeguarding motherhood," pp. 292–299; and "Editorial comment: the trend of modern obstetrics," *Am. J. Obst. & Gynec.*, 1938, *36*: 315.

69 See Alfred Hellman, "Better obstetrics and the Subcommittee on Maternal Welfare," *New York Medical Week*, July 22, 1939, *18*: 4; and Benjamin P. Watson, "Problems of maternity," in *Preventive Medicine in Modern Practice*, ed. James Alexander Miller et al. (New York: P. B. Hoeber, 1942), p. 176.

70 One difference between the New York and Philadelphia reports lay in the definition of preventable deaths. A death was preventable according to the New York definition, if the "best" possible skill of the community had been available, while preventability, to the Philadelphians, referred to a "reasonable" degree of physician skill. The Philadelphia study summarized four major causes of maternal mortality: self-induced, criminal abor-

tions; errors of judgment on the part of the medical profession; lack of appreciation of the need of prenatal care by lay people; and failure of hospitals, organized medicine, and allied agencies to grasp their responsibilities. Abortions, with resulting septicemia, were the largest single cause of puerperal death in Philadelphia. In its report, the committee spoke of the "overwhelming" evidence of the advisability of abortion legalization, based on the example of the Soviet experience, and called for an impartial analysis to be made of the question. Philadelphia County Medical Society, *Maternal Mortality in Philadelphia, 1931–1933* (Philadelphia, 1934), pp. 127–133; Philip Williams, "The preventive aspects of maternal mortality," *J. Mich. St. Med. Soc.*, 1943, *42*: 25–26.

71 Philip Williams, "Graduate education in obstetrics," *Am. J. Obst. & Gynec.*, 1942, *43*: 529; and P. Williams, "The responsibility of the hospital obstetric staff conference in maternal welfare," *Med. Ann. District of Columbia*, 1942, *11*: 298.

72 Thaddeus L. Montgomery, "The maternal welfare program in Philadelphia," *Proceedings of the First American Congress on Obstetrics and Gynecology, 1938*, p. 542.

73 "After office hours: a visit with Dr. Philip F. Williams," *Obst. & Gynec.*, 1956, *8*: 121–122; and Williams, "The preventive aspects of maternal mortality," p. 30.

74 Jose G. Marmol, Alan L. Scriggins, and Rudolph F. Wollman, "After office hours: history of the maternal mortality study committees in the United States," *Obst. & Gynec.*, 1969, *34*: 126.

75 See, for example, James Knight Quigley, "Maternal welfare, what are its fruits?" *Am. J. Obst. & Gynec.*, 1940, *39*: 349–353; Williams, "The preventive aspects of maternal mortality," p. 25; and Watson, "Problems of maternity."

76 Quigley, "Maternal welfare, what are its fruits?" p. 351; Sam Shapiro, Edward R. Schlesinger, and Robert E. L. Nesbitt, *Infant, Perinatal, Maternal and Childhood Mortality in the United States* (Cambridge, Mass.: Harvard Univ. Press, 1968), pp. 145–146.

77 Marjorie Gooch, "Ten years of progress in reducing maternal and infant mortality," *The Child*, 1945, *10*: 77–81.

78 Frank G. Dickinson and Everett L. Welker, "Maternal mortality in the United States in 1949," *J.A.M.A.*, 1950, *144*: 1395–1400.

79 Yerushalmy, "Infant and maternal mortality in the modern world," p. 139.

80 Reasons for the decline in maternal mortality after 1933 are suggested in Quigley, "Maternal welfare, what are its fruits?" p. 350; Gooch, "Ten years of progress in reducing maternal and infant mortality," p. 80; Dickinson and Welker, "Maternal mortality," p. 1398; Shapiro et al., *Infant, Perinatal, Maternal and Childhood Mortality in the U.S.*, pp. 145–146; and in Nicholas Eastman and Louis M. Hellman, *Williams' Obstetrics*, 13th ed. (New York: Appleton-Century Crofts, 1966), pp. 8–9.

81 Dickinson and Welker, "Maternal mortality," p. 1399.

82 Cited in Marmol et al., "History of the maternal mortality study committees," p. 133.

83 Williams, "Graduate education in obstetrics," pp. 528, 532.

84 The role of the academy report in lowering mortality rates throughout the nation was commented upon in 1974 by Dr. George Baehr, president of the New York Academy of Medicine. Baehr noted that corrective action taken by communities after release of the New York study resulted in a 66 percent decline in maternal mortality rates throughout the country (from 6.6 deaths per 1,000 live births in 1931 to 2.2 deaths in 1946), thus, by the way, achieving the academy goal that two-thirds of maternal deaths were preventable. The fact that the decline in New York City, where rates fell 80 percent over the same period of time (from 6.0–6.2 deaths per 1,000 live births in 1930–32 to 1.4 deaths in 1946), far exceeded that in other cities indicated to Baehr the catalytic role of the academy report in effecting obstetric improvement. George Baehr, *Maternal Death: A Problem in Preventive Medicine, The New York Academy of Medicine's Study of Fifteen Years Ago* (New York: N.Y.A.M., 1947).

85 Katherine Fayville, "Maternity care in New York City from the public health point of view," *Proceedings of the First American Congress on Obstetrics and Gynecology, 1939*, pp. 533–534. However, in 1931, the Maternity Center Association, a private organization, initiated a home delivery service and nurse-midwifery school, the Lobenstine Midwifery Clinic. Over the next decades, the school trained a small but growing number of public health nurses from many different states in midwifery. Three of the school's original incorporators, Drs. George Kosmak, Benjamin Watson, and John O. Polak, were members of the Obstetric Advisory Committee to the New York Academy of Medicine's study of maternal mortality. Dr. Kosmak became chairman of the Medical Board of the Maternity Center Association in 1931, serving in this capacity until his death.

86 During the next decade, the distribution of live births, according to persons in attendance, increased only for in-hospital deliveries by physicians

(from 36.9 percent of births in 1935 to 84.8 percent in 1947), and declined significantly for out-of-hospital births attended by physicians (from 50.6 percent of births in 1935, to 10.1 percent in 1947). *Vital Statistics*, Special Reports, Feb. 8, 1949, *31* (1), cited by Richard Bolt, "Maternal infant and pre-school health," in *Nelson New Loose Leaf Medicine*, 1941, 7: 762.

Politics

If epidemics, which brought terror and death to American cities in the 18th and 19th centuries, had any positive effect, it was in stimulating public health activities and the development of ameliorative institutions. John Duffy illustrates this point in showing how yellow fever and cholera stirred cities to spend money for such needed, yet expensive, projects as sewerage and water-supply systems and garbage disposal works. Without the high degree of fear engendered by an epidemic, lethargic city governments would never have spent such large sums of money on projects of such magnitude. On occasion, epidemics also increased the power of public officials to control infectious diseases, permitting them, for example, forceably to remove to isolation hospitals patients deemed dangerous to the public health.

But epidemics did not always produce such positive results. Judith Walzer Leavitt offers one illustration of an epidemic that had retrogressive effects: an outbreak of smallpox in Milwaukee in 1894 left that city's health department with fewer powers than it had possessed before the epidemic.

Many factors determined whether an epidemic would have positive or negative impact and whether health issues in general would benefit or suffer. Existing medical knowledge defined the limits of health activity, but that alone did not determine what would happen. Because appropriations had to pass through city councils and thus be debated in the public arena, politicians had to be convinced that health measures were both expedient and popular. Economic considerations, class and ethnicity, timing with regard to elections, and personalities all played a part in their decisions and determined how a particular city would respond to a given threat to the public health. These same nonmedical factors also influenced the way in which cities responded to *endemic* diseases. Daniel M. Fox shows how an astute health officer manipulated the city's political machinery to begin tuberculosis control in New York.

Today, nonmedical factors continue to affect the success of public health activities, even in situations where medicine has proven efficacious. Penicillin, for example, can cure most forms of syphilis and gonorrhea, yet venereal diseases exist in epidemic proportions. Individual modesty or fear, sexual morality, the reluctance of physicians to report cases, and the question of individual rights all influence the incidence and spread of these diseases. Medicine does not act in a vacuum.

28

Social Impact of Disease in the Late 19th Century

JOHN DUFFY

The late 19th century witnessed the bacteriological revolution, without doubt one of the most significant events in the history of medicine. Prior to this, epidemic and endemic diseases were as inextricable and mysterious to man as they had been to his most primitive forebears. A few empirical discoveries, such as vaccination for smallpox, had led to some improvement in conditions of health, but the origin and transmission of diseases were as obscure as ever. Acrimonious debates characterized medical meetings as late as the 1880s as theory vied with theory, and theorist with theorist. The greatest advance in knowledge of infectious diseases until then had come from the general recognition that such diseases flourished in filthy, overcrowded conditions. This development, for which the medical profession deserves only partial credit, resulted in the movement for sanitation, which began reducing the urban death rate well before bacteriology provided health officials with a sound rationale.

Although the movement for public and personal hygiene was firmly established in the second half of the 19th century, and Pasteur, Koch, and their colleagues were unveiling the tangled skein of bacteriology, communicable diseases still remained the leading health problem. The health records of every city show that tuberculosis, diphtheria, scarlet fever, whooping cough, enteric disorders, measles, smallpox, and even malaria were endemic. Infant mortality — largely attributed to such vague causes as summer fever and diarrhea, teething, colic, and convulsions — was a major component of the high total death rate. The loss of so many children, however, was accepted as the inexorable working of fate.

JOHN DUFFY is Priscilla Alden Burke Professor of History, University of Maryland, College Park, Maryland.

Reprinted with permission from the *Bulletin of the New York Academy of Medicine*, 1971, *47*: 797–811.

Smallpox, the one disease for which a fairly effective preventive measure was available, should have created no difficulty, yet it continued to flare up in every American city. A series of outbreaks in New York City during the 1870s caused 805 deaths in 1871, 929 in 1872, 484 in 1874, and 1,280 in 1875.[1] During three of these same years the annual death toll from smallpox in New Orleans was more than 500, and Dr. Joseph Jones, president of the Louisiana State Board of Health, later declared that 6,432 residents of New Orleans had died of smallpox in the years from 1863 to 1883. As late as the winter of 1899–1900, 3 of 12 medical students at Tulane University, infected during a widespread outbreak, died of the disease.[2]

Compared with other communicable infections such as diphtheria, for which little could be done, smallpox was only a minor cause of death. Diphtheria, a fearful disorder with an equally high fatality rate, was a major epidemic disease throughout most of this period. Earlier, during the 1850s and 1860s, it had been merely one of many children's complaints, but its incidence took a startling upturn in the 1870s. From 1866 to 1872 diphtheria deaths in New York averaged about 325 per year. In 1873 the figure jumped to 1,151, increased to more than 1,600 in 1874, and then reached a new high of 2,329 in 1875. From 1800 to 1896 the annual deaths from diphtheria never fell below 1,000; on three occasions the total was well in excess of 2,000. The peak period for diphtheria in New York City came during the 1890s, the years when throat cultures and antitoxin therapy were introduced. New York's problems with diphtheria were in no sense unique.[3] In New Orleans a health official informed a joint meeting of the city's two medical societies in 1887 that diphtheria had long existed there, but never before had it been "so widespread and abundant as now."[4] By this date diphtheria had spread throughout America, ravaging town and country alike. Since many deaths from diphtheria went unrecorded, and the hundreds of infant deaths attributed to croup and other vague causes undoubtedly included some cases of diphtheria, the actual toll was probably larger than the statistics of mortality show.

The most surprising aspect of diphtheria was that it aroused so little concern. One of the few newspaper editorials about it came after an 1873–1874 epidemic which killed 1,344 people in New York City. On this occasion the editor of the *New York Times* declared: "Had a tithe of the number died from anything resembling cholera or yellow fever we should have had a public scare which would have compelled such a cleaning out of tenements, flushing of sewers, and clearing away of street filth as had not been witnessed for many years."[5] Occasional discussions can be found in medical journals and transactions of societies but these centered chiefly around methods of treatment. The casual public reaction to diphtheria contrasts sharply with the attitude of colonists a century or so earlier. When a virulent form of the disease suddenly burst upon western Europe and the American colonies in the 1730s, it aroused widespread apprehension. By the 1870s, however, diphtheria was a familiar disorder to which the population had become accustomed, and its annual toll among the young had come to be taken as a matter of course. The doctors could do little about it, and the public attitude was one of resignation.

This same fatalistic attitude also characterized the public reaction to scarlet fever, tuberculosis, typhoid, and the other perennial disorders. Dr. Abraham Jacobi, reporting for the Committee on Hygiene of the New York County Medical Society, pointed out that between 1866 and 1890 about 43,000 residents of New York had died of diphtheria and croup and that more than 18,000 had succumbed to scarlet fever. Despite this enormous mortality, the city had made virtually no public provision for the sick. Nine years before, in 1882, he continued, the municipal hospital facilities were so crowded with cases of smallpox, typhus, and typhoid that there had been no room for patients with diphtheria or scarlet fever. Since that time nothing had been done except to open one hospital with 70 beds. Almost in despair, Dr. Jacobi exclaimed: "Seventy beds, and twenty-five hundred cases are permitted to die annually."[6] Dr. Jacobi's statement takes on added significance when one considers that New York City had one of the best health departments in the United States.

In terms of mortality, two diseases, phthisis, or consumption (tuberculosis of the lungs), and pneumonia, should have caused the greatest outcry. Both, however, were considered "constitutional" diseases, and their very frequence dispelled the fears one might expect to be associated with them. In 1870 tuberculosis of the lungs was responsible for about 4,000 deaths in New York City; this figure rose steadily in the ensuing years until about 1890, when almost 5,500 deaths were reported. Deaths from pneumonia rose even more sharply — from 1,836 in 1870 to 6,487 in 1893. Despite their enormous death toll, these familiar and chronic complaints lacked the drama of the great pestilences, and they went largely unnoticed by the general public.[7]

Although most of these statistics have been drawn from New York and New Orleans, the conditions that they reflect prevailed in all major American cities. New Orleans and other southern urban areas differed from the North only with respect to malaria and yellow fever. As in the North, tuberculosis and the respiratory diseases were the number one killers, while diphtheria, scarlet fever, smallpox, measles, and other disorders contributed to the general mortality.

Although gradually receding southward, malaria was a major problem in the United States throughout the 19th century. In New York City 457 deaths were attributed to malaria during 1881, and it was 1895 before the city's annual number of deaths from the disease fell below 100.[8] In terms of total mortality, malaria was of little significance to New York and most northern cities, but it was a major factor in the South. In 1888 Dr. Stanford Chaillé surveyed the causes of death in New Orleans and concluded that tuberculosis, malaria, and dysentery were the chief culprits. Bearing out Dr. Chaillé's statement, the records of the New Orleans Charity Hospital for 1883 show that 45 percent of the 8,000 patients admitted were treated for malaria. But malaria, too, was an old and familiar complaint, and in those areas where it was endemic its recurrence each spring and fall was accepted almost as inevitable as the seasonal cycle itself.[9]

In sharp contrast to this casual acceptance of the diseases mentioned thus far was the public reaction to Asiatic cholera and yellow fever. Although both disorders had reached their peak in the 1850s and henceforth were only a minor cause of morbidity and mortality, they dominated newspaper stories relating to health, preoccupied a good share of the time of the medical profession, and were important factors in promoting public health measures. Had either disease gained a permanent foothold in the United States, it might well have been among the ranking causes of mortality and morbidity, but at the same time it would have become familiar and in the process would have lost its capacity to inspire terror. As it was, outbreaks of cholera in any part of the world or the appearance of a case of cholera or yellow fever in quarantine was enough to arouse the newspapers, medical societies, and civic authorities in every American port.

Of the two diseases, yellow fever had a much longer history in the United States. It first appeared in the late 17th century in Boston and then plagued every American port from Boston southward until the beginning of the 19th century. After a series of major epidemics from 1793 to 1805, the northeastern section of the United States was virtually free of the disease. Attacks on the South Atlantic and Gulf Coast areas, however, intensified in the first half of the 19th century and reached their peak in the 1850s. The number and intensity of the outbreaks, with one or two exceptions, tapered off sharply after the Civil War, although the disease continued to be a real threat to every southern port.[10]

Yellow fever is a fatal and frightening disease; its attacks on the cities of the eastern seaboard from 1793 to 1805 left a vivid imprint upon the public mind. Throughout the remainder of the century, memories of this pestilence were constantly revived by grim accounts of the recurrent outbreaks in southern ports. Moreover, the disease was endemic in the West Indies, and it was a rare summer when one or more cases were not discovered by northern quarantine officials. In 1856 lax enforcement of quarantine laws resulted in more than 500 cases of yellow fever on Staten Island and the western end of Long Island. The New York City quarantine station was located on Staten Island at this time, and outraged local residents barricaded all entrances to it. When the New York authorities responded in 1857 by buying a new site several miles away, an armed mob vandalized the buildings. The following summer, when additional yellow fever patients were landed, another mob burned the quarantine hospital to the ground. Determined opposition by local citizens at all proposed new sites forced the quarantine officials to buy an old steamer to use as a floating hospital for yellow fever.[11] Although the fever never gained a foothold in Manhattan, every summer New York newspapers carried stories of its ravages in the South, and they rarely failed to editorialize upon its danger whenever cases were reported on incoming vessels.

In southern ports it was not necessary to revive old memories, since most residents had experienced close contact with the disease. In 1866–1867 the fever struck coastal towns from Wilmington and New Bern in North Carolina all the way to Brownsville, Texas. Desultory attacks continued until 1878, when the disease was once again widespread. On this occasion it traveled up the Mississippi Valley as far as St. Louis, Chattanooga, and Louisville. Aside from a major outbreak in Florida during 1888, only scattered cases were reported until 1897–1899 and 1905, when minor epidemics occurred in New Orleans and the surrounding areas. The 1878 outbreak, by far the most severe in the postwar years, resulted in 27,000 cases and over 4,000 deaths in New Orleans and wiped out almost 10 percent of the populations of Memphis and Vicksburg.[12]

Considering these statistics, it is not to be wondered that rumors of yellow jack or the "saffron scourge," as it was sometimes called in New Orleans, was enough to cause panic. When a reported outbreak of yellow fever in Ocean Springs, Mississippi, in 1897 led the New Orleans Board of Health to proclaim a quarantine against all Gulf Coast towns, a panic-stricken mob of New Orleans residents vacationing in one of the resorts seized control of a train and brought it to the Louisiana state line. Here the train was held up until the health officials, recognizing the hungry and desperate condition of the passengers, reluctantly permitted them to enter New Orleans. This act of mercy by the Board of Health was assailed bitterly and was a factor in the subsequent resignation of the entire board.[13]

When the disease appeared in New Orleans, the mayor arranged for one of the schools to be used as a temporary yellow fever hospital. The following night an armed mob, objecting to the presence of a hospital in their neighborhood, set fire to the building. When firemen arrived, onlookers cut the hoses, precipitating a fight between the mob and the firemen and policemen. Even as late as 1905 the reaction to the presence of yellow fever was one of profound shock. The president of the local medical society in New Orleans wrote: "When the first knowledge reached our city of the presence of this dread disease in our midst, there was almost a panic — stocks and bonds went begging, a pall seemed to be thrown on all things, a general exodus of those who could afford it took place, and the commercial interests seem paralyzed."[14]

Asiatic cholera, the most feared of all diseases in the 19th century, arrived in the western world as a by-product of the industrial revolution. Because of its short incubation period and rapid course, the disease was restricted to the Far East almost until the advent of steam power and rapid transportation. At the same time, industrialism brought massive urbanization with all its concomitant problems: crowded slums, limited and contaminated water supplies, hopelessly ineffectual methods for eliminating sewage and garbage, and city governments ill-equipped to deal with the explosive growth of population. Thus the industrial revolution provided both the rapid transportation necessary for spreading the disease and seed beds where it could flourish in the crowded cities.

Improvements in communication contributed further to enhancing the role played by cholera, for no disease in American history was so widely heralded at its first appearance (1832). The introduction of cheap newspapers and journals had made it possible for the American public to follow the disastrous course of this pestilence as it advanced through Russia, eastern Europe, and pushed northwestward to the Atlantic. The accounts of its destructive progress built up growing apprehensions which were intensified by urgent warnings from health authorities and medical societies that the filthy state of American communities had already set the stage for explosive outbursts of disease. Cholera struck the United States first in 1832 and returned in 1848–1849. On both occasions it swept through cities and towns within a few weeks, killing thousands. In 1866 and 1873 the disease again threatened, but prompt sanitary measures limited its effect. Without knowing precisely why, health authorities recognized that the infection was spread through the feces of infected persons, and they resorted successfully to disinfecting procedures.[15]

Unlike yellow fever, which periodically demonstrated the reality of its threat, Asiatic cholera was never more than a potential danger in the years which followed the Civil War, yet it received an inordinate amount of attention from newspapers and journals in all sections of the United States. Most of the civic cleanups and sanitary campaigns were sparked by what was considered to be the imminent danger from this disease. It shared with yellow fever the capacity for creating panic and brutalizing decent citizens. Victims of Asiatic cholera were often dumped ashore by crews and passengers of river boats, much to the dismay of local residents, who occasionally left them there to die. When the disease appeared in Pittsburgh in 1849 and the Sisters of Mercy opened their hospital to its victims, meetings were held by indignant neighborhood residents and local newspaper correspondents attacked the sisters bitterly. In nearby Allegheny the same situation held true for the Reverend Passavant when he, too, offered help to cholera patients.[16]

The reaction of Americans to a threatened cholera outbreak in 1873 shows how the apprehensions aroused by earlier epidemics carried over into the postwar years. As the disease began spreading into Europe, the newspapers were filled with cholera stories, and the *New York Times* editorialized on "cholera panics." The editor of a medical journal declared that in the United States cholera was the "all-absorbing topic." Responding to demands from newspapers and medical societies, the New York City Health Department promptly began a major effort to alleviate the worst sanitary conditions within the city.[17]

A few years later, when cholera broke out in Toulon and Marseilles, American newspapers once again carried daily front-page reports of the disease. In July 1884 President Chester Arthur reflected national concern by issuing a proclamation warning state officials to be on guard. Throughout the following winter cholera continued to preoccupy public attention. In January a group of New York businessmen organized the Sanitary Protective Society to mobilize all existing health agencies within the city. As the public clamor for action increased, the city board of health secured a special appropriation of $50,000. When the expected epidemic did not materialize, the board was given permission to retain the fund for future use. The following year Asiatic cholera was reported in Italy, and President S. Grover Cleveland was requested to prohibit all Italian immigration until the danger was over.[18]

The last major cholera scare came in 1892. Once again a state of alarm characterized the entire American seaboard. Daily front-page stories reported enormous casualties in Russia and hinted of comparable figures in western European cities. Municipal authorities, collaborating with health officials, initiated massive sanitary campaigns, checked on food and water supplies, and made preparations for the expected assault. In New York the city health department retained its summer corps of 50 physicians on an emergency basis; the St. John's Guild lent its "floating hospital" for the use of cholera cases; J. P. Morgan offered the use of a steamship to house cabin passengers from immigrant vessels during the quarantine period; and the directors of St. Mark's Hospital organized a volunteer medical and nursing corps. On the national scene President Benjamin Harrison responded to the crisis by ordering all immigrant vessels to perform a minimum 20-day quarantine. To facilitate the procedure of quarantine, the state of New York leased buildings on Fire Island for the use of healthy cabin passengers during the quarantine period. On hearing this news, the local board of health promptly deputized all citizens and prepared to resist. An armed mob lined the pier, and it was not until the governor mobilized the National Guard that the mob dispersed and passengers were able to land without being molested.[19]

Since most societies tend to operate on a crisis basis, the diseases which were most effective in precipitating social change were those with the greatest shock value. In this category it is clear that Asiatic cholera and yellow fever stood by themselves, with smallpox a poor third, and the other disorders ranking well behind. The outbreaks of yellow fever which struck the eastern seaboard from 1793 to 1795 had the immediate effect of bringing into existence temporary boards of health, which had surprisingly wide powers. In New York City, for example, the Board of Health was given the authority and funds to evacuate large sections of the city and to provide food, housing, and medical care for the poor. A permanent result of these outbreaks was the creation of the office of City Inspector, a forerunner of New York's health department. Throughout the century yellow fever scares continued to give impetus to health reform. The outbreaks in the 1850s in New Orleans and the southern states had repercussions in every eastern port and greatly strengthened the position of reformers fighting for permanent boards of health.

In the southern states, which bore the brunt of the attacks in the 19th century, yellow fever provided the chief stimulus to health reform. Two major epidemics in Louisiana in 1853 and 1854, the first of which killed almost 9,000 residents of New Orleans and the second another 2,500, were directly responsible for the creation of the Louisiana State Board of Health, the first such agency in the United States.[20] Successive epidemics strengthened this board until 1897, when the consternation aroused by the reappearance of yellow fever after an absence of several years forced the members of the board to resign and led to a reorganization of the state board and the establishment of a separate board of health for New Orleans. In 1878 the disastrous outbreak, which affected almost every major town on the South Atlantic and Gulf coasts and spread far up the Mississippi Valley, aroused the entire nation. In Memphis, a city which had not recovered from the Civil War, the loss of 3,500 residents to yellow fever brought a major social and political upheaval.[21] On the national scene, Congress reacted by passing the first national quarantine act. As the full impact of the 1878 epidemic was felt, health reformers were able to secure from Congress a second measure creating the National Board of Health. Neither of these laws proved effective; the quarantine law was weak, and the National Board of Health, after a stormy existence, virtually disappeared in 1883 when Congress eliminated its appropriation. Nonetheless, during its brief lifetime the National Board of Health did help to arouse a public health consciousness, and it paved the way for the creation of the United States Public Health Service a few years later.

Asiatic cholera, because it constituted a threat to all areas, was possibly even more significant than yellow fever. The first two waves of this disorder, 1832–1835 and 1848–1855, struck at the coastal cities and then followed the unexcelled waterways of North America. In their wake they left not only a trail of death and suffering but also a host of temporary health boards. During the first attack on Pittsburgh, for example, a ten-man sanitary board was appointed and given an appropriation of $10,000. The following year the funds were reduced to $6,000 and, as the threat of cholera receded, the board disappeared and the funds for sanitation were virtually eliminated from the municipal budget.[22] The second wave of Asiatic cholera at the mid-century coincided with the emerging sanitary movement and the peak years of yellow fever. The two diseases were largely responsible for the organization of the National Sanitary Conventions which met from 1856 to 1860. These gatherings of state and municipal health officials and representatives of medical societies were the first attempts to devise national quarantine and public health programs, and they helped lay the basis for the subsequent establishment of the American Public Health Association.

The second and third waves of Asiatic cholera played a significant role in the establishment of the Health Department of New York City. More than 5,000 New Yorkers died of cholera during 1849 and several hundred more died of it in 1854. Since sanitationists argued that cholera was the product of crowding, and the filth-and-quarantine faction believed that it was a specific communicable disease which could be kept out of the city, cholera supplied both factions in the health movement with ammunition in their effort to obtain a permanent health agency for the city. In the years following the cholera outbreaks of 1849–1854, campaigns to educate the public gradually gained momentum. Several health bills for New York City were introduced into the state legislature during the early 1860s but they all failed. At this stage the third epidemic wave of Asiatic cholera appeared, and its threat in the winter of 1865–66 led to the passage of a Metropolitan Board of Health Act for New York City. The first problem confronting the Metropolitan Board was to deal with the imminent danger from cholera. An energetic sanitary campaign combined with rigid isolation, quarantine, and disinfection measures kept the number of cases to a minimum. This 1866 attack on the United States was relatively mild and probably would have had a minor effect on New York City. New Yorkers, remembering the 5,000 deaths a few years earlier, gave full credit to the Metropolitan Board of Health. This auspicious start left a residue of good will which resulted in strong public support for the health department for many years.[23]

Repeated cholera scares continued to remind New York officials and the general public of the need for a strong health department, but it was not until 1892 that the disorder again made a permanent impact on the city. The widespread alarm touched off by cholera in that year has already been mentioned. For several years prior to it Drs. Hermann M. Biggs and T. Mitchell Prudden had been advocating the establishment of a bacteriological laboratory. Capitalizing on the general apprehension, Dr. Biggs won his point with the city Board of Estimate and, in September 1892, New York City established the first laboratory to be used for the routine diagnosis of disease.

Possibly more important than the direct effect of epidemic diseases upon social and political reform was their indirect impact. The middle and upper classes sought to insulate themselves from the deplorable condition of the working class, but for those members who encountered the appalling infant mortality and the ravages of disease among the lower economic groups the experience was often traumatic. Moreover, as conditions in the urban slums worsened, the diseases of the poor could not be contained, and public health became a matter of concern for all the people.

Members of the medical profession were among the first to encounter the disease and misery of the poor. It was recognized that clinics and dispensaries catering to the poor were essential to medical training and research, and young physicians and surgeons were thrown into direct contact with the realities of poverty. Not surprisingly, in America physicians were among the leading advocates of public health. More significantly, since the integral relation between poverty and disease was all too obvious, they were also among the leaders of social reform.

During the terrible epidemics of Asiatic cholera and yellow fever, volunteer groups of all sorts came in contact with dire poverty, and many individuals seeking to help the deserving poor gradually came to realize that even the undeserving poor were the product of their brutalizing environment. In the South a notable example of the volunteer groups was the Howard Association, named after John Howard, the famous English reformer. Originating in New Orleans during a yellow fever epidemic in 1837, its program gradually spread to other southern cities and towns. The members were young businessmen who volunteered their services during major epidemics. The Howards, as they were called, organized massive relief programs to provide medical care for the sick poor and housing and food for their families. The willingness of these men to volunteer for work with the Howard Association evidences some degree of social conscience, but their intimate contact with poverty created a new awareness of social needs.

As far back as the 16th century it had been argued that a country's population was a major form of wealth. By the mid-19th century demography was emerging as a science, and improvements in the collection of vital statistics began to reveal the high morbidity and mortality rates in urban areas. One of the major arguments used by health and social reformers was the economic cost of sickness and death. Estimating the productivity per adult worker, they calculated the loss of productivity caused by the many deaths and added to it the cost of medical care for the sick. The validity of this argument was demonstrated clearly by the repeated epidemics of yellow fever which effectively closed down southern cities and brought all economic activities to a halt. Throughout the 19th century most physicians and laymen believed that epidemic diseases were either propagated or nurtured in conditions of dirt and overcrowding. This environmental concept led to an assault on the atrocious tenement conditions, nuisance trades, deplorable working conditions, and other abuses.

Late in the century the bacteriological revolution turned the medical profession away from environmentalism and focused its attention upon pathogenic organisms. The germ theory had the beneficent effect of awakening the upper classes to the realization that bacteria were no respecters of economic or social position and that a man's health was dependent to some extent on the health of his fellowmen. The knowledge that the diseases of the workers who sewed clothes in their filthy tenement homes or who processed food could be spread to decent, clean, and respectable citizens served as a powerful incentive to the reform of public health. Since public health could not be separated from social conditions, the net result was an attack on poverty.

The best evidence that a concern for public health underlay much of the effort for social reform is to be found in the multiplicity of volunteer sanitary associations which sprang up in the late 19th century. In every city private groups worked to establish or improve water and sewerage systems, to clean streets, to provide pure milk for the infant poor, to remedy abuses in municipal hospitals and other institutions, and to establish dispensaries, clinics, and hospitals. Examples of these groups in New York City were the Association for Improving the Condition of the Poor, the New York Sanitary Reform Society, the Ladies Health Protective Association, the St. John's Guild, the Sanitary Protective League, the Sanitary Aid Society, and the New York Society for the Prevention of Contagious Diseases. Of the many voluntary organizations operating in New York during this period, some sought only one immediate objective and disbanded after a brief existence, others created organizations that survived for many years. What they all shared in common was the belief that a healthy population was basic to a sound society.

In glancing back over the 19th century one can safely conclude that the rapid expansion of urban areas provided fertile grounds for communicable diseases, and that these diseases were both a cause and effect of the desperate poverty which characterized so many of the cities. At the same time the frightening sickness and death rates drew attention to the deplorable condition of the poor. Dramatic outbreaks of yellow fever and cholera profoundly stirred public opinion and directly and indirectly contributed to the growth of public health institutions. Meanwhile statistical evidence was developing which showed an even heavier toll from chronic and endemic disorders. The net effect, as shown by even the most cursory reading of late-19th-century newspapers, was that public health and sanitary reform became major public issues. And for nearly all social reformers, whether their concern was with infant welfare, tenement conditions, or even political reform, the elimination of sickness and disease became a major aim.

NOTES

1 See the *Annual Report of the New York City Health Department, 1871–75* (the title varies, sometimes designated as the *Annual Report of the Board of Health. . . .*).

2 *The Rudolph Matas History of Medicine in Louisiana*, ed. J. Duffy, 2 vols. (Baton Rouge, 1958), II, 438, 442–443.

3 *Annual Report N.Y.C. Health Dept., 1866–1896.*

4 *New Orleans Med. & Surg. J.*, 1887–1888, *15*: 470–474.

5 *New York Times*, July 14, 1874.

6 A. Jacobi, "The unsanitary condition of the primary schools of the City of New York," *Sanitarian*, 1892, *28*: 331–324.

7 *Annual Report N.Y.C. Health Dept., 1870–1893.*

8 *Ibid.*

9 S. E. Chaillé, "Life and death rates; New Orleans and other cities compared," *New Orleans Med. & Surg. J.*, 1888–1889, *16*: 85–100. *Ibid.*, 1884–1885, *12*: 716–717.

10 J. Duffy, "Yellow fever in the continental United States during the nineteenth century," *Bull. N.Y. Acad. Med.* 1968, *54*: 687–701.

11 J. Duffy, *A History of Public Health in New York City, 1625–1866* (New York, 1968), pp. 101–123, 440–460.

12 Duffy, "Yellow fever in the continental United States," pp. 639–696.

13 *The Rudolph Matas History of Medicine in Louisiana*, ed. Duffy, II, 430.

14 G. Augustin, *History of Yellow Fever* (New Orleans, 1909), pp. 1061–1062.

15 For an excellent account, see C. E. Rosenberg, *The Cholera Years: The United States in 1832, 1849 and 1866* (Chicago, 1962).

16 J. Duffy, "The impact of Asiatic cholera on Pittsburgh, Wheeling, and Charleston," *Western Penn. Hist. Mag.*, 1964, *58*: 199–211.

17 *Sanitarian*, 1873, *1*: 228–229.

18 This material was taken from chapter 7 of the author's second volume on the public health history of New York City: *A History of Public Health in New York City, 1866–1966* (New York, 1974).

19 *Ibid.*

20 J. Duffy, *Sword of Pestilence: The New Orleans Yellow Fever Epidemic of 1853* (Baton Rouge, 1966), pp. 139, 167.

21 J. H. Ellis, "Memphis' sanitary revolution, 1880–1890," *Tenn. Hist. Quart.*, 1964, *23*: 59–72.

22 Duffy, "Impact of Asiatic cholera on Pittsburgh, Wheeling, and Charleston," pp. 202–203.

23 Duffy, *History of Public Health in New York City, 1625–1866*, pp. 441–446.

29

Politics and Public Health: Smallpox in Milwaukee, 1894–1895

JUDITH WALZER LEAVITT

Smallpox was to Milwaukee what cholera and yellow fever were to other 19th-century American cities. It was an infrequent visitor, but when it came, smallpox caused major disruptions of city life and generated fear and panic among the residents. The effects of smallpox epidemics were typically to increase the powers and effectiveness of the Health Department. John Duffy, Charles Rosenberg, and others, have indicated this pattern with regard to cholera and yellow fever epidemics.[1] I have found it also explains the impact of smallpox in Milwaukee. As a result of five 19th-century smallpox epidemics, health officials greatly increased their authority to control infectious diseases in Milwaukee.[2]

However, the smallpox epidemic which hit Milwaukee in the summer and fall of 1894 interrupted this pattern. As a direct result of that epidemic, the powers of the Health Department were significantly diminished, and its reputation in the city sank to an all-time low. This 1894 example, I think, serves to dramatize the relationship between politics and public health and to remind us that medical factors do not alone determine the course of public health events.

The 1894 Milwaukee smallpox epidemic illustrates the dependence of 19th-century public health on political circumstances. Moreover, it shows that epidemics could have had — and occasionally did have — retrogressive as well as progressive effects on the development of the public health movement.

A frightening disease, with ugly physical manifestations, smallpox attacked all ages and, exacerbated by unsanitary conditions and overcrowding, spread quickly through a city. Victims who did not succumb to the disease were often left disfigured and pockmarked for life. But in the 19th century, smallpox was a preventable disease, since vaccination with cowpox virus was available. Thus one would not expect smallpox still to be a disease of dread. However, although vaccination was quite widely used, it was not universally accepted in the medical community or among the lay public. Most medical practitioners advocated vaccination, but many thought it an inadequate protection against the disease; some antivaccinationists claimed it to be more harmful than the disease itself.[3]

Milwaukee newspapers aired the disagreements within the medical community over vaccination and about treatment of smallpox, and the result was a confusion which seemed to grow as the century wore on. The presence of a large immigrant community in the city, among whom the efficacy of vaccination was most frequently questioned, merely increased dissension.[4]

The infrequent appearance of the disease and the confusion about medical theory account for a large part of the reaction Milwaukeeans had to smallpox. But the particular political circumstances which greeted the outbreak of an epidemic in the city also generated fear. Divided opinion among the people about how to react to the disease, and over whether or not to vaccinate occasionally furthered already existing political and ethnic divisions in the city. In 1894, the Milwaukee Health Department found it difficult to control a medical situation because of its political ramifications.

Milwaukee in the 1890s was a bustling commercial and industrial city. Its population jumped

---

JUDITH WALZER LEAVITT is Assistant Professor, History of Medicine Department, University of Wisconsin, Madison, Wisconsin.

Reprinted with permission from the *Bulletin of the History of Medicine*, 1976, *50*: 553–568.

from 20,000 at mid-century to 115,000 by 1880, and to 285,000 at the turn of the 20th century. By 1910, Milwaukee was the twelfth largest city in the United States. Contrary to popular belief, its economy was based only partly on beer; other heavy and light industries also flourished.[5] Milwaukee contained members of almost every ethnic group which migrated to this country, with Germans and Poles predominating. Many have noted the German character of 19th-century Milwaukee.[6] Although most of its population lived in single-family, or two- to three-family dwellings, Milwaukee was very much an urban metropolis in the 1890s. Like all other cities in the United States during the period, it wrestled with the problems of housing congestion, street sanitation, and disposal of wastes.

In 1894, a Republican victory at the polls led to the appointment of a new Health Commissioner, Walter Kempster, a Republican and a nationally known physician and psychiatrist. Although best known for his work with the insane, Kempster had spent much time studying how Europeans dealt with contagious diseases, especially cholera, and the new mayor felt that a man of such stature would be an asset to the city.[7]

The Common Council immediately questioned Kempster's appointment. Democrats might have been expected to oppose a Republican appointee as a matter of course; but Kempster's strongest opposition came from fellow Republicans, most vociferously from aldermen Robert Rudolph and Charles Kieckhefer, both representing German wards.[8] Both men criticized the fact that Kempster was new to Milwaukee and unfamiliar with the city and its problems. They opposed his appointment initially because they had supported other local physicians for the job. Kempster's English heritage and national reputation acted against him in the minds of those who sought a familiar, and possibly ethnic, representative of Milwaukee's population. But the majority of the council was willing to give Kempster a chance, and confirmed his appointment by a vote of 23 to 13.[9]

With the nation and the city in the middle of a severe economic depression in 1894, the 26 patronage jobs controlled by the Health Commissioner assumed great significance. Although Kempster was a Republican, he was not susceptible to the influences of fellow party members. In fact, when he announced his appointees, he completely ignored the party's suggested lists. Council members immediately challenged the appointments over which they had consent powers, and vetoed some of them, early establishing the pattern which was to typify Kempster's relations with the legislative body.[10]

As a result of this episode, tension existed between the Health Department and the Common Council in June 1894 when the incidence of smallpox began to increase and an epidemic threatened. The atmosphere of cooperation, necessary to cope successfully with an emergency situation, was missing. Smallpox became the weapon with which certain members of the Common Council, led by South Side saloon-keeper Robert Rudolph, fought the Health Commissioner. The Polish and German immigrant groups most hard hit by the epidemic furnished the movement's political strength.

Dr. Kempster's reaction to smallpox in the city was similar to that of health commissioners before him. He at once hired extra physicians to launch a widespread vaccination campaign. He moved swiftly to isolate those patients reported to have the disease by removing them to the Isolation Hospital in the Eleventh Ward, acting under the 1892 ordinance giving him the power to do this forcibly if necessary. And he enforced a strict quarantine on those allowed to remain at home. The department also carried on extensive patient education campaigns and made wide use of the city's disinfecting van.[11]

The reaction of citizens to the Health Department's offensive was initially similar to the response during previous outbreaks. They cooperated with everything but vaccination, which the German and Polish areas of the city resisted. The Health Department had no authority to force vaccinations on anyone who did not want them, although nonvaccinated children could be refused admission to the public schools. Since the epidemic began just when the public schools were closing for the summer, this restraint was not particularly effective.[12]

During June and July, smallpox appeared in all sections of the city, keeping the Health Department busy vaccinating and isolating reported cases. Kempster was confident that his procedures were effective, and that an epidemic would not materialize. But by mid-July it was evident that a significant number of people were not cooperating with the health authorities. Many cases of smallpox went unreported. Discontent with Health Department policy grew when smallpox seemed to localize in the South Side wards. The one hardest hit by the contagion was the Eleventh Ward, site of the Isolation Hospital and home of Alderman Rudolph.

At first Kempster denied that there was a seat of infection in the South Side, but the numerous cases discovered there belied his assertions. Significant numbers of parents refused to allow their children to be examined or vaccinated by health officials, contributing to the rapid spread of the disease.[13] The immediate focus of the people's wrath was the Isolation Hospital in the crowded Eleventh Ward. Despite the renovations that had recently transformed the institution into what health authorities called a "modern facility," residents in the neighborhood still viewed it as a "pesthouse" and the source of their trouble. They claimed that it was a "menace to the health of citizens" and a "slaughterhouse" where patients "were not treated like human beings." Health officials maintained that the hospital was in good condition and offered good service to the sick poor who were admitted.[14] Whatever the actual condition of the hospital in July and August 1894, southsiders were convinced that it was a death house for those who went there as patients and that its presence infected the nearby districts.[15]

A crisis was reached on August 5 when a crowd of neighbors successfully resisted an attempt by the Health Department to take a sick two-year-old to the hospital. About 3,000 "furious" people armed with clubs, knives, and stones assembled in front of the child's house. The family had recently lost a child after it had been removed to the hospital, and the mother was frantic with fear and determined not to let the city "kill" (as she put it) another of her children. "I can give it better care and nourishment here than they can give it at the hospital. I will not allow my child to be taken to the hospital." Faced with the violent mob, and unable to control the situation, the ambulance on this occasion beat a hasty retreat.[16]

There is no evidence that Alderman Rudolph was in any way connected with the initial outburst on the night of August 5. But by the next day his name was being intimately linked with the South Side "rioters," and he was participating actively to organize and mold the political force unleashed in his ward. On August 6, he introduced a resolution in the Common Council to remove the power of the Health Commissioner to take patients to the hospital against their will. Although the resolution had no effect against the ordinance which gave the power, its adoption was seen as a vote of support of the southsiders.[17] Rudolph appeared as a leader at public rallies, and on August 7, when a crowd gathered to protest the night burial of a smallpox victim, Rudolph addressed them with a speech that "was not entirely free from incendiarism." With his support, southsiders continued actively to protest Health Department activities.[18]

Dr. Kempster reacted by stiffening the official position, insisting that if smallpox spread it was not due to Health Department negligence but rather to the rioters themselves spreading the contagion through the South Side wards. He carefully defended every argument leveled at the department, and told a reporter, "But for politics and bad beer, the matter would never have been heard of."[19] This belittlement of an issue as crucial as life itself to the South Side residents did little to ease tensions between the Health Department and that section of the city. In fact, it emphasized the differences — class and ethnic — between Kempster and the immigrant South Side residents. Showing little compassion, Kempster remained firm during the entire episode, never bending to the southsiders, never recognizing that their concerns may have been legitimate. "I am here to enforce the laws," he said, "and I shall enforce them if I have to break heads to do it. The question of the inhumanity of the laws I have nothing to do with."[20]

The situation on the South Side clearly aided the spread of smallpox in that region of the city. Daily, crowds of people took to the streets, seeking out health officials to harass. Quarantine officials watching guard over houses were frequently the object of the mob's attack. With thousands of people roaming the streets and entering houses infected with smallpox, the contagion was destined to spread throughout the district. Case reports, despite the many concealed from authorities, indicate that the South Side wards 11 and 14 were most severely hit during the summer and fall of 1894 (Fig. 1).[21]

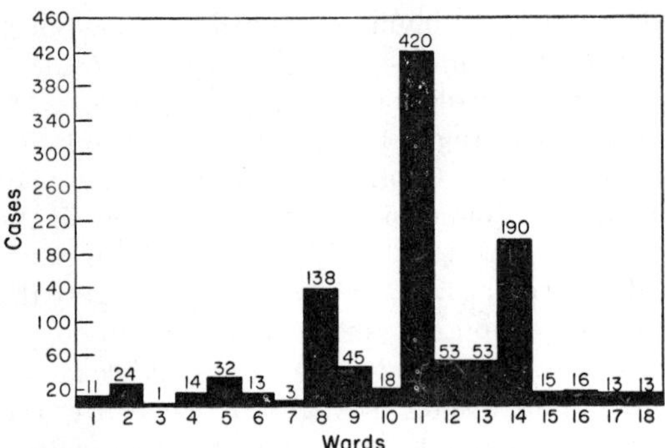

Fig. 1. Milwaukee smallpox epidemic, 1894–1895: ward distribution. Wards 5, 8, 11, 12, 14, and 17 were on the South Side.

The focus of the crowds' hatred was Dr. Kempster. He symbolized arbitrary governmental authority which was subverting immigrant culture and threatening personal liberty. Calling for his execution, crowds demanded that the "people's rights were paramount and should be protected, if need be, at the point of a pistol."[22] Women played a particularly important part in the disturbances. Since police were reluctant to use their clubs on "feminine shoulders," women were effective at maintaining disorder. Armed with clubs and stones, they assaulted the city police sent to preserve order. They threw stones and scalding water at the ambulance horses in an effort to stop officials from removing any patients. As one newspaper observed the situation: "Mobs of Pomeranian and Polish women armed with baseball bats, potato mashers, clubs, bed slats, salt and pepper, and butcher knives, lay in wait all day for . . . the Isolation Hospital van" (Fig. 2).[23]

City officials met daily to try to determine a course of action which would stem the riots and the spread of smallpox. They consulted the State Board of Health. Despite their efforts, the disturbances continued intermittently through August and into September.[24]

In addition to governmental meetings, South Side citizen groups met to try to regain the image of that section as a peaceable place, safe for business. Deeply regretting "the notoriety which has been recently thrust upon that section of the city," one such meeting blamed the carelessness of the people for spreading the disease. Even the moderate groups, however, were not in sympathy with the Health Department, which, it was felt, had lost the confidence of the people and was thus no longer competent to deal with health emergencies.[25]

The activity in the Eleventh Ward diminished the effectiveness of the Health Department. Kempster himself admitted that although smallpox had been under control before the riots, quarantine was impossible and the spread of the disease inevitable since the mobs began roaming the streets.[26] Vaccinations, although freely available, were often rejected. During the violence on the South Side the daily work of the Health Department virtually came to a halt. Patients could not be removed to the hospital in the face of weapon-wielding mobs; patients from other wards in the city could not be transported to the hospital through the hostile Eleventh Ward.[27] Kempster was denounced for attempting to remove patients to the hospital, and further denounced when failure to remove such patients resulted in the spread of the epidemic.

To a meeting of concerned physicians and businessmen, he voiced his frustrations:

> The laws are not enforced because the Common Council has prevented me. Not a single proposition that I have made . . . has been acted upon. . . . Proposition after proposition has been made to revise the laws as they now are. This has caused opposition among the people. We come to a house to remove a patient and are resisted. They tell us that their alderman informed them that next week the laws will be changed and they need not go. I have been tied hand and foot with investigations, injunctions and work that is never finished.[28]

At the beginning of September, with the opening of school, the coming of cooler weather, and increased police action against the rioters, the roving mobs on the South Side became less visible. The focus of the anti-Kempster movement changed from street action to the Common Council, as that body took up the battle in earnest.

Alderman Rudolph maintained a hold on his constituency and leadership of the mass movement against the Health Department by his actions and inflammatory rhetoric within the Common Coun-

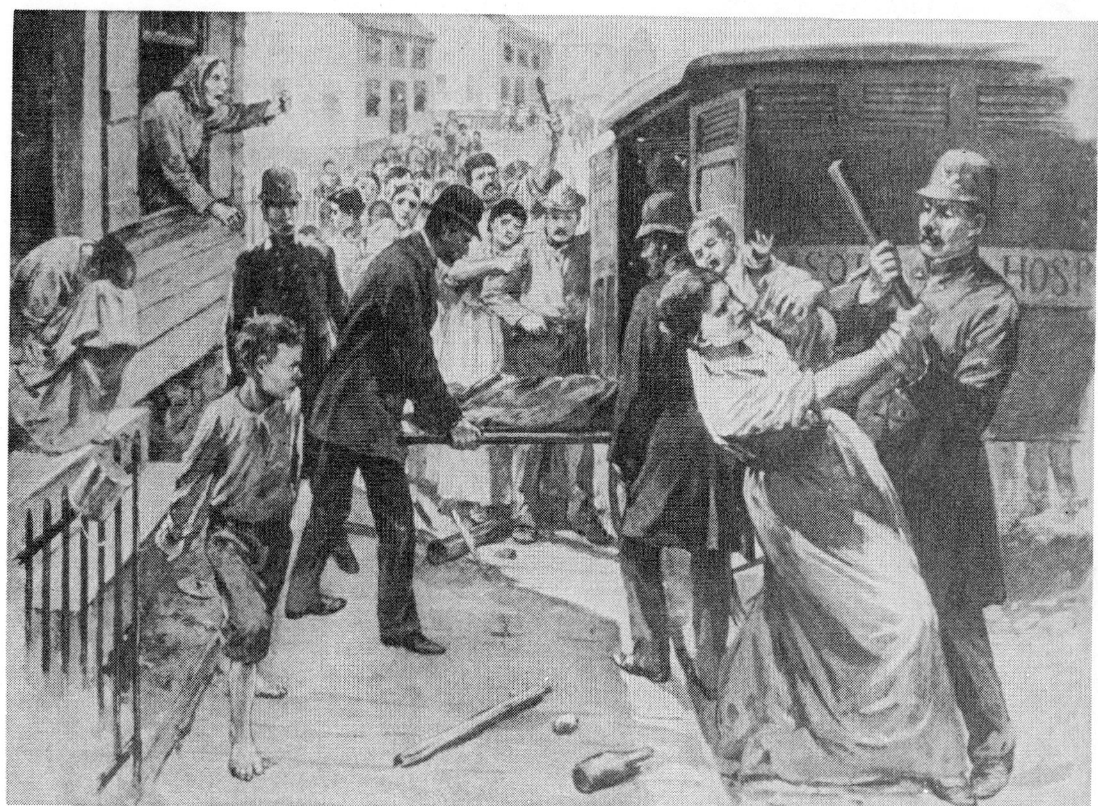

State Historical Society of Wisconsin

Fig. 2. "Smallpox troubles in Milwaukee." From *Leslie's Weekly Illustrated Newspaper*, Sept. 27, 1894, *79*: 207. I am grateful to Martin S. Pernick and Janet S. Numbers for help in locating this illustration.

cil. There he introduced resolution after resolution and ordinance after ordinance, each one concerned with limiting the power of the Health Department and Walter Kempster. As a member of the Council Health Committee and as a close friend of Council President William G. Rauschenberger, Rudolph had considerable influence over health measures in the council.

Beginning with the measures introduced on August 6 attempting to limit Kempster's power to remove patients to the hospital, Rudolph's actions crescendoed as the epidemic itself increased in intensity. In early September, he introduced an ordinance designed to accomplish what his earlier resolution could not: legally to tie the hands of the Health Commissioner by not allowing him to remove patients without their consent. The ordinance, revised slightly, passed the council and became law.[29]

Part of Rudolph's success in passing this ordinance was due to his scare tactics. The only member of the council in daily touch with the rioters, he promised renewed violence if the council did not pass his measure. He emoted loud and long on the injustices of tearing a child from its mother's breast. And he convinced his fellow politicians that voters would not be happy unless this measure passed. Council President Rauschenberger, who also thought Kempster incapable of handling the epidemic, actively supported Rudolph.[30]

In October, with the epidemic still raging about the city, Rudolph called for a special investigating committee to inquire into Kempster's activities, listing 34 charges against him.[31] The main charges were that Kempster had been negligent of his duties in the management of the Isolation Hospital, that he showed ignorance of quarantine methods, that patients were removed from their homes when they could have been better taken care of at their residences, and that the Health Department had grown tyrannical.[32] Twenty-eight physicians, including some of the more "prominent" physicians in the city, signed testimonials of misconduct on the part of the Health Commissioner.[33] Rudolph's charges were a serious matter.

Rudolph himself was appointed chairman of the council's committee to investigate the charges. The impeachment proceedings were front-page news in all the city's newspapers. Although most English-language papers declared that the investigation was a "farce" since it was led by so prejudiced a man, even the friendly *Sentinel* agreed that there was a need to clear the air.[34] The German-language press, on the other hand, endorsed Rudolph from the start and fully supported the impeachment proceedings.[35]

Rudolph's allies included the Anti-Vaccination Society, the German-language press, and the South Side activists. There were many physicians among this group. Their leader was Dr. Emil Wahl, a German physician with a successful South Side practice. Dr. Wahl was a member of the Milwaukee Medical Society (although he resigned from that organization when it accepted Kempster as a member), and his accusations that Kempster was incompetent to deal with the epidemic could not be dealt with lightly.[36]

There were genuine differences among physicians about the treatment of smallpox patients, as there had been on the vaccination issue. The division in the medical community was one between men of good faith, similarly trained, who used the tools of their profession to come to opposing conclusions. Dr. Wahl may or may not have been politically motivated to speak publicly against Dr. Kempster, but this does not necessarily mean that his medical disagreements were less real. His arguments were serious ones, which the medical community seriously debated. Wahl's principal complaint was that Kempster was responsible for discharging patients from the hospital while they were still contagious, thus aiding the spread of the disease. The debate centered on the condition of the smallpox pustule at the various stages.

The epidemic reached its height during the month of October, when the impeachment hearings began. South Side physicians, led by Emil Wahl, gave testimony about patients who had been prematurely dismissed from the hospital. Kempster's cross-examination of these witnesses attempted to show their lack of familiarity with the disease and their inability to recognize its contagious states.[37] Witnesses also included South Side families who felt wronged by the Health Department because it had attempted to remove their relatives to the hospital. It was claimed that Kempster had attempted to remove one patient who was not even ill with smallpox. A nurse who had served at the Isolation Hospital charged that the institution was mismanaged, that screens were not kept on the windows, and that its water supply was not adequate. In answering the charges against him, Kempster continued to deny any wrongdoing. The testimony of many leading physicians, including officers of the State Board of Health, supported him. The Milwaukee Medical Society also backed Kempster during the investigation. The Health Commissioner was obviously better able to withstand the public condemnations because of his medical colleagues' approval.[38]

Judging that nine of the original 34 charges were sustained by the testimony, the investigation committee recommended conviction. Speculation ran high in the city about the council vote on the impeachment question, with newspapers predicting the decision. Daily shifts of various aldermen were front-page headlines. The council heard the relevant testimony for three days and nights consecutively. The exhausted aldermen were eager to be finished with the whole business. As the council neared the vote, its president complained: "I am at a loss to know whether we are attending a circus or a session of the Common Council." Excitement ran high, interruptions were frequent, and disorder was rampant. Finally, in February 1895, with the epidemic not yet over, the council voted 22 to 14 to dismiss the Health Commissioner.[39]

Although the impeachment vote did not divide along party lines, the move against Kempster was nonetheless political. Patronage, class, and ethnic divisions were responsible for a significant part of the opposition to Kempster in the city. Physicians who sought his post or appointments within the Health Department were disappointed and resentful of the man who held office, and Republican politicians were bitter because of their loss of influence in department appointments.[40] From the beginning of his tenure in office, Kempster had labored against a vocal opposition. When the epidemic struck the city, the opposition had a weapon to use to successfully resist the health officer. The issue of the Isolation Hospital was one which carried with it a tradition of anxiety and fear and was easily employed to gather support against Kempster. The issue of forcible removal of children from their homes was one that pulled at the heartstrings of every immigrant parent.

The *Sentinel* termed the movement against Kempster a "cabal," and although it might be hard to document such a conspiracy, there is no question that Kempster's position in Milwaukee, while it may have been medically sound, was politically untenable. He had few friends and many enemies on the Common Council.[41]

Ethnic divisions in the city were evident from the differences in reactions between the English-language papers which supported Kempster and the German-language press which rejoiced over his dismissal.[42] Analysis of the impeachment vote shows that the ethnic divisions within the city held. Those wards which contained large numbers of German and Polish immigrants, or their descendants, were those which sustained the impeachment vote. Those wards which were largely populated by American-born, or by immigrant groups other than German and Polish, voted for Kempster. Party affiliations did not determine the vote, since both Democrats and Republicans on the council were split. Figure 3 illustrates the close correlation between German and Polish ethnicity and the vote against Kempster.[43]

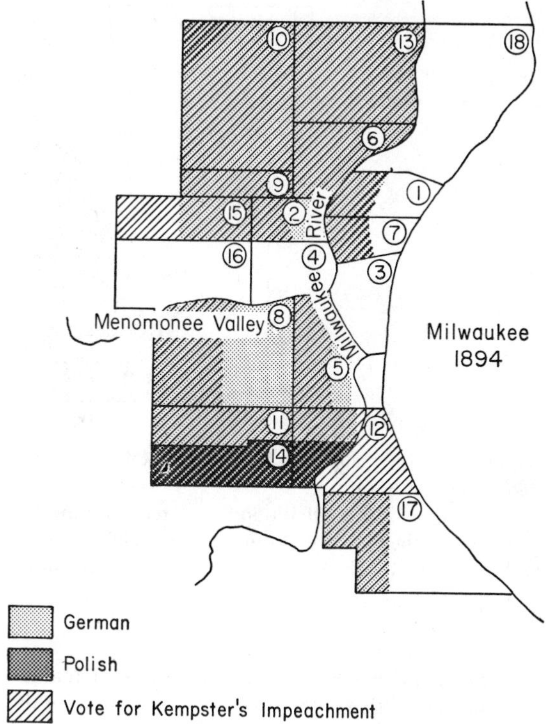

Fig. 3. Ethnic vote for Kempster's impeachment.

The smallpox epidemic of 1894 severely divided the city of Milwaukee, causing political conflicts and resentments which were long lived. Most significantly for our interest, it had a retrogressive effect on public health in Milwaukee. Traditionally, epidemics were times when health authorities increased their powers. This had been true in Milwaukee and in other American cities. In 1894 in Milwaukee the opposite happened. During the height of the epidemic, with fear running high, the council repealed those health measures which were seen as effective in halting the spread of the disease and fired the physician who supported those techniques. As Figure 4 illustrates, the moves against Kempster were all initiated while the epidemic was still raging in the city. Within the space of the ten months from May 1894, when Dr. Kempster took office, to February 1895, when he was dismissed, the Common Council deprived the Health Department of some of the powers important for it to be effective, and ultimately deprived the Health Commissioner of his job. Kempster appealed the impeachment decision and was reinstated as Health Commissioner after one year. The episode, however, affected the Health Department permanently. It never regained powers lost during the tumultuous 1894 smallpox epidemic.[44]

Milwaukee's history with the disease illustrates the political nature of the issue of smallpox control. Slowly through the century the Health Department had gained confidence and control over the treatment of smallpox, until by 1894 it felt secure in its powers. But in that year, during a severe epidemic, the Common Council challenged and in part took away the most traditional of all Health Department functions — the ability to control epidemic diseases. Political issues, only some of which were directly related to smallpox, determined how the municipal government handled the medical emergency.

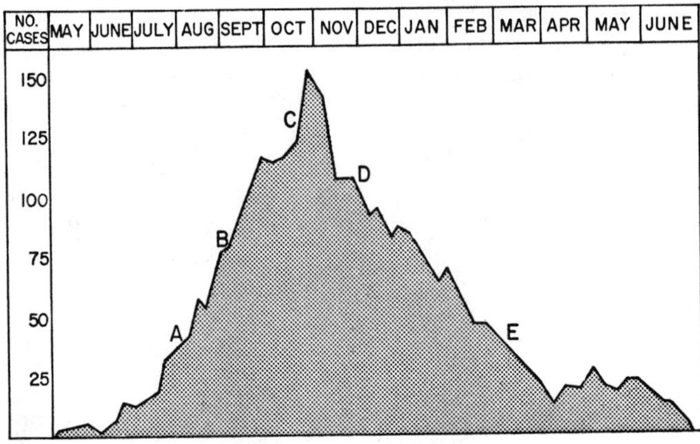

Fig. 4. Cases of smallpox in Milwaukee, 1894–1895, and moves against Kempster.

A. August 6, 1894. Resolution on forcible removal.
B. September 4, 1894. Ordinance on forcible removal.
C. October 15, 1894. Resolution for impeachment investigation; revised ordinance on forcible removal.
D. November 26, 1894. Revised ordinance on forcible removal passed.
E. February 21, 1895. Common Council impeaches Health Commissioner.

NOTES

This is a revised version of a paper presented at the annual meeting of the American Association for the History of Medicine, Philadelphia, Pennsylvania, May 1, 1975. The research was aided in part by a Maurice L. Richardson Fellowship from the University of Wisconsin.

1 Charles Rosenberg, studying the effects of cholera epidemics on American cities, noted: "The cholera epidemics of the nineteenth century provided much of the impetus needed to overcome centuries of governmental inertia and indifference in regard to problems of public health . . . . It is not surprising that the growing public health movement found in cholera an effective ally." *The Cholera Years: The United States in 1832, 1849 and 1866* (Chicago: Univ. of Chicago Press, 1962), pp. 2–3. See also John Duffy, who posits that cholera and yellow fever were "important factors in promoting public health measures," because of their "crisis" presentation. "Social impact of disease in the late nineteenth century," *Bull. N.Y. Acad. Med.*, 1971, *47*: 800 [see pp. 395–402 in this book]. Although Duffy saw smallpox running a poor third to cholera and yellow fever, in Milwaukee smallpox took the place of the former two diseases, which did not threaten the city after 1850. I make the parallel with cholera and yellow fever despite the major differences between those diseases and smallpox, the availability of a preventative for one and not the others. While vaccination raises interesting differences between the examples used here, those differences did not affect the public reaction evoked in each case: fear and panic and an immediate governmental response to alleviate conditions.

2 Smallpox first appeared in Milwaukee in 1843, and reappeared three years later in virulent form. A major epidemic occurred in 1868, immediately after the Board of Health was established, and was responsible for establishing certain power patterns which were to remain throughout the century. During the 1870s Milwaukee suffered two major outbreaks of smallpox. Despite the fact that smallpox was never a major cause of death in Milwaukee, it aroused more interest on the part of the public authorities and was responsible for more public health legislation than any other disease.

3 See Martin Kaufman, "The American antivaccinationists and their arguments," *Bull. Hist. Med.*, 1967, *41*: 463–478. Kaufman describes most antivaccinationists as irregular practitioners, and identifies the movement with sectarian medicine. It is not clear to me that that division holds in Milwaukee, where many regularly trained physicians were hesitant about the protective value of vaccination throughout the 19th century.

4 *Ibid.*, p. 474. Kaufman also noticed the prevalence of strong antivaccinationist sentiment among the immigrants, specifically among the German immigrants. Not only were immigrants in Milwaukee vocal against vaccination, but other governmental

health activities also drew their wrath. Placarding a home containing an infectious disease, removing sick to an isolation hospital, requiring private night burials, were all seen by newly arrived Germans and Poles as direct infringements on their personal liberties and were vigorously resisted in Milwaukee. For more on this reaction of Milwaukee immigrants, see my Ph.D. dissertation, "Public health in Milwaukee 1867–1910" (Univ. of Chicago, 1975). The reaction was found throughout the state of Wisconsin. See, for example, the *6th Annual Report of the State Board of Health of Wisconsin, 1881*, pp. 116, 120; and the *15th Annual Report of the State Board of Health of Wisconsin, 1894–1895*, pp. 138–139, 163.

5 For more on Milwaukee's economy see Bayard Still, *Milwaukee: The History of a City* (Madison: The State Historical Society of Wisconsin, 1965) and Roger David Simon, "The expansion of an industrial city: Milwaukee, 1880–1910," (unpublished Ph.D. dissertation, Univ. of Wisconsin-Madison, 1971).

6 On the German population of Milwaukee and its assimilation, see Gerd Korman, *Industrialization, Immigrants and Americanizers: The View from Milwaukee 1866–1921* (Madison: The State Historical Society of Wisconsin, 1967) and Kathleen Neils Conzen, "The German Athens: Milwaukee and the accommodation of its immigrants, 1836–1860," (unpublished Ph.D. dissertation, Univ. of Wisconsin-Madison, 1972).

7 Walter Kempster had only small ties of any kind to the city of Milwaukee. He had a national reputation as physician to the insane and had held posts at the State Lunatic Asylum at Utica, New York, and at the Northern Hospital for the Insane, at Oshkosh, Wisconsin. He had testified for the prosecution in the Guiteau case. He had moved to Milwaukee in 1890, but since that time had been on two missions abroad studying cholera and investigating Jewish emigration from Russia. His tenure in the city of Milwaukee, his critics were quick to point out, had been short indeed. For biographical material on Walter Kempster see the *Dictionary of American Biography* (New York: Charles Scribner's Sons, 1933) X, 324–325; Howard Kelly and Walter Burrage, *American Medical Biographies* (Baltimore: The Norman, Remington Co., 1920), pp. 652–653; and most thoroughly, F. M. Sperry, *A Group of Distinguished Physicians and Surgeons of Milwaukee* (Chicago: J. H. Beers & Co., 1904), pp. 56–69. See also Kempster's obituary, *Milwaukee Sentinel*, Aug. 23, 1918, and the *New York Times*, Aug. 23, 1918, p. 9. Kempster was buried in Arlington National Cemetery.

8 *Milwaukee Sentinel*, April 17, 18, 24, 30, 1894.

9 Eight Republicans opposed and five Democrats supported Kempster. Without Democratic support, the Republican nominee would not have been confirmed. Milwaukee *Common Council Proceedings*, April 30, 1894. See also the *Milwaukee Sentinel*, May 1, 1894.

10 *Milwaukee Sentinel*, June 12, 26, 1894; Milwaukee *Common Council Proceedings*, June 11, 1894, p. 132; May 14, 1894, p. 61.

11 *17th Annual Report of the Milwaukee Health Department, 1894*, pp. 26–32; *19th Annual Report of the Milwaukee Health Department, 1895*, pp. 10–12; *18th and 19th Annual Report of the Health Department, 1895*, pp. 35–39; *Milwaukee Sentinel*, June 28, July 4, 1894. Physicians were urged to cooperate with health officials in reporting the disease. The Health Commissioner closed schools when he thought it necessary. See the *Milwaukee Sentinel*, Sept. 2, 3, Nov. 3, 13, 24, 1894. See also the Milwaukee *School Board Proceedings*, Nov. 6, 1894, pp. 124–125.

12 At least two German-language newspapers argued that vaccination did not protect against smallpox and that its effects were often worse than the disease it was to prevent. The Anti-Vaccination Society disseminated its information through pamphlets widely circulated in three languages. *Milwaukee Sentinel*, Aug. 1, 1894.

13 *Milwaukee Sentinel*, July 23, 1894. See also, July 24, 1894.

14 *Milwaukee Sentinel*, Aug. 3, 4, 6, 1894. The antihospital sentiment expressed by residents of the South Side reopened a familiar Milwaukee debate about moving the hospital outside the city limits. The issue flared up, encompassed much time for the city's legal staff, and was finally dropped at the end of the summer. Most physicians were against removal from the city limits, as long-distance travel was not seen as beneficial to an acutely ill patient, nor was it convenient for physicians.

15 The theory of air-borne contagion is not yet disproved as one way in which the smallpox virus might travel. It has also been shown that flies have acted as vectors in spreading the disease. See Cyril W. Dixon, *Smallpox* (London: J & A Churchill, 1962), p. 264. This theory was supported at the time because the Eleventh Ward was, in fact, the main seat of infection in the city. Certainly, popular opinion very strongly blamed the Isolation Hospital for the large number of smallpox cases on the South Side. See the *Milwaukee Sentinel*, Aug. 4, 1894.

16 The mother is quoted in the *Milwaukee Sentinel*, Aug. 6, 1894. For more on the episode, see the *18th and 19th Annual Report of the Milwaukee Health Department, 1895*, pp. 42–43. For a brief popularized account of the riots, see Richard L. Stefanik, "The smallpox riots of 1894," *Historical Messenger*, December 1970, pp. 123–128.

17 Milwaukee *Common Council Proceedings*, Aug. 6, 1894, p. 326. See also the *Milwaukee Sentinel*, Aug. 7, 1894; and the *18th and 19th Annual Report of the Milwaukee Health Department, 1895*, pp. 41–42. The initial ordinance had been passed in reaction to a cholera scare in the city in 1892, and had never been used.

18 For more on the August 7 rally, see the *Milwaukee Daily News*, a workingman's newspaper, which tended to support the rioters, but not the riots in early August. "There is reason to believe that there has been some basis for the many criticisms . . . made" (Aug. 8, 1894). The *Sentinel*, however, was quick to blame the "ignorance of the people" in not following existing health regulations and in defying authorities (Aug. 8, 1894).

19 *Milwaukee Sentinel*, Aug. 7, 1894.

20 Quoted in the *Milwaukee Daily News*, Aug. 11, 1894.

21 Out of a total of 1,074 cases, 846 were from South Side Wards — half of these were from the Eleventh Ward.

22 *Milwaukee Sentinel*, Aug. 9, 1894.

23 *Milwaukee Sentinel*, Aug. 30, 1894. For more on the role of women in the rioting, see the *Sentinel*, Aug. 10, 12, 1894; and the *Milwaukee Daily News*, Aug. 10, 1894.

24 For details about the involvement of the State Board of Health, see the *Wisconsin State Board of Health Report, 1893–1894*, "Report of the Executive Committee relative to the smallpox situation in the City of Milwaukee," pp. 56–69; U. O. B. Wingate, "Smallpox in Wisconsin from January 1894 to June 1895," *Public Health: Papers and Reports of the American Public Health Association*, 1896, *21*: 268–272; and the *18th and 19th Annual Report of the Milwaukee Health Department, 1895*, pp. 49–58; and the *Milwaukee Sentinel*, Aug. 11, 12, 14, 1894.

25 *Milwaukee Sentinel*, Aug. 12, 14, 1894.

26 *Milwaukee Sentinel*, Aug. 12, 1894.

27 *Evening Wisconsin*, Aug. 29, 1894.

28 Quoted in the *Sentinel*, Oct. 23, 1894.

29 Milwaukee *Common Council Proceedings*, Sept. 4, Oct. 1, Nov. 26, 1894. See a copy of the ordinance as passed in the Appendix to the 1894–1895 *Proceedings*, pp. 22–23. Section I provided: "The commissioner of health shall not remove to any Isolation Hospital in said city any child or person suffering from any such disease who can be nursed and cared for during such illness in his or her home during the continuance of the disease except upon the recommendation and advice of the said commissioner of health or one of the assistant commissioners of health, and the physician, if any, attending upon such child or person, not being a member of the health department of said city; and in case such commissioner, or assistant commissioner and such physician shall be unable to agree as to the advisability of removing such child or person, then they shall call in and appoint another physician not a member of the health department, and the decision of the majority of such physicians and commissioner or assistant commissioner shall be decisive of the question. The third physician called in, as above provided, shall not receive or be entitled to any fees from the city for consultation or service in the decision of the case submitted to such board of physicians." The conditions were so burdensome they effectively tied the hands of a health commissioner attempting to act swiftly to stem an epidemic.

30 *Milwaukee Sentinel*, Sept. 4, 5, Oct. 2, 6, 7, 9, Dec. 2, 1894. *Evening Wisconsin*, Oct. 8, 1894. See also *18th and 19th Annual Report of the Milwaukee Health Department, 1895*, p. 69; and the Milwaukee *Common Council Proceedings*, Sept. 4, 1894.

31 Milwaukee *Common Council Proceedings*, Oct. 15, 1894, pp. 524–531. Although the two actions discussed here, ordinances for the removal of patients and impeachment, were not the only ones Alderman Rudolph initiated against the Health Commissioner, they were the most important, and thus form the focus of the discussion here. For additional measures the council considered at Rudolph's initiation, see *Common Council Proceedings*, Aug. 20, 1894, pp. 364–365; Sept. 4, 1894, pp. 374–375; Oct. 15, 1894, p. 497; Oct. 29, 1894, p. 571; Nov. 12, 1894, p. 583. See also the *Milwaukee Sentinel*, Aug. 21, Sept. 1, Oct. 2, 13, 1894.

32 *Milwaukee Sentinel*, Oct. 16, 1894.

33 Of the 28, at least 19 were members of the local medical society, the State Medical Association or the American Medical Association. See the membership list of the Milwaukee Medical Society and the local A.M.A. members in the archives of the Milwaukee Academy of Medicine. The membership list of the State Medical Society was in the *Wisconsin Medical Journal*, 1903–1904, pp. 196–208. At least two of the physicians had been brought to court by Kempster, charged with not reporting smallpox, which might account for their hostile position.

34 See the *Milwaukee Sentinel, Daily News*, and *Evening Wisconsin*, *passim*, Oct. 15, 1894, to Feb. 21, 1895. See, for example, editorial of Jan. 5, 1895, in the *Sentinel* entitled, "The farce continued." Other newspapers voiced similar sentiments. The (Milwaukee) *Catholic Citizen* ridiculed the matter of putting the "prosecuting attorney on the bench as the judge of the case" (Oct. 20, 1894).

35 See, for example, *Seebote* and *Herold*, *passim*, in these months.

36 For biographical material on Emil Wahl, see Louis Frank, *The Medical History of Milwaukee 1834–1914*

(Milwaukee: Germania Press, 1915), p. 72. He appears on the membership list of the Milwaukee Medical Society, having joined the organization in 1888. For more on Wahl's resignation, see the Milwaukee Medical Society minutes, Jan. 22, 1895, and Feb. 12, 1895, in the archives of the Milwaukee Academy of Medicine.

37 *Milwaukee Sentinel*, Nov. 15, 16, 17, 28, 29; Dec. 4, 5, 1894; Jan. 4–16, 1895. See also the *Milwaukee Journal*, Jan. 4–10, 1895.

38 At a joint meeting, Medical Society members and business leaders hissed Rudolph's name while loudly cheering Kempster's. See the *Sentinel*, Oct. 23, 1894. The transcripts of the impeachment proceedings are, unfortunately, lost, and it is impossible to discern the technical aspects of the medical debate from the newspaper accounts.

39 For the press assessment of how the vote would be, see the *Sentinel*, Feb. 14, 15, 16, 18, 1895; *Journal*, Feb. 18, 1895; and the *Daily News*, Feb. 18, 1895. See a description of the final session in the *Journal*, Feb. 21, 1895; *Sentinel*, Feb. 21, 1895.

40 For contemporary arguments along these lines, see the *Milwaukee Sentinel*, Aug. 30, 31, Sept. 2, 4, 1894, Feb. 20, 22, 1895, Jan. 21, 1896; *Daily News*, Aug. 31, 1894; *Journal*, Feb. 19, 1895; *Catholic Citizen*, Sept. 8, 1894.

41 *Milwaukee Sentinel*, Feb. 22, 1895.

42 See, for example, the editorial in the *Herold*, Feb. 22, 1895, in which it noted: "The decision of the Common Council . . . will be received by the great majority of the population with satisfaction. It is the confirmation of many months' experience and the conviction that [Kempster] is not the right man to execute those measures necessary in the case of an epidemic . . . . [He] is not master of the situation and could not awaken the general trust which is, after all, in such a case, a necessary prerequisite." I am grateful to Edith Hoshino Altbach for help in translating this editorial.

43 The sources of ethnicity were the *Eleventh United States Census*, 1890, and the 1895 *Wisconsin State Census*. Precise population figures by ethnic group were not available by ward.

44 See the *Milwaukee Sentinel*, Jan. 18, 1896. For a copy of the judge's decision, see the *18th and 19th Annual Report, 1895*, pp. 81–85.

30

Social Policy and City Politics: Tuberculosis Reporting in New York, 1889–1900

DANIEL M. FOX

In 1901, Dr. Robert Koch of Berlin complained to Dr. Hermann Biggs of New York about opposition among German physicians to a proposed law requiring "compulsory reporting of such cases of tuberculosis as are in a communicable state." Nineteen years after isolating the tubercle bacillus, Koch found the implications of his research for public policy better developed in New York City than in his own country. "I wish to cite the example of the free American people," he told Biggs, a dominant figure in public health in New York, "who of their own free will accepted the limitation of their own liberties in the interest of the public health."[1]

Similarly, Sir Robert Philip, a leader in tuberculosis control in the United Kingdom, recalled that, in 1890, "I pressed strongly for compulsory notification of tuberculosis . . . . Yet more than twenty years passed before compulsory notification became the law of the land." Nowhere "has a more thorough plan of action been instituted than in the city of New York," Sir Robert said in 1908.[2]

By the 1890s Americans were accustomed to praise and envy from abroad for their enterprise, invention, and, increasingly, for achievements in science, scholarship, and the arts. It is not surprising to historians, just as it did not surprise contemporaries, that New York, the second largest city in the world, received attention for establishing the first diagnostic research laboratory in bacteriology administered by an agency of government. The laboratory was a superb technical innovation, a medico-scientific and political counterpart to the Brooklyn Bridge. But the innovation in public social policy praised by Koch and Philip and used as a model in the United States and abroad is not explained by conventional views of American society and public life.

American municipal government in the 1890s usually excited scorn, not envy, from leading men of science and public affairs at home and abroad. New York City in particular was generally held to be dominated by the limited and venal goals of the Tammany political machine led by Richard Croker. It is unusual to discover New York City pioneering in the use of the coercive power of government to protect citizens' health. The story of tuberculosis notification in New York suggests that American municipal reformers and their subsequent historians have too readily accepted James Bryce's supercilious judgment that municipal government constituted the most conspicuous failure in America.[3]

To public health advocates in the 1890s, notification for contagious or communicable disease was a necessary first step in effective social policy to protect the public's health. Notification provided essential epidemiological data and information about the acceptance of bacteriology among physicians. More important, the reports triggered subsequent activities by either private or public organizations. In tuberculosis control these activities included regular investigation and disinfection of sickrooms, education of patients and their families, removal of patients to sanatoria or hospitals, and supervision of sanitary precautions in factories and shops. Private physicians would provide or coordinate these services for more affluent citizens, particularly when threatened with public assumption of neglected responsibilities. The State, it was gen-

---

DANIEL M. FOX is Professor of Humanities in Medicine and Assistant Vice President for Academic Affairs, Health Sciences Center, State University of New York at Stony Brook.

Reprinted with permission from the *Bulletin of the History of Medicine*, 1975, *49*: 169–195.

erally agreed, was only obligated to provide direct services to the poor.[4]

The usual explanation for the primacy of New York City in tuberculosis control is derived from the concept of an idea whose time has come. A generation after Koch's discovery, public policy in Europe and the United States was based on the need to discover, report, and control the bacillus. The inevitable happened first in New York mainly because of the statesmanship of Dr. Hermann M. Biggs and a few of his medical colleagues.[5] A corollary interpretation contrasts the sorry state of general government in New York with the "unyielding integrity and forward looking altruism" of a group of physicians "waging a crusade for public health." The corrupt men who ran all of city government except the Health Department were either baffled or impressed by these virtuous men of science.[6]

This interpretation, caricatured for argument, is suspect on analytical and factual grounds. It is anachronistic to read the 20th-century consensus about the etiology of tuberculosis into the events of the 1890s. Reasonable men disagreed about the validity and, more important, the interpretation of the research stimulated by Koch's discovery. Moreover, the eventual acceptance of compulsory notification as part of public social policy everywhere does not explain how and why New York City took precedence by more than a decade. Similar debates had different political results in other places.

The implication that scientific medicine neutralized the political process is suspect. Scientific knowledge is not transformed into policy and administrative arrangements without the conflict and bargaining that generally characterize the governmental process. It is difficult to explain why the control of some diseases, some hazards to health, should be placed above or aside from general politics while other concerns should, to the dismay of reformers, be part of the calculus of political interests. Tuberculosis, it may be urged, was exceptional: a major killer, a constant cause of anxiety. But so were alcoholism, adulterated food, and unsafe and unsanitary streets. Perhaps these evils are different from tuberculosis less because the disease agent is not a bacillus than because of differences in the strategies of political and community organization brought to the issues since the 1890s.

The conventional interpretation is also contradicted by data. Biggs' influence was a result of skillful use of the tools of conventional politics. With jobs and money to supplement the appeal of scientific medicine, he led an expanding constituency among New York physicians. The medical opponents of compulsory notification were similarly adept. The struggle for position, place and policy around the issues raised by tuberculosis control is of historical interest because it exemplifies the use of the techniques of the closed politics of bureaucracies and professional organizations to achieve measures for the general welfare.

I

In May 1889, Commissioner of Health Dr. Joseph Bryant asked the department's consulting pathologists, Drs. Biggs, T. Mitchell Prudden, and Horace P. Loomis to report on tuberculosis. The report was timed to take advantage of the appointment of a new, sympathetic, and politically astute president of the Board of Health, Charles G. Wilson, an eminent corporation lawyer. The pathologists asserted the validity of Koch's findings and declared tuberculosis both a "distinctly preventable disease" and "in very many cases a distinctly curable affection."[7]

Prevention and cure required Health Department action to inspect cattle, educate citizens in preventive methods, and disinfect rooms occupied by tuberculous patients. Compulsory notification of the department by physicians who diagnosed cases of the disease was advocated by the pathologists in an early draft of the report. But the proposal was dropped, on Bryant's advice, after informal political and medical screening of the idea by several leading physicians indicated intense opposition.[8] The final report was accepted without significant controversy by the leading medical organizations in the city and both the professional and lay press.[9] Ten thousand copies were circulated.

Compulsory notification for cases of pulmonary tuberculosis diagnosed in public institutions was instituted four years later, in the winter of 1893–94. Physicians in private practice were "requested to notify" the department of all cases of the disease. A special group of medical inspectors to administer the new regulations were appointed by the department the following year.[10] More important, the municipal laboratory, under the direction of Biggs and Dr. William Hallock Park, began to offer free sputum examinations to induce physicians to report suspected cases.[11] As in 1889, there was general praise for these innovations among the physicians quoted in the press and active in professional organizations.[12]

When notification of the department by physicians was made compulsory for all cases of pulmonary tuberculosis in January 1897, strong protests were made at medical meetings and in the press. Patients' rights and physicians' obligations and livelihoods were threatened, it was alleged, by this abuse of the police power of the state. Resolutions were passed; threats were made about legislative combat to restrict the powers of the Health Department; personal slurs on Biggs and his associates were spoken more publicly than is customary in medical politics.[13] At the height of the controversy, Prudden described the opposition to Dr. E. G. Trudeau, as the "little scattering gang of purps" who longed for the "good old times when a patient with tuberculosis could be lulled into a sense of security for a few months more."[14] Biggs, always aggressive but usually restricting his attacks to physicians' ideas rather than their personal traits, ascribed the opposition to "timidity, selfishness, ignorance" — a trinity he later softened to "tradition, prejudice, and sentiment."[15]

A compromise which both deferred and made inevitable the achievement of compulsory notification was negotiated by Prudden and his successor as president of the Academy of Medicine, Dr. E. G. Janeway. The compromise included delay in the enforcement of compulsory notification and more formal and frequent consultation between the Department of Health and leaders of the medical profession. Penalties for failure to notify were enforced selectively over the decade.[16] By 1907, when the Board of Health extended the notification requirement to all forms of tuberculosis, the achievements of the public health physicians and their supporters, and the international recognition they received, were matters of pride and self-congratulation to the medical profession of New York City.[17]

Notification did not impose severe administrative burdens on physicians and only violated the confidentiality of their relationship with low-income patients. Initial and yearly follow-up reports were made on postcards supplied by the Health Department. Inspectors were sent only on physicians' request, or when the patient lived in a tenement or lodging house. When cases were reported by citizens or by employees of other departments and charitable organizations, the department's inspector first tried to locate and confer with the patients' physicians.[18]

Enforcement of compulsory notification was cautious and selective, as specified in the Prudden-Janeway compromise. The strategy was "to continually increase the strictness of enforcement," Biggs recalled in 1909. Physicians who failed to report cases which appeared as tuberculosis on death certificates received letters calling attention to the law and asking for an explanation of the discrepancy. Several physicians were summoned before the Board of Health to explain their negligence.[19] Apparently a few were "defiant." During the first decade of the compulsory notification, Biggs reported in 1907, six recalcitrant physicians were fined between 50 and 200 dollars each.[20]

The public health advocates were satisfied that reporting was increasingly accurate as a result of the spread of scientific knowledge among physicians and patients, gentle peer pressure, and the inducement of free sputum examinations. In the 1897 controversy, the advocates of notification ignored charges that even dispensary physicians disregarded the 1893 regulations. By 1902, the department claimed that two-thirds of the cases in Manhattan and the Bronx were reported. In 1908, Biggs estimated that reporting was 90 percent accurate. Both estimates were, however, speculative.[21]

Notification was generally justified by citing encouraging statistics about the number of cases reported and the decline in the death rate from tuberculosis. The number of new cases reported increased from 8,559 in 1898 to 32,065 in 1910, when the total of known cases was 70,260, the highest ever recorded in the city. The number of sputum examinations increased from 2,920 in 1898 to approximately 40,000 in 1910. During this time the total population of the city increased by a smaller percentage, about one-third. More important, the death rate from tuberculosis maintained the decline that had begun around 1880 and appeared to have accelerated because of the public health campaigns of the 1890s. Historians and epidemiologists are uncertain about the causes of the declining incidence of tuberculosis in the 20th century. But public officials and leaders of voluntary associations at the turn of the century had good reason to take most of the credit for it.[22]

Statistical data, combined with new bacteriological knowledge, encouraged strategists in the first campaigns against tuberculosis in New York to press for measures for the general welfare of all social and ethnic groups in the city rather than special measures for the poor. In 1890, the year after the Department of Health declared the disease to be both preventable and curable, the disease was the most destructive killer in the city. In that year, 5,500 people died of tuberculosis; compared with 5,000 from pneumonia and just under 1,000 from cancer. Tuberculosis struck the young disproportionately; only a quarter of those dying of the disease were over 45 years of age. The most threatened group was males between the ages of 30 and 35.[23] Although the death rate declined steadily after 1880, population growth brought a steady increase in the total number of deaths from tuberculosis in the city. Not until 1925 did the total number of deaths from the disease in the city clearly begin to decline. Moreover, the ratio of deaths from tuberculosis to total deaths increased or remained constant until the second decade of this century.[24]

While tuberculosis threatened everyone in the city, the death rate in the poorest areas was almost twice what it was for the city as a whole. There was, however, considerable ethnic variation, a result less of degrees of poverty than of the resistance developed through exposure to the disease in the past generations. Black New Yorkers were most in jeopardy; Jews least. The Irish, Scottish, Bohemian, and Scandinavian groups were considerably more endangered than Italians. But native-born whites were more likely to succumb than either Hungarians or Russian Jews.[25]

Epidemiological statistics were useful for political arithmetic only if the perceptions of tuberculosis among physicians and laymen were also taken into account. When Koch announced the isolation of the bacillus in Berlin in 1882, many New York physicians were not convinced he had found the cause of a specific disease. The two leading medical colleges in the city taught contradictory doctrines: at one it was argued that the "development of tubercles was merely a symptom of various diseases"; at the other that tuberculosis was a single disease.[26] Many physicians were not impressed when, in 1883, T. Mitchell Prudden at the College of Physicians and Surgeons and Austin Flint, Sr., William H. Welch, and Biggs at the Bellevue Hospital Medical School published findings which confirmed Koch's work.[27]

There were strong arguments for the opinion that tuberculosis was a result of inherited constitutional traits. In the absence of agreement about the frame of reference with which to view clinical evidence, data that would later be regarded as confirming the bacterial origin of the disease were interpreted in support of the opposing view. These data included the presence of the disease in several generations of a family, the freedom from infection of many employees in hospitals for tuberculous patients, the transmission of the disease to spouses, and the lack of human infection from direct contact with meat from tuberculous cattle.[28]

Competing views of the etiology of tuberculosis provide a partial explanation for the debate among medical men about appropriate public policy to prevent and control the disease. The bacterial view meant, as contagionism had throughout history, state intervention in the lives of citizens: reporting, inspection, isolation — the administrative devices by which citizens are deprived of liberties in the interests of society. The hereditary view of the transmission of tuberculosis, on the other hand, justified public restraint. Tuberculosis, long a stigmatizing disease, seemed even more punishing to its victims as a result of the bureaucratic interference that followed from the theories of Koch and his followers.[29]

For middle- and working-class citizens of New York City in the 1890s the debate over compulsory notification involved major anxieties of daily life. They had to balance their instinctive contagionism, the traditions of folk medicine confirmed by science and popularized in the press, against their fear of the police power of the State. They weighed the desire to have all possible actions taken against the disease as early as possible against the fear that acknowledged tuberculosis, because it was an exclusion in most life insurance policies, would leave families destitute.[30]

The issues were equally intense for physicians. The controversy threatened present and future livelihood — not just income but the organization of medical practice and the perceptions of laity from which income, status, and self-esteem were derived. At a time when their incomes were declining and the profession was fluid to the point of chaos, the new public policy was threatening. Patients might shop for physicians who either did not report or, more likely, gave optimistic diagnoses.[31] City medical inspectors, checking on a physician's report or failure to report, might ask questions that would cause patients to question his judgment — questions leading, in at least one instance, to nonpayment of fees.[32] The impersonal laboratory would review and challenge judgments made on the basis of years of training and practice.[33] Patients and the fees physicians had earned from attending them at home would be absorbed by the growing apparatus of hospitals and sanatoria.[34] Privileged communication between physicians and patients, protected by a much-admired New York statute, might be eroded by administrative lawmaking.[35] Finally, in this atmosphere of anxiety and threat, there were grounds for general practitioners, more than 2,000 in the city, to fear that their incomes and freedom were under siege from a growing coalition of specialists, medical college faculty, and experts in public health.

II

The medical profession in New York in the 1890s was under both external and internal stress. The years 1893 to 1897, when the notification controversy was most bitter, were a time of severe economic depression. In 1893, the year voluntary reporting by private physicians was instituted, some 500 banks and 16,000 businesses failed across the nation. Estimates of unemployment in the winter of 1893–94 averaged about two million.[36] In New York the Board of Health reported 314 suicides, a record number.[37] More threatening to the collection of physicians' fees, Professor Richmond Mayo-Smith, a conservative statistician at Columbia University, reported to Mayor Thomas Gilroy in February 1894 that 48,681 families, made up of 206,701 individuals, reported one or more members of the household out of work. According to Mayo-Smith, 67,592 New Yorkers were unemployed.[38] In addition, 20,000 homeless vagrants strained the accommodations of police stations and philanthropic shelters. Less than a quarter of the manufacturing plants in the city operated at full capacity.[39]

Anxious physicians, feeling their status slipping as their incomes diminished, saw in tuberculosis reporting another example of what, in direct analogy to contemporary developments in the organization of commerce and industry, they regarded as vertical and horizontal combinations in restraint of trade. This attitude was a constant theme in addresses to medical organizations. "The improved condition of the public health," in particular the "eradication or limitation of disease by the Health Department of this City" contributed to the decline in physicians' incomes, Dr. Charles Phelps told the State Medical Association in 1898. Moreover, the public health physicians and their allies on the medical school faculties increasingly dominated public hospitals and dispensaries and even many small hospitals. Clinics, by eliminating means tests, were an artful abuse of charity designed to pauperize the affluent and distribute the best care below market cost. It was "naked application to the practice of medicine of the principle upon which mercantile trusts are founded." A recurrent American image, the welfare cheat, was evoked for medical audiences. Where phantom Cadillacs would later park, "dispensary patients leave their carriages and servants around the nearby corner of a street."[40] According to the president of the New York County Medical Society, 737,171 New Yorkers, 39 percent of the population, received free care in 1895.[41]

The general practitioners, or at least their spokesmen, also blamed their anxieties on the condition of the national economy, competition from unlicensed practitioners, fraternal undercutting of fees and unethical dispensing of pharmacists. The great medical coalition of the early 20th century cannot easily be discerned in the 1890s: the temporary union of academics, specialists and generalists to limit the size of the profession by reducing the number — or, to the same end, raising the quality — of medical schools.

New York medicine on the eve of the 20th century was fluid, chaotic, and riddled with factions. This disorganization may have been more influential than the mystique of modern science in enabling the innovations in tuberculosis control to occur.

The number of regular physicians in the city in any year in the 1890s can only be estimated. For 1894–1895, for example, most New York medical leaders claimed some 3,000 practitioners. More likely they meant the metropolitan area, since the *Medical Register: New York, New Jersey and Connecticut* lists that number for the area, but only about 2,000 as practicing in the city, then limited to Manhattan and the Bronx.[42]

The *Medical Register* reveals more of the fluidity of the profession than the carefully chosen words of the leaders of medical organizations and factions. The physicians listed included everyone eligible for membership in either of the two regulars' organizations, the County Society and the County Association. About 10 percent of the physicians in the city left New York, retired, or died each year in the decade. In 1895, for example, 195 physicians gave up practices in the city; 104 of these, about 5 percent, had not communicated their present addresses to their organizations or to the *Register*.[43]

The fluidity and uncertainty caused by turnover and disappearance was increased by the antagonism between the society and the association, at both county and state levels. The break, which lasted from 1882 to 1896, was, on one level, the result of disagreement about the consultation clause in the American Medical Association Code of Ethics. The A.M.A. code, reflecting its origin in the controversies of mid-century, prohibited consultation with sectarian practitioners. By the 1880s many New York physicians felt it to be both economically and therapeutically necessary to consult and be consulted by homeopaths. The state society liberalized the prohibition in 1882. As a result its delegates were refused seats at the annual meeting of the A.M.A. The leadership of the society was, however, ahead of the members: a subsequent mail ballot indicated that those physicians who voted preferred the A.M.A. code by a margin of two to one. But the numbers in each group were sufficient to sustain two state organizations and their county affiliates for 20 years.[44]

The organizers of the statewide challenge to the A.M.A., members of the New York County Society's Committee on Ethics were, however, playing for larger stakes than consultation with homeopaths. The New York City men sought to trade freedom to consult with homeopaths for more restraint on physicians' advertising and sale of proprietary secret remedies. They felt that legitimizing existing consultation practices was a small price to pay for greater control over the public behavior of physicians. Though the later stages of the controversy seemed to be entirely about homeopathy, the first resolutions introduced to the state society made the ethics of consultation secondary to the issue of restraining commercialization.[45]

The division between the society and the association, in addition to further fragmenting the profession, demonstrated a political principle that was valuable in the battle for notification of tuberculosis. In professional politics, a strong minority with access to sufficient patronage and publicity to sustain its members' livelihoods and respectability could achieve its goals just as surely as a majority coalition can in open politics. Professional stalemate makes prudent legislators neutral. There could be no intervention on behalf of the general public interest when even the New York Academy of Medicine, the most prestigious group of regular physicians in the state, first gave unequivocal support to the A.M.A. code and then, under intense pressure, tacitly accepted the dual organization of the profession.[46] Among those whose later behavior indicated understanding of the power of a well-organized professional minority was Dr. Joseph Bryant, a member of the County Society's Committee on Ethics in the early 1880s, sponsor of the first report on tuberculosis as Commissioner of Health in 1889, and a leading architect of the notification compromises of the 1890s.

III

Medical and general politics were interdependent in the controversy over compulsory notification. Tuberculosis control was more important in New Yorkers' lives than whether physicians were free to consult practitioners whom their patients freely consulted. Medical advertising was more immediately painful to physicians than to the public. Notification and its consequences required the expenditure of public funds and, because of the sanitary and therapeutic measures that followed from it, entailed costs for families and institutions.

The debate about compulsory notification was, however, conducted primarily within the medical profession and around competing interpretations of science, technology, and professional ethics. Problems in the administrative control of disease could not easily be dramatized to compete successfully for broad public attention. Moreover, the scientific and professional issues were matters of deep conviction to many members of the medical profession. The politics of tuberculosis was rooted in serious philosophical and scientific controversy.

Although the philosophical controversy was not unique to New York, the achievement of compulsory notification was. Rather than risk interpretations which require the assertion that physicians and public officials in New York City were more enlightened or more public-spirited than their counterparts in, for example, Berlin, or Edinburgh, or Paris, it is useful to ask how the city differed from other places. An essential difference was that the techniques of American municipal politics, at a particularly high level of development in New York City in the 1890s, were available for a wide variety of goals. Through the skillful manipulation of patronage and prestige, the medical profession in the city was organized to support, tolerate, or passively resist notification some years before conversion to the scientific basis of notification occurred.

The public health innovators faced a difficult political challenge. They had to create sufficient support for compulsory notification within the city to prevent the state legislature from restricting the powers of the Board of Health. The board's power to make social policy in the form of amendments to the Sanitary Code was derived from the legislature. The legislature, dominated by Republicans, was eager for opportunities to discredit agencies of the city's government, as a way to diminish Tammany's power. If the medical enemies of notification could present it as a power grab by a band of arrogant radicals who did business with Tammany, the legislature would intervene. If, on the other hand, the notification controversy became a dispute among learned and respectable physicians, all of whom had loyal patients, prudent Republicans would look to other issues.

Biggs, Prudden, and their allies avoided antagonizing laymen. The Health Department offered useful services to tuberculous citizens and their families without challenging any interest group except physicians. The department was especially sensitive to the anxieties of a city population 80 percent foreign born or first generation. Circulars were printed in a variety of languages. Department personnel who visited the homes of tubercular patients were multilingual or accompanied by interpreters. Patients were not hospitalized without careful consideration of the economic and emotional effects on their families.[47]

Making it difficult for physician opponents to build a lay constituency was essential but not sufficient to institutionalize reform. Physicians had to be involved in the process of notification and control, whether voluntarily or grudgingly, for the new measures to have any significant effect on citizens' health. Moreover, it would be difficult to maintain lay support if the legitimacy of the new measures was eroded by constant medical attack.

Lay support was maintained and solidified by mutually satisfactory relationships with the dominant factions in general politics. These same relationships provided tools to build a sufficiently solid medical constituency to achieve more effective control of tuberculosis than in any other political jurisdiction in the world at that time.

The New York public health innovators in the 1890s were intensely political and selectively partisan. The intersection of medical, bureaucratic, and partisan politics was as fast and dangerous in the 90s as at any time in the 20th century. Later claims to apolitical status by the managers of public health innovation and their historians have obscured the strategies and tactics of institutional change on behalf of disease control in the 1890s.

The innovations for which the Health Department received international recognition were made, with one exception, when city government was controlled by Tammany Hall, led by Richard Croker. The first pathologists' report was written in the administration of Mayor Hugh Grant; the bacteriological laboratory and programs to control diphtheria and tuberculosis were instituted under Mayor Thomas Gilroy. Only the 1897 regulation notification for tuberculosis was issued with a reform mayor, William Strong, in office. There is no evidence that Strong or men identified with him were involved in the controversy, which concluded with the consolidation of the measures envied by Robert Koch and Robert Philip during the administrations of Tammany mayors Robert Van Wyck and George B. McClellan, Jr.

The public health physicians were in touch with the major partisan actors. Joseph Bryant had ties to the state Democratic organization; serving, for example, in the ceremonial role of surgeon-general to Governor Flower.[48] Dr. Alvah H. Doty, a veteran of the Health Department staff and a medical power as Health Officer of the Port of New York, was close enough to Senator Thomas Platt's regular Republican organization for Theodore Roosevelt to enlist his support in his campaign to be appointed assistant secretary of the navy.[49] Prudden had ties to anti-Tammany reformers but, like most physicians in the public health coalition, avoided public identification with the organized reformers, whose support could generally be counted on throughout the decade of the 90s.[50] Biggs himself had a warm personal and professional relationship with Charles F. Murphy, then a Tammany District Leader.[51]

If Murphy assisted Biggs during the 90s it must have been as a strategist, not as a protector. Murphy, generally regarded as the ablest of Tammany leaders, did not become County Leader until 1902 or the "dominant factor in the politics of New York State" until 1906. Throughout the 90s, he led the Tammany organization in the working-class Gas House district, removed in geographic and social distance from Biggs' consulting practice on West Fifty-eighth Street and the arena of medical politics at the New York Academy on West Forty-third. Both Biggs and Murphy were young and ambitious in the nineties; in their 30s, energetic, with highly developed technical skills, and eager to take advantage of opportunities.[52]

Whether or not Biggs and Murphy collaborated in public health innovation, Biggs was adept at practicing Murphy's principles of "thorough political organization and all year round work."[53] Dr. James Alexander Miller, a young Health Department physician in the late 90s, recalled him as a "practical realist who turned conditions as he found them to his own purposes with uncanny skill." In addition, Biggs had flexible scruples. Both Miller and William Hallock Park were recruited by Biggs. Both received civil service appointments after taking examinations engineered by Biggs to ensure that they would be selected. Miller, at the suggestion of Biggs and Park, arranged a false address in the city to qualify for his job.[54] Park himself had gained some independence from Biggs by refusing to allow him to take credit for work Park had done.[55]

Biggs used his political skill to define issues during the decade of controversy about tuberculosis notification. Although the results of notification were of greatest immediate benefit to the poor, Biggs refused to alienate potential support by taking sides in the controversies of the decade about society's responsibility to the poor. Notification was presented as a measure for the general welfare: debates about heredity and environment, self-help and charity, and the fit and the unfit were left to others. Similarly, Biggs and his colleagues never advocated regulations to require inspection and publication of health abuses in places of employment.

In his public statements, Biggs decorously sought to find physicians' price for acquiescence in compulsory notification. He generally offered incentives rather than punishment, praise rather than criticism. Free sputum examinations were designed to assist physicians in diagnosing their patients. Biggs was apologetic about not paying a fee for each case report, as was done for some contagious diseases in Europe. He offered services instead.[56] In the Health Department's 1893 report, physicians were exonerated of the charge of participating in insurance fraud in order to collect their fees through a brilliant exercise in specious epidemiological logic. Writing for a medical journal a year later, however, Biggs described the way physicians falsified death certificates for victims of tuberculosis so that claims could be made on industrial life insurance policies. Enforcement of notification through legal penalties was gradual and selective, done more to caution than to punish.[57]

Most important, the Health Department became a source of financial benefit for an increasing number of New York physicians through the decade of the 90s. Amid a national depression and fears that oversupply of physicians contributed to declining income, the department's importance to the medical economy of New York City grew steadily. Departmental patronage — an average of a quarter million dollars a year in full and part-time salaries — was undoubtedly dispensed to qualified men who were loyal to the party in power.[58] The patronage was, moreover, dispensed by a medical-bureaucratic leadership that had policy goals as well as skill at political organization. The combination of shared policy goals, intraprofessional loyalty, and superb use of patronage enabled physicians with allegiance to competing political parties and factions to work together in the Department of Health. Most of the growth in personnel during the decade was incremental. There was relatively little turnover in the Health Department, in a period when an estimated 12,000 city jobs were made available to the faithful after each election. The only well-publicized political purge of the department during the 1890s left most of the senior leadership in charge.[59]

The Board of Health, the four-member body that officially made policy for the department and the city, was continuous in personnel and responsiveness to the policy interests of the public health innovators throughout the decade. Charles G. Wilson remained as President of the Board from 1889 to 1897. Bryant, Commissioner of Health from 1889 to 1893, was replaced from within the department by Dr. Cyrus Edson. His successor, Dr. George Fowler, was a department veteran. The third member of the board, the Health Officer of the Port, changed three times in the decade. During the critical 1896–1897 period the office was held by Dr. Alvah H. Doty, a former staff member of the department. The fourth member was the President of the Board of Police, *ex officio*; a post held throughout the decade by men who, with the exception of Theodore Roosevelt (1895–1896), could be counted on to mind Tammany's business. And Tammany's business, the circumstantial evidence indicates, was to help Biggs and his allies to try to control pulmonary tuberculosis.

Good science and good health made good politics when, to paraphrase Tammany sage G. W. Plunkitt, the public health physicians saw their opportunities and took them. It was useful to avoid dealing with poverty as a general issue, to avoid exploring the ways in which exploitative employment and housing practices contribute to tuberculosis. This avoidance was also good pathology, as Biggs told the humanitarian readers of *The Forum* in 1894. Tuberculosis rates in the United States were lower than those in Europe because the poor lived under better sanitary conditions in this country. More important, after conducting countless autopsies in the city hospitals, Biggs was convinced that in "a considerable proportion of cases of incipient tuberculosis even among persons living under the most unfavorable conditions the disease becomes stationary or retrogressive." Thus environmental conditions, while significant, do not inevitably determine the outcome of the disease.[60] Biggs welcomed support from *The Forum's* constituency; he saw no reason to join it. Similarly, despite the clear relationship between tuberculosis and standards of living, Biggs and the New York innovators, unlike, for example, L. E. Flick and his Philadelphia associates, separated the antidisease from the antipoverty constituencies. For the New Yorkers it was sufficient that tuberculosis lesions appeared uptown. As Prudden wrote in *Harper's Magazine* in 1894, bacilli thrived in the "thick pile carpets" of the rich and others who accepted the "tyranny of things."[61]

The health of school children, always a grave concern, became a matter of good politics in the troubled winter of 1897. As the leadership of the County Medical Society and the Academy of Medicine made copy for the general and medical press with attacks on the Health Department for requiring notification for tuberculosis, the department recruited 192 physicians — 150 of them residents of Manhattan and the Bronx — as School Inspectors. Each physician spent 40 minutes a day in neighborhood schools examining children thought to be ill and referring them either to private physicians or dispensaries. For this work each physician was paid 30 dollars a month; a cost to the city of about $75,000 for the year.[62] Most of these physicians surely found it prudent to support the Board of Health's regulatory and reporting policies. Moreover, on their first day at work, they examined 4,225 children and found 14 cases of diphtheria, 3 of measles, and 55 of parasitic diseases.[63]

IV

After almost a decade of preparation, advocates of compulsory notification took their greatest risk on January 19, 1897, when the Board of Health announced that "It shall be the duty of every physician in this city to report . . . in writing the name, sex, occupation and address" of every patient suspected of pulmonary tuberculosis.[64] Biggs, Prudden, and their allies had reason to be gratified by the results of their efforts up to that date. The Health Department's achievements were attracting international attention. Within the city, the past year had been encouraging. In May 1896 the board adopted New York's first antispitting ordinance. A month earlier, the State Board of Health had adopted a plan, prepared by Doty, Biggs, and Prudden, to control bovine tuberculosis. Support was growing for a municipal tuberculosis hospital.[65]

There was, moreover, empirical evidence that the medical profession was beginning to accept tuberculosis as a communicable disease and the analysis of sputum as a diagnostic tool. Although the number of deaths from tuberculosis in the city increased in 1895, two years after the first reporting regulations, the rise was attributed to the high incidence of influenza in 1894 and 1895.[66] The reporting regulations may also have stimulated greater honesty among physicians in filling out death certificates — particularly physicians serving charitable institutions, who were legally obligated to report cases. The number of cases reported by public institutions increased from 3,985 in 1894 to 7,349 in 1896. Perhaps more significant, the number of cases voluntarily reported by private physicians increased from 278 in 1894 to 985 in 1896.[67] Biggs wrote jubilantly to Park in October of that year: "The tuberculosis work has increased very much — sometimes fifteen or twenty specimens a day."[68]

Political considerations may have contributed to timing the decision to require notification. The presidency of the Academy of Medicine was about to pass from one friend of public tuberculosis control, Joseph Bryant, to another, E. G. Janeway. Academy elections in these years were hard fought; the moment of victory was a time of exhaustion for the defeated faction.[69] Moreover, the imminent hiring of school medical inspectors meant new patronage for the Health Department. In addition, Greater New York would be created within a year under a recently revised city charter, adding the practitioners of three additional counties to the calculations of public health strategists.

At the end of 1896, the leading men in the Department of Health had a sure sense of whom they did and did not need to achieve their ends. Although reformer William Strong was still mayor, they could count on his constituency to support tuberculosis control on moral and scientific grounds. Other groups were less certain. An early draft of the department's report for 1896, in which the prose of some naive enthusiast was edited for political impact by an unknown superior, demonstrates the expertise with which the public health advocates entered the critical days, just ahead, of the struggle for compulsory notification. References to "business and civil service principles" and "public approval" were deleted. A boast about the immunity achieved because free smallpox vaccine was distributed to the poor was softened. Statements about the department's production of diphtheria antitoxin were eliminated, in order to avoid irritating physicians who criticized the department for engaging in the practice of medicine. A discussion of "important statistical information in respect to the tenement house population" was deleted; so was a statement that the department could name the owners of unsanitary buildings.[70] The reasoning which guided the editorial changes reveals mastery of the craft of political administration in the United States: avoid irritating individuals and groups you might need; do not flatter constituencies with nowhere else to go, in this case reformers, philanthropists, and civil service reformers.

Opposition to compulsory notification was, as had been expected and prepared for, immediate and intense. Two days after publication of the regulations, on January 21, 1897, there was a long and bitter debate about them at a regular meeting of the Academy. At the close of the meeting, Prudden tried to take full advantage of his faction's strength. He moved that a committee of eight be appointed by the chair (Joseph Bryant), of which the incoming president (E. G. Janeway) would be chairman, "To consider and report to the academy upon tuberculosis and its relationship to the public welfare and the measures which should be adopted to curtail its ravages."[71] Privately Prudden was less polite. Writing to Trudeau the next day, he described the meeting: "Of course the Fool was there in force, and went through his usual wailings over the aggressive tyrannies of the Health Board . . ."[72]

Compulsory notification was blasted as "offensively dictatorial," by Dr. George Shrady in a lead

Moreover, Shrady in a lead editorial in the nation-Moreover, Shrady, a former Department of Health insider, called the regulations a result of a conspiracy of "a few workers in the Board to alarm the public unduly." Lashing out at Biggs, he accused the board of "unduly magnifying the importance of its bacteriological department" even if tuberculosis was "in a very limited way . . . contagious."[73]

Three years earlier, Shrady had endorsed the first notification regulations, praising Biggs and hoping that "a more comprehensive scheme" would be instituted.[74] Why Shrady changed sides is not clear. But his vituperation reflected the views of a considerable faction — as did the *Medical Record's* dramatic silence about notification in the second half of 1897 and all of 1898. The only clue to Shrady's favorable attitude in 1893 was his obligation to the board for hiring him as a consulting physician just a few months before his editorial; and less than a year after he had broken with the department in protest against "political" (i.e., Tammany) interference in hiring policy.[75] Presumably he was an outsider again by 1897.

Other journals, medical and lay, were more favorable. The *Medical News*, for example, praised the decision to provide medical inspection for school children in a lead editorial the week after the new reporting requirements were announced. In March, before the academy or the Medical Society took action, the *News* supported the board's policy as "wise and judicious." The *Medical Journal*, with the largest national circulation, was favorable but guarded. The lay press was generally favorable: the *Times*, for example endorsing the board in January, the *Herald* in February.[76]

On March 18, 1897, the New York Academy addressed the issue postponed for maximum bargaining advantage by Prudden in January. The Committee of Eight, with Prudden and Janeway as spokesmen, suggested that the Board of Health "might wisely delay the enforcement of compulsory notification but should adopt more stringent measures for the care of all sputum . . . ." The academy accepted their motion that the board delay enforcement of — but not rescind — compulsory notification for tuberculosis.[77]

Concurrently, an academy Committe of Five — which included Bryant, Janeway, and Dr. Stephen Smith, architect of the legislation creating the Board of Health three decades earlier — addressed the central issue raised by notification. Ostensibly reviewing the proposal to create a Greater New York Health Department, the committee noted that the department's powers had been "extraordinary" because the Board of Health had not used them in "injudicious" or "unwarranted" ways. The powers were "tolerated" because the board had been "chary" of their use.

The message was clear. A compromise had been arranged. With Shrady leading a faction of outraged physicians advocating prior clearance of all Board of Health measures by the academy and the Medical Society on one side, and Biggs leading a faction supporting notification on the other, the medical elite had decided to temporize one step beyond the *status quo*, leaving new but gently enforced regulations on the books.[78] By 1898 an official consulting board, chosen by the academy, was providing advice to the Health Department.[79]

The County Medical Society reinforced the compromise negotiated by the academy's leaders. The president of the society in 1897 and 1898 was Dr. Arthur M. Jacobus, a trustee of the academy who two years earlier had nominated Bryant for its presidency.[80] On March 3, the society received a report from its Committee on Hygiene endorsing compulsory notification, provided department inspectors did not communicate with patients without the consent of their attending physicians.[81] At the society meeting of March 22, however, the society rejected its committee's report, declaring by unanimous vote that compulsory notification was "unnecessary, inexpedient, and unwise."[82]

Jacobus attacked the Health Department in his presidential address to the society in November, perhaps to assuage the general practitioners, who had more power in the society than in the academy. The Health Department, Jacobus fumed, was "usurping the duties, rights, and privileges of the medical profession," not only by notification for tuberculosis, but also by offering free care to affluent patients, free vaccinations to everyone, and free examinations to school children without regard to their parents' wealth. He assured his audience that the society, represented by himself, and two other physicians — one of whom supported notification — had met with the board and been assured that there would be "more stringent rule for the guidance of inspectors and other employees in their relations with practitioners and the patients of such."[83]

Reasserting the Prudden-Janeway compromise and encouraging physicians with grievances to put them in writing to the board, Jacobus continued talking loudly and carrying a small stick. Rhetoric subtracted, the board had promised consultation and condemned the "abuse of power" but did not repeal the requirement for notification. Finally, Jacobus called on the state legislature to restrict the powers of the Health Department. A legislative committee was appointed which included Shrady, apparently to give credence to the society's commitment to punish the department.[84]

Jacobus, as a member of the ruling group in the academy, probably knew that the legislative action was a charade. Only a token effort was made, and the attempt to restrict the powers of the Health Department was quickly dropped. A prominent member of the Medical Society, Dr. Frank Van Fleet, was accused of sabotaging the legislation but he, as was perhaps intended, though threatened with expulsion from the society, survived to become chairman of its Board of Censors in 1900 and to represent it in merger negotiations with the Medical Association in 1904.[85]

The appeal to the legislature has considerable historiographic interest, however. Biggs later believed, or wanted others to believe, that he led a successful counter attack in Albany in 1898 and 1899. In 1900, to start the legend, he told a Philadelphia audience that the Medical Society had staged a "determined but unsuccessful" legislative effort.[86] An official history of the antituberculosis movement, written two decades later by Dr. S. Adolphus Knopf and submitted to an editorial committee which included Biggs, declared: "During the legislative session of 1898 and 1899, Dr. Biggs spent much of the winter in Albany fighting" bills to restrict the Health Department's powers. Knopf continued that, following this struggle, Biggs arranged the Prudden-Janeway compromise approved by the Academy of Medicine.[87] Biggs' biographer, C.-E. A. Winslow, quoted Knopf's description of Biggs' Albany campaign while quietly restoring the academy compromise to 1897, where it belonged.[88] Neither Knopf nor Winslow, though later close to Biggs, worked with him in 1897 and 1898. James Alexander Miller, who did, recalled in 1943 that, "The County Medical Society . . . tried to have a law passed in Albany which would prevent Biggs doing what he wanted to do . . . ." But Miller's recollection was heavily dependent on what "Biggs told me personally on several occasions" in later years.[89]

The County Medical Society's Committee on Legislation tried to explain the political issue in its report on the "unfavorable" year of 1898 — when it could not obtain a quorum at any meeting. "Some few of our profession have not been in accord with the wishes of the majority and legislators are in the habit of asking for united action."[90] There was no profit and much risk for legislators to take sides in an intraprofessional dispute in which the public's stake was not explicit. The legislators, experts in political arithmetic, knew that the "few members" who opposed the majority were a considerable faction.

Political arithmetic, a difficult task at any time, is even riskier in hindsight. It is clear which interest groups in the medical profession supported compulsory notification by 1897 and 1898. But it is also evident that, in New York medical politics of the 1890s, leadership was not hierarchical. The profession was fluid: membership shifted; two societies competed for membership; illicit practitioners flourished; physicians were anxious about their incomes.

The public health innovators had, at a cautious estimate, a constituency of at least 1,000 physicians; a third to almost a half, depending on whose total is accepted, of the regular physicians in the city. Constituency in this context has a narrow definition: physicians who had a financial reason to either support the Health Department or to remain neutral when it was attacked. The number 1,000 is computed as follows: at least 50 physicians who derived most of their income from the department; about 250 who had welcome increases in income from school inspection or special summer work; a large proportion of the 950 who served for salary or other benefits in the hospitals and clinics staffed by the medical schools under a grant from the Board of Charities of city government or working in private hospitals or clinics which, because they treated the poor, had some dependency on city government.[91]

Leaving aside the ties particular Health Department leaders had to Tammany, upstate Democrats, and the Platt Republican organization, it is probable that few state legislators cared to risk being accused of meddling in the internal affairs of a learned profession; especially just five years after they had voted to give the medical profession extraordinary control of its own affairs. Friendly legislators and political advisers might have suggested to the angry members of the New York County Society that they could do worse than live with the compromise suggested by the Academy of Medicine.

Why did Biggs and his biographers fight an imaginary legislative battle? Perhaps they felt the double pressure of the apolitical mythology of organized medicine and the ideology of good government which spread among their social and economic peers in the early 20th century. Exaggerating a legislative battle in Albany left the implication that compulsory notification was protected by persuading Republicans to support it, not by using Tammany methods, money, and muscle to win friends and neutralize enemies. In the 20th century, public health became identified with sanctimonious politics; linked to a moral and scientific crusade against inefficiency, ignorance, and corruption. The valued skills became the ability to impress elites: marshalling evidence, excelling in debates, organizing for efficient administration. Political expertise, the ability to orchestrate self-interest across professional, class, and ethnic lines, was devalued as a strategy to achieve public social policy.[92]

The managers of public health innovation in the 1890s later claimed better reform credentials than they had. As early as 1901, Prudden wrote the newly elected Fusion mayor, Seth Low, urging him to retain Hermann Biggs in the Health Department. Apparently confident that Low was ignorant of the politics of public health, Prudden told him what he probably wanted to hear: ". . . until the advent of Tammany four years ago, the Health Department . . . had for several years led the way in this country in the adoption of new methods in the prevention of disease." Moreover, Prudden continued, Biggs almost decided "he should drop the work when Tammany came in" but decided to stay "in the hope that some of the hard won ground might be saved."[93] Prudden's plea was successful, if inaccurate, Biggs having served in three Tammany administrations since 1889.

Biggs chose to be remembered, a hand-corrected typescript from his later years indicates, as a man above partisan politics, unshakeably dedicated to principle. Although nominally a "Cleveland Democrat," he had been offered jobs by all parties. "An ardent believer in Civil Service," Biggs chose his associates "without regard to their political affiliations."[94]

In 1902, after New York public health innovators had begun to identify their achievements with general political reform, Dr. William Osler praised them at an international congress. Osler, a recent convert to compulsory notification, noted the "difficulties" the New Yorkers "had to deal with in manipulating Tammany."[95] Whether from diplomacy or distance, Osler missed the central point and fostered the subsequent mythology. If Tammany was manipulated, it was with its consent; if the physicians were allowed to manipulate, it was because they accepted the rules and ethics of political professionals.

Robert Koch, speaking at the international tuberculosis congress a year earlier, argued that Biggs' achievement was the creation of a superb public health organization rather than the reporting requirement. Noting that Norway and Saxony had also mandated compulsory notification, Koch "most urgently" recommended the New York model to the "study and imitation of all municipal sanitary authorities."[96]

In the 20th century, the New York model for the control of tuberculosis was widely praised for its structure and results. The model dominated medical and public debate so thoroughly that it helped to create an international medical and public consensus about the communicability of tuberculosis. But this consensus based on science, morality, and self-interest had little relationship to empirical evidence about how, to whom, and under what conditions the disease is communicable.[97] The model remains resistant to change, however. This resistance, whatever its later sources in bureaucratic territoriality, began when the New York model was sanctified as the inevitable result of scientific progress rather than as the skillful political response of concerned and ambitious men to hypotheses which appeared, for a time, to be in the interest of the public's health.

NOTES

Presented at the 47th annual meeting of the American Association for the History of Medicine, Charleston, South Carolina, May 4, 1974.

1 Robert Koch (Berlin) to Hermann M. Biggs (New York), May 26, 1901, quoted in C.-E. A. Winslow, *The Life of Hermann M. Biggs: Physician and Statesman of the Public Health* (Philadelphia: Lea & Febiger, 1929), p. 178.

2 Sir Robert W. Philip, *Collected Papers on Tuberculosis* (London: Oxford Univ. Press, 1937), pp. 412, 63.

3 James Bryce, *The American Commonwealth* (London, 1888), II, 281.

4 The most complete account is John S. Billings, *The Registration of Pulmonary Tuberculosis in New York City* (New York: Department of Health, 1912). The use of notification to measure support for scientific medicine among physicians in general practice is discussed in Hermann M. Biggs, "The administrative control of tuberculosis," reprinted from *The Medical News*, Feb. 20, 1904, p. 4. Biggs made this point on many occasions. In 1906, Philip, *Collected Papers*, pp. 78–79, noted that "tuberculosis differs from all other notifiable diseases . . . . Cases are often not detected until long after infection has occurred . . . the greatest practical difficulty in connection with notification is to achieve it sufficiently early."

5 Winslow, *The Life of Hermann M. Biggs*, *passim*; S. Adolphus Knopf, *A History of the National Tuberculosis Association* (New York, N.T.A., 1922), pp. 6–18. A general theory of innovation in public health in these terms is elaborated by George Rosen, *A History of Public Health* (New York: MD Publications, 1958), p. 150. Rosen posits a four-stage process: (1) A social evil is recognized by an individual or a small influential group; (2) individuals take the initiative to develop the issues through studies and experiments; (3) these actions "enlighten and mold public opinion" and attract government attention; (4) agitation leads to government action and "if successful to legislation." Rosen notes that the model is oversimple but maintains its general validity.

6 Wade W. Oliver, *The Man Who Lived for Tomorrow* (New York: Dutton, 1941), p. 418.

7 *Annual Report of the Board of Health of the Health Department of The City of New York for the Year Ending December 31, 1889* (New York, 1890), pp. 38–40. (Hereafter cited as Health Department, *Report*, year.) Wilson was appointed by Mayor Hugh J. Grant on May 2, 1889, amid public accusations — including a story in the *New York Times* that he was corrupt. New York City, Municipal Archives and Records Center, Early Mayors' Papers, Health, 1885–1890, contains revealing material about Wilson's political connections and skill. Biggs took sole credit for initiating the pathologists' report in "The registration of tuberculosis," reprinted from the *Philadelphia Med. J.*, Dec. 1, 1900, p. 1.

8 The earliest eyewitness account of the informal screening is Hermann M. Biggs and John H. Huddleston, "The sanitary supervision of tuberculosis as practiced by the New York City Board of Health," reprinted from *Am. J. Med. Sci.*, January, 1895, n.s. *109*: 17. Knopf, *A History*, p. 6, reports that Bryant communicated with 12 physicians of whom only 2, Drs. Frank P. Foster and E. G. Janeway, supported notification. Biggs gives the number canvassed as 24, of whom only 5 or 6 replied, all but 2 opposing notification.

9 "The germs of tuberculosis," *The New York Times*, editorial, June 7, 1889, p. 4; J. Hilgard Tyndale, "Pulmonary consumption and the Board of Health," *N.Y. Med. J.*, Oct. 18, 1890, *52*: 419–420.

10 Health Department, *Report, 1893*, pp. 38–40. The best secondary source for the details of the notification controversy is Winslow, *The Life of Hermann M. Biggs*, ch. IX.

11 Hermann M. Biggs, "Compulsory notification and registration of tuberculosis," discussion before the Advisory Council of the National Association for the Study and Prevention of Tuberculosis, Washington, D.C., May 6, 1907, p. 6. Philip, *Collected Papers*, p. 206, in 1913, stressed the frequency with which practitioners relying exclusively on signs and symptoms failed to diagnose tuberculosis.

12 Winslow, *The Life of Hermann M. Biggs*, pp. 131–137.

13 *Sanitary Code of the City of New York, 1897*, sec. 225; for documentation of the controversy see Winslow, *The Life of Hermann M. Biggs*, pp. 143–149 and below, notes 71–90.

14 T. Mitchell Prudden (New York City) to Edward Livingston Trudeau (Saranac Lake), Jan. 22, 1897, *Biographical Sketches and Letters of T. Mitchell Prudden, M.D.* (New Haven: Yale Univ. Press, 1927), p. 232.

15 Hermann M. Biggs, "Sanitary science, the medical profession and the public," reprinted from *Med. News, N.Y.*, Jan. 8, 1898, p. 10; Biggs, "The registration," p. 16.

16 See below, notes 19–20.

17 Winslow, *The Life of Hermann M. Biggs*, and Knopf, *A History*, *passim*; Charles V. Chapin, "History of state and municipal control of disease," in *A Half Century of Public Health*, ed. M. P. Ravenel (New York, 1921), p. 143.

18 Ernest J. Lederle and Hermann M. Biggs, "The ad-

ministrative control of tuberculosis," *Charities*, Dec. 12, 1903, *11*: 571–574.

19 Hermann M. Biggs, *The Administrative Control of Tuberculosis in New York City* (New York: Department of Health, 1909), p. 5.

20 Biggs, "Compulsory notification," p. 10. This statement contradicts Biggs' declaration to the British Congress on Tuberculosis in 1902 that no prosecutions were either made or, more important, intended. ("Notification of tuberculosis," *Transactions of the British Congress on Tuberculosis*, 1902, *1*: 10.) Presumably enforcement policy changed as notification became a source of New York medical pride.

21 Health Department, *Report*, 1896, p. 26; "Resolution of the Medical Board of the West Side German Dispensary," *Med. Rec.*, March 20, 1897, *51*: 431–432: ". . . now more than 50 percent of the physicians make no report." Lederle and Biggs, "Administrative control of tuberculosis," p. 570; Hermann M. Biggs, *Brief History of the Campaign Against Tuberculosis in New York City* (New York: Department of Health, 1908), p. 10.

22 Godias J. Drolet and Anthony M. Lowell, *A Half Century's Progress Against Tuberculosis in New York City, 1900–1950* (New York: Tuberculosis and Health Association, mimeo., 1952), pp. v, vi, xxxiii, xlviii; Lederle and Biggs, "Administrative control of tuberculosis," p. 570. Doubts about the efficacy of public action in the control of tuberculosis are expressed in Richard H. Shryock, *National Tuberculosis Association, 1904–1954* (New York: N.T.A., 1957), p. 306, and Anthony M. Lowell et al., *Tuberculosis* (Cambridge, Mass.: Harvard Univ. Press, 1969), p. 15.

23 Health Department, *Report, 1890*, p. 207.

24 Drolet and Lowell, *A Half Century's Progress*, pp. iii, xxvi; Lederle and Biggs, "Administrative control of tuberculosis," p. 571.

25 John Shaw Billings, *Vital Statistics of New York City and Brooklyn . . . Ending May 31, 1890*, 53rd Congress, 1st session, House Misc. Doc. (Washington, D.C., 1894), quoted by Drolet and Lowell, *A Half Century's Progress*, pp. li, lxiv.

26 C.-E. A. Winslow, *The Conquest of Epidemic Disease* (Princeton: Princeton Univ. Press, 1943; New York, 1967), p. 309.

27 H. R. M. Landis, "The reception of Koch's discovery in the United States," *Ann. Med. Hist.*, September, 1932, *4*: 533.

28 *Ibid.*, pp. 535–537. Leading New York physicians did not share the temporary optimism stimulated in 1890 when Koch announced that tuberculin could be used both to detect and to cure the disease. If tuberculin had met Koch's initial expectations, tuberculosis control might have been accomplished with a minimum of political and bureaucratic elaboration. But T. Mitchell Prudden early declared himself unconvinced by Koch's claims and Abraham Jacobi, an influential figure in New York medicine, conducted and published a thorough study which suggested that, although tuberculin produced mixed effects, it was most useful in treating incipient cases of the disease. Moreover, E. L. Trudeau argued cogently and with wide influence in New York that the results of treatment with tuberculin "even in selected cases are, on the whole, but little better than are usually obtained by the climactic and out-of-door plan." His research suggested that nutrition was a more important variable than treatment with tuberculin. In combination, these positions reinforced the arguments for compulsory notification. A. Jacobi, *Tr. Med. Soc. St. N.Y.*, 1891: 91–133. E. A. Trudeau, "Results of the employment of tuberculin and its modifications at the Adirondack Cottage Sanitarium," *Med. News, N.Y.*, 1856, *14*: 298–300.

29 Erwin H. Ackerknecht, *Medicine at the Paris Hospital, 1794–1848* (Baltimore: Johns Hopkins Press, 1967), pp. 156–160; Howard D. Kramer, "The germ theory and the early public health program in the United States," *Bull. Hist. Med.*, May-June 1948, *22*: 233–247.

30 Winslow, *Conquest*, pp. x–xi; Biggs and Huddleston, "Sanitary supervision," p. 10, for the most complete statement on insurance economics.

31 S. B. Taylor, "The duty of a physician to a tubercular patient and to the public," *Columbus Med. J.*, 1897, *18*: 18–19.

32 Letter to the editor, Stuyvesant F. Morris, M.D., *N.Y. Med. J.*, Dec. 2, 1893, *58*: 666.

33 George F. Shrady, "The health board and compulsory reports," *Med. Rec.*, Feb. 27, 1897, *51*: 305–306.

34 See below, notes 40–41.

35 "The physician-patient privilege," *Northwestern University Law Review*, May-June, 1961, *56*: 263–264.

36 Samuel Rezneck, "Unemployment, unrest and relief in the United States during the depression of 1893–97," *J. Polit. Econ.*, August 1953, *61*: 327–328.

37 Health Department, *Report, 1893*, p. 17.

38 Richmond Mayo-Smith to Seth Low, transmitted to Thomas Gilroy, Feb. 6, 1894, New York City Municipal Archives, Early Mayors' Papers, Box 6144.

39 James B. Lane, "Jacob A. Riis and scientific philanthropy during the progressive era," *Social Service Review*, March 1973, *47*: 37.

40 Charles Phelps, "The causes of a decline in the average income of general practitioners," *Med. News, N.Y.*, 1897, *71*: 528–531.

41 Landon Carter Gray, "Inaugural Address of Presi-

dent," Minutes, The Medical Society of the County of New York, Nov. 23, 1896, p. 138, New York Academy of Medicine Library.

42 *Medical Register, New York, New Jersey and Connecticut*, 1895–1896, *33*: *passim*.

43 *Ibid.*, pp. lxv–lxvi.

44 James J. Walsh, *History of the Medical Society of the State of New York* (Brooklyn: Published by the Society, 1907), pp. 205–206; H. G. Piffard, "The status of the medical profession in the State of New York," *N.Y. Med. J.*, 1883, *37*: 400–404, 456–457, 484–487, 567–571, 589–593; 1883, *38*: 372–377, 568–574.

45 *N.Y. Med. J.*, 1883, *38*: 567 ff.

46 *Ibid.*, pp. 375, 573; Philip van Ingen, *The New York Academy of Medicine* (New York: Columbia Univ. Press, 1949), pp. 181–190.

47 The most complete summaries of department strategies are Lederle and Biggs, "Administrative control of tuberculosis," pp. 572–573, and Biggs, *Administrative Control*, pp. 1–11.

48 Gordon Atkins, "Health, housing and poverty in New York City, 1865–1898" (unpublished Ph.D. dissertation, Columbia Univ., 1947), p. 252.

49 *The Letters of Theodore Roosevelt*, ed. Elting E. Morison (Cambridge, Mass.: Harvard Univ. Press, 1951–1954), I, 587–588.

50 T. M. Prudden to Seth Low, Nov. 11, 1901, in *Biographical Sketches*, pp. 287 ff.

51 Winslow, *The Life of Hermann Biggs*, p. 188; James Alexander Miller, "The beginnings of the American antituberculosis movement," *Am. Rev. Tuberculosis*, 1943, *48*: 374.

52 M. R. Werner, *Tammany Hall* (New York, 1928), pp. 485, 516.

53 "A tribute to Plunkitt by the Leader of Tammany Hall," Charles F. Murphy, in William L. Riordan, *Plunkitt of Tammany Hall* (New York: Dutton, 1906, 1963), p. xxvi.

54 Miller, "American antituberculosis movement," pp. 374–375.

55 Oliver, *Man Who Lived for Tomorrow*, p. 90.

56 Hermann M. Biggs, "Sanitary science, the medical profession and the public," reprinted from *Med. News, N.Y.*, Jan. 8, 1898, p. 14.

57 Health Department, *Report, 1893*, p. 16; Biggs and Huddleston, "Sanitary supervision," p. 9.

58 There is considerable evidence to suggest the involvement of the department in partisan patronage. Perhaps the most compelling is the testimony to the Mazet Committee of the state legislature in 1899. (Report of the Special Committee of the Assembly, Appointed to Investigate the Public Offices and Departments of the City of New York, 5 vols. [Albany, 1900], pp. 917, 3807–3814, 4012, 5198.)

59 Staff lists are printed in the Health Department *Reports* for most years in the 1890s. The most detailed account of the purge of 1892, developed mainly from Republican sources, is Atkins, "Health, housing, and poverty in New York City," pp. 251–253. *The Medical Journal* covered the story circumspectly in its news columns (e.g. "The City Board of Health," *55*, April 23, 1892). Two months later, a pseudonymous physician wrote the *Medical Journal* that it has been "an open secret for years" that medical jobs, on the police force, Board of Health, visiting staffs of municipal hospitals were "matters of political influence" (July 9, 1892). The most penetrating analysis of New York patronage politics is Theodore Lowi, *At the Pleasure of the Mayor* (New York: Free Press of Glencoe, 1964). Although Lowi's research begins in 1898 it is reasonable to apply his analysis to the immediately preceding years. Thus he makes the conventional, but somewhat misleading, remark that the Board of Health has never been a "Party enclave" (pp. 40–41), and then documents the way the board's patronage has been used for partisan ends (e.g. pp. 80–85). The point is not that the board was above partisan politics, but rather that it was influenced by more than one party, since patronage had to serve the ends of medical as well as general politics.

60 Hermann M. Biggs, "To rob consumption of its terrors," *The Forum*, 1894, *16*: 758–767.

61 T. Mitchell Prudden, "Tuberculosis and its prevention," *Harper's Magazine*, March 1894, *88*: 630–637.

62 Health Department, *Report, 1898*, p. 43.

63 A. W. Smith, "The economic worth of the physicians," *N.Y. Med. J.*, 1897, *66*: 827.

64 The full text of the recommendations approved by the board was reprinted in the *Medical Journal*, Jan. 23, 1897, *65*: 130–132.

65 Winslow, *The Life of Hermann M. Biggs*, pp. 140–143.

66 Health Department, *Report, 1895*, p. 82.

67 Health Department, *Report, 1896*, p. 26.

68 Oliver, *Man Who Lived for Tomorrow*, pp. 154–155.

69 New York Academy of Medicine, Minutes of meetings, *passim*, for bitterness of annual elections.

70 New York City Municipal Archives, "Memoranda—Health Department, 1896."

71 New York Academy of Medicine, Minutes of meetings, Jan. 21, 1897, p. 509.

72 T. Mitchell Prudden to Edward L. Trudeau, Jan. 22, 1897, in *Biographical Sketches*, p. 235.

73 George F. Shrady, "The health board and compulsory reports," *Med. Rec.*, Jan. 23, 1897, *51*: 126–127.

74 [George F. Shrady], "The health department and pulmonary tuberculosis," *Med. Rec.*, Dec. 23, 1893, *44*: 817.

75 *N.Y. Med. J.*, April 22, 1893, *57*: 621.

76 "The tuberculosis question in New York," *Med.*

News, March 13, 1897, *70*: 341; Editorial, *N.Y. Med. J.*, Jan. 23, 1897, *55*: 124; Editorial, *New York Herald*, *30*, Feb. 26, 1897; "Fighting consumption," *New York Times*, Jan. 25, 1897, p. 6.

77 New York Academy of Medicine, Minutes of meetings, March 18, 1897, p. 521; cf. van Ingen, *New York Academy of Medicine*, pp. 263–264.

78 New York Academy of Medicine, Minutes, March 18, 1897, p. 521.

79 Health Department, *Report*, n.p., list of members of "Consulting Board to the Board of Health." Iago Galdston wrote James Alexander Miller, April 5, 1943, to challenge the conventional interpretation of Biggs's righteousness and the academy's opposition (New York Academy of Medicine, MSS of Miller). In Galdston's interpretation, the Prudden-Janeway compromise becomes even more important for institutional change: "It is my impression that the Academy has been libelled on this score. Actually, the Academy Committee only asked for a delay in the application of the law. Furthermore, when you read the original law, you see that it was a thoroughly Prussian proposition, including all sorts of fines and dire threats. The spirit of the law was not unlike Biggs." Miller replied, April 7, 1943, disagreeing with Galdston, but basing his views solely on Biggs' statements to him.

80 New York Academy of Medicine, Minutes of meetings, December 1895.

81 "To stay consumption," *New York Times*, March 4, 1897, p. 12.

82 Minutes, Medical Society of the County of New York, March 22, 1897, pp. 159–160.

83 Minutes, Medical Society, Nov. 22, 1897, pp. 209–214. Dr. W. H. Katzenbach, who chaired the Committee on Hygiene and later served as a consultant to the Department of Health, supported notification.

84 *Ibid.*, pp. 217–220.

85 Minutes, Comitia Minora, The Medical Society of the County of New York, May 21, 1898, p. 3941; Minutes, Medical Society, Oct. 24, 1898, p. 249; Report of the Joint Committee of Conference . . . Consolidating the Medical Society of the State of New York and the New York State Medical Association (1904), New York County Society Papers, New York Academy of Medicine.

86 Biggs, "The regisration," p. 15. The claim was repeated in Biggs, *Administrative Control*, p. 5.

87 Knopf, *A History*, pp. 8–9.

88 Winslow, *The Life of Hermann M. Biggs*, pp. 148–149.

89 Miller to Galdston, note 79, above: cf. Billings, *The Registration*, p. 11. The alleged legislative battle is mentioned neither in the index to the *New York Times*, which covered with great care proposed legislation affecting the city, nor in *The Letters of Theodore Roosevelt*. Neither is it mentioned in the most thorough secondary source on New York government in the period, G. Wallace Chessman, *Governor Theodore Roosevelt: The Albany Apprenticeship, 1898–1900* (Cambridge, Mass.: Harvard Univ. Press, 1965).

90 Minutes, Medical Society, Oct. 24, 1898, p. 268.

91 *Ibid.*, 1896, n.p., noting the transfer of appointing power from the city's Board of Charities to the medical schools. The Medical Society protested, arguing that physicians appointed to municipal and charitable hospitals ought to be regulated by civil service. The society's resolution emphasized the economic nexus by asking that even unsalaried physicians be under civil service. The number 950 (949) is in *ibid.*, Nov. 23, 1896, p. 138. The number 300 for the Health Department is based on staff lists in the *Report* for 1896. Testimony to the Mazet Committee (above, n. 58) indicated the total number of health department inspectors was over 600, but only a minority were physicians.

92 Among the most helpful discussions of the politics of public health in the 20th century are James H. Cassedy, *Charles V. Chapin and the Public Health Movement* (Cambridge, Mass.: Harvard Univ. Press, 1962); Rosen, *A History*; Shryock, *National Tuberculosis Association*; and Walter I. Trattner, *Homer Folks* (New York: Columbia Univ. Press, 1968).

93 Prudden to Low, above, n. 50.

94 "Herman M. Biggs," Anonymous typescript biographical sketch corrected in Biggs' own hand, New York Academy of Medicine, n.d., c. 1920; cf. Winslow, *The Life of Hermann M. Biggs, passim.*

95 *Transactions of the British Congress on Tuberculosis*, 1902, *1*: 14. Osler equivocated in a widely reprinted debate on notification in 1894 (*Proceedings*, College of Physicians of Philadelphia, Jan. 12, 1894; reprinted in *N.Y. Med. J.*, Feb. 17, 1894, *59*: 221–222). But Osler emphatically supported compulsory notification by 1900; "On the study of tuberculosis," *Philadelphia Med. J.*, Dec. 1, 1900, *6*: 1029–1030. L. E. Flick was bitter about Osler's opposition, which he ascribed to Osler's "working in the interest of his friends," but grateful for his public apology, at a dinner in Paris in 1905; Ella M. E. Flick, *Beloved Crusader* (Philadelphia: Dorrance, 1944), pp. 15–16, 205, 228.

96 Robert Koch, "The suppression of tuberculosis" (Paper read at the British Congress on Tuberculosis, July 23, 1901) reprinted in *Scient. Am. Suppl.*, Aug. 17, 1901, *52*: 21–34.

97 I am grateful to Drs. Paul Diamond and Marvin Kuschner for calling my attention to current uncertainty about the communicability of tuberculosis.

A Guide to Further Reading

Books and articles listed in this Guide are arranged under the following headings: *General, Allied Professions, Diseases, Domestic and Folk Medicine, Education, Faith Healing and Quackery, Hospitals, Hygiene, Image and Income, Mental Health, Military, Minority Medicine, Practice, Public Health: Colonial, Public Health since 1776, Research, Sanitation, Sectarians,* and *Women.*

GENERAL

Bonner, Thomas N. *The Kansas Doctor: A Century of Pioneering.* Lawrence: University of Kansas Press, 1959.

Bonner, Thomas N. *Medicine in Chicago, 1850–1950: A Chapter in the Social and Scientific Development of a City.* Madison, Wis.: American History Research Center, 1957.

Brieger, Gert H., ed. *Medical America in the Nineteenth Century: Readings from the Literature.* Baltimore: Johns Hopkins Press, 1972. A collection of primary documents.

Cowen, David L. *Medicine and Health in New Jersey: A History.* Princeton: D. Van Nostrand Co., 1964.

Duffy, John. *The Healers: The Rise of the Medical Establishment.* New York: McGraw-Hill Book Co., 1976. The most recent survey of American medical history.

Duffy, John, ed. *The Rudolph Matas History of Medicine in Louisiana.* 2 vols. Baton Rouge: Louisiana State University Press, 1958, 1962.

Grob, Gerald. "The social history of medicine and disease in America: problems and possibilities." *Journal of Social History,* 1977, *10*: 391–409. Overview and prospects.

Kett, Joseph F. *The Formation of the American Medical Profession: The Role of Institutions, 1780–1860.* New Haven: Yale University Press, 1968. A study of medical licensing, education, organization, and sectarianism in five states.

Lerner, Monroe, and Anderson, Odin W. *Health Progress in the United States, 1900–1960.* Chicago: University of Chicago Press, 1963. A helpful compilation of health statistics.

McKeown, Thomas. *The Modern Rise of Population.* New York: Academic Press, 1976. A provocative study emphasizing the importance of diet in reducing infectious diseases in England and Wales.

Rosen, George. *Preventive Medicine in the United States, 1900–1975: Trends and Interpretations.* New York: Prodist, 1976. A valuable introduction by the leading historian of public health.

Rothstein, William G. *American Physicians in the 19th Century: From Sects to Science.* Baltimore: Johns Hopkins University Press, 1972. A controversial but informative sociological-historical study.

Shryock, Richard Harrison. *Medicine and Society in America, 1660–1860.* New York: New York University Press, 1960. Still the best introduction to American medicine.

Shryock, Richard Harrison. *Medicine in America: Historical Essays.* Baltimore: Johns Hopkins Press, 1966. Wide-ranging articles by the foremost historian of American medicine.

Stevens, Rosemary. *American Medicine and the Public Interest.* New Haven: Yale University Press, 1971. A history of the medical profession emphasizing specialization in the 20th century.

ALLIED PROFESSIONS

Ashley, JoAnn. *Hospitals, Paternalism and the Role of the Nurse.* New York: Teachers College Press, 1976. Surveys the difficulties faced by hospital training schools for nurses.

Burnham, John C. "The struggle between physicians and paramedical personnel in American psychiatry, 1917–41." *Journal of the History of Medicine and Allied Sciences,* 1974, *29*: 93–106.

A case study of the medical profession's attitude toward interlopers.

Gregg, James R. *The Story of Optometry*. New York: Ronald Press Co., 1965. A popular work that includes considerable American background.

Lewi, Maurice J. "Medicine and podiatry in New York State." *New York State Journal of Medicine*, 1954, *54*: 536–540. The story of how corncutters became health-care professionals, by the "father" of American podiatry.

McCluggage, Robert W. *A History of the American Dental Association: A Century of Health Service*. Chicago: American Dental Association, 1959. One of the few histories of dentistry by a historian.

Marshall, Helen E. *Mary Adelaide Nutting: Pioneer of Modern Nursing*. Baltimore: Johns Hopkins University Press, 1972. The first full-time professor of nursing in America.

Safier, Gwendolyn. *Contemporary American Leaders in Nursing: An Oral History*. New York: McGraw-Hill, 1977.

Schwartz, L. Laszlo. "The historical relations of American dentistry and medicine." *Bulletin of the History of Medicine*, 1954, *28*: 542–549. Briefly surveys the founding of the American dental profession.

Sonnedecker, Glenn. *Kremers and Urdang's History of Pharmacy*. 4th ed. Philadelphia: J. B. Lippincott Co., 1976. The standard text, of which Part Three is devoted to "Pharmacy in the United States."

DISEASES

Ackerknecht, Erwin H. "Anticontagionism between 1821 and 1867." *Bulletin of the History of Medicine*, 1948, *22*: 569–593. Pioneering essay on major 19th-century medical theories.

Ackerknecht, Erwin H. *Malaria in the Upper Mississippi Valley*. Baltimore: Johns Hopkins Press, 1945. Classic historical account of malaria in the Midwest.

Blake, John B. *Benjamin Waterhouse and the Introduction of Vaccination: A Reappraisal*. Philadelphia: University of Pennsylvania Press, 1957. A brief examination of America's reception of Jenner's vaccine.

Carrigan, JoAnn. "Privilege, prejudice and the 'Strangers Disease' in 19th century New Orleans." *Journal of Southern History*, 1970, *36*: 568–578. Yellow fever in a southern city.

Caulfield, Ernest. *A True History of the Terrible Epidemic Vulgarly Called the Throat Distemper which Occurred in His Majesty's New England Colonies between the Years 1735 and 1740*. New Haven: Beaumont Medical Club, 1939. Classic description of diphtheria devastation in the colonial period.

Crosby, Alfred W. Jr. *Epidemic and Peace, 1918*. Westport, Conn.: Greenwood Publishing Co., 1976. Provocative account of the 1918 influenza epidemic.

Dowling, Harry F. *Fighting Infection: Conquests of the Twentieth Century*. Cambridge, Mass.: Harvard University Press, 1977. The story of the control of infectious diseases since the turn of the century.

Duffy, John. *Sword of Pestilence: The New Orleans Yellow Fever Epidemic of 1853*. Baton Rouge: Louisiana State University Press, 1966. "Probably the worst single epidemic ever to strike a major American city."

Etheridge, Elizabeth. *The Butterfly Caste: A Social History of Pellagra in the South*. Westport, Conn.: Greenwood Publishing Co., 1972. Account of a disease that took many American lives.

Kaufman, Martin. "The American antivaccinationists and their arguments." *Bulletin of the History of Medicine*, 1967, *41*: 463–478. Explores some difficulties in applying medical knowledge.

Powell, J. H. *Bring Out Your Dead: The Great Plague of Yellow Fever in Philadelphia in 1793*. Philadelphia: University of Pennsylvania Press, 1949. Fullest narrative account of this classic epidemic.

Rosenberg, Charles E. *The Cholera Years: The United States in 1832, 1849, and 1866*. Chicago: University of Chicago Press, 1962. A thorough and excellent account of cholera in the United States; in fact, one of the best books in the history of American medicine.

Shryock, Richard Harrison. *National Tuberculosis Association, 1904–1954*. New York: National Tuberculosis Association, 1957. A study of the first national voluntary health society.

DOMESTIC AND FOLK MEDICINE

Hand, Wayland D., ed. *American Folk Medicine: A Symposium.* Berkeley: University of California Press, 1976. A collection of historical and anthropological essays.

Risse, Guenter B., Numbers, Ronald L., and Leavitt, Judith Walzer, eds. *Medicine without Doctors: Home Health Care in American History.* New York: Science History Publications, 1977. Five essays on domestic medicine.

Young, James Harvey. *American Self-Dosage Medicines: An Historical Perspective.* Lawrence, Kansas: Coronado Press, 1974. From quackery to semirespectability.

EDUCATION

Bell, Whitfield, J., Jr. *John Morgan: Continental Doctor.* Philadelphia: University of Pennsylvania Press, 1965. Founder of the first American medical school.

Blake, John B. "Women and medicine in antebellum America." *Bulletin of the History of Medicine*, 1965, *39*: 99–123. Brief survey of women's attempts to enter medicine.

Bonner, Thomas Neville. *American Doctors and German Universities: A Chapter in International Intellectual Relations, 1870–1914.* Lincoln: University of Nebraska Press, 1963. Approximately 15,000 American doctors continued their training abroad.

Fleming, Donald. *William H. Welch and the Rise of Modern Medicine.* Boston: Little, Brown, 1954. The first dean of the Johns Hopkins University Medical School.

Flexner, Abraham. *Medical Education in the United States and Canada.* New York: Carnegie Foundation, 1910. This epoch-making report is still worth reading.

Jones, Russell M. "American doctors and the Parisian medical world, 1830–1840." *Bulletin of the History of Medicine*, 1973, *47*: 40–65, 177–204. Nearly 700 American physicians studied in Paris.

Kaufman, Martin. *American Medical Education: The Formative Years, 1765–1910.* Westport, Conn.: Greenwood Press, 1976. A short history from the College of Philadelphia to Flexner.

Lippard, Vernon W. *A Half-Century of American Education: 1920–1970.* New York: Josiah Macy, Jr., Foundation, 1974. A brief outline of 20th-century developments.

Norwood, William Frederick. *Medical Education in the United States before the Civil War.* Philadelphia: University of Pennsylvania Press, 1944. An encyclopedic account of medical education in ante-bellum America.

Numbers, Ronald L., ed. *The Education of American Physicians.* Berkeley: University of California Press, 1979. Individual histories of the subjects taught in medical schools from 1765 to the present.

Stevens, Rosemary. "Trends in medical specialization in the United States." *Inquiry*, 1971, *8*: 9–19. The effects of specialization on the distribution of physicians.

Walsh, Mary Roth. *"Doctors Wanted: No Women Need Apply": Sexual Barriers in the Medical Profession, 1835–1975.* New Haven: Yale University Press, 1977. A study of women's struggles to become physicians.

FAITH HEALING AND QUACKERY

Cunningham, Raymond, J. "The Emmanuel movement: a variety of American religious experience." *American Quarterly*, 1962, *14*: 48–63. Nonsupernatural religious healing in the early 20th century.

Cunningham, Raymond J. "From holiness to healing: the faith cure in America, 1872–1892." *Church History*, 1974, *43*: 499–513. Faith healing and perfectionism in the Gilded Age.

Harrell, David Edwin, Jr. *All Things Are Possible: The Healing and Charismatic Revivals in Modern America.* Bloomington: Indiana University Press, 1975. A fascinating account of faith healing after World War II.

Young, James Harvey. *The Medical Messiahs: A Social History of Health Quackery in Twentieth-Century America.* Princeton: Princeton University Press, 1967. A readable account of the multi-billion-dollar quackery business.

Young, James Harvey. *The Toadstool Millionaires: A Social History of Patent Medicines in America before Federal Regulation.* Princeton: Princeton University Press, 1961. An excellent study of medical self-help and quackery.

HOSPITALS

Eaton, Leonard K. *New England's Hospitals, 1790–1833.* Ann Arbor: University of Michigan Press, 1957. The hospital comes to New England.

Rosenberg, Charles E. "And heal the sick: the hospital and the patient in 19th century America." *Journal of Social History*, 1977, *10*: 428–447. The day-to-day operation of hospitals during the first three-quarters of the century.

Williams, William H. *America's First Hospital: The Pennsylvania Hospital, 1751–1841.* Wayne, Pa.: Haverford House, 1976. Focuses on administration.

HYGIENE

Blake, John B. "Health reform," in *The Rise of Adventism: Religion and Society in Mid-Nineteenth-Century America*, ed. Edwin S. Gaustad, pp. 30–49. New York: Harper and Row, 1974. Sylvester Graham and his friends.

Blake, John B. "Mary Gove Nichols: Prophetess of Health." *Proceedings of the American Philosophical Society*, 1962, *106*: 219–234. A prominent hydropath and health reformer.

Cummings, Richard Osborn. *The American and His Food: A History of Food Habits in the United States.* Chicago: University of Chicago Press, 1941. Still the best introduction to the changing American diet.

Kirkland, Edward C. "'Scientific Eating': New Englanders prepare and promote a reform, 1873–1907." *Proceedings of the Massachusetts Historical Society*, 1974, *86*: 28–52. Turn-of-the-century nutrition and nutritionists.

Musto, David F. *The American Disease: Origins of Narcotic Control.* New Haven: Yale University Press, 1973. A history of drug addiction and cures.

Numbers, Ronald L. *Prophetess of Health: A Study of Ellen G. White.* New York: Harper and Row, 1976. The visions and health teachings of the founder of Seventh-day Adventism.

Whorton, James C. "'Christian Physiology': William Alcott's prescription for the millennium." *Bulletin of the History of Medicine*, 1975, *49*: 466–481. The evangelical ideology of health reform.

IMAGE AND INCOME

Anderson, Odin W. *The Uneasy Equilibrium: Private and Public Financing of Health Services in the United States, 1875–1965.* New Haven: College and University Press, 1968. A period-by-period survey.

Berlant, Jeffrey Lionel. *Profession and Monopoly: A Study of Medicine in the United States and Great Britain.* Berkeley: University of California Press, 1975. A sociological-historical analysis of professional control.

Branson, Roy. "The secularization of American medicine." *Hastings Center Studies*, 1973, *1*: 17–28. A quasi-historical account of the defrocking of American physicians.

Burns, Chester R. "Malpractice suits in American medicine before the Civil War." *Bulletin of the History of Medicine*, 1969, *43*: 41–56. An analysis of 27 suits between 1794 and 1861.

Burrow, James G. *AMA: Voice of American Medicine.* Baltimore: Johns Hopkins Press, 1963. An impartial history of the A.M.A. since its reorganization at the turn of the century.

Burrow, James G. *Organized Medicine in the Progressive Era: The Move Toward Monopoly.* Baltimore: Johns Hopkins University Press, 1977.

Hirshfield, Daniel S. *The Lost Reform: The Campaign for Compulsory Health Insurance in the United States from 1932 to 1943.* Cambridge, Mass.: Harvard University Press, 1970. The second debate over compulsory health insurance.

Numbers, Ronald L. *Almost Persuaded: American Physicians and Compulsory Health Insurance, 1912–1920.* Baltimore: Johns Hopkins University Press, 1978.

Rosen, George. *Fees and Fee Bills: Some Economic Aspects of Medical Practice in Nineteenth Century America.* Baltimore: Johns Hopkins Press, 1947. One of the few studies on the history of medical economics.

Rosenkrantz, Barbara G. "The search for professional order in 19th century American medicine." *Proceedings of the XIVth International Congress of the History of Science* No. 4, pp. 113–124. Tokyo and Kyoto, 1974. Argues that American physicians enjoyed "a remarkably prestigious professional status" during the first half of the 19th century.

Shryock, Richard H. *The Development of Modern*

Medicine: An Interpretation of the Social and Scientific Factors Involved. New York: Alfred A. Knopf, 1947. Ch. 13: "Public Confidence Lost," and Ch. 16: "Public Confidence Regained."

Shryock, Richard H. *Medical Licensing in America, 1650–1965.* Baltimore: Johns Hopkins Press, 1967. A short essay comparing the American and European experiences.

Stevens, Robert, and Stevens, Rosemary. *Welfare Medicine in America: A Case Study of Medicaid.* New York: Free Press, 1974. A careful analysis of one form of government health insurance.

MENTAL HEALTH

Burnham, John Chynoweth. *Psychoanalysis and American Medicine, 1894–1918: Medicine, Science, and Culture.* New York: International Universities Press, 1967. The impact of psychoanalysis on American medicine.

Caplan, Ruth B. *Psychiatry and the Community in Nineteenth Century America: The Recurring Concern with the Environment in the Prevention and Treatment of Mental Illness.* New York: Basic Books, 1969. From moral treatment to custodial care and subsequent reforms.

Dain, Norman. *Concepts of Insanity in the United States, 1789–1865.* New Brunswick, N.J.: Rutgers University Press, 1964. From religion to science.

Deutsch, Albert. *The Mentally Ill in America: A History of Their Care and Treatment from Colonial Times.* 2nd ed. New York: Columbia University Press, 1949. A standard survey.

Grob, Gerald N. *Mental Institutions in America: Social Policy to 1875.* New York: Free Press, 1973. An outstanding contribution to the history of mental health care.

Hale, Nathan G., Jr. *Freud and the Americans: The Beginnings of Psychoanalysis in the United States, 1876–1917.* New York: Oxford University Press, 1971. Explores the enthusiastic reception of Freud's theories in America.

Rosenberg, Charles E. *The Trial of the Assassin Guiteau: Psychiatry and Law in the Gilded Age.* Chicago: University of Chicago Press, 1968. A fascinating look at American psychiatry in the 1880s.

Rothman, David J. *The Discovery of the Asylum: Social Order and Disorder in the New Republic.* Boston: Little, Brown, 1971. A controversial interpretation downplaying the curative aspects of the 19th-century mental hospitals.

Tyor, Peter. "Denied the power to choose the good: sexuality and mental defect in American medical practice 1850–1920." *Journal of Social History*, 1977, *10*: 472–489.

MILITARY

Adams, George Worthington. *Doctors in Blue: The Medical History of the Union Army in the Civil War.* New York: Henry Schuman, 1952.

Breeden, James O. *Joseph Jones, M.D.: Scientist of the Old South.* Lexington: University Press of Kentucky, 1975. Medical scientist and Civil War surgeon.

Breeden, James O. "Military and Naval Medicine," in *A Guide to the Sources of United States Military History*, ed. Robin Higham, pp. 317–343. Hamden, Conn.: Archon Books, 1975. A bibliographical essay.

Cash, Philip. *Medical Men at the Siege of Boston, April, 1775–April, 1776: Problems of the Massachusetts and Continental Armies.* Philadelphia: American Philosophical Society, 1973.

Cunningham, H. H. *Doctors in Gray: The Confederate Medical Service.* Baton Rouge: Louisiana State University Press, 1958.

Shryock, Richard H. "A medical perspective on the Civil War." *American Quarterly*, 1962, *14*: 161–173. Theory and practice during one of the bloodiest wars of all time.

MINORITY MEDICINE

Haller, John S. "The Negro and the Southern physician: a study of medical and racial attitudes, 1800–1860." *Medical History*, 1972, *16*: 238–253. Science and prejudice in medical theory.

May, J. Thomas. "A 19th century medical care program for blacks: the case of the Freedmen's Bureau." *Anthropological Quarterly*, 1973, *46*: 160–171. Based on admissions data from a federally sponsored hospital in Louisiana.

Postell, William Dosite. *The Health of Slaves on Southern Plantations.* Baton Rouge: Louisiana

State University Press, 1951. A positive view of health care for slaves.

Savitt, Todd L. *Medicine and Slavery: The Health Care and Diseases of Blacks in Antebellum Virginia.* Urbana: University of Illinois Press, 1978.

Torchia, Marion M. "Tuberculosis among American Negroes: medical research on a racial disease, 1830–1950." *Journal of the History of Medicine and Allied Sciences*, 1977, *32*: 252–279. An essay on the ethnicity of disease.

Vogel, Virgil. *American Indian Medicine*. Norman: University of Oklahoma Press, 1970. Study of Native American medical practice.

PRACTICE

Atwater, Edward C. "The medical profession in a new society, Rochester, New York (1811–60)." *Bulletin of the History of Medicine*, 1973, *47*: 221–235. Shows the decline of professional standards and status.

Atwater, Edward C. "The physicians of Rochester, N.Y., 1860–1910: a study in professional history, II." *Bulletin of the History of Medicine*, 1977, *51*: 93–106. Emphasizes the centralization of professional power in the hospital staff.

Bell, Whitfield, J., Jr. *The Colonial Physician & Other Essays.* New York: Science History Publications, 1975. Sketches of colonial medicine by a distinguished historian.

Boorstin, Daniel J. *The Americans: The Colonial Experience.* New York: Random House, 1958. Part 8, "New World Medicine," stresses the democratizing effect of the American environment.

Brieger, Gert H. "Therapeutic conflicts and the American medical profession in the 1860's." *Bulletin of the History of Medicine*, 1967, *41*: 215–222. The debate over calomel.

Bryan, Leon S., Jr. "Blood-letting in American medicine, 1830–1892." *Bulletin of the History of Medicine*, 1964, *38*: 516–529. The decline of heroic therapy.

Horine, Emmet Field. *Daniel Drake (1785–1852): Pioneer Physician of the Midwest.* Philadelphia: University of Pennsylvania Press, 1961. Perhaps the greatest physician of the ante-bellum Midwest.

Kett, Joseph F. "Provincial Medical Practice in England, 1730–1815." *Journal of the History of Medicine and Allied Sciences*, 1964, *19*: 17–29. Emphasizes the absence of professional distinctions among physicians, surgeons, and apothecaries.

Riznik, Barnes. "The professional lives of early nineteenth century New England doctors." *Journal of the History of Medicine and Allied Sciences*, 1964, *19*: 1–16. A quantitative study of 896 physicians in six counties, 1790–1840.

Rosenberg, Charles E. "The therapeutic revolution: medicine, meaning, and social change in nineteenth-century America." *Perspectives in Biology and Medicine*, 1977, *20*: 485–506. The best introduction to 19th-century therapeutics.

PUBLIC HEALTH: COLONIAL

Beall, Otho T., Jr., and Shryock, Richard H. *Cotton Mather: First Significant Figure in American Medicine.* Baltimore: Johns Hopkins Press, 1954. A study of the man who introduced inoculation to America.

Blake, John B. *Public Health in the Town of Boston, 1630–1822.* Cambridge, Mass.: Harvard University Press, 1959. One colonial town's response to diseases.

Blake, John B. "Yellow fever in eighteenth century America." *Bulletin of the New York Academy of Medicine*, 1968, *44*: 673–686. Overview of yellow fever and critique of Ackerknecht's view about the influence of politics in the contagionism-anticontagionism split.

Cassedy, James H. *Demography in Early America: Beginnings of the Statistical Mind, 1600–1800.* Cambridge, Mass.: Harvard University Press, 1969. Vital statistics in the colonial period.

Crosby, Alfred W., Jr. *The Columbian Exchange: Biological and Cultural Consequences of 1492.* Westport, Conn: Greenwood Publishing Co., 1972. What Columbus brought to America and took home again.

Duffy, John. *Epidemics in Colonial America.* Baton Rouge: Louisiana State University Press, 1959. Standard work on colonial diseases.

Duffy, John. "The passage to the colonies." *Mississippi Valley Historical Review*, 1951–52, *38*: 21–38. America was settled by sickly people.

Duffy, John. "Smallpox and the Indians in the American colonies." *Bulletin of the History of Medicine*, 1951, *25*: 324–341. The effects of smallpox on native groups.

PUBLIC HEALTH SINCE 1776

Cassedy, James H. *Charles V. Chapin and the Public Health Movement.* Cambridge, Mass.: Harvard University Press, 1962. Biography of major public health figure.

Cassedy, James H. "The roots of American sanitary reform, 1843–1847: seven letters from John H. Griscom to Lemuel Shattuck." *Journal of the History of Medicine and Allied Sciences*, 1975, *30*: 136–147. Letters from one public health reformer to another in useful historical context.

Duffy, John. *A History of Public Health in New York City.* 2 vols. New York: Russell Sage Foundation, 1968, 1974. An encyclopedic account of public health in the nation's largest city.

Ellis, John. "Business and public health in the urban South during the nineteenth century: New Orleans, Memphis, and Atlanta." *Bulletin of the History of Medicine*, 1970, *44*: 197–212, 346–371.

Galishoff, Stuart. *Safeguarding the Public Health: Newark, 1895–1918.* Westport, Conn.: Greenwood Press, 1975. Turn-of-the-century Newark's achievements.

Griscom, John C. *The Sanitary Condition of the Laboring Population of New York.* New York: Harper Brothers, 1845. Doctor's view of the urban environment; important in fostering public health movement.

Jordan, Philip D. *The People's Health: A History of Public Health in Minnesota to 1848.* St. Paul: Minnesota Historical Society, 1953. Narrative of a Midwestern state's efforts to accomplish health reforms.

Kramer, Howard. "Early municipal and state boards of health." *Bulletin of the History of Medicine*, 1950, *24*: 503–529. Early events in public health movement.

Rosen, George. "Political order and human health in Jeffersonian thought." *Bulletin of the History of Medicine*, 1952, *26*: 32–44. Valuable article for understanding medical and political ideological interactions.

Rosen, George. "Politics and public health in New York City." *Bulletin of the History of Medicine*, 1950, *24*: 441–461. Patronage in the pre-Metropolitan Board of Health era.

Rosenkrantz, Barbara. "Cart before horse: theory, practice, and professional image in American public health, 1810–1920." *Journal of the History of Medicine and Allied Sciences*, 1974, *29*: 55–73. Explores the relationships between physicians and nonmedical sanitarians in the public health movement.

Rosenkrantz, Barbara Gutmann. *Public Health and the State: Changing Views in Massachusetts, 1842–1936.* Cambridge, Mass.: Harvard University Press, 1972. An analytical study of the Massachusetts State Board of Health.

Shattuck, Lemuel. *Report of the Massachusetts Sanitary Commission.* Boston: Dutton and Wentworth, 1850. Landmark document in promoting public health movement.

Sigerist, Henry. "The cost of illness to the City of New Orleans in 1850." *Bulletin of the History of Medicine*, 1944, *15*: 498–507. A distinguished historian examines economic motivations for health reform.

Whorton, James. *Before Silent Spring: Pesticides and Public Health in Pre-DDT America.* Princeton: Princeton University Press, 1974. An excellent case study of shifting public health concerns.

RESEARCH

Benison, Saul. *Tom Rivers: Reflections on a Life in Medicine and Science.* Cambridge, Mass.: M.I.T. Press, 1967. An oral history of a pioneer virologist.

Rosen, George. "Patterns of health research in the United States, 1900–1960." *Bulletin of the History of Medicine*, 1965, *39*: 201–221. From foundations and universities to the federal government.

Shryock, Richard H. *American Medical Research: Past and Present.* New York: The Commonwealth Fund, 1947. A basic survey.

Strickland, Stephen P. *Politics, Science, and Dread Disease: A Short History of United States Medical Research Policy.* Cambridge, Mass.: Harvard University Press, 1972. Focuses on cancer research.

Swain, Donald C. "The rise of a research empire:

NIH, 1930 to 1950." *Science*, 1962, *138*: 1233–1237. The growth of federal support of biomedical research.

SANITATION

Blake, John B. "Lemuel Shattuck and the Boston water supply." *Bulletin of the History of Medicine*, 1955, *29*: 554–562. Explores how politics influenced one important health reformer.

Blake, Nelson. *Water for the Cities*. Syracuse: Syracuse University Press, 1956. Important for understanding the evolution of urban water systems.

Galishoff, Stuart. "Drainage, disease, comfort and class: a history of Newark's sewers." *Societas*, 1976, *6*: 121–138.

Larson, Lawrence. "Nineteenth century street sanitation: a study of filth and frustration." *Wisconsin Magazine of History*, 1968, *52*: 239–247. A descriptive account of efforts to clean up dirty streets.

Tarr, Joel. "Urban pollution — many long years ago." *American Heritage*, 1971, *22*: 65–69ff. Nineteenth-century urban environments.

Waserman, Manfred J. "Henry L. Coit and the Certified Milk movement in the development of modern pediatrics." *Bulletin of the History of Medicine*, 1972, *46*: 359–390. Explores aspects of the movement to provide clean raw milk to turn-of-the-century Americans.

SECTARIANS

Berman, Alex. "Neo-Thomsonianism in the United States." *Journal of the History of Medicine and Allied Sciences*, 1956, *11*: 133–155. Thomsonians seeking scientific respectability.

Berman, Alex. "The Thomsonian movement and its relation to American pharmacy and medicine." *Bulletin of the History of Medicine*, 1951, *25*: 405–428, 519–538. The basic account of this early sectarian movement.

Kaufman, Martin. *Homeopathy in America: The Rise and Fall of a Medical Heresy*. Baltimore: Johns Hopkins Press, 1971. Focuses on the relationship between homeopaths and regular physicians.

Legan, Marshall Scott. "Hydropathy in America: a nineteenth century panacea." *Bulletin of the History of Medicine*, 1971, *45*: 267–280. An introduction to the water-cure movement, although Legan has it cresting prematurely.

Numbers, Ronald L. "The making of an eclectic physician: Joseph M. McElhinney and the Eclectic Medical Institute of Cincinnati." *Bulletin of the History of Medicine*, 1973, *47*: 155–166. A look at America's largest eclectic medical school during its heyday.

WOMEN

Bullough, Vern, and Voght, Martha. "Women, menstruation, and nineteenth century medicine." *Bulletin of the History of Medicine*, 1973, *47*: 66–82. Victorian perception of menstruation as an illness.

Donegan, Jane B. *Women and Men Midwives: Medicine, Morality and Misogyny in Early America*. Westport, Conn.: Greenwood Press, 1978.

Gordon, Linda. *Woman's Body, Woman's Right: A Social History of Birth Control in America*. New York: Grossman Publishers, 1976. A prize-winning book on an important subject.

Haller, John S., and Haller, Robin M. *The Physician and Sexuality in Victorian America*. Urbana: University of Illinois Press, 1974. Describes the relations between the sexes in Victorian America, concentrating on the physicians' role in defending the status quo.

Litoff, Judy Barrett. *American Midwives: 1860 to the Present*. Westport, Conn.: Greenwood Press, 1978.

Mohr, James C. *Abortion in America: The Origins and Evolution of National Policy*. New York: Oxford University Press, 1977.

Morantz, Regina Markell. "The lady and her physician." In *Clio's Consciousness Raised: New Perspectives on the History of Women*, ed. Mary S. Hartman and Lois Banner, pp. 38–53. New York: Harper and Row, 1974. Critique of Ann Douglass Wood and others.

Reed, James. *From Private Vice to Public Virtue: The Birth Control Movement and American Society Since 1830*. New York: Basic Books, 1978.

Sklar, Kathryn Kish. *Catharine Beecher: A Study in American Domesticity*. New Haven: Yale University Press, 1973. An excellent biography of a water-cure enthusiast and popular writer on women's health problems.

Smith-Rosenberg, Carroll, and Rosenberg, Charles E. "The female animal: medical and biological views of woman and her role in 19th century America." *Journal of American History*, 1973, *60*: 332–356. Excellent account of Victorian medicine's view of women.

Smith-Rosenberg, Carroll. "Puberty to menopause: the cycle of femininity in nineteenth-century America." *The Journal of Interdisciplinary History*, 1973, *4*: 25–52.

Wertz, Richard W. and Dorothy C. *Lying-in: A History of Childbirth in America*. New York: Free Press, 1977.

Wood, Ann Douglass. "The fashionable diseases: women's complaints and their treatment in nineteenth century America." *The Journal of Interdisciplinary History*, 1973, *4*: 25–52. A controversial survey of "female invalidism" relying heavily on literary sources.

Abbreviations of Journal Titles

Am. Architect & Bldg. News (*American Architect and Building News*)
Am. Hist. Rev. (*American Historical Review*)
Am. J. Clin. Med. (*American Journal of Clinical Medicine*)
Am. J. Insanity (*American Journal of Insanity*)
Am. J. Med. Sci. (*American Journal of the Medical Sciences*)
Am. J. Nursing (*American Journal of Nursing*)
Am. J. Obst. & Dis. Women & Children (*American Journal of Obstetrics and Diseases of Women and Children*)
Am. J. Obst. & Gynec. (*American Journal of Obstetrics and Gynecology*)
Am. J. Pharm. (*American Journal of Pharmacy*)
Am. J. Psychiatry (*American Journal of Psychiatry*)
Am. J. Psychoth. (*American Journal of Psychotherapy*)
Am. J. Public Hlth. (*American Journal of Public Health*)
Am. Law Rev. (*American Law Review*)
Am. Medico-Surg. Bull. (*American Medico-Surgical Bulletin*)
Am. Med. Monthly (*American Medical Monthly*)
Am. Med. Times (*American Medical Times*)
Am. Quart. (*American Quarterly*)
Am. Rev. Tuberculosis (*American Review of Tuberculosis*)
Am. Veg. (*American Vegetarian*)
Ann. Am. Acad. Polit. & Soc. Sci. (*Annals of the American Academy of Political and Social Science*)
Ann. Chim. Phys. (*Annales de chimie et de physique*)
Ann. Med. Hist. (*Annals of Medical History*)
Ann. N.Y. Acad. Sci. (*Annals of the New York Academy of Sciences*)
Arch. Med. (*Archives of Medicine*)
Arch. pathol. Anat. (*Archiv für pathologische Anatomie und Physiologie*)
Arch. Pediat. (*Archives of Pediatrics*)
Arch. Sexual Behavior (*Archives of Sexual Behavior*)
Arch. Surg. (*Archives of Surgery*)
Berl. klin. Wchnschr. (*Berliner klinische Wochenschrift*)
Birth Control Rev. (*Birth Control Review*)
Boston J. Hlth. (*Boston Journal of Health*)
Boston Med. & Surg. J. (*Boston Medical and Surgical Journal*)
Boston Med. Magazine (*Boston Medical Magazine*)
Brit. & Foreign Med. Rev. (*British and Foreign Medical Review*)
Brit. J. Med. Psychol. (*British Journal of Medical Psychology*)
Brooklyn Med. J. (*Brooklyn Medical Journal*)
Buffalo Med. & Surg. J. (*Buffalo Medical and Surgical Journal*)
Buffalo Med. J. & Monthly Rev. (*Buffalo Medical Journal and Monthly Review*)
Bull. et mém. Soc. méd. hôp. Paris (*Bulletin et mémoires de la Société médicale des hôpitaux de Paris*)
Bull. Hist. Med. (*Bulletin of the History of Medicine*)
Bull. N.Y. Acad. Med. (*Bulletin of the New York Academy of Medicine*)
Bull. Soc. Med. Hist. Chicago (*Bulletin of the Society of Medical History* [*of Chicago*])
Charleston Med. J. & Rev. (*Charleston Medical Journal and Review*)
Chicago Med. Exam. (*Chicago Medical Examiner*)
Chicago Med. J. (*Chicago Medical Journal*)
Chicago Med. J. & Exam. (*Chicago Medical Journal and Examiner*)
Columbia Univ. Quart. Suppl. (*Columbia University Quarterly Supplement*)
Columbus Med. J. (*Columbus Medical Journal*)
Deutsche med. Wchnschr. (*Deutsche medizinische Wochenschrift*)
Eclectic Med. J. (*Eclectic Medical Journal*)
Edinburgh Med. J. (*Edinburgh Medical Journal*)
Galveston Med. J. (*Galveston Medical Journal*)
Graham J. Hlth. & Long. (*Graham Journal of Health and Longevity*)
Hosp. Admin. (*Hospital Administration*)
Iowa Med. J. (*Iowa Medical Journal*)
J.A.M.A. (*Journal of the American Medical Association*)
J. Am. Hist. (*Journal of American History*)

J. Anat. & Physiol. (*Journal of Anatomy and Physiology*)
J. Assn. Am. Med. Colls. (*Journal of the Association of American Medical Colleges*)
J. Chron. Dis. (*Journal of Chronic Diseases*)
J. Econ. Issues (*Journal of Economic Issues*)
J. Exper. Med. (*Journal of Experimental Medicine*)
J. Gynec. Soc. Boston (*Journal of the Gynecological Society of Boston*)
J. Hist. Ideas (*Journal of the History of Ideas*)
J. Hist. Med. (*Journal of the History of Medicine and Allied Sciences*)
J. Hyg. & Herald Hlth. (*Journal of Hygiene and Herald of Health*)
J. Infect. Dis. (*Journal of Infectious Diseases*)
J. Interdisc. Hist. (*Journal of Interdisciplinary History*)
J. Med. Educ. (*Journal of Medical Education*)
J. Med. Soc. N.J. (*Journal of the Medical Society of New Jersey*)
J. Mental Sci. (*Journal of Mental Science*)
J. Mich. St. Med. Soc. (*Journal of the Michigan State Medical Society*)
J. Nerv. & Ment. Dis. (*Journal of Nervous and Mental Disease*)
Johns Hopkins Hosp. Bull. (*Johns Hopkins Hospital Bulletin*)
J. Polit. Econ. (*Journal of Political Economy*)
J. Soc. Hist. (*Journal of Social History*)
J. Western Soc. Engrs. (*Journal of the Western Society of Engineers*)
Lib. Hlth. (*Library of Health*)
Long Island Med. J. (*Long Island Medical Journal*)
Los Angeles J. Eclectic Med. (*Los Angeles Journal of Eclectic Medicine*)
Maryland Med. Recorder (*Maryland Medical Recorder*)
Mass. Med. J. (*Massachusetts Medical Journal*)
Med. & Surg. Reptr. (*Medical and Surgical Reporter*)
Med. Ann. District of Columbia (*Medical Annals of the District of Columbia*)
Med. Comm. Mass. Med. Soc. (*Medical Communications of the Massachusetts Medical Society*)
Medico-Legal J. (*Medico-Legal Journal*)
Med. J. & Rec. (*Medical Journal and Record*)
Med. Life (*Medical Life*)
Med. News Libr. (*Medical News Library*)
Med. News, N.Y. (*Medical News [New York]*)
Med. Press & Circular (*Medical Press and Circular*)
Med. Rec. (*Medical Record*)
Med. Rec. in N.Y. (*Medical Record [in New York]*)
Med. Rev. Rev. (*Medical Review of Reviews*)
Med. Times & Gaz., London (*Medical Times [and Hospital Gazette], London*)
Med. Times & Long Island Med. J. (*Medical Times and Long Island Medical Journal*)
Med. Woman's J. (*Medical Woman's Journal*)
Milbank Mem. Fund Quart. Bull. (*Milbank Memorial Fund Quarterly Bulletin*)
Miss. Valley Hist. Rev. (*Mississippi Valley Historical Review*)
Modern Hosp. (*Modern Hospital*)
Modern Med. (*Modern Medicine*)
Nation's Hlth. (*Nation's Health*)
Neurol. Bull. (*Neurological Bulletin*)
New Eng. J. Med. (*New England Journal of Medicine*)
New Orleans Med. & Surg. J. (*New Orleans Medical and Surgical Journal*)
New Orleans Med. J. (*New Orleans Medical Journal*)
New Orleans Med. News & Hos. Gaz. (*New Orleans Medical News and Hospital Gazette*)
N.Y. Hist. Soc. Quart. (*New York Historical Society Quarterly*)
N.Y. J. Gynec. & Obst. (*New York Journal of Gynaecology and Obstetrics*)
N.Y. J. Med. (*New York Journal of Medicine*)
N.Y. Med. Gaz. (*New York Medical Gazette*)
N.Y. Med. Gaz. & J. Hlth. (*New York Medical Gazette and Journal of Health*)
N.Y. Med. J. (*New York Medical Journal*)
N.Y. Rev. (*New York Review*)
N.Y. St. J. Med. (*New York State Journal of Medicine*)
North Am. Arch. Med. & Soc. Sci. (*North American Archives of Medical and Social Science*)
North Am. Rev. (*North American Review*)
North Carolina Med. J. (*North Carolina Medical Journal*)
North-Western Med. & Surg. J. (*North-Western Medical and Surgical Journal*)
Obst. & Gynec. (*Obstetrics and Gynecology*)
Ohio Med. & Surg. J. (*Ohio Medical and Surgical Journal*)
Ohio State Archaeol. & Hist. Quart. (*Ohio State Archaeological and Historical Quarterly*)
Pacific Med. & Surg. J. (*Pacific Medical and Surgical Journal*)
Peninsular J. Med. & Collateral Sci. (*Peninsular Journal of Medicine and the Collateral Sciences*)
Penn. Mag. Hist. & Biography (*Pennsylvania Magazine of History and Biography*)
Penn. Med. J. (*Pennsylvania Medical Journal*)
Perspect. Biol. & Med. (*Perspectives in Biology and Medicine*)

Philadelphia Med. J. (Philadelphia Medical Journal)
Physn. & Bull. Medico-Legal Soc. (Physician and Bulletin of the Medico-Legal Society)
Proc. Am. Inst. Homoeopathy (Proceedings of the American Institute of Homoeopathy)
Proc. Am. Pharm. Assn. (Proceedings of the American Pharmaceutical Association)
Proc. Am. Phil. Soc. (Proceedings of the American Philosophical Society)
Proc. Am. Soc. Civil Engrs. (Proceedings of the American Society of Civil Engineers)
Proc. Nat. Conf. Charities & Correction (Proceedings of the National Conference of Charities and Correction)
Richmond & Louisville Med. J. (Richmond and Louisville Medical Journal)
Rocky Mount. Social Sci. J. (Rocky Mountain Social Science Journal)
St. Louis Clin. Rec. (St. Louis Clinical Record)
St. Louis Med. & Surg. J. (St. Louis Medical and Surgical Journal)
St. Louis Med. Reptr. (St. Louis Medical Reporter)
St. Paul Med. J. (St. Paul Medical Journal)
Saturday Rev. (Saturday Review)
Scient. Am. (Scientific American)
Scient. Am. Suppl. (Scientific American Supplement)
Social Security Bull. (Social Security Bulletin)
Southern J. Med. Sci. (Southern Journal of the Medical Sciences)
Southern Med. & Surg. J. (Southern Medical and Surgical Journal)
Southern Med. J. (Southern Medical Journal)
Southern Med. Rep. (Southern Medical Reports)
Tenn. Hist. Quart. (Tennessee Historical Quarterly)
Texas Hlth. J. (Texas Health Journal)
Texas Med. News (Texas Medical News)
Texas Med. Practitioner (Texas Medical Practitioner)
Tr. A.M.A. (Transactions of the American Medical Association)
Tr. Am. Gynec. Soc. (Transactions of the American Gynecological Society
Tr. Am. Hosp. Assn. (Transactions of the American Hospital Association)
Tr. Am. Laryng. Assn. (Transactions of the American Laryngological Association)
Tr. Am. Ophth. Soc. (Transactions of the American Ophthalmological Society)
Tr. Am. Soc. Civil Engrs. (Transactions of the American Society of Civil Engineers)
Transylvania J. Med. (Transylvania Journal of Medicine and the Associated Sciences)
Tr. Coll. Physicians Phila. (Transactions and Studies of the College of Physicians of Philadelphia)
Tr. Homoeopathic Med. Soc. St. N.Y. (Transactions of the Homoeopathic Medical Society of the State of New York)
Tr. Homoeopathic Med. Soc. St. Penn. (Transactions of the Homoeopathic Medical Society of the State of Pennsylvania)
Tr. Indiana St. Med. Soc. (Transactions of the Indiana State Medical Society)
Tr. La. St. Med. Soc (Transactions of the Louisiana State Medical Society)
Tr. Med. Assn. St. Ala. (Transactions of the Medical Association of the State of Alabama)
Tr. Med. Soc. St. N.J. (Transactions of the Medical Society of the State of New Jersey)
Tr. Med. Soc. St. N.Y. (Transactions of the Medical Society of the State of New York)
Tr. Med. Soc. St. N.C. (Transactions of the Medical Society of the State of North Carolina)
Tr. Med. Soc. St. Penn. (Transactions of the Medical Society of the State of Pennsylvania)
Tr. Med. Soc. St. Va. (Transactions of the Medical Society of the State of Virginia)
Tr. Southern Surg. & Gynec. Assn. (Transactions of the Southern Surgical and Gynecological Association)
U.C.L.A. Forum Med. Sci. (University of California at Los Angeles Forum of Medical Science)
U.S. Mag. & Democ. Rev. (United States Magazine and Democratic Review)
Veg. World (Vegetarian World)
Verhand. d. Cong. Inn. Med. (Verhandlungen des Congresses für innere medizin)
Water-Cure J. (Water-Cure Journal)
Western J. Med. (Western Journal of Medicine)
Western J. Med. & Phys. Sci. (Western Journal of the Medical and Physical Sciences)
Western J. Med. & Surg. (Western Journal of Medicine and Surgery)
Western Med. Gaz. (Western Medical Gazette)
Western Penn. Hist. Mag. (Western Pennsylvania Historical Magazine)
Wien. med. Presse (Wiener medizinische Presse)
William & Mary Coll. Quart. (William and Mary College Quarterly Historical Magazine)
Wis. Med. J. (Wisconsin Medical Journal)
Woman's Med. J. (Woman's Medical Journal)
Yale J. Biol. & Med. (Yale Journal of Biology and Medicine)
Zentralbl. Bakt. (Zentralblatt für Bakteriologie)
Ztschr. Tiermed. (Zeitschrift für Tiermedizin)

Index

Abbott, Grace, 376
Abbott, Simon, 89
Abrams, Albert, 98–99
Achard, Emile, 283
Ackerknecht, Erwin, 13
Adams, Charles Francis, 259
Adams, John G., 57
Addams, Jane, 31, 33, 187
Addiction, 13
Agnew, C. R., 57
Alcoholism, 13
Alcott, William, 315, 317, 317–18, 320, 321, 323, 324, 326
Alleghany County Medical Society, 223
Alms House (New York), 62
American Association for Labor Legislation, 139–41
American Association of Milk Commissions, 285, 288
American Board of Obstetrics and Gynecology, 386
American College of Surgeons, 386
American Committee on Maternal Welfare, 386
American Hospital Association, 208, 211, 213, 386
American Medical Association, 107; Bureau of Investigation, 99; changes view on voluntary health insurance, 143; Code of Ethics, 420; Committee on Medical Ethics, 65; defends Calomel, 82; opposition to compulsory health insurance, 139, 141, 142, 144, 145–47; struggle for reform of medical education, 108–9, 110, 135
American Nurses' Association, 207, 208, 211
American Public Health Association, 400

WILLIAM J. ORR, JR., prepared the Index

American Red Cross, 192, 193, 194, 208
American Vegetarian Society, 315
Amory, Thomas C., Jr., 174, 175
Anderson, Odin W., 142
Antibiotics, 8; in milk, 290
Aranow, Harry, 379
Arnstein, Elizabeth, 380
Arthur, Chester, 399
Aspinwall, William, 43, 49
Association of American Medical Colleges, 108, 109, 110
Astor, John Jacob, Jr., 364
Astor House, 339
Asylums, 28, 29, 155

Bache, Benjamin Franklin, 244
Baker, C. Alice, 120
Baker, Josephine S., 375
Baker, Paul de Lacy, 118
Baltimore City Health Department, 194
Baltimore College of Dental Surgery, 201
Bang, Bernhard, 283
Bard, John, 47
Bard, Samuel, 47
Barron, Clarence W., 285
Bartholow, Robert, 82, 83
Bartlett, Josiah, 50
Bartley, E. H., 285
Barton, Benjamin Smith, 243, 246
Bathing, 331–40; before 1800, 333–38; frequency of, 313, 331; in New York City, 352; 19th-century, 338–40
Baylor University Hospital Plan, 142
Beach, Wooster, 89
Beard, George M., 25, 26, 27, 28, 29, 30–31, 32, 33, 34, 35
Beatty, John, 50
Beaumont, William: on cholera, 258; researches cited in support of vegetarianism, 321–22
Bell, Luther, 319, 320, 321
Bellevue Hospital, New York, 57, 62, 63, 379
Bellevue School of Midwives, 217, 379, 387
Bellevue Yorkville Health Demonstration, 194, 196
Belmont, August, 364
Bennett, Hughes, 81
Bennett, J. H., 83
Bensaude, Raoul, 283
Bernard, Claude, 83
Bible Christian Church, 317
Biddle, Nicholas, 337
Bigelow, Henry J., 163
Bigelow, Jacob, 63, 81, 85
Biggs, Hermann M., 194, 305, 310, 400, 415, 416, 417, 418, 421, 422, 423, 424, 425, 426, 427
Billings, J. S., 108
Billroth, Christian Albert Theodor, 206
Bingham, William, 250
Bird, Seth, 47
Blacks, 3, 5, 208, 213
Blackwell, Elizabeth, 103, 117, 120–21, 123
Blackwell, Emily, 117, 123
Blakeman, W. M., 57
Bloodletting, 87; deprecation of, 79–80; in New York, 64; reason for abandonment of, 80–82
Bloomer, Amelia, 313
Blossom Street Health Unit, 192
Blue, Rupert, 140
Blue Cross, 142
Boerhaave, Herman, 21, 47, 48, 77
Bohune, Lawrence, 42
Boole, Francis I. A., 367
Bordley, John Beale, 244
Boston, 3, 4; hospitals in, 173–81; smallpox in, 231–37
Boston City Hospital, 30, 174, 175, 176, 178
Boston Dispensary, 157, 158, 159, 162, 163

Boston Lying-in Hospital, 175, 177, 222
Bouchelle, Peter, 44
Boussingault, Jean-Baptiste, 323
Bowditch, Henry I., 79, 306
Bowditch, H. P., 108
Bowling Green Neighborhood Association, 191
Boylston, Zabdiel, 41; efforts to promote inoculation, 232, 233, 234
Brackett, Joshua, 46
Bradford, William, 46
Brett, John, 47
Brewster, Mary, 187
Brill, A. A., 33
British Nurses Association, 207
Brooklyn Dispensary, 159
Brooks, John, 50
Broussais, François, 78, 257; cited in support of vegetarianism, 316, 320, 321
Brown, Andrew, 244, 249
Brown, Baker, 18, 19, 21, 22
Brown, Brockden, 332-33
Brown, John, 19, 22, 64
Browne, John, 46, 48
Brunton, Thomas Lander, 83
Bryant, Joseph, 416, 420, 422, 424
Buck, Gurdon, 57
Budd, William, 262
Budin, Pierre, 189
Burke, John, 60
Burnett, Waldo, 263
Byrne, Bernhard, 259-60

Cabot, Richard, 165, 186
Cadet Nursing Corps, 209
Caldwell, Charles, 257
California Medical Association, 144
Calomel, 64, 78, 79, 87; dosages of, 133; Hammond orders removal of, 82-83, 86; repudiation of, 83, 84
Cancer, 5, 10
Carey, Henry, 339
Carey, Matthew, 244, 245, 250
Carnegie Foundation, 109
Carson, John, 243
Carson, Joseph, 337
Cartwright, Samuel, 259
Catesby, Mark, 41
Cathrall, Isaac, 243
Central Medical College, 117
Cerebrovascular disorders, 5, 10
Chabert, Xavier, 263-64
Chadwick, Edwin, 305, 306, 307, 311
Chaillé, Stanford, 396
Chalmers, Lionel, 41
Chamberlin, Joseph, 177
Chapin, Charles V., 305, 311
Chapin, Henry Dwight, 282
Chapin, John P., 296
Charcot, Jean-Martin, 28
Charity Hospital (New Orleans), 16, 17
Charity Hospital (New York), 57, 62
Charity Organization Society, 187
Chesbrough, Ellis Sylvester, 293-302; construction of Chicago water and sewerage system, 294-301; in Boston, 294
Chesney, J. P., 121
Chew, Benjamin, 244
Cheyne, George, 317
Chicago: sanitation in, 293-302. *See also* Chesbrough, Ellis Sylvester
Chicago Board of Public Works, 298
Child Welfare Commission, 189, 190
Childbirth, 13, 176. *See also* Death rates, maternal; Midwives; Obstetrics
Children's Hospital (Boston), 174, 178, 180
Chiropractors, 75
Cholera, 4, 8, 229, 257-67, 397; atmospheric theory on origins of, 258-59, 261, 265; compared with smallpox and other diseases, 257-58, 262; contagion theory of, 259-60; incidence of in United States, 398-99; microorganism theory on origins, 262-64, 266; promotes health reforms, 400
Cincinnati: health center in, 190-91
Cincinnati Anti-Tuberculosis League, 190
Cirrhosis, 10
Citizens' Association, 364
Clark, Alonzo, 57
Clark, Henry G., 265
Clarke, E. H., 120
Clarkson, Matthew, 241, 248, 250
Cleaves, Margaret, 32, 37
Cleveland, Emmeline, 121, 123
Cleveland, Grover S., 399
Cleveland Medical College, 117
Clitoridectomy, 18, 19
Cobbett, William "Porcupine," 244, 247
Coit, Henry Leber, 283-84, 285
Colden, Cadwallader, 132
Coleman, Ruffin, 122
Colman, Benjamin, 233, 235
Columbia University, 103
Colwell, N. P., 109
Consumptives' Hospital Department, 192
Cooke, John Esten, 78
Cooper, Peter, 361, 364
Cooper, William, 233, 234, 234-35
Corwin, Edward, 165
Cowles, Edward, 29
Croker, Richard, 421
Cullen, William, 48, 77, 279
Currie, William, 243, 244

DDT, 290
Dalhonde, Lawrence, 232, 237
Danforth, Samuel, 44, 48
Darlington, Thomas, 281, 287
Dartmouth College, 103
Davis, Michael M., 142, 165, 188, 193, 195
Davis, N. S., 110
Death rates, 3, 6, 8, 9; comparative statistics for different cities in 19th century, 364; from diphtheria, 395-96; from malaria, 396-97; from pneumonia, 396; from tuberculosis, 396
— maternal: 217, 220, 378; causes of, 380-82; in New York City, 379, 384; in Philadelphia, 385; in United States, 375-76, 386; reasons for drop in, 386-87; relation of midwifery to, 377, 384-85
— New York City: from cholera infantum, 288-89; from typhoid fever, 288; in hospitals, 62
Delevan, Daniel E., 363
Demilt Dispensary (New York), 61-62, 157
Denise, Nicholas, 336

Dentistry: desire to include in medical curriculum, 201
Devèze, Jean, 243, 244, 246, 249
Devine, Edward T., 187
Diabetes, 10
Diagnosis, in New York City, 63
Dickson, Samuel Henry, 263
Dingell, John, 145
Dinwiddie, Courtenay, 190
Diphtheria, 3, 4, 5, 6; death rate from, 8, 395–96
Diseases: social impact of, 395–402. *See also* names of specific diseases
Dispensaries, 155, 157–67; budget of, 158; charitable associations, 159; decline of, 165–67; in New York, 61–62; origin and growth of, 157; prescriptions from, 158–59; reasons for existence of, 159–62; specialization in, 159
Dix, Dorothea, 155
Dock, Lavinia, 206
Dolley, Sarah Adamson, 123
Doty, Alvah H., 422, 423
Douglass, William, 5, 42, 47, 132; as anti-inoculationist, 232, 233, 234, 236–37
Downing, Richard, 360
Drake, Daniel, 88, 258, 259
Dress reform, 313
Drinker, Elizabeth, 334, 335, 336, 337, 338
Drinker, Mrs. Henry, 203
Drown, Ruth, 99–100
DuPonceau, Peter S., 49
Dysentery, 3, 8

East Harlem Health Center, 194
East River Medical Society, 60, 65
Eastern Dispensary (New York), 157, 158, 346
Eastern Health District, 194
Eaton, Dorman B., 366, 368
Eberth, Carl Joseph, 283
Eddy, Mary Baker, 333
Edinburgh University, 41
Edson, Cyrus, 423
Education, medical; 103*ff*; in New York, 66; of women, 103, 117; postgraduate training, 107–9, 173–74; role of dispensaries in, 160–61; training abroad, 108
Ellis, John, 91
Elmer, Jonathan, 50
Elsberg, Louis, 65
Emerson, Haven, 192, 379
Emetics, 64, 87
Emmett, Thomas Addis, 66
Ethics, medical, 58
Evans, John, 261

Farnham, Marynia, 380
Fenno, John, 244, 245, 247
Finlay, Carlos, 311
Fish, Hamilton, 364
Fishbein, Morris, 143, 146
Fisher, Abel F., 336
Fitz, Reginald, 110
Flexner, Abraham, 103, 105, 107, 109, 110, 111
Flick, L. E., 423
Fliess, Wilhelm, 17
Flint, Austin, 57, 59, 63, 64, 418; disagrees with contagion theory, 263, 364
Food and Drug Administration, 99, 100, 101
Forand, Aime, 147
Forbes, John, 81
Fothergill, John, 48
Fowler, George, 423
Fox, Harry, 296
Francis, John W., 260
Frank, Johan Petrias, 277
Franklin, Benjamin, 155; and bathing, 332
Franklin, James, 233, 237
Fraser, Thomas Richard F., 83
Freeman, Nathaniel, 46, 50
Freneau, Philip, 242, 243, 245, 249
Freud, Sigmund, 17, 26
Friendly Botanic Society, 87
Frontier Nursing Service in Kentucky, 386
Fuller, Samuel, 42

Gallup, I. A., 78
Garbage, 9
Gardner, Augustus K., 279
Garrison, Fielding H., 50, 51
Gastritis, 5
General practitioners: role in childbirth, 377
Genêt, Citizen, 242, 246, 249
Geneva Medical College, 117
George, Henry, 186
Germans, in Milwaukee, 404, 406, 408, 409
Gilman, Charlotte Perkins, 31, 33, 125
Gilroy, Thomas, 421
Girard, Stephen, 244, 246, 248
Glenn, Georgiana, 122
Godman, John D., 346
Goldwater, S. S., 140, 165, 188, 191
Gompers, Samuel, 141
Goodrich, Chauncey, 246
Gorgas, William Crawford, 311
Graham, James, 45
Graham, Sylvester, 313, 315, 316, 317, 318, 319, 323; contribution to bathing, 340; his death, 325–26; interest in Beaumont's experiments, 321–22
Gray, Samuel, 307
Graydon, Alexander, 246
Green, Frederick R., 140, 141
Green, John Jr., 49
Green, Thomas, 44
Gregory, John, 44
Gregory, Samuel, 117
Griffitts, Samuel P., 243
Griscom, John H., 264–65, 345–49, 351, 353, 359–60, 361, 364
Gross, Samuel D., 80, 81, 82, 85
Gunn, John, 87

Hack, George, 42
Hahnemann, Samuel, 89, 90
Hamill, Samuel M., 191
Hamilton, Alexander (American statesman), 242, 247, 249
Hamilton, Dr. Alexander, 44, 45, 49
Hamilton, Frank H., 364
Hamilton, James, 77, 84
Hamilton, John, 308–9
Hammond, Surgeon General W. A., 82
Hampton, Isabel, 207
Hand, Edward, 50
Harris, Elisha, 361, 364, 365
Harris, Robert, 43
Harrison, Benjamin, 399
Hartley, Robert M., 345, 349–52, 353; opposition to "swill milk" trade, 277–80, 350
Hartwell, J. S., 383
Harvard University, 103
Havana, 310
Havers, Clopton, 231
Haynie, M. L., 133
Hazard, Ebenezer, 244, 248
Health insurance, 139–49; initial physician support for, 146;

physician opposition to, 140–41, 143, 144, 146–47
Heart disease, 10
Hebrew Federated Charities, 192
Hempel, Charles J., 91
Henderson, Thomas, 50
Henry Street Settlement, 187, 207
Hering, Constantine, 90
Hering, Rudolph, 307, 308
"Heroic" medicine, 133–34
Hersey, Abner, 47
Hersey, Ezekiel, 48
Hill-Burton Act, 195
Hippocrates, 15
Hoffmann, John T., 367
Hollingsworth, Levi, 244, 245, 248
Holmes, Oliver Wendell, 58, 59, 81, 90, 91
Holten, Samuel, 46
Homeopathic Medical College of Pennsylvania, 91
Homeopathic Medical Society (New York), 56
Homeopathic New York Medical College for Women, 117
Homeopaths, 68, 75, 80, 90–91, 420. *See also* Hahnemann, Samuel; Sectarians
Homeopathy, 81, 89–91
Homosexuality, 13
Hooker, Ransom S., 379
Hooker, Worthington, 77
Hopkins, Lemuel, 48
Hosack, David, 49, 51, 359
Hospitals: expansion of, 155; in New York, 62; role in medical education, 62, 173–74
— in Boston: 173–81; character of women patients, 176–77; class and ethnic character of patients, 175–76; public view of, 177–78; treatment of children, 178–80
House of Refuge, 346
Howard, Horton, 88, 89
Howard, John, 401
Howard Association, 401
Howell, W. H., 108
Hudson, Henry, 275
Hull House, 187
Humphreys, Frederick, 91
Huntington, J. L., 220–21, 222
Hurlbut, James, 49
Husted, S. L., 280
Hutchinson, James, 44, 243
Hutchinson, Jonathan, 17
Hydropathy, 91–93
Hypochondria, 29

Immigrants, 163–64, 176; hostility to, 186; incidence of tuberculosis among, 418; social work among, 186–87. *See also* specific ethnic groups
Infant mortality, 4, 7, 155; and milk consumption, 285; in 19th-century New York, 55
Infant's Hospital, 62
Influenza, 3, 4
Inoculation, 6; first instances of, 231
— opposition to: in Boston, 233, 234, 235; in Milwaukee, 406
Insanity, 28
Instructive District Nursing Association, 192
Irish, 164, 176
Irvine, William, 50
Israel, Israel, 248, 250

Jackson, Hall, 44
Jackson, James Caleb, 93
Jackson, J. Hughling, 28
Jacobi, Abraham, 57, 65, 67, 284, 396; promotes pasteurization, 286
Jacobi, Mary Putnam, 120, 122, 124, 125
Jacobus, Arthur M., 425–26
James, William, 31, 34
Janet, Pierre, 26
Janeway, E. G., 417, 424
Jarvis, Charles, 46
Jefferson, Thomas, 242, 244, 245, 249
Jeffries, John, 50
Jenner, William, 229
Jervis, John, 294
Johns Hopkins School of Hygiene and Public Health, 194
Johns Hopkins University, 108, 110–11
Johnson, Benjamin, 244
Johnson, Thomas, 336
Jones, John, 336
Jordan, Philip D., 89

Kaiser-Permanente Foundation, 195
Kearsley, John, 334
Kellogg, John Harvey, 93
Kempster, Walter, 404, 405, 406, 407, 408, 408–9
Kennedy, John F., 147
Kieckhefer, Charles, 404
Kimball, Justin F., 142
Kings County Psychiatric Hospital, 210
Kings County Pure Milk Commission, 285
Kirkwood, James B., 307
Klebs, T. A. E., 283
Knapp, Hermann, 65
Knight, John, 262
Knopf, S. Adolphus, 426
Koch, Robert, 266, 283, 415, 416, 418, 422, 427
Koelliker, R. A., 83
Kosmak, George, 377, 379, 380, 384
Krackowizer, Ernst, 57, 65
Kraker, Florence E., 219
Kuhn, Adam, 243, 248

Ladies Health Protective Association, 401
LaGuardia, Fiorello, 194
Lambe, William, 317
Lambert, Alexander, 140
Lambert, S. W., 383
Latrobe, Benjamin, 293
Law, Sylvia, 142
Lawrence, Amos, 174
Lawrence, William R., 174
Lederle, Ernest J., 287
Lee, Joseph, 186
Leeuwenhoek, Anton van, 283
Leib, Michael, 242, 246
Leidy, Joseph, 263
Leslie, Frank, 280
Levy, Julius, 220, 222
Lice, 333–34
Licensing, medical, 109–10; opposition to during 19th century, 135
Liebig, Justus von: excites interest among vegetarians, 323, 324–25
Liebreich, Matthias Eugen Oscar L., 83
Life expectancy, 3, 4, 6, 149
Lloyd, James, 43, 44
Lobenstine, Ralph W., 379
Logan, Deborah, 259
Logan, George, 246, 248
Longshore, Hannah, 122–23
Longshore, Joseph, 117, 121, 122

Loomis, Horace P., 416
Louis XIV (King of France), 333
Louis, Pierre Charles Alexandre, 81, 82, 83
Louisiana State Board of Health, 399
Low, Seth, 427
Lozier, Clemence, 117
Ludlam, Henry, 336

McClellan, George B., Jr., 422
McClurg, James, 44
McCready, Benjamin W., 359, 360
McKean, Robert, 45
McKissack, William, 49
McLean Asylum (Boston), 29, 180
McNulty, John, 360
Magendie, François: cited by vegetarians, 322, 323
Malaria, 3, 13; death rates from, 396–97; treatment of with quinine, 85
Martin, H. N., 108
Massachusetts General Hospital, 30, 34, 174, 175, 176, 178, 180
Masturbation, 13, 15–23, 32; diseases attributed to, 16, 17; etiology of, 17, 18; nosology of, 17; treatment of, 18–20
Matas, Rudolph, 213
Maternity Center Association of New York, 379, 386, 387
Mather, Cotton, 6, 131; efforts to promote smallpox inoculation, 231–32, 235, 236
Mather, Increase, 233, 235, 236, 237
Mattson, Morris, 88
May, Franz, 204
Mayo, Charles H., 208, 210
Mayo Clinic, 39
Mayo-Smith, Richmond, 419
Means, Alexander, 78, 79
Medicaid, 147–49
Medical and Surgical Society (New York), 56, 65, 66
Medical Journal Society (New York), 57
Medical Milk Commission, 284, 285, 288
Medical Society of the County of New York, 57, 59
Medicare, 147–49
Medicine, domestic, 87–94
Meigs, Grace, 376
Memphis, Tennessee: yellow fever epidemic of 1878, 308, 399
Mercer, Hugh, 50
Mercury, 77
Mesmer, Franz Anton, 97
Metcalfe, William, 317
Metropolitan Board of Health (New York), 57, 368, 400
Metropolitan Health Bill, 368, 400
"Miasmatic" theory, 273
Middleton, Peter, 47, 133
Midwives, 217–24; decline of, 223–24; high standards for in Britain and Germany, 219–20; in New York City, 56, 223; number of births handled by, 217, 219, 377; physicians' attitudes toward, 218*ff*, 377
Mifflin, Thomas, 243, 244
Milk: adulteration of, 280, 281, 283; "certified," 284–85; consumption in colonial times, 276; distribution of to infants, 189; earliest regulations, 277, 281; goat's, 290; grading of, 287–88; "loose," 288; pasteurization of, 286–87; production in distilleries, 277–81; recent improvements in provision of, 289–90
Milk and Baby Hygiene Association, 192
Milk Commission (Medical Society of the County of New York), 285
Miller, Edward, 78
Miller, Elizabeth Smith, 313
Miller, James Alexander, 422
Mills, Hiram, 307
Miln, John, 132
Milwaukee, 403–10; establishment of child health program in, 189–90; smallpox in, 403, 404–5, 408, 409, 410
Milwaukee Common Council, 404, 405, 406, 408, 409
Milwaukee Health Department, 403, 404, 406, 408, 409
Milwaukee Medical Society, 408
Miner, Thomas, 78
Minot, C. S., 108
Mitchell, John, 41
Mitchell, John Kearsley, 262
Mitchell, S. Weir, 26, 28, 29, 30, 31, 33, 34, 35
Mitchell, T. D., 78
Moffatt, Thomas, 47
Monson, Aeneas, 46
Montagu, Lady Mary Wortley, 231
Montgomery, Thaddeus, 385
Morgan, Benjamin, 250
Morgan, John, 42, 43–44
Morgan, J. P., 399
Morrill Act, 105
Morris, Anthony, 337
Mortality: causes of, 7–8. *See also* Death rates
Morton (New York City Inspector), 360
Mosher, Eliza, 123
Mosler, F., 83
Mott, Valentine, 57, 346, 364
Mountin, Joseph W., 195
Muhlenberg, Heinrich Melchoir, 44–45, 46
Mullaly, John, 280
Munsell, Joel, 259
Murchison, Charles, 307
Murray, James, 145
Mussey, Reuben, 315, 321
Mussey, W. H., 263

Nasse, H., 83
National Board of Health, 399–400
National League of Nursing, 213
National League of Nursing Education, 210
National Sanitary Association, 400
National Social Unit Organization, 190
Neighborhood health centers, 185–97
Neurasthenia, 13, 17, 25–38; and sex, 31–32; care of, 32–33, 34; causes of, 25–26; class character of, 29–30, 34; diagnosis of, 26, 34; why concept arose, 27–29
Neurologists, 28
Neurology, 28
New England Female Medical College, 117
New England Hospital for Women and Children, 117, 205
New Haven Health Center Demonstration, 196
New Jersey Medical Society, 41, 45
New Orleans, 3, 4, 401; yellow fever in, 397–98
New Orleans Charity Hospital, 396
New York Academy of Medicine, 57, 346, 420; concern about ma-

ternal mortality, 379; on milk, 279, 281; stand on tuberculosis reporting, 423, 424, 425; study of maternal mortality, 383–84, 387; urges better health laws, 360; views on cholera, 264
New York Association for Improving the Condition of the Poor, 189, 279, 345, 349, 351–52, 379, 401
New York City, 3–4; health center in, 191–92, 194; milk trade in, 275–90 *passim*; movement toward safe maternity in, 379–84; physicians in, 56–58, 60–61, 65–67, 420; population growth, 276; sanitary conditions in, 348–49, 359–60, 365; struggle for sanitary reform in, 359–68; tuberculosis reporting in, 417–18, 419, 421, 423–27; yellow fever in, 397
New York City Board of Health, 288, 361, 399, 421, 423, 425; and tuberculosis reporting, 423–24
New York City Health Department, 192, 194, 281–82, 283, 380, 398, 421, 422–23, 425, 426
New York City Inspectors Department, 361; Stephen Smith's attack on, 362–63, 366
New York City Temperance Society, 350
New York City Tract Society, 350
New York Commissioners of Health, 361
New York County Medical Society, 380, 419, 420, 425, 426
New York Dispensary, 161, 346
New York Eye and Ear Infirmary, 62
New York Hospital, 346
New York Infirmary, 119
New York Infirmary for Women and Children, 205
New York Medical and Surgical Society, 346
New York Medical Journal Club, 57, 67
New York Medical Society, 425
New York Milk Committee, 189, 191
New York Obstetrical Society, 380, 383
New York Ophthalmic Hospital, 62
New York Pathological Society, 57, 67
New York Polyclinic, 107
New York Sanitary Association, 352; fights for health legislation, 361
New York Sanitary Reform Society, 401
New York State Medical Association, 419
Newark, 220
Nichols, Mary Gove, 92, 93, 122
Nichols, William R., 307
Nicholson, W. R., 219
Nightingale, Florence, 119, 204–5, 212
Noeggerath, Emil, 65
Northern Dispensary (New York), 157, 163
Northern Dispensary (Philadelphia), 157, 159, 162
Northwestern Dispensary (New York), 62, 157
Norwood, W. F., 107
Nurses' Settlement, 187
Nursing, 203–14; blacks in, 208, 213; efforts to improve status of, 210–12; growth of colleges of, 209; growth of schools of in 19th century, 205–6; improvement of standards, 208, 211; salaries, 211, 212; supply of, 208, 209, 210, 211, 213
Nutrition, 10

Obesity, 13
Obstetrics: advances in, 378; low state of profession in early 20th century, 218, 377–78. *See also* Midwives
Odell, Jonathan, 45
Oldmixon, John, 132
Olmstead, Frederick Law, 305, 306
Opdyke, George, 363
Ophthalmologists, 201
Opium, 78
Optometrists, 201
Ordronaux, John, 349
Orne, Joseph, 47
Osgood, Samuel, 368
Osler, William, 108, 427
Osteopaths, 75
Otis, Fessenden, 57
Owen, Griffith, 42

Paine, A. K., 222
Paris, John Ayrton, 320
Park, William Hallock, 285, 310, 417, 422
Parke, Thomas, 43, 243
Parker, Willard, 364
Passavant, William A., 398
Pasteur, Louis, 286; and pasteurization, 283
Peabody, Nathaniel, 48
Pennington, S. H., 260
Pennsylvania Bureau of Medical Education and Licensure, 219
Pennsylvania Hospital, 41, 43, 155, 165
Pepys, Samuel, 333
Percy, Samuel R., 281
Perkins, Elisha, 97
Perkins Jacob, 279
Pettenkoffer, Max Joseph von, 264, 265, 266, 307
Pharmacists: in New York City, 56; relation to physicians, 64–65, 201
Phelps, Charles, 419
Philadelphia, 3, 4, 42; bathing in, 331–40 *passim*; colonial medical practice in, 133; movement toward safe maternity in, 385; yellow fever in, 241–52
Philadelphia College of Physicians, 245
Philadelphia County Medical Society, 80, 81, 384
Philadelphia Dispensary, 157, 158, 162, 165
Philadelphia Medical Society, 43
Philip, Sir Robert, 415, 422
Phillips, Elsie Cole, 189, 190
Phillips, Wilbur C., 189, 190, 191
Phthisis. *See* Tuberculosis
Physicians: billing and charges, 139; colonial, 41–53, 131–33; image and status of, 129, 131–36; income of, 57, 129, 140, 142, 148; in New York City, 56–58, 60–61, 65–67, 420; opposition to women in profession, 118–20; specialization of, 39, 56, 65–66
— women: attitude toward childbirth, 378–79; specialization of, 124

— nineteenth century; 133–35; hostility to, 134
Pickering, Timothy, 244, 248
Pietism, and sanitary reform, 345–53
Plunkitt, G. W., 423
Pneumonia, 3, 4
Podiatry, 201
Polak, John O., 379, 380
Poles, in Milwaukee, 404, 406, 409
Pott, John, 42
Potter, James, 42, 43
Practitioners Club of Newark, New Jersey, 284
Prescott, Samuel, 50
Priessnitz, Vincent, 92
Prince, Thomas, 233
Privies, 9
Prudden, T. Mitchell, 310, 400, 416, 417, 418, 421, 422, 423, 424, 425, 426
Public health movement, 8
Pullman, George, 297
Pylarinus, Jacobus, 231, 232, 235

Quackery: device, 97–101; in colonial times, 45
Quacks, 75, 97–101
Quen, Jacques, 97

Ramsey, Cyrus, 367
Rand, Isaac, 44
Rauch, John, 106
Rauschenberger, William G., 407
Raymond, Henry, 366
Read, William, 265
Reed, Walter, 242, 311
Riddell, John L., 262
Riesman, David, 107
Robb, Isabel Hampton, 208
Rockefeller, John D., 111
Rockwell, A. D., 26
Roman Catholic Carney Hospital (Boston), 174
Roosevelt, Franklin Delano, 143
Roosevelt, Theodore, 422, 423
Rotch, Francis M., 281
Rubinow, Isaac M., 140
Rudolph, Robert, 404, 405, 406–8
Rush, Benjamin, 13, 41, 46, 48, 49, 50, 51, 77, 133, 241, 244, 245, 249, 250, 251, 306; therapy for yellow fever, 246–47; views on origin of yellow fever, 242–43
Russell Sage Foundation, 219
Rutgers Medical College, 346
Rutherford, William, 83

St. John's Guild, 399, 401
St. Luke's Hospital, 62
St. Mark's Hospital, 399
St. Martin, Alexis, 321
Salmon, Daniel, 305
Sanche, Hercules, 98
Sanitary Protection Association of Newport, 309
Sanitary Protective League, 401
Sanitation, in Chicago, 293–302
Savage, Samuel, 50
Say, Benjamin, 246
Sayre, Lewis A., 66, 367
Scarlet Fever, 4, 396
Schools, medical: course of instruction, 107; entrance requirements, 105–6; low quality of in 19th century, 135; subjects taught, 107. *See also* Education, medical
Scott, George, 83
Seaman, Valentine, 204
Sectarians, 75; conflict with regular medical profession, 134, 135, 420. *See also* Homeopaths; Hydropathy; Thomsonians
Selleck, Thaddeus, 279
Sevigné, Madame de, 333
Sewall, Samuel, 234
Sewerage, 9
Shattuck, Benjamin, 47
Shattuck, Lemuel, 3, 305
Shelley, Percy Bysshe, 317
Shelmire, J. B., 19
Sheppard-Towner Act, 224, 376–77
Sherbon, Florence B., 124
Shew, Joel, 92
Shiga, Kiyositi, 283
Shipman, George E., 90
Shippen, William, 43, 246, 248
Shippen, William Jr., 44
Shrady, George, 424–25
Shryock, Richard, 105
Sibble, Philip George, 45–46
Simon, John, 307
Simon, Joseph, 338
Sims, J. Marion, 57
Sisters of Mercy, 398
Smallpox, 3, 4, 5, 6, 9; in colonial times, 229, 231–37; in Milwaukee, 403, 404–5, 408, 409, 410; in New Orleans, 395; in New York City, 395
Smith, Elias, 88
Smith, Joseph M., 361, 364
Smith, Southwood, 306
Smith, Stephen, 110, 349, 359, 361, 364, 425; struggle for sanitary reform, 361–66, 368
Smith, Theobald, 283, 305
Smith, William, 45, 245, 248, 334
Snow, Edwin, 264, 265, 266
Social Security Act. 386
Society for the Prevention of Pauperism, 346
Society of German Physicians (New York), 57
Sondern, Frederic E., 379
Southern Dispensary (Philadelphia), 157
Spencer, Herbert, 110
Spring, Marshall, 47–48
Stanton, Edwin, 83
State Medical Society of Wisconsin, 144
Sternberg, George, 305
Stevens, Alexander, 261
Stillé, Alfred, 83
Storer, D. H., 263
Strauss, Nathan, 189, 283–84, 286
Streptomycin, 6
Strong, William, 421–22, 424
Strontium 90, 290
Sulphonamides, 8
Sutcliff, Robert, 338
Swaim, William, 340
Swanwick, John, 244, 246, 249
Sydenham, Sir Thomas, 77, 132

Taft, Robert A., 145
Thernstrom, Stephan, 175
Thomas, T. Gaillard, 64
Thoms, William, 61
Thomson, Samuel, 87
Thomsonians, 79, 80, 87–89, 110; hostility to, 134
Timonius, Emanuel, 231, 232, 235
Tissot, S. A., 15–16, 21
Todd, Robert Bentley, 82, 85
Townsend, Amos, 325
Townsend, Peter S., 134
Trall, Russell T., 92, 280, 315, 321

Transylvania University Medical School, 134
Tremont House, 339
Trudeau, E. G., 417
Truman, Harry S., 145, 146
Tuberculosis, 4, 5, 6, 415, 416; death rates from, 396, 418; incidence of, 417–18, 424; reporting of in New York City, 417–18, 419, 421, 423–27
Tuberculosis League of Pittsburgh, 191
Tucker, St. George, 336
Tully, William, 78
Typhoid fever, 4, 396
Typhus, 4, 396

U.S. Children's Bureau, 376, 377, 380
U.S. Food and Drug Administration, 290
U.S. Public Health Service, 195, 209
University of Pennsylvania, 107
University of Pennsylvania School of Medicine, 346

Van Fleet, Frank, 426
Van Ingen, Philip, 379
Van Wyck, Robert, 422
Vaux, Calvert, 305
Vegetarianism, 315–27; argument from nature, 319–20; longevity argument, 325–26; physiological argument for, 320–25; religious basis of, 316–17, 318
Venereal disease, 68, 393
Vignal, M., 83
Virchow, Rudolf, 28
Visiting Nurses' Association, 187

Wagner, Robert F., 143, 145
Wahl, Emil, 408
Wald, Lillian, 186, 187, 207
Walsh, James J., 123
Wansey, Henry, 335
Waring, George E., Jr., 305–11; and "filth" theory of disease, 306–7; as advocate of "earth" and water closets, 306; as commissioner of street cleaning in New York, 309; efforts to promote improved sewerage, 307–8; death, 310
Warren, John, 50
Water Supplies, 9. *See also* Chesbrough, Ellis Sylvester
Waterhouse, Benjamin, 49, 229
Watson, Benjamin P., 379, 380, 383, 384
Watson, Sir Thomas, 260, 262
Watterson, Helen, 125
Watts, John, 132–33
Weatherly, J. S., 119
Webb, John, 233
Webster, Noah, 306
Welch, William, 66, 108, 194, 305, 418
Wetherill, Samuel, 250
White, Andrew D., 366, 367
White, Ellen G., 93
White, Frances Emily, 125
White, George Robert, 192
White, William (Bishop), 244, 248
White, William C., 191
White House Conference on Child Health and Protection, 382
Wilbur, Ray Lyman, 143
Wilder, Charles W., 79
Wile, Ira S., 220
Wilinsky, Charles F., 188
Williams, J. Whitridge, 218, 378
Williams, John, 235, 237
Williams, Philip, 384, 385, 387
Williams, Pierce, 142
Willing, Thomas, 244
Wilson, Charles G., 416, 423
Winslow, C. E. A., 192
Wolcott, Oliver, 244
Woman's Hospital (Philadelphia), 205
Woman's Medical College of Pennsylvania, 117, 119, 122
Women, 3, 20, 29, 31, 56; appeal of homeopathy to, 90; appeal of hydropathy to, 92; as physicians, 117–25. *See also* Midwives; Nursing; Physicians, women
Women's City Club, 379
Wood, Fernando, 360
Wood, George B., 77–78
Wood, H. C., 77
Woods, Robert A., 189
Woodward, John, 231
Woolf, Leonard, 26
Woolf, Virginia, 30
Wynne, Shirley W., 288

Yellow fever, 3, 4, 229; epidemic in Memphis, Tennessee, 308; eradication of, 311; incidence of in United States, 397–98; tends to strengthen health boards, 399
—epidemic in Philadelphia, 18th century: 241–52; debate over cure, 246–47; viewed as kind of retribution, 245–54; views on cause of, 242–46
Young, J. Van D., 221

Zakrzewska, Marie, 117, 123, 124, 125
Ziegler, Charles, 221, 222–23, 224

DESIGNED BY EDGAR J. FRANK
COMPOSED BY THE NORTH CENTRAL PUBLISHING COMPANY, ST. PAUL, MINNESOTA
MANUFACTURED BY GEORGE BANTA COMPANY, INC., MENASHA, WISCONSIN
TEXT AND DISPLAY LINES ARE SET IN BASKERVILLE

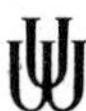

Library of Congress Cataloging in Publication Data

Main entry under title:
Sickness and health in America.
Bibliography: p.
Includes index.
1. Medicine—United States—History—Addresses, essays, lectures.
2. Public health—United States—History—Addresses, essays, lectures.
I. Leavitt, Judith Walzer. II. Numbers, Ronald L.
[DNLM: 1. History of medicine, Modern—United States—
Collected works. 2. Public health—History—United States—
Collected works. WZ70 AA1 S481]

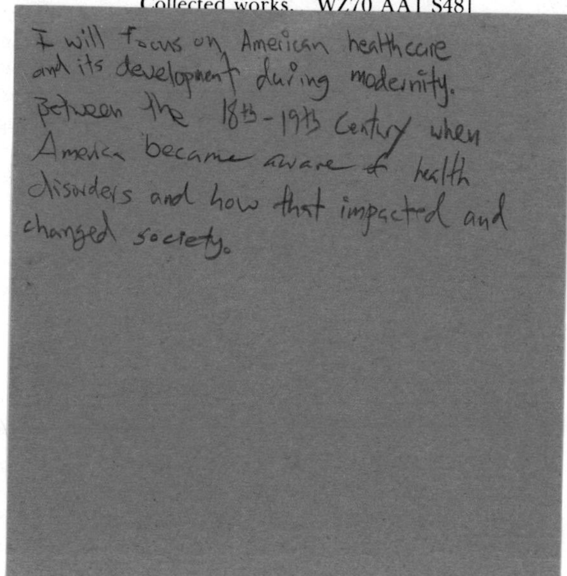
I will focus on American healthcare
and its development during modernity.
Between the 18th - 19th Century when
America became aware of health
disorders and how that impacted and
changed society.